Advances in Implantation Otology

Prawin Kumar • Niraj Kumar Singh
Mohnish Grover • Sunil Narayan Dutt
Editors

Advances in Implantation Otology

Springer

Editors
Prawin Kumar
Department of Audiology
All India Institute Speech and Hearing
Mysore, Karnataka, India

Niraj Kumar Singh
Department of Audiology
All India Institute Speech and Hearing
Mysore, Karnataka, India

Mohnish Grover
ENT and Head Neck Surgery
SMS Medical College
Jaipur, Rajasthan, India

Sunil Narayan Dutt
ENT and Head Neck Surgery
Apollo Hospital
Bangalore, Karnataka, India

ISBN 978-981-96-8670-4 ISBN 978-981-96-8671-1 (eBook)
https://doi.org/10.1007/978-981-96-8671-1

This Springer imprint is published by the registered company Springer Nature Singapore Pte Ltd.
The registered company address is: 152 Beach Road, #21-01/04 Gateway East, Singapore 189721, Singapore

Foreword

Medicine is an ever-evolving field—rooted in science, refined by evidence, and practiced with compassion. The journey from foundational knowledge to clinical expertise is paved with rigorous study, critical thinking, and a commitment to lifelong learning. This textbook stands as a testament to that journey, offering readers a comprehensive and current guide to the core principles and emerging advancements that shape modern applications of implant technology in otology.

The authors and contributors of this volume bring together years of clinical experience, academic rigor, and pedagogical insight. Their dedication to clarity, accuracy, and relevance ensures that this text not only informs but also inspires. From fundamental concepts to complex clinical scenarios, the content is crafted to support learners at various stages of their medical education—whether in the lecture hall, at the bedside, or in preparation for critical examinations.

In a time when medical knowledge is expanding at an unprecedented pace, resources like this textbook are indispensable. It does more than transmit facts—it fosters the analytical mindset and ethical grounding that define true professionalism in healthcare.

It is with great respect and enthusiasm that I commend this work to students, educators, and practitioners alike. May it serve not only as a source of knowledge but as a catalyst for curiosity, competence, and compassionate care.

Elina Kari

Associate Professor, Director, Cochlear Implant Program,
Division of Otology and Neurotology, Department of
Otolaryngology-Head and Neck Surgery
University of California, San Diego, School of Medicine,
La Jolla, CA, USA

Preface

Being able to hear is a bliss of God. The great Helen Keller in her own admission once said, "Blindness separates people from things; deafness separates people from people." However, the physical distance between people would never end, but for the ability for unsupported movement, which allows them to walk to meet and greet each other. In fact, together, the auditory and vestibular systems help us understand and navigate the world around us, contributing to our ability to communicate, engage in social interactions, and maintain physical stability. When either of these systems becomes impaired, the impact on a person's quality of life can be profound. Fortunately, bionic auditory and vestibular implants offer hope, providing individuals with the opportunity to regain at least some degree of lost function.

The field of auditory and vestibular implants has seen remarkable advancements. From the groundbreaking cochlear implant to the emerging possibilities of vestibular implants, this book examines the technical foundations, clinical applications, and ongoing developments in these areas. This book encompasses chapters related to a variety of implant types designed to address the challenges faced by individuals with different forms of auditory and vestibular dysfunction. The chapters of this book cover six key categories of implants: middle ear implants, cochlear implants, bone conduction implants, auditory brainstem implants, auditory midbrain implants, and vestibular implants. They also highlight the multidisciplinary approach required for successful implantation and rehabilitation, as well as the miraculous impact these technologies have on patients' lives.

This book is a comprehensive resource for anyone interested in the science, technology, and clinical applications of auditory and vestibular implants. Whether you are a clinician, researcher, or someone affected by hearing or balance disorders, we hope to provide valuable insights into the remarkable world of sensory restoration. The rapid advancements in implant technology are reshaping the way we think about sensory disabilities, offering hope and new possibilities for individuals worldwide. As we continue to push the boundaries of what is possible, the future of auditory and vestibular implants promises to be filled with even greater innovations and transformative outcomes.

Mysore, Karnataka, India Prawin Kumar
Mysore, Karnataka, India Niraj Kumar Singh
Jaipur, Rajasthan, India Mohnish Grover
Bangalore, Karnataka, India Sunil Narayan Dutt

Acknowledgments

This book is a result of the collective efforts, support, and guidance of many individuals, to whom we are deeply indebted.

First and foremost, we extend our sincere gratitude to Dr. M. Pushpavathi, Director of All India Institute of Speech and Hearing, Mysore, India, for her unwavering support and encouragement in the creation of this book. Her leadership and vision played a crucial role in fostering academic excellence and research at the Institute.

We are in deep appreciation for the supportive environment the officials at the University of Mysore, Mysore, India, provide.

We would also like to express our heartfelt appreciation to Dr. N. Devi, Head of the Department, Department of Audiology, All India Institute of Speech and Hearing, Mysore, India, for providing an enriching academic environment that nurtures learning, research, and clinical excellence. The support of our colleagues, mentors, and students within the department has been invaluable in the development of this book.

We are also grateful and indebted to the contributing authors of various chapters, whose expertise and hard work have enriched this book. Their dedication to sharing knowledge and advancing the field of implantable hearing and vestibular devices has made this a comprehensive and valuable resource. We especially thank you all for standing by us and remaining patient for the duration of this work. But for your support, this book would not have seen the light of the day.

Special words of gratitude go to the patients and their families, who have been our greatest teachers and placed immense trust in us. Their willingness to share their time and experience has provided us with invaluable clinical and research insights and reinforced the significance of our work. Their stories serve as a powerful reminder of the real-world impact of the implantable hearing and vestibular devices.

We would also like to acknowledge the hard work of Rajesh Kumar Raveendran, Archisman Shubhadarshan, Sivasankaran Kumar, B. Gangu Chengappa, Nayana M, and Sachika S. Bharadwaj, whose assistance in editing, reviewing, and formatting has been invaluable. We sincerely appreciate the efforts of Aditya Harishchandra Deokar for his exceptional talent and dedication in illustrating the figures for this book. Their behind-the-scenes contributions have played a crucial role in bringing this book to completion.

Finally, we are deeply grateful to our families for their unwavering support, patience, and encouragement. Their belief in us has been a source of strength throughout this journey, and we could not have completed this book without them.

"Alone we can do so little; together we can do so much." —Helen Keller

With heartfelt appreciation,

Prawin Kumar
Niraj Kumar Singh
Mohnish Grover
Sunil Narayan Dutt

Contents

Contributors

Kumari Apeksha MarThoma College of Special Education, Kerala University of Health Sciences, Kasaragod, Kerala, India

Debadeep Bagchi State Cancer Institute, Guwahati, Assam, India

Sanjay Kumar Behera Department of ENT, All India Institute of Medical Sciences (AIIMS), Bhubaneswar, India

Prabuddha Bhatarai Department of Audiology, All India Institute of Speech and Hearing, University of Mysore, Mysore, India

The University of Texas at Dallas, Dallas, TX, USA

Department of Speech, Language and Hearing Sciences, The University of Texas at Dallas, Richardson, TX, USA

Kranti Bhavana Department of Oto-rhino-laryngology, All India Institute of Medical Sciences, Patna, Bihar, India

Preetam Chappity Launceston General Hospital, Launceston, TAS, Australia

Monita Chatterjee Center for Hearing Research, Boys Town National Research Hospital, Omaha, NE, USA

The Roxelyn and Richard Pepper Department of Communication Sciences & Disorders, Northwestern University, Evanston, IL, USA

Kayla Cormier Speech Language and Hearing Science, University of Colorado Boulder, Boulder, CO, USA

Meghna Deepak All India Institute of Speech and Hearing, University of Mysore, Mysore, Karnataka, India

Rashmi Deshpande Listen Learn and Communicate, HSLS (Hearing Speech and Language Services), Bengaluru, Karnataka, India

Elke M. J. Devocht Division of Balance Disorders, Maastricht University Medical Centre, Maastricht, The Netherlands

Sandhya Dharmarajan Department of ENT, JSS Medical College & Hospital, Mysore, India

Sunil Narayan Dutt Department of ENT, Apollo Hospital, Bengaluru, India

Angélica Perez Fornos Geneva University Hospital, Geneva, Switzerland

Shezeen Abdul Gafoor Kasturba Medical College, Mangalore, India

Sumit Kumar Gaur Department of ENT, Apollo Hospital, Bengaluru, India

Mohnish Grover Department of ENT, SMS Medical College and Hospital, Jaipur, Rajasthan, India

Nils Guinand Geneva University Hospitals, Geneva, Switzerland

Gaurav Gupta Department of Oto-rhino-laryngology, Sardar Patel Medical College, Bikaner, Rajasthan, India

Priyanjali Harit Army Hospital Research & Referral, New Delhi, Delhi, India

Divya Jangid SMS Medical College and Hospital, Jaipur, Rajasthan, India

Akshay Kamath Department of Audiology, All India Institute of Speech and Hearing, Mysore, Karnataka, India

Mustafa Karabulut Division of Balance Disorders, Department of Otorhinolaryngology and Head and Neck Surgery, School for Mental Health and Neuroscience, Maastricht University Medical Center, Maastricht, The Netherlands

Sreenivas Kamath Kasargod Krishna Hospital, Kasargod, Kerala, India

Nirnay Kumar Keshree Sri Aurobindo Institute of Speech & Hearing, Sri Aurobindo University, Indore, Madhya Pradesh, India

Milind V. Kirtane Department of ENT, P. D. Hinduja Hospital and Medical Research Centre, Mumbai, Maharashtra, India

Ameet Kishore Department of ENT, Indraprastha Apollo Hospital, Sarita Vihar, New Delhi, Delhi, India

Apurva Kumar Ashadeep ENT Centre & Apollo Hospital, Bangalore, India

Prabhash Kumar Brahmnaad Speech and Hearing Clinic, New Delhi, Delhi, India

Pranav Kumar Department of Neurosurgery, Indraprastha Apollo Hospital, Sarita Vihar, New Delhi, India

Prawin Kumar Department of Audiology, All India Institute of Speech and Hearing, University of Mysore, Mysore, India

Sandy Magallan Doctor's Hospital at Renaissance, Ear Nose & Throat Institute, McAllen, TX, USA

Saji Maruthurkkara Cochlear Limited, Macquarie University, Sydney, Australia

Rupali Mathur Shabda Brahma Speech and Hearing Clinic and Cochlear Implant Centre, Ahmedabad, Gujarat, India

Gaurav Medikeri Medikeri Super Speciality ENT Centre, Bangalore, India

Shankar Medikeri Medikeri Super Speciality ENT Centre, Bangalore, India

Aanchal Aggarwal Mittal Department of ENT, Apollo Hospital, Bengaluru, India

Banumathy Nagamani Department of Otolaryngology-Head and Neck Surgery, Post Graduate Institute of Medical Education and Research (PGIMER), Chandigarh, Punjab and Haryana, India

Neevita Narayan SpHear Speech & Hearing Clinics, G-32, New Delhi, India

Anindya Nayak Department of ENT, Medanta Medicity Hospital, Gurugram, Haryana, India

Gyanaranjan Nayak Department of Otolaryngology-Head and Neck Surgery, Post Graduate Institute of Medical Education and Research (PGIMER), Chandigarh, India

Naresh Panda Department of Otolaryngology-Head and Neck Surgery, Post Graduate Institute of Medical Education and Research (PGIMER), Chandigarh, India

Prem Ranjan MEDEL Pvt Ltd, Innsbruck, Austria

Chandan Saha Decibel Audiology and Speech Clinic Pvt Ltd, Kolkata, India

Krithika Iyengar Saha Decibel Audiology and Speech Clinic Pvt Ltd, Kolkata, India

Ashima Saxena Soni Hospital, Jaipur, Rajasthan, India

Kara C. Schvartz-Leyzac Department of Otolaryngology-Head and Neck Surgery, Medical University of South Carolina, Charleston, SC, USA

Neha Shakrawal Department of Oto-rhino-laryngology, Dr. Sampurnanand Medical College, Jodhpur, Rajasthan, India

Anu Sharma Speech Language and Hearing Science, University of Colorado Boulder, Boulder, CO, USA

Arpit Sharma Department of ENT, PD Hinduja Hospital and Medical Research Centre, Mumbai, India

Kapil Sikka Department of ENT, All India Institute of Medical Sciences (AIIMS), New Delhi, India

Niraj Kumar Singh Department of Audiology, All India Institute of Speech and Hearing, University of Mysore, Mysore, India

Sachchidanand Sinha Pt. Jawaharlal Nehru Memorial Medical College and associated Dr. Bhim Rao Ambedkar Memorial Hospital, Pt. Deen Dayal Upadhyay Memorial Health Sciences and Ayush University of Chhattisgarh, Raipur, Chhattisgarh, India

Sujeet Kumar Sinha Department of Audiology, All India Institute of Speech and Hearing (AIISH), Mysore, India

Joost J. A. Stultiens Division of Balance Disorders, Department of Otorhinolaryngology and Head and Neck Surgery, School for Mental Health and Neuroscience, Maastricht University Medical Cente, Maastricht, The Netherlands

Anurita Swarup Department of ENT, All India Institute of Medical Sciences (AIIMS), Bhubaneswar, India

Viral D. Tejani Department of Otolaryngology-Head and Neck Surgery, University of Iowa Hospitals and Clinics, Iowa City, IA, USA

Department of Communication Sciences and Disorders, University of Iowa, Iowa City, IA, USA

Department of Otolaryngology-Head and Neck Surgery, University Hospitals Cleveland Medical Center/Case Western Reserve University, Cleveland, Cleveland, USA

Ajith Kumar Uppunda Department of Audiology and Center for Hearing Sciences, All India Institute of Speech and Hearing (AIISH), Mysore, Karnataka, India

Swathi Vadlamani Department of ENT, Apollo Hospital, Bengaluru, India

Raymond van de Berg Division of Balance Disorders, Department of Otorhinolaryngology and Head and Neck Surgery, School for Mental Health and Neuroscience, Maastricht University Medical Center, Maastricht, The Netherlands

Alexander van Soest Division of Balance Disorders, Department of Otorhinolaryngology and Head and Neck Surgery, School for Mental Health and Neuroscience, Maastricht University Medical Cente, Maastricht, The Netherlands

Sangeeta Varty Department of ENT, P. D. Hinduja Hospital and Medical Research Centre, Mumbai, Maharashtra, India

Chandrakant Vishwakarma Shabda-Brahma Speech, Hearing & Vertigo Clinic, Ahmedabad, India

Abbreviations

3DVR	3-Dimensional Volume Rendering
A1	Primary Auditory Cortex
ABC	Activity Balance Confidence
aBCI	Active Bone Conduction Implant
ABI	Auditory Brainstem Implant
ABR	Auditory Brainstem Response
AC	Air Conduction
AC-cVEMP	Air Conduction Cervical Vestibular Evoked Myogenic Potential
ACE	Advanced Combination Encoder
ACh	Acetylcholine
ACIP	Advisory Committee on Immunization Practices
AC-oVEMP	Air Conduction Ocular Vestibular Evoked Myogenic Potential
ADRO	Adaptive Dynamic Range Optimization
AGC	Automatic Gain Control
AGF	Amplitude Growth Function
AIM	Active Insertion Monitoring
ALD	Assessment of Language Development
AMPA	Amplitude Modulation
AMPA	A-Amino-3-Hydroxy-5-Methyl-4-Isoxazole Propionic Acid
ANSD	Auditory Neuropathy Spectrum Disorder
APCEI	Acceptation, Perception, Comprehension, Oral Expression, Speech Intelligibility
APHAB	Abbreviated Profile of Hearing Aid Benefit
ART	Auditory Response Telemetry
ASC	Auditory Skills Checklist
ASC	Auto-sensitivity Control
ASHA	American Speech-Language Hearing Association
ASHA	Audio Streaming for Hearing Aids
ASL	American Sign Language
A-SSCC	Ampullated End Superior Semicircular Canal
ASSR	Auditory Steady State Response

ATP	Adenosine Triphosphate
ATT	Aided Threshold Test
AVC	Automatic Volume Control
AVCN	Anteroventral Cochlear Nucleus
AVT	Auditory-Verbal Therapist
BAHA	Bone-Anchored Hearing Aids
BB	Bonebridge
BBS	Berg Balance Scale
BC	Bone Conduction
BC-cVEMP	Bone Conduction Cervical Vestibular Evoked Myogenic Potential
BCD	Bone Conduction Device
BC-FMT	Bone Conduction Floating Mass Transducer
BCI	Balance Control Index
BCI	Bone Conduction Implant
BC-oVEMP	Bone Conduction Ocular Vestibular Evoked Myogenic Potential
BKB-SIN	Bamford-Kowal-Bench Speech-In-Noise
BLE	Bluetooth Low Energy
BOT	The Bruininks-Oseretsky Test of Motor Proficiency
BPPV	Benign Paroxysmal Positional Vertigo
BT-C	Basal Turn of Cochlea
BTE	Behind-The-Ear
BVP	Bilateral Vestibulopathy
C/M	Maximum Comfortable Loudness Level
CA–PA	Cochlear Aqueduct Petrous Apex Segment
CA-MO	Cochlear Aqueduct Medial Orifice
CA	Compressed Analog
CAA	Congenital Aural Atresia
CA-LO	Cochlear Aqueduct Lateral Orifice
CA-OC	Cochlear Aqueduct–Otic Capsule Segment
CAP	The Categories of Auditory Performance
CAPE-V	Consensus Auditory-Perceptual Evaluation of Voice
CASLLS	Cottage Acquisition Scales for Listening and Spoken Language
CC	Crus Commune
CCIQ	Comprehensive Cochlear Implant Questionnaire
CDC	Centre for Disease Control and Prevention
CDP	Computerized Dynamic Posturography
CDR	Current Density Source Reconstruction
CELF-4	Clinical Evaluation of Language Fundamentals
CF	Characteristic Frequency
CHL	Conductive Hearing Loss
CI	Cochlear Implant
C-ICA	Cavernous Segment of the Internal Carotid Artery
CIFI	Cochlear Implant Function Index
CIQoL-35	Cochlear Implant Quality of Life
CIS	Continuous Interleaved Sampling

CISS	Constructive Interface Steady State
CISS	Continuous Interface in Steady State
CL	Current Levels
CLA	Complete Labyrinthine Aplasia
CN/CN VIII	Cranial Nerve/Cochlear Nerve
CN IX	Glossopharyngeal Nerve
CN V	Trigeminal Nerve
CN VII	Facial Nerve
CN X	Vagus Nerve
CNC	Consonant Nucleus Consonant/Cochlear Nucleus Complex
CND	Cochlear Nerve Deficiency
CNS	Central Nervous System
COP	Center of Pressure
COSI	Client-Oriented Scale of Improvement
CP	Cochleariform Process
CPR	Cardiopulmonary Resuscitation
CROS	Contralateral Routing of Signal
CSF	Cerebrospinal Fluid
CSRD	Checklist to Screen Children with Reading Difficulty
CT	Computed Tomography
CT2	2nd Turn of Cochlea
CTOPP	Comprehensive Test of Phonological Processing
CU	Current Units
cVEMP	Cervical Vestibular Evoked Myogenic Potential
Cz	Vertex
DCN	Dorsal Cochlear Nucleus
DDHS	Direct Drive Hearing System
DGI	Dynamic Gait Index
DHI	Dizziness Handicap Inventory
DICOM	Digital Imaging and Communications in Medicine
DPOAE	Distortion Product Otoacoustic Emissions
DSL	Desired Sensation Level
DT	Device Telemetry
DTT	Digit Triplet Test
DVA	Dynamic Visual Acuity
E	Excitatory
eABR	Electrically Evoked Auditory Brainstem Response
EAC	External Auditory Canal
EAM	External Auditory Meatus
EAS	Electric-Acoustic Stimulation
ECAP	Electrically Evoked Compound Action Potential
ECochG	Electrocochleography
EDR	Enhanced Data Rate
EEG	Electroencephalography
ELF	Early Listening Function for Infant and Toddlers

ELST	Early Literacy Screening Tool
eMLR	Electrically Evoked Middle Latency Response
EP	Evoked Potentials
ERS	Early Reading Skills
ESP	Early Speech Perception
ESRT	Electrical Stapedius Reflex Threshold
ET	Eustachian Tube
F0	Fundamental Frequency
FAPI	Functional Auditory Performance Indicators
FC-L	Facial Canal (Labyrinthine Segment)
FDA	Food and Drug Administration
FHSS	Frequency Hopping Spread Spectrum
FIESTA	Fast Imaging Employing Steady-state Acquisition
FM	Frequency Modulation
fMRI	Functional MRI
FMT	Floating Mass Transducer
FN – M	Facial Nerve Mastoid Segment
FOV	Field of View
FSP	Fine Structure Processing
GABA	Gamma-Aminobutyric Acid
GBI	Glasgow Benefit Inventory
GG	Geniculate Ganglion
GHABP	Glasgow Hearing Aid Benefit Profile
GHADP	Glasgow Hearing Aid Differences Profile
GST	Gaze Stabilization Test
HA	Hearing Aids
HDSS	Hearing Device Satisfaction Scale
HEAR-QL	Hearing Environments And Reflection on Quality of Life
Hib	*H. influenzae* Type B Conjugate
HINT	Hearing In Noise Test
HIT	The Head Impulse Test
HRCT	High-Resolution Computed Tomography
HUI-3	Health Utilities Index
I	Inhibitory
IAC	Internal Acoustic/Auditory Canal
IAM	Internal Auditory Meatus
IC	Inferior Colliculus
ICF	International Classification of Functioning, Disability and Health
ICU	Intensive Care Unit
IDR	Input Dynamic Range
IHC	Inner Hair Cell
IID	Interaural Intensity Difference
IIDR	Instantaneous Input Dynamic Range
IJV	Internal Jugular Vein
ILD	Interaural Level Difference

IPC	Integrated Processor Coil
ISD	Integrated Scales of Development
IT-MAIS	Infant-Toddler Meaningful Auditory Integration Scale
IV	Intravenous
IVN	Inferior Vestibular Nerve
K^+	Potassium
LAN	Lateral Ampullary Nerve
LED	Light-Emitting Diode
LNT	Lexical Neighborhood Test
LSO	Lateral Superior Olive
MAC	Mastoid Air Cells
MAIS	The Meaningful Auditory Integration Scale
MAP	Mapping
MCCI	Music in Children with Cochlear Implants
MCDI	MacArthur Communicative Development Inventories
MEI	Middle Ear Implant
MET	Middle Ear Transducer
MF	Meatal Foramen
MIP	Maximum and Minimum Intensity Projection
MLNT	Multisyllabic Lexical Neighborhood Tests
MLU	Mean Length of Utterance
MNTB	Medial Nucleus of the Trapezoid Body
MOCB	Medial Olivocochlear Bundle
MPI	Masker Probe Interval
MPO	Maximum Power Output
MPR	Multiplanar Reformatting
MR	Magnetic Resonance
MRI	Magnetic Resonance Imaging
MSO	Medial Superior Olive
MSTB	Minimum Speech Test Battery
MUSS	Meaningful Use of Speech Scale
MV	Master Volume
MVBT	Master Volume, Bass and Treble
Na^+	Sodium Ion
NAL-NL	National Acoustics Laboratory-Non-linear
NCIQ	Nijmegen Cochlear Implant Questionnaire
NF2	Neurofibromatosis Type 2
NMDA	N-Methyl-D-Aspartate
NRI	Neural Response Imaging
NRT	Neural Response Telemetry
NWSST	North Western Syntax Screening Test
OAE	Otoacoustic Emissions
OHC	Outer Hair Cells
OMS	Occipito-Mastoid Suture Line
OPD	Outpatient Department

OTE	Off the Ear
oVEMP	Ocular Vestibular Evoked Myogenic Potential
P	Ponticulus/Promontory
PAA	Posterior Auricular Artery
PABI	Penetrating Electrode ABI
PALSA	Phonological Awareness Literacy Screening Assessment
PAN	Posterior Ampullary Nerve
PAQ	Play Assessment Questionnaire
PARC	Placement And Readiness Checklist
PAS	Play Assessment Scale
pBCI	Percutaneous Bone Conduction Implant
PBS	Pediatric Balance Scale
PC	Personal Computer
P-CTSIB	Postural-Computerized Dynamic Posturography Test
PCVN	Posteroventral Cochlear Nucleus
PEACH	Parent Evaluation of Aural/Oral Performance of Children
PedsQL™	Pediatric Quality of Life Inventory
PET	Positron Emission Tomography
P-ICA	Petrous Internal Carotid Artery
PIECES	Play In Early Childhood Evaluation System
PIHA	Partially Implantable Hearing Aid
PLS-5	Preschool Language Scale
PLSI	Pragmatic Language Skills Inventory
PMMA	Gordon's Primary Measures of Music Audiation
PMSTB	Pediatric Minimum Speech Test Battery
PORP	Partial Ossicular Replacement Prosthesis
PP	Pyramidal Process
PPSV	Pneumococcal Polysaccharide Vaccine
PPV23	23-Valent Pneumococcal Polysaccharide Vaccine
PSCC-A	Ampullated End of the Posterior Semicircular Canal
PSCC	Posterior Semicircular Canal
PSI	Pediatric Speech Intelligibility
PSI	Parenting Stress Index
PTA	Pure Tone Audiometry
PVC7	Pneumococcal Conjugate Vaccine
PVSQ	Pediatric Vestibular Symptom Questionnaire
QOL	Quality of Life
RCT	Rotational Chair Test
RDLS	Reynell Developmental Language Scales
RECD	Real Ear to Coupler Difference
RF	Radio Frequency
RS	Receiver Stimulator
RW	Round Window
RWM	Round Window Membrane
RWN	Round Window Niche

SAN	Superior Ampullary Nerve
SAT	Speech Awareness Threshold
SCC	Semicircular Canal
SECS	Scales for Early Communication Skills
SG	Spiral Ganglion
SGN	Spiral Ganglion Neurons
SHA	Sinusoidal Harmonic Acceleration
SIFTER	Screening Instrument for Targeting Educational Risk
SIR	Speech Intelligibility Rating
SLP	Speech-Language Pathologists
SNHL	Sensorineural Hearing Loss
SNR	Signal to Noise Ratio
SOC	Superior Olivary Complex
SOT	Sensory Organization Test
SP	Speech Processor
SPEAK	Spectral Peak Coding
SPV	Slow Phase Velocity
SRT	Speech Reception Threshold
SS	Sigmoid Sinus
SSCC	Superior Semicircular Canal
SSD	Shaded Surface Display
SSD	Single Sided Deafness
SSEP	Somatosensory Evoked Potentials
SSQ	Speech, Spatial, and Qualities
SSQ-C	Speech Spatial Qualities Questionnaire-Comparative
SSTT	Syntax Screening Test in Tamil
ST	Sinus Tympani
STA	Superficial Temporal Artery
STS	Sliding Thin Slab Reconstruction
SV	Sway Velocity
SVA	Static Visual Acuity
SVN	Superior Vestibular Nerve
SVV	Subjective Visual Vertical
T	Threshold Level
TASK	Test for Acquisition of Syntax in Kannada
tBCI	Transcutaneous Bone Conduction Implant
TBVL	Total Bilateral Vestibular Loss
tEABR	EABR Threshold
tECAP	ECAP Threshold
TEEM	Test for Examining Expressive Morphology
TICA	Totally Implanted Cochlear Amplifier
TMJ	Temporo-Mandibular Joint
TONI-4	Test of Nonverbal Intelligence Fourth Edition
TOPEL	Test of Preschool Early Literacy
TORP	Total Ossicular Replacement Prosthesis

T-PAS	Test for Pre-academic Skills
TT	Tensor Tympani Muscle
TUG	Timed Up and Go
UNHS	Universal Newborn Hearing Screening
VA	Vestibular Aqueduct
VCI	Vestibulocochlear Implant
VCN	Ventral Cochlear Nucleus
VCR	Vestibulocollic Reflex
VEP	Visual Evoked Potential
vHIT	Video Head Impulse Test
VI	Vestibular Implant
VOR	Vestibulo-Ocular Reflex
VORP	Vibrating Ossicular Prosthesis
VRISD	Visual Reinforcement Infant Speech Discrimination
VSB	Vibrant Sound Bridge
VSR	Vestibulospinal Reflex
WDRC	Wide Dynamic Range Compression
WHO	World Health Organization
WNR	Wind Noise Reduction

Chapter 1
Anatomy and Physiology of Peripheral Auditory System

Sandhya Dharmarajan, Sreenivas Kamath Kasargod, and Sujeet Kumar Sinha

Abstract The ear is a complex sensory organ responsible for hearing and balance. It is housed in the temporal bone and comprises the external, middle, and inner ear. The external and middle ears play an important role in the transmission of sound to the inner ear. The tympanic membrane is situated at the junction of the external and middle ear and plays a vital role in sound transmission. The middle ear cavity is also called the tympanic cavity and contains the three ossicles. The facial nerve runs through the middle ear. The facial recess forms the route of entry into the middle ear during the posterior tympanotomy approach of Cochlear implantation. Understanding the inner ear's anatomy is essential for successful cochlear implantation. Variations in the size, shape, and orientation of the cochlea can influence how and where the electrode array is inserted. A good understanding of normal anatomy of the inner ear will help understand the cochlear ossifications or malformations during the cochlear implant surgery. Understanding ear anatomy is crucial for diagnosing and treating auditory and balance disorders, and in-depth knowledge is essential for auditory implant surgeries.

Keywords Temporal bone · Sound transmission · Tonotopic organization · Hair cell transduction

S. Dharmarajan
Department of ENT, JSS Medical College & Hospital, Mysore, India

S. K. Kasargod
Krishna Hospital, Kasargod, Kerala, India

S. K. Sinha (✉)
Department of Audiology, All India Institute of Speech and Hearing (AIISH), Mysore, India

P. Kumar et al. (eds.), *Advances in Implantation Otology*,
https://doi.org/10.1007/978-981-96-8671-1_1

Anatomy of External Ear

Brief Temporal Bone Anatomy

Temporal bone is the most complicated bone of the skull. It is a paired structure and forms the lateral and inferior walls of the skull. It contains the labyrinth (cochlea and vestibule) and cranial nerves such as the Vestibulocochlear (CN VIII), Facial nerve (CN VII), Trigeminal nerve (CN V), Vagus nerve (CN X), Glossopharyngeal nerve (CN IX). The Internal carotid artery also courses through the temporal bone. Hence, the knowledge of the anatomy of the temporal bone and its physiology plays a vital role in learning the art of otologic surgeries.

Temporal bone consists of 5 parts, namely squamous, tympanic, petrous, mastoid, and styloid part (Fig. 1.1). Each of these parts holds significance to those dealing with otology.

The squamous part forms the lateral wall of the skull. The superficial temporal line (Fig. 1.1a) seen on its lateral side guides the surgeon on the expected lower limit for the middle cranial fossa (Dural plate) while doing mastoid surgeries. It can also be used for identifying the surface landmark for the transverse sinus while doing surgery for implantable bone conduction devices.

The squamous part, along with the tympanic part, forms the bony external auditory canal (EAC). Halt in the development of the bony EAC can lead to congenital aural atresia with or without associated pinna abnormalities. Children with aural atresia are probable candidates for implantable bone conduction devices.

The petrous portion of the temporal bone (Fig. 1.1b) forms the floor of the middle cranial fossa as well as the anterior wall of the posterior cranial fossa. This part harbors the vital components of the temporal bone.

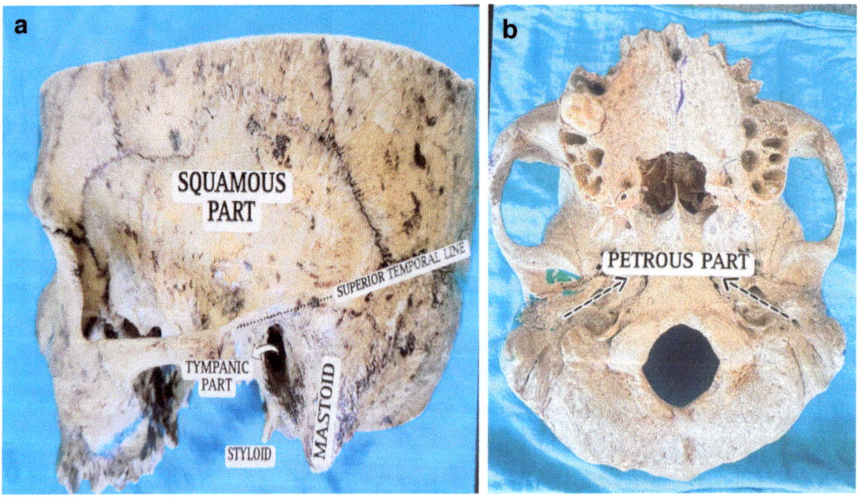

Fig. 1.1 Anatomical divisions of the temporal bone: (**a**) lateral view; (**b**) inferior view

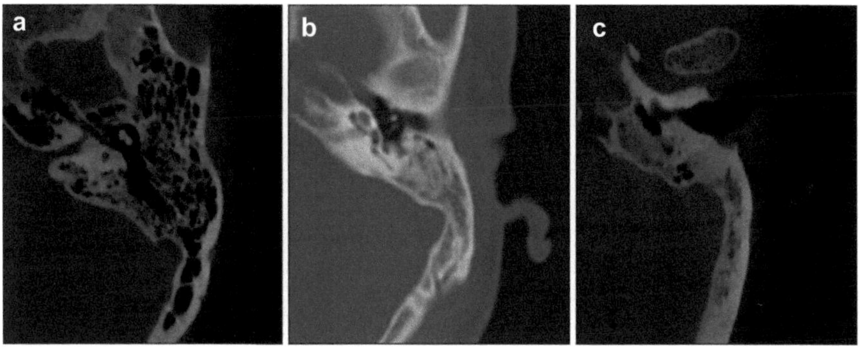

Fig. 1.2 Types of mastoid pneumatization: (**a**) well pneumatized; (**b**) diploic pneumatization; (**c**) sclerosed pneumatization

The mastoid portion forms the posterior part of the temporal bone. This part of the bone has numerous foramina amongst which the largest is called mastoid foramen. The mastoid foramen transmits the mastoid emissary vein to the transverse sinus. It also transmits a branch of the occipital artery to the meninges. The mastoid bone is often pneumatized to varied extents and contains mastoid air cells. The pneumatization is often classified into three types- well pneumatized (1.a), diploic (1.2b), and sclerosed (1.2c) (Fig. 1.2). The degree of pneumatization can play a crucial role in otologic surgeries due to the ease of access to the middle ear because the space for instrumentation depends on this.

The styloid part is a slender projection seen on the inferior surface of the temporal bone. It gives attachment to two ligaments (stylohyoid and stylomastoid ligaments) and 3 muscles (styloglossus, stylopharyngeus, and stylohyoid muscles).

After a brief overview of the temporal bone that houses the ear, let us shift the attention back to the ear itself. For ease of understanding, the ear can be divided into three parts—the external, middle, and inner ear. While the vestibule is also a part of the inner, it will not be discussed in this chapter. This book has a separate chapter on the vestibular system's anatomy and physiology (Chapter 3).

(a) The external ear—The pinna, external auditory canal, tympanic membrane
(b) The middle ear- ossicles, middle ear mucosa and spaces.
(c) The inner ear- the cochlea, vestibule and semicircular canal.

The External Ear

Pinna is a funnel-shaped complex 3-dimensional structure made of a single unit of cartilage, except for the lobule, which is mainly composed of adipose tissue (rich in fat content). Pinna is characterized by ridges and depression unique to each individual (Fig. 1.3). The pinna consists of 3 complexes- the Conchal complex, the Helix-Antihelix complex, and the Lobule. The Conchal complex consists of Cymba

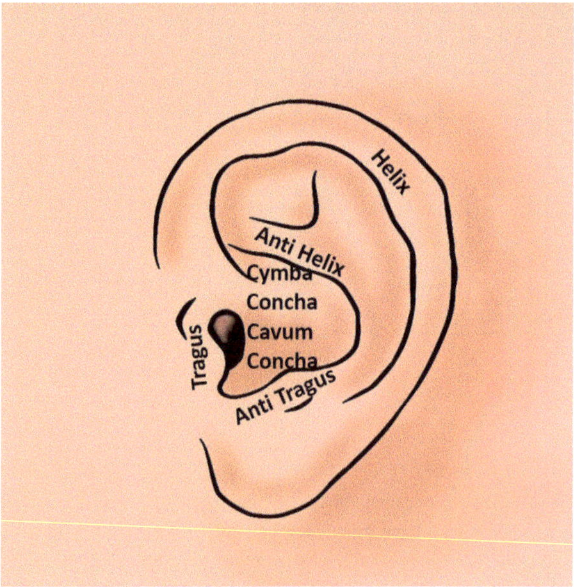

Fig. 1.3 A line diagram of the Pinna showing its various parts

concha and Cavum concha. The Helix-Antihelix complex consists of the Helix, which is the outer rim of the pinna, and the Antihelix, which is a Y-shaped cartilaginous ridge of the conchal cartilage that splits into two (Superior crus and Inferior crus) at the upper end of the pinna enclosing a space called the Triangular fossa. The space between the Helix and Antihelix is called the Scaphoid fossa. The soft inferior part of the pinna, which is made of fat, is called the Lobule. The cartilage of the pinna is an elastic cartilage, which is strong yet flexible. The gap between the Tragus and root of the Helix (Incisura terminalis) lacks cartilage and is, hence, the area used to place incisions for endaural surgeries (including the veria technique of cochlear implantation). The skin of the pinna is tightly adherent over the underlying cartilage except for the Lobule's helical margins. The Tragal and Conchal cartilage are often the donor sites for harvesting cartilage for various purposes of ear surgeries.

The pinna attains the normal adult size (5–6.5 cm length and 1.5–2.0 cm width) by the age of 13–15 years. The congenital aural atresia and microtia are classified by many authors. Readers can refer to Weerda's classification, De la Cruz's classification, and Jahrdorfer's classification. The basic principle of these classifications is to grade the microtia and atresia according to the severity of the abnormality, mild being close to the normal anatomy and severe being anotia. The implantable bone conduction device is a surgical option for hearing habilitation for those with poor grading on Jahrdorfer's outcome scoring.

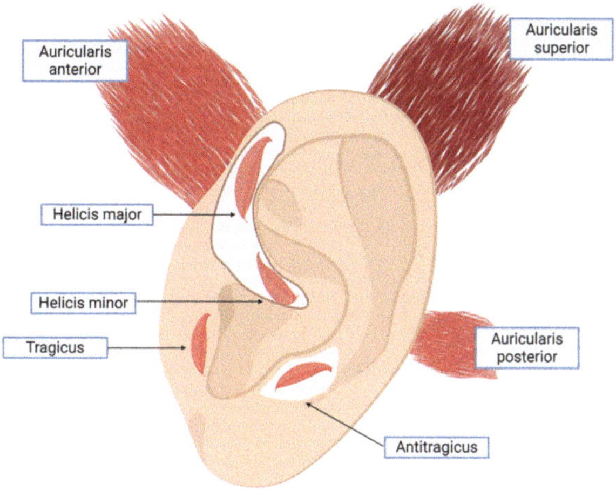

Fig. 1.4 Various intrinsic and extrinsic muscles of the pinna

Muscles of the Pinna

The muscles of the pinna are grouped as extrinsic and intrinsic based on their attachments. In all, there are 3 extrinsic muscles (Anterior, Posterior, and Superior). These muscles are responsible for some amount of movement of the pinna. There are 6 intrinsic muscles (Helicis major, Helicis minor, Tragicus, Antitragicus, Transverse auricular, and Oblique muscles) which are vestigial muscles and are not shown to play any known functions (Fig. 1.4).

Blood Supply of Pinna

The pinna is mainly supplied by the Superficial temporal artery (STA) and the Posterior auricular artery (PAA). The STA runs anterior to the pinna and gives off branches to supply the anterior surface of the pinna. In most people, the STA gives three perpendicular branches- the superior, middle, and anterior-inferior auricular branches. The branching and territory supplied can vary from one person to another. The posterior or medial surface is supplied by the PAA. The PAA can have up to 7 branches; these branches are also found to pierce and supply the auricular cartilage from its posterior aspects (perforators of the PAA) and also supply the anterior surface of the pinna. Although rarely, the arterial arcades of the STA and PAA seem to communicate with each other over the helical margins in a few individuals.

Nerve Supply of Pinna

The sensory innervation of the pinna is a contribution of several nerves. The Greater auricular nerve supplies the lower two-thirds of the pinna, including both surfaces. The Lesser occipital nerve supplies the upper one-third of the pinna, including the medial portion near the mastoid. The Auriculotemporal Nerve supplies the anterior portion of the upper half of the pinna, and the roof and anterior wall of the external auditory canal. The auricular branch of the Vagus nerve, also known as Arnold's nerve, supplies the posterior wall and floor of the external auditory canal and the skin of the concha. The Facial nerve supplies sensory fibers to the external auditory canal and pinna. The motor innervation for the muscles of the pinna is through the posterior auricular branch of the Facial Nerve (CN VII).

Lymphatic Drainage

The medial surface drains to the postauricular/ mastoid lymph nodes, the lateral surface, tragus and root of helix drain to the preauricular/peri parotid group of lymph nodes, and the rest of the anterior surface drains to an upper deep cervical group of lymph nodes.

External Auditory Meatus (EAM)

The conduit between the pinna and tympanic membrane, which measures approximately 24–28 mm, is the External auditory meatus (EAM). Elsewhere, it is also called the External auditory canal (EAC). It is made up of an outer cartilaginous part and an inner bony part. The outer one-third part of the canal, which is cartilaginous, is the continuation of the pinna cartilage. The cartilaginous portion has the ceruminous and sebaceous glands and also contains the hair follicles, all of which have protective functions in the ear. The medial two-thirds of the EAC is bony, and the skin lining this part of the canal is thin, has very little subcutaneous tissue, and lacks any hair or glands. It is the tympanic part of the temporal bone, along with the mastoid and squamous part, which form the bony canal of the EAC. This anatomy is evident with the presence of the suture lines- the Tympanosquamous and Tympanomastoid suture lines. Clinically important while elevating the tympanomeatal flap, care should be taken near this site where the flap is usually tightly adherent. The EAC can have two deficiencies- one which is noted in the cartilaginous part (Fissure of Santorini) and another in the bony part (Foramen of Huscke), which can act as routes of infection to and from the parotid space.

Relationship of EAC

Anteriorly, the EAC is related to the Temporomandibular joint and its capsule, posteriorly to the Mastoid air cells, superiorly to the Middle cranial fossa, and inferiorly to the Parotid gland.

Blood Supply of EAC

The blood supply to EAC is mainly from the External carotid artery. The anterior wall is supplied by the auriculotemporal branch of the Superficial temporal artery, and the posterior wall is supplied by the branches from the Posterior Auricular Artery.

Innervation of EAC

The nerve supply is similar to that of the pinna. EAC receives innervation from the Auriculotemporal nerve in its anterior wall, whereas the posterior wall is supplied by the Facial nerve and Vagus nerve.

Tympanic Membrane

The Tympanic membrane (TM) is a 0.1 mm thick membrane that separates the middle ear from the external auditory canal. It is obliquely set, ovoid in shape with 9–10 mm length in the posterosuperior to anteroinferior dimension and 8-9 mm width. It forms an angle of about 55° with the floor of the EAC. In general, it is a three-layered structure- the outer epithelial layer, the middle fibrous layer, and the inner mucosal layer.

TM is divided into- Pars tensa and Pars flaccida. This part is tenser than the Pars flaccida due to the unique arrangement of the fibrous layer into the radial, circular, and parabolic fibers. These fibers of different directional orientations condense in the TM's periphery to form a thick fibrocartilaginous ring called the Annulus (not completely absent in the superior aspect), which sits in the tympanic sulci. The posterior aspect of the Annulus forms the lateral boundary during the posterior tympanotomy and has to be carefully identified and preserved to avoid the formation of cholesteatoma in cochlear implanted patients in the future. The tip of the Malleus is attached to the medial surface of the Pars tensa causing a depression in its lateral surface called the Umbo. The Pars flaccida/ Shrapnell's membrane lies superior to the Pars tensa. It is attached to the Notch of Rivinus, anterior and posterior Malleolar folds, and the lateral process of the Malleus.

Blood Supply of TM

The lateral aspect of the TM is supplied by the Deep auricular artery, which is a branch of the Internal maxillary artery that branches from the External carotid artery. The medial surface is supplied by the Anterior tympanic artery (again, a branch of the Internal maxillary artery), and the Stylomastoid artery (a branch of the Posterior auricular artery). The blood vessel arcades in the periphery of the TM, whose congestion gives a cartwheel appearance clinically.

Innervation of TM

The nerve supply in the lateral aspect of the TM is by the auriculotemporal nerve anteriorly and by the Facial and Vagus nerve posteriorly. The medial aspect of the TM is supplied by Jacobson's nerve.

Anatomy of Middle Ear (Tympanic Cavity)

The middle ear cavity, also called the Tympanic cavity, is a mucosal-lined air-filled space medial to the Tympanic membrane. The Tympanic cavity, along with the Eustachian tube, Aditus ad antrum, and Mastoid air cells, form the middle ear cleft. It contains 3 ossicles which are suspended by different ligaments and wrapped with various mucosal folds.

A tympanic cavity can be grossly divided into three spaces based on its relation with the tympanic Annulus. The part of the middle ear cavity above the Annulus is called the Epitympanum, the part medial and at the level of the Annulus is called the Mesotympanum, and the part below the level of the Annulus is called the Hypotympanum (Fig. 1.5). The Mesotympanum extends laterally from Pars tensa to the Promontory medially and from the Eustachian tube opening anteriorly till the Pyramidal process and Sinus tympani posteriorly.

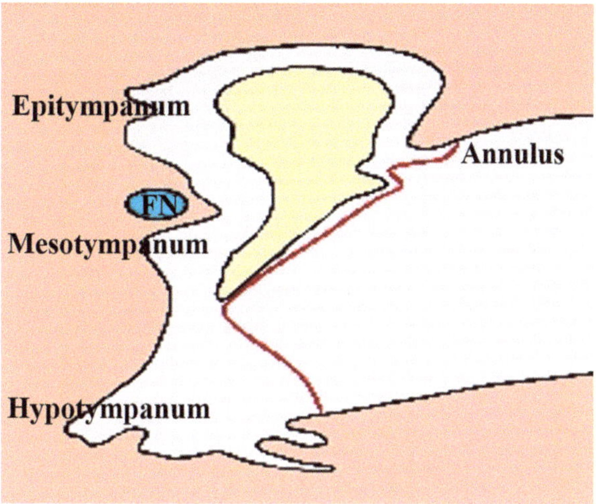

Fig. 1.5 The anatomical divisions of the tympanic cavity

Boundaries/ Walls of Tympanic Cavity

The tympanic cavity is a three-dimensional space with 6 walls (like that of any box) (Fig. 1.6).

Each wall is peculiar in its own way, with various anatomical landmarks. The various walls and their anatomy are described in the sub-sections below.

Anterior Wall

The anterior wall is the wall of the Tympanic cavity that separates the middle ear from the Internal carotid artery and also connects it to the Nasopharynx via the Eustachian tube. This wall also contains the opening for the Tensor tympani muscle superomedial to the Eustachian tube and the Caroticotympanic vessels in its inferior aspect. Dehiscent Carotid artery in this region has been reported in 4.9–35.2% of the cases (Pauna et al., 2017). The average distance between the Carotid and cochlear basal turn is approximately 1–2 mm. Understanding this relation is crucial when a basal turn drill-out procedure is planned.

Posterior Wall

The wall that separates the middle ear space from the mastoid air cells, except in the superior aspect, where it communicates with the mastoid antrum via aditus ad antrum, is the posterior wall. This wall also separates the middle ear from the vertical segment of the Facial nerve. This wall contains many ridges, eminences, and

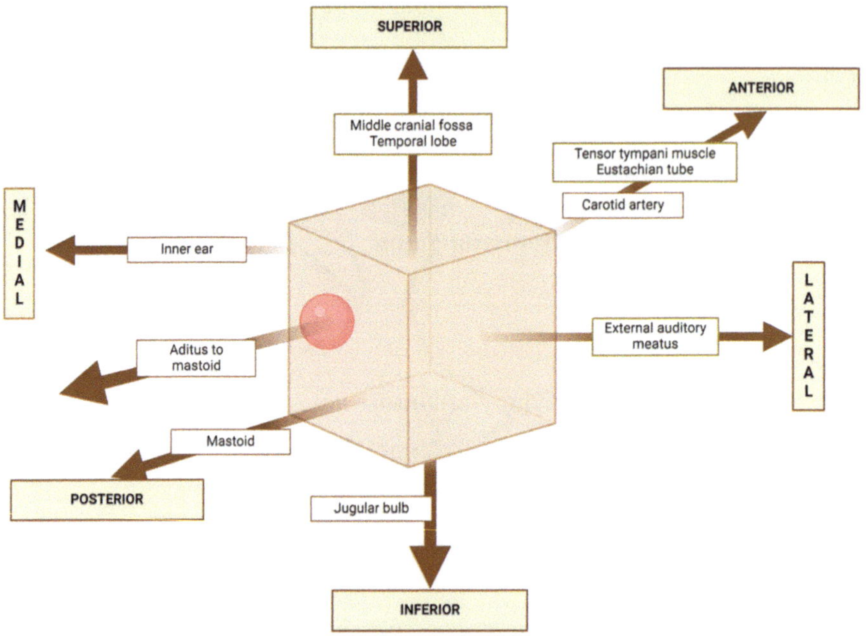

Fig. 1.6 Schematic representation of the tympanic cavity with six walls

various spaces. This complicated arrangement is amongst the most important anatomy that needs to be mastered by any individual planning to pursue a career as an Otologist/Implant surgeon. There are three eminences -- the Styloid eminence, Chordal eminence, and Pyramidal eminence.

The Pyramidal eminence harbors the Stapedius muscle; the tendon emerges out from the tip of this eminence. Surgically, this eminence is often drilled to expose the Stapedius muscle and tendon to perform the electrical stapedius reflex telemetry. Several ridges divide the retro tympanum into various spaces, such as the Sinus tympani, Posterior tympanic sinus, Facial recess, and Lateral tympanic sinus. Among these spaces, for implantation otology, the Facial recess plays an important surgical role. It is bounded by the Facial nerve medially, Chorda tympani and the Annulus laterally, and the Fossa incudis superiorly. The Facial recess is the route used in the posterior tympanotomy technique to approach the middle ear in the transmastoid approach. It is of adult size in the newborn and has an average size of 2 mm near the round window. In case of narrow facial recess, the drilling can be carried out further down by sacrificing the chorda tympani in what is called as extended facial recess approach.

Medial Wall

The medial wall separates the middle ear from the inner ear (Fig. 1.6). The upper one-third of the medial wall, which forms the medial boundary of the Epitympanum, is devoid of specific landmarks and is, therefore, smoother than its lower two-thirds. The lower two-thirds contains the important structures such as the Oval window, Promontory, and Round window. We also find the Cochleariform process, a spoon-shaped bony structure on the medial wall of the Tympanic cavity. It acts as a fulcrum for the Tensor tympani muscle tendon and can be used as a surgical landmark to identify the Facial nerve. The Facial nerve is posterosuperior in relation to the Cochleariform process. The Cochleariform process is also a landmark to identify the second turn cochleostomy, which is often performed inferior and posterior to it. Cochlear promontory represents the bulge of the basal turn of the cochlea. The Oval window is an opening behind and above the Promontory that connects the middle ear cavity with the Scala vestibuli. It is closed by the footplate of the Stapes and the Annular ligament. The Oval window roughly measures 3.25 mm long and 1.75 mm wide, although a great deal of variation in the sizes exists in nature.

The Round window on the medial wall is of prime importance for the implant surgeon. The Round window membrane is covered by a bony projection from the promontory called as the Round window niche. The Round window in human is ovoid in shape and reaches to adult dimensions early during the fetal life. This is situated approximately 2 mm below the oval window. The thickness of the membrane covering the Round window, called the Round window membrane, varies between 50 μm and 100 μm, and its size is about 2.3 mm × 1.87 mm (Proctor et al., 1986). The anterior pillar of the Round window continues further inferiorly to the Jugular bulb as the funiculus and the posterior pillar continues inferiorly to the Styloid process as fustis. At the anteroinferior margin of the Round window lies the hook region, also called the Crista fenestrae. This can cover the Round window membrane to a variable degree. This projection can misdirect the electrode towards the Modiolus during Round window insertion of the cochlear implant. Hence, the removal of this hook region during surgery would not only improve the surgical view but also reduce the resistance to the electrode insertion. A standard electrode array with a maximum diameter of 1.0 mm can be inserted through the Round window (Rask-Andersen et al., 2012). Several cochlear implant electrodes at present have dimensions of less than 1.0 mm. The Round window membrane visualization intraoperatively is graded by St. Thomas Hospital classification to guide the surgeon on the extent of drilling needed for smooth electrode insertion. Figure 1.7 shows the schematic representation of the extent of visualization of the round window membrane according to different grades (Table 1.1).

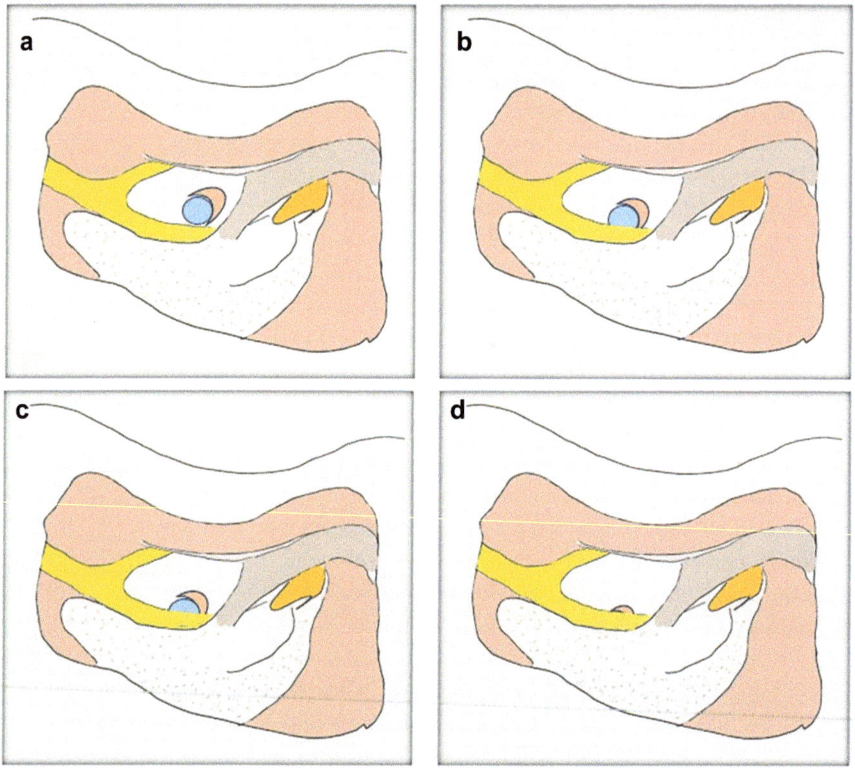

Fig. 1.7 Schematic representation of the extent of visualization of the round window membrane according to different grades: (**a**) Grade I, (**b**) Grade IIa, (**c**) Grade IIb, (**d**) Grade III

Table 1.1 The St. Thomas Hospital classification of intraoperative visualization of the Round window membrane after drilling the niche

Grade	Extent of visualization of the round window membrane
Grade I	The complete (100%) Round window membrane is visualized
Grade IIa	When visualization of the Round window is less than 100% but more than 50%
Grade IIb	When the visualization of the Round window is less than 50% but more than 0%.
Grade III	The Round window membrane is not visible

Lateral Wall

The lateral wall is formed primarily by the Tympanic membrane and rest by the bony wall covering the Epitympanum. There is a thin bony projection pointing medially near the junction of the lateral bony wall and the roof of EAC, called the Spine of Henle. Its clinical significance emanates from the attic cholesteatoma patients in whom the Spine of Henle is the first structure eroded.

Superior Wall

The bony wall that separates the middle ear cavity from the overlying middle cranial fossa is the superior wall. This wall is also called as the Tegmen tympani.

Inferior Wall

The inferior wall consists of a thin plate of bone, which separates the middle ear space from the Jugular bulb and Internal carotid artery. The inferior tympanic canaliculus is noted in the inferior wall, it transmits the Jacobson's branch of the Glossopharyngeal nerve and the Inferior tympanic artery to the middle ear. High riding Jugular bulb is defined when the bulb is seen to be above the level of the inferior rim of the tympanic Annulus. This can obliterate the Round window and may cause difficulty during cochlear implantation. Clinically, the high riding Jugular bulb can be suspected from the otoscopic finding of a bluish mass behind the TM or from the Computerized tomographh (CT) evaluation.

Mucosal Folds and Middle Ear Spaces

Within the middle ear, the mucosal folds pass from the walls to the middle ear contents. These middle ear mucosal folds also create different compartments (spaces) within the middle ear. The understanding of these folds and spaces are important for a clear understanding of various middle ear pathologies, such as dysventilation and cholesteatoma spread. However, the anatomy descriptions of these are beyond the scope of this chapter.

Ossicles

Middle ear ossicles, namely Malleus, Incus, and Stapes, are the key components of sound transmission from the Tympanic membrane to the inner ear. To accomplish effective sound transmission, the ossicles are suspended freely from the bony walls of the middle ear by their ligaments and mucosal covering. Any fixation of ossicles to the nearby walls can cause significant conductive hearing loss.

Embryologically, the head of the Malleus and body of the Incus develop from the Meckel's cartilage (a derivative of the first brachial arch), whereas the rest of the Incus and Malleus and most of the Stapes, except the footplate, develop from the Reichert's cartilage (a derivative of the second brachial arch). The footplate of the Stapes originates from the mesenchyme of the otic capsule, probably the reason for the common involvement of the footplate of stapes in otosclerosis (a condition of the otic capsule).

The Malleus is the largest of the three ossicles. It measures up to 9 mm in length. The different parts of the Malleus are shown in Fig. 1.8. The Malleus is tightly adherent to the Tympanic membrane over the Umbo. While the rest of the handle of the Malleus is free from the Tympanic membrane's surface, it is actually attached to TM with a mucosal fold. Hence, when the prosthesis is crimped over the middle portion of the handle of Malleus, it would rarely come in contact with the TM and has rare chances of extrusion.

The Incus, between the Malleus and Stapes, is the second ossicle in the ossicular chain. The different parts of the Incus are shown in Fig. 1.8. The short process of the incus runs from the posterior aspect of the body of the Incus and lies inferiorly in the aditus in the Fossa incudis. This knowledge is vital to cochlear implantation. The short process of incus points towards the second genu and can be used as a surgical landmark for drilling during the posterior tympanotomy. The long process runs medially to articulate with the Stapes supra structure. The lenticular process is

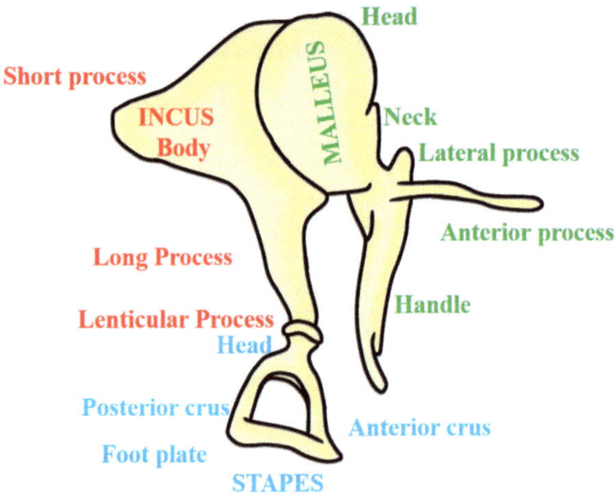

Fig. 1.8 Middle ear ossicles and their parts

characterized by a lack of arterial arcade and is supplied by end arteries, which explains why chronic otitis media and tight crimping of the prosthesis over it easily causes erosion in the long process of the Incus.

The Stapes is the medial most and smallest of the three ossicles. It consists of a head, neck, anterior and posterior crura, and a footplate. The average dimensions of the footplate are 3 mm long and 1.4 mm wide. It sits over the Oval window and transmits the ossicular vibration to the inner ear. The parts of the Stapes are shown in the Fig. 1.8.

Middle Ear Muscles

There are two muscles situated in close relation with the middle ear, the Tensor tympani and the Stapedius. The Tensor tympani is the larger of the two middle ear muscles. The Tensor tympani take its origin from the cartilage of the Eustachian tube, the greater wing of the Sphenoid, and the petrous part of the temporal bone. It runs towards the Cochleariform processes where it takes a lateral turn to insert on the neck of the Malleus. This muscle is a derivative of first brachial arch and derives its nerve supply from the Trigeminal nerve. The muscle plays crucial role in the opening of the Eustachian tube and a minor role in dampening of the acoustic transmission to the Cochlea by drawing the Malleus and TM medially thereby increasing the impedance at the TM.

The Stapedius muscle, the smallest striated muscle in the human body, arises from the posterior wall of the Tympanic cavity. Its tendon emerges from the Pyramidal eminence and attaches near the Incudostapedial junction closer to the posterior crus of the Stapes. The Stapedius muscle is a second arch derivative and derives its nerve supply from the Facial nerve. It plays an important role in acoustic reflex, a reflexive contraction of the Stapedius muscle in response to loud sound, which is ensured due to stretching of the Annular ligament, which in turn dampens the energy reaching the inner ear, reducing its further stimulation.

Blood Supply

The major blood supply to the middle ear is accomplished by multiple branches originating from the External carotid artery, with a minor contribution from the branches of the Internal carotid artery via Caroticotympanic arteries. The major arterial branches contributing to the blood supply of the middle ear are mainly the Anterior tympanic artery which supplies the anterior wall, and the anterior part of the medial wall of the Tympanic cavity. The Inferior tympanic artery is a branch of the Ascending pharyngeal artery that supplies the medial wall of the middle ear and anastomoses with other tympanic arteries. The Superior tympanic artery which is a small branch of the Middle meningeal artery and supplies the Tensor tympani muscle and the canal of the Tensor tympani. The Superficial petrosal artery, which is also a branch of the Middle meningeal artery, supplies the Geniculate ganglion and the tympanic segment of the Facial nerve. Caroticotympanic branches, which are branches of the Internal Carotid artery and Stylomastoid artery, supplies the lateral, posterior, and inferior walls of the Tympanic cavity.

Nerve Supply

The innervation of the middle ear cavity is through the tympanic plexus, which has contributions from the tympanic branch of the Glossopharyngeal nerve (also called the Jacobson's nerve), which supplies the middle ear, Eustachian tube, and the Mastoid antrum. The Caroticotympanic nerves from the carotid plexus carry the sympathetic innervation.

Anatomy of the Inner Ear

Anatomy of the Bony and Membranous Labyrinths

The inner ear is contained within the petrous portion of the temporal bone. The outer covering of the inner ear is bony, called the bony labyrinth, which houses the membranous portion of the inner called the membranous labyrinth. The inner ear is divided into three sections: the Cochlea, the Vestibule, and the semicircular canals. The Stapes footplate is connected to the oval window lying just over the inner ear's Vestibule portion (Fig. 1.9). Three semicircular canals (superior/anterior, lateral/horizontal, and posterior) and two otolith organs (utricle and saccule) together constitute the vestibular system. You will learn more about the otolith organs and semicircular canals (the Vestibular system) in Chapter 3.

The Cochlea, a coiled (snail-shaped) structure, is the organ of hearing. It lies anteriorly and inferiorly to the Vestibule. The human Cochlea curls to complete approximately 2 ¾ turns (Hardy, 1938). It is about 3.5 cm long. It is broader at the base, with a diameter of about 9 mm, and narrower towards the apex, which has a diameter of about 5 mm. The outer cochlear wall has a mean length of about 42 mm, while the first turn is 22.6 mm, representing 53% of the total length. The apical turn, with its narrow lumen, prevents the full insertion of the electrode array right until the cochlear tip. Even otherwise, such deep electrode insertion is unnecessary as the human spiral ganglion extends only up to 1¾ turns. An otic capsule surrounds the human cochlea. The otic capsule is a compact, bony structure and is the hardest bone in the body. Because of the hardness of the bone, the fluids inside the cochlea are not reflected or absorbed by the temporal bone. The otic capsule appears to be yellow in color.

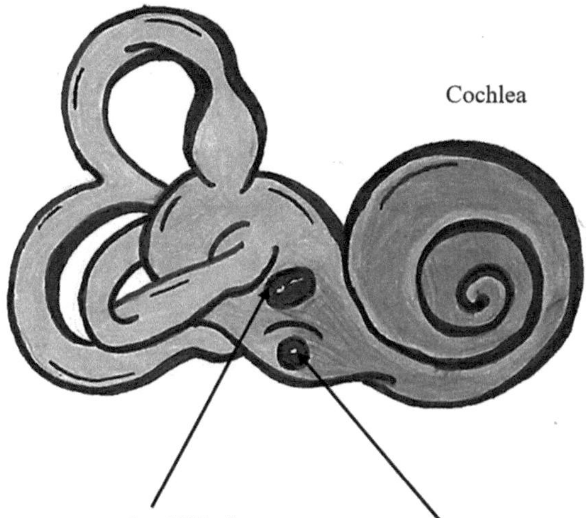

Fig. 1.9 A line diagram of the inner ear showing its major components (divisions)

The cochlea coils around a bony, hollow, cone-shaped shaft called the Modiolus. The Modiolus is a thin yet multi-layered porous bone (Rask-Andersen et al., 2012; Mei et al., 2020). It forms a cone with a base diameter of nearly 9 mm and a height of almost 5 mm (Hawkins, 2024). The modiolus contains multiple openings that allow the passage of fibers from the cochlear branch of the acoustic nerve. The nerve fibres in the lower one-and-a-half turns travel through the Tractus spiralis foraminosus, while the fibres in the apical turn pass through the Foramen centrale. The canals of the Tractus spiralis foraminosus ascend through the modiolus, curving outward to reach the Osseous spiral lamina. At this point, they enlarge and, by coming together, form the spiral canal of the Modiolus, which follows the Osseous spiral lamina and houses the Spiral ganglion (Corti's ganglion). The Modiolus gradually decreases in size from the second coil onwards. The characteristic porous nature of the Modiolus indicates that the fluid within the perineural and perivascular spaces within the modiolus could be traveling to Scala tympani and Scala vestibuli, and the fluid within these cochlear partitions could be traveling to the perineural and perivascular spaces within the Modiolus (Kucuk et al., 1991; Rask-Andersen et al., 2006).

The cochlear Spiral lamina is a slender bony structure that extends from the Modiolus, dividing the cochlear canal into two major compartments; the lower compartment is called Scala tympani, and the upper one is termed Scala vestibuli. At the apex of the Cochlea, the Spiral lamina terminates in a hook-like projection known as the Hamulus laminae spiralis, or simply the Hamulus, which plays a role in forming the Helicotrema. The Foramen centrale extends into a canal running through the Modiolus toward its apex.

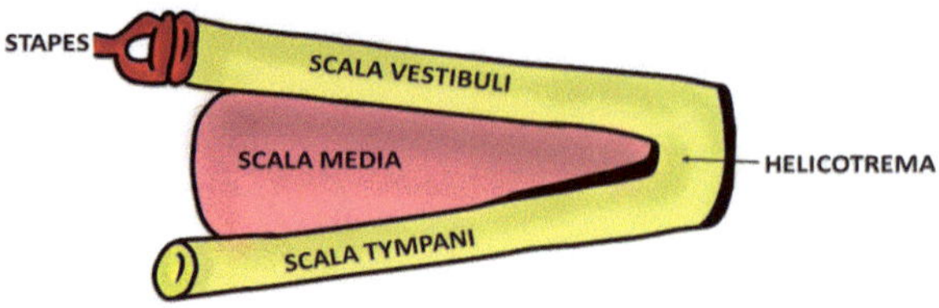

Fig. 1.10 A schematic diagram of an imaginary uncoiled cochlea showing its three major compartments

The Spiral limbus is a thickened layer of periosteum found on the uppermost layer of the osseous Spiral lamina. The Spiral limbus contains a C-shaped concavity known as the internal Spiral sulcus. The upper extremity of the "C" is known as the Vestibular lip and hangs over the concavity. The lower lip of the concavity is called the Tympanic lip. From this endpoint, the Tectorial membrane extends across the cochlear duct. The Tympanic lip also allows for the passage of cochlear nerve filaments via small canals known as the Habenula perforata. In the lower aspect of the Spiral limbus, the Tympanic labia, Cochlear nerve fibers are given passage to communicate with the specialized hair cells in the organ of Corti through the Habenula perforata. Additionally, the Spiral limbus also receives the insertion of the Basilar membrane, and therefore, it is involved in supporting the Basilar membrane. The membranous Cochlea has three compartments: the Scala media, Scala tympani, and Scala vestibuli. If we uncoil the cochlea, it is easy to visualize the three compartments. The three compartments can be seen in Fig. 1.10.

The Scala vestibuli and Scala tympani communicate with each other at the apex of the cochlea through a small opening called as Helicotrema. The Scala vestibuli and Scala tympani contain identical extracellular fluid called Perilymph. The Scala media does not communicate with the Scala vestibuli or Scala tympani. It contains another type of extracellular fluid called Endolymph. The Perilymph has a high concentration of sodium and a very low concentration of potassium, whereas the Endolymph has a high concentration of potassium and a low concentration of sodium. The Reissener's membrane separates the Scala vestibuli from Scala media, and the Basilar membrane separates the Scala media from Scala tympani.

Organ of Corti

The organ of Corti (Fig. 1.11) is the sensory organ within the Cochlea, which resides over the Basilar membrane and runs along the entire length of the cochlear duct within the Scala media. It consists of two types of sensory hair cells: Inner hair cells (IHC) and Outer hair cells (OHC). The Inner hair cells appear like flask, whereas the Outer hair cells are cylindrically shaped. There are four rows of Outer hair cells (approximately 12,000 in number) and one row of Inner hair cells (approximately 3000–3500) in number. On the top of the hair cells, there is a cuticular plate, which has bundles of sensory hairs known as Stereocilia. The Stereocilia of the Outer hair cells are embedded in the Tectorial membrane. The Stereocilia are made up of actin

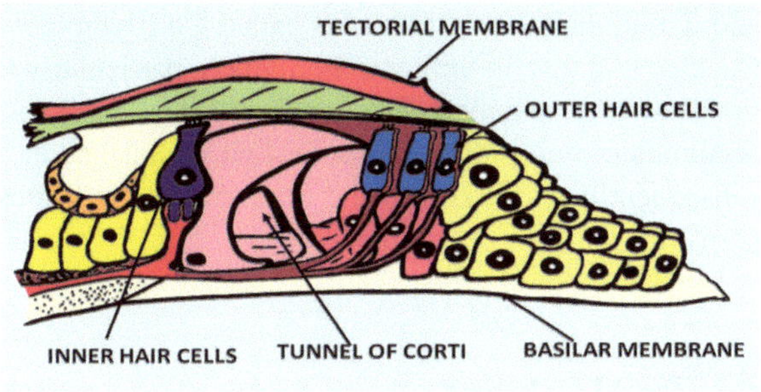

Fig. 1.11 A cross-section of the scala media showing the organ of Corti

filaments and are housed in a plasma membrane. The Stereocilia are arranged in a W-shaped pattern on the OHC and either a U- or W-shape on the IHC. The Stereocilia progressively reduce in thickness from the apex to the base. In response to a stimulus, the Stereocilia bend from the base (Flock et al., 1977). The Kinocilia, the largest of all Steriociliae on a particular hair cell, vary in length from the base to the apex. The length of the Kinocilia is about 4–5 μm at the base and 7–8 μm at the apex. The length of the Outer hair cells also varies from base to apex. At the base, the length of an Outer hair cell is <2 μm, whereas it is approximately 8 μm at the apex. The length of the Inner hair cells does not vary along the cochlear length. Total number of the Stereocilia on the inner hair cells are also fixed (approximately 50–70 on top of each Inner hair cell at the base and about 100 at the apex). Apart from the differences in shape and the innervation (dealt in detail later in this chapter), an important difference between the IHCs and OHCs is the arrangement of the endoplasmic reticulum and the presence of contractile proteins. It is known that the OHCs contain contractile proteins in the cell body (actin, myosin, tubulin) (Flock, 1980; Flock et al., 1982, 1986; Slepecky et al., 1988). The studies in the early to middle 1980s had demonstrated the capability of mechanical deformations in the OHCs when they were electrically stimulated at acoustic frequencies (Brownell, 1983; Brownell et al., 1985). Ever since, several studies have shown evidence for OHCs altering their size when stimulated with appropriate mechanical or electrical stimuli (Ashmore, 1987; Dallos et al., 1991; Santos-Sacchi, 1992).

The IHCs and OHCs are surrounded by several types of supporting cells which are connected with the Basilar membrane. The OHCs are supported by Dieter's cells, whereas the IHCs are supported by the Phalangeal cells. These Phalangeal cells hold the round base of the IHC like a cup. There are several rows of supporting cells lying lateral to the Dieter's cells, known as Hensen's cells. Further lateral to the Hensen's cells is another set of cells called the Cladius cells. The Cladius cells continue laterally to the Spiral ligament and the Stria vascularis. Between the Inner hair cells and the Outer hair cells, there are two types of pillar cells. These pillar cells meet each other at the top, forming a tunnel below called the tunnel of Corti. The cochlear nerve fibers travel across the tunnel of Corti to innervate the Outer hair cells.

The space of Nuel, a vital physiological entity, encircles the lateral surfaces of the OHCs and the phalangeal processes of the Deiters' cells. The fluid in this area and within the tunnel of Corti is called Cortilymph, whose composition, when the Cochlea is at rest, is similar to Perilymph, particularly in terms of the K+ concentration; however, it undergoes changes during sound stimulation as extracellular K+ accumulates due to hair cell activation (Johnstone et al., 1989). The excess K+ is subsequently recycled into the Stria vascularis through a connexin gap junction network.

Basilar Membrane

The Basilar membrane, anchored between the osseous Spiral lamina and the basilar crest of the Spiral ligament, plays a pivotal role in cochlear functioning. The length of the Basilar membrane is about 32 mm and has a variable width across the length of the Cochlea (Bekesy, 1960). It is about 0.5 mm (0.42–0.65 mm) wide at the apex and tapers down to 0.1 mm (0.08–0.16 mm) width near the base (Brugge & Howard, 2002; Oghalai, 2004). It is also thinner and has higher flaccidity at the cochlear apex than at its base. These characteristics of the Basilar membrane increase the risk of its perforation when attempting a deep insertion of the cochlear implant electrode array. The Basilar membrane serves as the initial frequency analyzer for the incoming complex auditory signals in addition to the transduction mechanism that converts mechanical vibrations into neural impulses for subsequent processing. High frequencies are mapped at the base and the low frequencies at the apex of the Basilar membrane (Brodal, 2004; Robles & Ruggero, 2001), as the resonant frequency of the membrane is influenced by its width and stiffness rather than the cochlea's diameter at specific points. A portion of the Basilar membrane between the tunnel of Corti and the osseous Spiral lamina forms a continuous membrane with small apertures for the passage of nerve fibers to the organ of Corti called the Habenula perforata. The parallel strands peripheral to this area are free to vibrate. Towards the Scala tympani, a cellular layer of tympanic covering cells with phagocytic properties adheres to the thick matrix of the Basilar membrane. These cells react with the cochlear implant electrode and form a fibroblast cover encasing the cochlear implant electrode. Proliferations of these fibroblasts may lead to an increase in electrode impedance, which in turn may result in lower performance with the cochlear implant (Rask-Andersen et al., 2012).

Due to being anchored between two rigid structures, the basilar membrane was believed to be mobile only at the tympanic surface of the cochlear partition (Wever, 1954; Geisler, 1998; Pickles, 2013). However, recent research has provided evidence that the osseous Spiral lamina itself moves in response to sound in the cochlear base of human temporal bones and that the movement of the Basilar membrane alone accounts for only 27–43% of the total cochlear partition's volume displacement, rather than the 100% assumed in the classical models (Raufer et al., 2019). In fact, this study revealed the presence of a soft tissue bridge between the Basilar membrane and the osseous Spiral lamina in humans, and that the peak motion of the cochlear partition occurs near the attachment of this bridge to the Basilar membrane. This bridge is absent in laboratory animals and is not considered in existing cochlear models (Raufer et al., 2019).

Reissener's Membrane

The Reissener's membrane separates the Scala media from the Scala vestibuli. Like the Basilar membrane, Reissner's membrane is also a multilayered structure. Towards the Scala media, the Reissener's membrane has an epithelial cell layer of ectodermal origin, whereas the epithelial layer towards the Scala vestibuli is of mesodermal origin. The basement membrane layer separates the epithelial layers, forming a barrier between the endolymph and the perilymph. The epithelial cells facing the Endolymph exhibit an irregular shape yet a smooth surface. They are tightly packed together and exhibit high ATP-ase activity. In contrast, the epithelial cells facing the Perilymph have a flattened appearance with oval-shaped nuclei within them. Scanning electron microscopy reveals that both sides of the membrane possess microvilli on the cell surfaces and pinocytotic vesicles in the cytoplasm, suggesting that the Reissner's membrane has a potential role in regulating the ionic balance between the Endolymph and Perilymph. Using the patch-clamp technique, Yeh et al. (1997) identified three types of ion channels on the apical membrane of the epithelial cells facing the Endolymph in isolated Reissner's membranes from guinea pigs: stretch-activated nonselective cation channels, chloride channels, and potassium channels. Studies using immunolabeling have shown evidence for the expression of various aquaporins in the Reissner's membrane, potentially working together to regulate the electrochemical equilibrium of the Endolymph and maintain homeostasis within the inner ear (Zhong & Liu, 2003; Huang et al., 2002). In instances of obstructed or ossified Scala tympani, it is not uncommon for cochlear implantation to be performed with electrode insertion into the Scala vestibuli. However, such attempts bring the risk of damage to the Reissener's membrane, which can cause a loss of the endocochlear potentials and, ultimately, the loss of residual hearing.

Tectorial Membrane

The Tectorial membrane of the inner ear is a ribbon-like extracellular matrix structure that spans the full length of the Cochlea in a spiral manner. It is formed by four genetically distinct types of collagens (Types 2, 5, 9 & 11) and three glycoproteins (α-tectorin, β-tectorin, & otogelin) (Cohen-Salmon et al., 1997; Legan et al., 1997; McGuirt et al., 1999; Richardson et al., 1987; Shpargel et al., 2004; Thalmann et al., 1987; Thalmann, 1993). The upper surface of the Tectorial membrane curves outwards, whereas the lower surface is flat and smooth, thereby creating its uneven shape. It is anchored along its medial edge to the Spiral limbus, extends across the Spiral sulcus, and rests on the surface of the organ of Corti, where it attaches to the tips of the Outer hair cell bundles. The size of the Tectorial membrane varies across the length of the Cochlea. The radial width and the cross-sectional area of the Tectorial membrane is more towards the apical area compared to the basal area (Weaver & Schweitzer, 1994). The radial stiffness of the Tectorial membrane is more than the longitudinal stiffness (Abnet & Freeman, 2000). Previously, the Tectorial membrane was considered to function primarily as a rigid beam that pivoted at its attachment point to the Spiral limbus, with the relative motion between the organ of Corti and the Tectorial membrane causing shear forces that drive the hair bundles in response to sound-induced vibrations of the Basilar membrane. However, Ghaffari et al. (2007) have proved that the Tectorial membrane has more intricate behaviours, including its ability to support traveling waves at audio frequencies along its length. The Tectorial membrane resonates at frequencies lower than the Basilar membrane. This mechanism provides an efficient mass load to the Stereocilia at the best characteristic frequency (Allen, 1980). The Tectorial membrane vibration at a given place in the Cochlea is dominated by the radial or the transverse components depending upon the frequency (Richardson et al., 2008). The Tectorial membrane can influence the sensitivity and the frequency tunning properties of the Cochlea in many ways. The Tectorial membrane ensures the optimal gain and timing of the traveling wave.

Reticular Lamina

The Reticular lamina, also called the Reticular membrane or Apical cuticular plate, is constituted by the apical portions of hair cells and supporting cells. It stretches from the Outer hair cells to the Hensen's cells. It is pivotal for the maintenance of the ionic separation between the Endolymph and perilymph (Gulley & Reese, 1976). The forces induced by oscillations place significant strain on the junctions between Deiters' cells and the motile OHCs. This cell-cell interface is distinctive in that the connection between OHCs and Deiters' cells forms a hybrid junction, combining characteristics of both tight and adherens junctions (Nunes et al., 2006). Therefore, it also withstands the mechanical forces exerted on the organ of Corti. Disruption of this ionic barrier can lead to alterations in cell morphology and electrical properties, as well as the disruption of synaptic activity, ultimately leading to significant hearing loss (Duvall & Rhodes, 1967; Konishi & Kelsey, 1973; Marcus et al., 1981).

Spiral Ligament and Stria vascularis

Located within the lateral aspect of the cochlea, the crescentic-shaped Spiral ligament is a band of thickened periosteum and a large fibrous structure found on the lateral aspect of the cochlear duct, making up a large majority of the cochlear outer wall (Dorland, 2011). It consists of intertwined fibers that attach to the bony cochlear wall, the Basilar membrane, and the base of the Stria vascularis. It contains numerous fibrocytes of various morphologies, which are likely involved in the production and maintenance of these fibres. The classification of fibrocytes is based on their location within the Spiral ligament, as well as their size, structure, and orientation (Standring, 2016). The Spiral ligament inserts the Basilar membrane at the basal (or spiral) crest, a triangular projection. Its upper and lower regions are closely associated with the Scala vestibuli and Scala tympani, respectively. Because of its attachment to the Basilar membrane, the Spiral ligament plays a direct role in stabilizing the orientation of the Basilar membrane, contributing to the coordinated mechanical processes of the Cochlea. Additionally, it helps maintain consistent tension across the Basilar membrane, likely through structural fibers resembling stress fibers produced by the fibroblasts of the Spiral ligament. The Spiral ligament is also vital for the functioning and health of the Stria vascularis. The Spiral ligament is important for the generation and absorption of the Perilymph. The Spiral ligament consists of Na^+/K^+ ATPase pumps, thus has an important role in maintaining the K^+ ion balance in the Cochlea. A decrease in the expression of transport molecules within the ligament can impair potassium ion recycling, leading to disruptions in the endocochlear potential (Doherty & Linthicum, 2004). The tip of the cochlear implant electrode reaches at the spiral ligament between the lower and the upper basal turn junction. This is important during the insertion of the cochlear implant electrode as it can damage the spiral ligament.

The Stria vascularis, located adjacent to the Spiral ligament on the lateral wall of the cochlear duct, is a complex epithelial structure. This specialized stratified epithelium is richly vascularized with a dense network of capillaries interspersed between the three epithelial cell layers: the marginal cells, intermediate cells and the basal cells. The marginal and basal cells are true epithelial cells, while the intermediate cells resemble melanocytes. The marginal cells line the cochlear duct (Scala media) side of the Stria vascularis. The basal cells are situated deepest within the Stria vascularis and have connections with the Spiral ligament. The marginal cells have descending cytoplasmic extensions, while the intermediate and basal cells have cytoplasmic extensions that project upward toward the marginal cells (Standring, 2016). The Stria vascularis plays a crucial role in the production of Endolymph by facilitating ion transport, which is essential for generating the distinctive ionic composition of Endolymph and maintaining its electrical potential. Therefore, it is responsible for maintenance of the endocochlear potential within the Scala media.

The Cochlear Innervation

Two types of nerve fibers innervate the inner ear: afferent and efferent. The majority (nearly 90–95%) of afferent nerve fibers are connected to the Inner hair cells, whereas a vast majority of the efferent fibers (nearly 90–95%) are connected to the Outer hair cells (Spoendlin, 1966, 1969, 1971; Liberman, 1982). Further, each afferent neuron innervates a single IHC; nonetheless, a single IHC receives innervation from 20 to 30 afferent neurons. In contrast, one afferent neuron innervates 20 OHCs. Although the OHCs have a share of 5–10% in the afferent innervation, there is no clarity on the physiological significance of this innervation, as these fibers seem unresponsive to sound stimulation (Robertson, 1983). The afferent auditory nerve fibers innervating the cochlear Inner hair cells are bipolar cells. The cell bodies of the afferent auditory nerve are located in the Spiral ganglion cells. The Spiral ganglion cells are located in the bony Rosenthal's canal. The auditory nerve fibers enter the Cochlea through the Habenula perforata before they get connected to the Inner hair cells. The afferent auditory nerve is unmyelinated inside the Habenula perforata.

There are approximately 30,000 afferent auditory neurons. There are two types of auditory affrent neurons: Type-I afferent neurons and Type-II afferent neurons. Type-I neurons are myelinated neurons and are connected to the Inner hair cells. Type-I neurons have large cell bodies and constitute 95% of the afferent neurons. Type-II neurons have small cell bodies and constitutes 5% of the afferent auditory neurons. The afferent auditory neurons get connected to the Inner hair cells and the Outer hair cells via different types of synapses. Each of the Inner hair cells receives approximately 20 Type-I afferent auditory neurons, whereas Type-II neurons connect to many Outer hair cells.

The efferent auditory pathways start from the olivocochlear bundles. There are two types of efferent auditory pathways: medial olivocochlear nundle (MOCB) and the lateral olivocochlear bundle (LOCB). The medial efferent fibers originate from the Medial superior olivary complex, whereas the lateral efferent auditory pathways originate from the Lateral superior olivary complex. The medial olivocochlear bundles are crossed pathways. The medial efferent pathways terminate on the contralateral Outer hair cells. Each Outer hair cell receives many efferent fibers. The MOCB fibers are myelinated fibers and have large cell bodies. The LOCB fibers have small cell bodies and are unmyelinated fibers. The lateral olivocochlear efferent fibers are supplied to the inner hair cells ipsilaterally. The medial efferent fibers are connected directly to the Outer hair cells whereas the lateral efferent fibers are not directly connected to the Inner hair cells. The lateral efferent fibers connect to the Type-I fibers connected to the Inner hair cells. Thus, the medial efferent pathway influences the activity of the Outer hair cells directly, whereas, the lateral efferent fibers influence the nerve activity (Fig. 1.12).

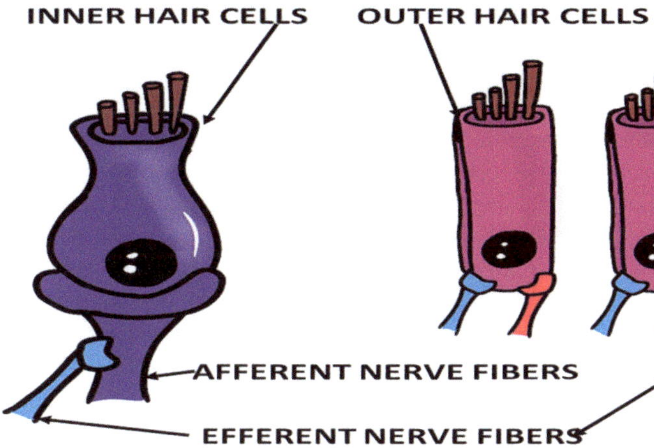

Fig. 1.12 Schematic drawing of innervation of Inner and Outer hair cells by auditory nerve fibers

Blood Supply to the Cochlea

The Labyrinthine artery, also called the Internal auditory artery, is the sole artery supplying the human inner ear. In 83.6% of people, the Labyrinthine artery arises from the Anterior inferior cerebellar artery (AICA), as opposed to the Basilar artery in 12.3% or the Vertebral artery in 4.1% (Zhang et al., 2002). In 2–3% of the cases, the Labyrinthine artery is a branch of the Posterior inferior cerebellar artery (PICA), and although rarely, it can also arise from the Superior cerebellar artery (Hausler & Levine, 2000). Dos Santos et al. (2020) described three different distributions of the terminal branches of the Labyrinthine artery after its origin in AICA. The distribution of its terminal branches is 53.42% uni-arterial, 44.31% bi-arterial, and 2.27% tri-arterial systems. In the uni-arterial system, the Labyrinthine artery takes an anterior superior path to the Cochlear nerve, and its terminal branches originate in the gap between the Cochlear nerve and the inferior part of the Vestibular nerve. In the bi-arterial system, the Anterior labyrinthine artery is located anterior and superior to the Cochlear nerve, while the Posterior labyrinthine artery appears postero-superior to the superior part of the Vestibular nerve. In the tri-arterial system, the terminal branches originate directly from the AICA loop. In most individuals, two primary branches, the Cochleo-vestibular artery and the Cochlear artery, enter the Internal auditory meatus through the fundus region. A third branch, the Anterior vestibular artery, provides blood to the vestibular end organs in conjunction with the vestibular branch of the Cochleo-vestibular artery (Nabeya, 1923; Siebenmann, 1894). The Cochlear arteries supply blood to the Spiral lamina, Limbus, and lateral cochlear wall tissues, including the Stria vascularis. These vessels also supply the Modiolus and Spiral ganglion neurons within the Rosenthal canal. Interestingly, the sensory epithelium, including hair cells, lacks direct vascularization, suggesting that their metabolic needs may be met through surrounding fluids and cells (Axelsson, 1968). The Cochleo-vestibular artery bifurcates into cochlear and vestibular branches. The cochlear branch follows the spiral course of the Modiolus and forms anastomoses with the Cochlear artery (Nabeya, 1923; Siebenmann, 1894; Charachon, 1961), creating vascular arcades. However, in some anatomical variations, the Cochlear artery may be absent, in which case the cochlear branch of the Cochleo-vestibular artery supplies the entire Cochlea. Both the cochlear and vestibular branches are thought to supply the capillary regions of the human Spiral ganglion. Overall, the cochlear blood supply mainly feeds three regions. The lateral region, which includes Stria vascularis and Spiral ligament, receives 57–80% of the total blood supply to the Cochlea, whereas the medial region, mainly consisting of the organ of Corti and the modiolar region, which encompasses the Spiral ganglions, receives 9–19% and 9–24% of the blood volume flow to the cochlea; however, the proportion tend to vary between the animal species (Neng et al., 2015; Nikolakopoulou et al., 2019). Figure 1.13 has a schematic depiction of the blood supply to the inner ear.

The venous drainage system is even more complex than the arterial supply. The venous drainage in the inner ear occurs through the Vestibular and Cochlear aqueducts, which is an atypical arrangement, as it does not follow the same pattern as the arterial system (Nabeya, 1923; Axelsson, 1968). Although there are possibilities of inter-subject variability, the venous blood drainage of the inner ear takes place through three major veins: (i) the Vein of the cochlear aqueduct, also known as the Vein of the cochlear canaliculus; (ii) the Vein of the vestibular aqueduct; and (iii) the Labyrinthine vein, also called the Internal auditory vein (Gray & Carter, 2008; Moller, 2006; Toro et al., 2018). The Vein of the cochlear aqueduct runs alongside the cochlear aqueduct, draining blood from the basal turn of the Cochlea, Saccule, and a part of the Utricle before emptying into the superior bulb of the Internal jugular vein. The Vein of the vestibular aqueduct, which may sometimes present as two

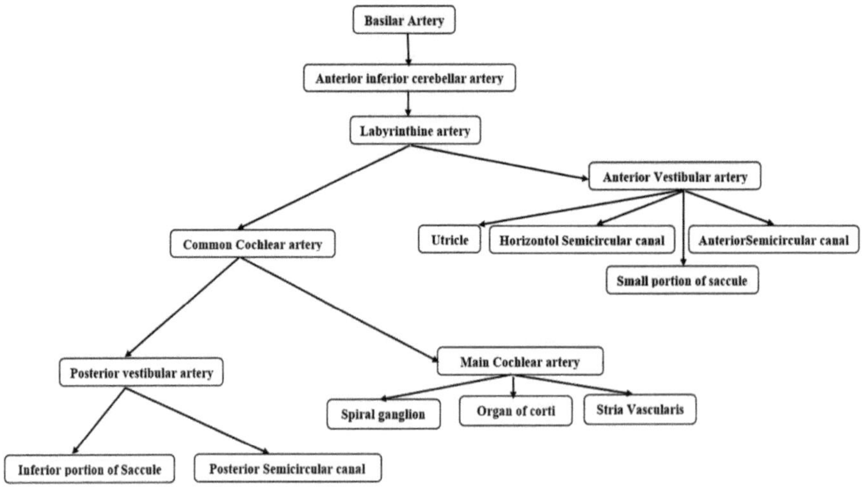

Fig. 1.13 Block diagram of the blood supply to the inner ear

separate branches, the Anterior and Posterior vestibular veins, drains blood from the Semicircular canals and the Utricle. These veins converge into the Vein of the cochlear aqueduct, which follows the path of the Vestibular aqueduct and runs parallel to the endolymphatic duct, draining into the Inferior petrosal sinus or the Jugular bulb.

However, the Anterior and Posterior vestibular veins are not always present in the vasculature of the inner ear. Blood from the Vestibular aqueduct is primarily drained by the Labyrinthine vein, which runs alongside the Labyrinthine artery. This vein collects venous blood from both the cochlear and vestibular structures and drains into the Sigmoid sinus, Superior petrosal sinus, or Transverse sinus. According to Perlman and Kimura (1957), venous obstruction leads to cochlear changes, such as a reduction in ganglion cells within 2 weeks in animal models, suggesting limited collateral drainage between the cochlear and vestibular regions. These findings, alongside the observation that the Inferior petrosal vein runs superficially along the floor of the Scala tympani near the Round window (Mei et al., 2018), have clinical implications. They indicate that large cochlear implant electrodes could obstruct this critical vein, potentially leading to nerve degeneration. Additionally, a 3D analysis has identified the Vein of the round window, which could be damaged during cochleostomy drilling. The inferior petrosal vein also has collateral veins draining from the middle ear, with one such vein originating from a small "infundibulum" on the floor of the Round window niche (Atturo et al., 2018). Watanabe et al. (1988) suggested that these vessels may serve as collateral pathways in cases of acute venous congestion within the inner ear.

Neurotransmitters in the Cochlea

Inner hair cells are the main sensory cells responsible for transmitting sound signals to the auditory nerve. Outer hair cells, on the other hand, amplify and fine-tune sound signals within the Cochlea. These cells are in close contact with nerve fibers from the cochlear Spiral ganglion, forming synapses where neurotransmitters are released. When sound waves enter the inner ear, they cause mechanical vibrations of the Basilar membrane, which in turn deflects the Stereocilia of the hair cells. This deflection results in a change in the electrical potential of the hair cells, leading to the release of neurotransmitters that trigger action potentials in the Auditory nerve fibers, allowing for the transmission of auditory information to the brain.

Glutamate is the primary neurotransmitter involved in cochlear synaptic transmission, particularly at the synapses between the Inner hair cells and the Auditory nerve fibers. When the Inner hair cells depolarize in response to sound-induced deflection, they release Glutamate at their synaptic junctions. This release of Glutamate binds to specific receptors on the postsynaptic membrane of the Auditory nerve fibers, primarily *N*-methyl-d-aspartate (NMDA)-type and α-amino-3-hydroxy-5-methyl-4-isoxazole propionic acid (AMPA)-type Glutamate receptors. Both NMDA and AMPA receptors have distinct roles in controlling synaptic strength. AMPA receptors contribute to short-term modifications in synaptic strength, while NMDA receptors control the genes necessary for the long-term preservation of these alterations. Activation of NMDA and AMPA receptors leads to the generation of action potentials in the Auditory nerve, which is then relayed to the brainstem and higher auditory centres in the brain for sound processing. Glutamate is crucial for encoding sound information and ensuring accurate transmission of auditory signals. However, excessive Glutamate release or prolonged Glutamate activity can lead to excitotoxicity. In this condition, the overstimulation of nerve cells causes cellular damage or death, contributing to hearing loss or cochlear dysfunction. Therefore, regulation of Glutamate release is essential for maintaining cochlear health.

Acetylcholine (ACh) is another important neurotransmitter in the Cochlea, primarily involved in the modulation of cochlear sensitivity. ACh neurotransmitter is primarily located in the efferent auditory pathways. The Medial olivocochlear bundle descends down from the brainstem to provide a synapse to the contralateral Outer hair cells. ACh is released at the junction of the MOCB fibers and Outer hair cells. The release of ACh can produce either inhibitory or excitatory effects, depending on the specific receptors it interacts with on the Outer hair cells. Activation of muscarinic receptors by ACh inhibits Outer hair cell motility, resulting in decreased sound amplification in the Cochlea. Conversely, when ACh binds to nicotinic receptors, it promotes Outer hair cell motility, boosting cochlear amplification. By adjusting cochlear amplification, acetylcholine helps optimize hearing sensitivity and improves the ability to discriminate sounds in noisy surroundings (Jasser & Guth, 1973; Kitcher et al., 2022).

Dopamine is yet another neurotransmitter that plays a role in cochlear function. Dopamine is released by dopaminergic efferent fibers that also synapse on Outer hair cells and other cochlear structures. The dopaminergic system is involved in modulating both cochlear blood flow and the release of Glutamate from Inner hair cells. Dopamine receptors in the Cochlea are involved in the regulation of the cochlear microcirculation, which in turn influences cochlear health and function. Additionally, Dopamine has been shown to modulate synaptic activity and influence the responsiveness of cochlear cells to sound stimuli. Dopamine's role in cochlear modulation is especially relevant in the context of protecting the Cochlea from damage caused by excessive noise or harmful stimuli. It is believed that dopaminergic modulation can reduce the sensitivity of hair cells to excessive excitatory input, thus helping to prevent cellular damage under stressful conditions.

Gamma-aminobutyric acid (GABA) is the major inhibitory neurotransmitter in the central nervous system, and it also plays a role in cochlear function. GABA immunoreactive fibers and the terminals are primarily located in the apical portion of the Cochlea. GABA is involved in the regulation of synaptic activity in both Inner and Outer hair cells. GABA receptors in the Cochlea help balance the excitatory input from Glutamate, contributing to the inhibition of excessive neuronal firing and maintaining homeostasis within the cochlear environment (Altschuler et al., 1986).

Adenosine triphosphate (ATP) is another important signalling molecule in the cochlea. ATP acts as a purinergic neurotransmitter, and its role in cochlear function involves regulating hair cell activity and cochlear blood flow. ATP is released by hair cells and other cochlear cells and interacts with purinergic receptors to modulate cellular responses. ATP release has been implicated in the regulation of cochlear ion homeostasis and in mediating cell-to-cell communication within the Cochlea. ATP's role in cochlear function is still being investigated. However, it is thought to contribute to the regulation of cochlear microcirculation, cellular metabolism, and the overall homeostasis required for optimal auditory processing (Altschuler et al., 1986).

Physiology of the Ear

The sound from the source to the inner ear can be conducted via two mechanisms: via the tympanic membrane and ossicular levers (air conduction) or directly via the temporal bone vibrations (bone conductions).

The Physiology of Conduction of Sound via TM and Middle Ear

The sound is conducted from its source through the air medium into the inner ear via the external ear and middle ear structures. Each component of the external and middle ear influences this sound conduction to some degree. This will be dealt with in detail in the following section.

Head and Pinna's Position on the Head

Head is vital to the creation of the directional cues on which the brain relies to detect the direction of incoming sound. The head blocks the transmission of the sound wave to the opposite ear (Head shadow effect), which in turn results in different sound pressure being transmitted to the opening of two external auditory canals. The effect of head on free field sound results in higher sound pressure at the ear in line with the sound source (baffling effect) and lower sound pressure (shadowing effect) in the ear opposite. This is a frequency (wavelength) dependent mechanism.

Physics Behind the Directional Hearing at the Level of EAC

Directional cues processed by the central auditory system from EAC are

- The difference in intensity of sound arriving at the EAC, also called the inter-aural intensity difference (IID) or inter-aural level difference (ILD), is in turn dependent on the frequency (wavelength) of the sound. This difference is thought to help in directional hearing (localization) of high-frequency sounds.
- The difference in time of arrival of sound at EAC, also called inter-aural time difference (ITD), is thought to be more important for low-frequency sounds. The ITD increases with the increase in angle where the sound source is placed along the azimuth. It peaks at 90° and then returns to minimum at 180° (sound behind the head).

Physiology of the External Ear

The external ear is known to contribute to two important aspects of sound conduction: (a) directional cues and (b) sound pressure gain.

The funnel-shaped arrangement of the pinna and the EAC was previously thought to have no role in the physiology of hearing. But many researchers have thrown light to its neglected role in direction cues and sound pressure gains. The large pinna collects sounds and directs them toward EAC, which acts like a resonating chamber. This amplified sound hits on the TM. This mechanism is expected to bring about a gain of 15–20 dB compared to the original sound. Although each structure has its own resonant frequency, the overall gain in sound pressure is noted between 2 and 7 kHz, with resonance from the EAC in the 2.5–2.7 kHz region and from Concha in the region of 5–6 kHz (Howarth & Shone, 2006). However, the amount of gain provided by the concha resonance also depends on the azimuth at which the sound source is located.

As for the directional cues, the elevations and depressions on the pinna is thought to play active role. It is thought that sound waves are reflected from these elevations and depression to the Concha, which in turn directs them to EAC. When the sound waves from the source and these reflected waves are out of phase, they are thought to cancel each other out and result in reduced sound pressure level. This change in the intensity gives directional cues to the brain along with the difference in the latency of sound.

Physiology of Middle Ear

Middle ear plays an important role in not just the conduction of sound from the external ear to the inner ear but also helps in impedance matching. The sound in the external ear is conducted in an air medium (less impedance), and it has to be transferred to the inner ear fluid (high impedance). The ratio of the impedance of the air to fluid medium is approximately 1:4000. If sound were to be transferred to the inner ear as such, there would be a loss of a significant amount of energy, approximately 99.9%. When converted to sound pressure, this would equate to approximately 30 dB of loss while getting transferred.

Middle ear also has a role in inner ear fluid mechanic. Of the two openings in the Otic capsule (Oval window and Round window), only one should be the entry point for the sound. The cochlear fluid will be set into wave-like motions only if pressure is transferred through one opening.

Middle Ear Impedance Matching Mechanism

The middle ear impedance matching is accomplished by mainly three factors (Fig. 1.14): (A) the ratio of the surface area of the Tympanic membrane to the Oval window (Stapes footplate), (B) the middle ear ossicle lever mechanism, and (C) the curved membrane mechanism, also known as Buckling effect.

A. *Area ratio of TM to Stapes footplate:* The ratio of the effective surface area of the Tympanic membrane (about 55 mm^2) to that of the Stapes footplate (about 3.2 mm^2) is approximately 17:1. This results in concentration of the energy falling on the TM to a 17 times smaller stapes footplate, providing a gain of around 24.7 dB.
B. *The ossicular lever mechanism:* The handle of the Malleus and the long process of Incus form the two arms of the lever that have a difference in their lengths. The handle of Malleus is approximately 1.3 times longer than the long process of Incus. This is expected to bring about a 2.28 dB gain.

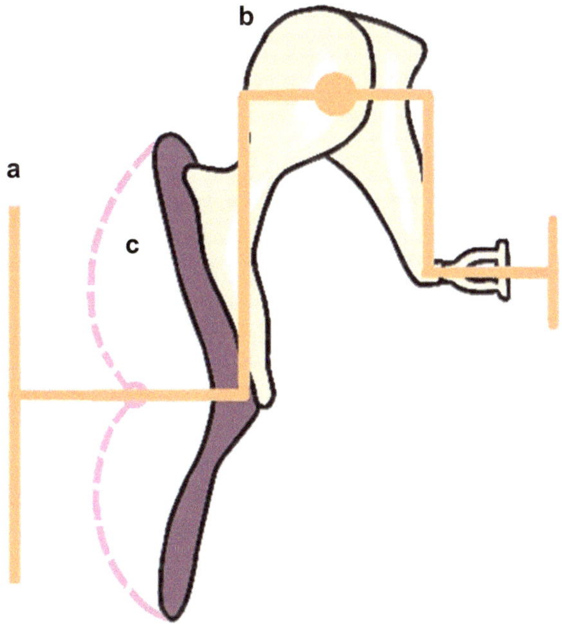

Fig. 1.14 Different mechanisms of middle ear impedance matching: (A) area ratio effect, (B) ossicular lever mechanism, and (C) curved membrane (Buckling) effect

C. *Buckling effect:* When air pressure hits the TM from the ear canal, it causes deformation (buckling) of the TM, with different parts of the membrane moving at different distances, making the TM's action like a double lever. This buckling motion increases the force fourfold and focuses sound waves onto the malleus. The gain produced by the Buckling effect is about 2.5 dB.

The middle ear transformer action is variable across the range of acoustic frequencies. As the frequency increases, the contribution of the transformer action decreases. The above calculation is appropriate for sound frequencies below 1 kHz. For frequencies of 1–3 kHz, the gain due to the transformer action is in the range of 20–25 dB, whereas the frequencies above 3 kHz have even lower gain, typically around 10–15 dB for 5 kHz.

Middle Ear Protective Reflexes

The two middle ear muscles, the Stapedius muscle, and the Tensor tympani muscle, increase the stiffness of the ossicular chain by way of their reflexive contraction in response to loud sounds of 70 dB SPL or higher, and hence dampens the sound conduction to the inner ear. This helps in protecting the inner ear structures against harmful loud sounds. The contraction of the Stapedial muscle in response to loud acoustic stimuli is called the Stapedial reflex. The reflexive contraction can also be achieved in response to high-amplitude electrical stimulation. The electrically evoked stapedial reflex can be used as a cue during surgery as well as in the postoperative period as an objective measure of auditory response via the implant.

Role of Middle Ear in Bone Conduction Physiology

The conduction of the sound via the bone is explained to occur via three main mechanisms: Compressional mode, Inertial mode, and Osseotympanic mode. The Inertial mode of bone conduction utilizes the inertia of the ossicular chain suspended within the middle ear cavity. When the temporal bone is vibrated by a vibrating object or by loud sounds, the middle ear ossicles lag behind the vibration due to inertia. This results in relative movement of the Stapes footplate; hence, vibrations are transmitted to the inner ear. The same vibration of the temporal bone can also lead to the vibration of the air column within the EAC, which can cause the movement of the TM, which transmits the energy via the ossicular chain to the Cochlea, resulting in contribution to hearing by the bone conduction modality. While the Inertial mode contributes to hearing in the frequencies below 800 Hz, the Osseotympanic mode does so in the frequencies below 1500 Hz. Therefore, the middle ear contributes to bone conduction hearing in the low frequencies, typically below 1500 Hz.

Physiology of the Inner Ear (Cochlea)

The sound energy is converted to mechanical energy when it reaches the Cochlea via the middle ear. The ultimate goal of the Cochlea is to transform these complex mechanical vibrations into neural impulses. The mechanical vibrations transmitted to the Cochlea from the middle ear by the piston-like movement of the Stapes footplate at the Oval window propagates from the base to apex within the Scala vestibuli. The pressure wave then passes through the Helicotrema to the Scala tympani and travels back to the base, where the pressure is relieved due to compensatory movement of the Round window membrane at the basal end of the Scala tympani (Lim & Brichta, 2016). The movement of pressure wave within these two ducts results in the formation of crest and trough on the Basilar membrane. Because the Outer and Inner hair cells are located on the Basilar membrane, the Basilar membrane's movement causes the hair cells to move too. The Stereocilia located atop the hair cells can bend as the Basilar membrane moves. This bending of the Stereocilia causes changes in the intracellular potentials of the hair cells. When the shorter Stereocilia move towards the longest stereocilia, depolarization occurs; conversely, when the longest Stereocilia move towards the shorter Stereocilia, hyperpolarization happens. Depolarization triggers the generation of action potentials in the Auditory nerve, which are then propagated through the central auditory pathway to the auditory cortical areas.

Sensory Transduction

Stereocilia is the essential site for sensory transduction. The longest Stereocilia atop the Outer hair cells are in contact with the Tectorial membrane. The hair cells are specialized epithelial cells, and as with all surface epithelial cells, the plasma membrane of the hair cells is polarized into apical and basolateral portions. Sensory hair cells are activated when their Stereocilia bend in a specific direction, and inhibition occurs when they bend in the opposite direction. More specifically, activation results in an increase in the firing rate of the Auditory nerve. Though cochlear hair cells do not have Kinocilium, they have an analogous structure known as the Basal body at the base of the 'W' shaped stereocilia. The base of the 'W' faces the cochlear duct away from the Modiolus. When the shorter Stereocilia bends towards the Basal body, in other words, away from the Modiolus, hair cells depolarize. Bending the Stereocilia towards the Modiolus (away from the Basal body) compresses the tip links, leading to inhibition.

The Stereocilia of hair cells bend when they are sheared between the Tectorial membrane above the Reticular lamina. The hair cells are located on the Basilar membrane with the Reticular lamina on the top. The shearing effects occur as the Tectorial and Basilar membranes hinge at two different places. The Basilar membrane extends from the bottom of the osseous Spiral lamina, and the Tectorial membrane hinges at the upper limb of the Limbus. As the axis of rotation is different for the Tectorial and Basilar membranes, they move relative to each other.

Both Inner hair cells and Outer hair cells have resting membrane potentials. The resting membrane potential is the difference in charge between the inside and outside of the cells when the cells are not in a depolarised condition. The resting membrane potential is maintained by the differential distribution of the Na+ and K+ ions inside and outside the membrane. The resting membrane potential is around −70 mV. The electrochemical gradients between the inside and outside of the Inner hair cell are maintained by the Na^+/K^+ ATPase pump, which pumps sodium out of the cell and potassium into the cell. The resting membrane potential of the Outer hair cell is around −60 mV. The resting membrane potential of the Outer hair cell is dependent upon the electrochemical gradient of K + ion.

At the tip of the Stereocilia, there are filamentous structures known as Tip links. The Tip links connect the tips of the Stereocilia on the hair cells. As the Stereocilia move away from the Modiolus, the transducer channels open, leading to a change in the membrane potential. When sound-induced vibrations cause deflection of the Stereocilia on the hair cells, the Tip links stretch and open the mechanically gated ion channels located at the tips of the Stereocilia. This opening allows K^+ ions (and some Ca^{2+} ions) to flow from the Endolymph into the hair cells, as the electrochemical gradient for K^+ favors this influx. The influx of positively charged ions depolarizes the hair cell. During the depolarisation of the hair cell, the cell becomes less negative (more positive) inside, leading to a change in membrane potential. This depolarization triggers the release of Glutamate from the IHCs, activating Auditory nerve fibers and sending the sound signal to the brain. In the active process, upon sound stimulation, when a low-intensity stimulus is given, there is a resultant Stereocilia movement on the OHC, which leads to mechanical to electrical transduction and depolarizes the OHC. Upon depolarization, an electrical to mechanical transduction correspondingly changes the OHC length. The Reticular lamina is stiff; therefore, the change in the OHC length pulls the BM, which in turn moves the Stereocilia on the IHC, leading to IHC depolarization and neural discharges to the Auditory nerve fibres.

Frequency Selectivity in Cochlea

Bekesy (1949) first described the presence of frequency tuning in the Cochlea using a binocular microscope. He found that the frequency selectivity of the Basilar membrane is greater at lower intensities than at higher intensities. This implies that the Basilar membrane vibrates differently at various intensities and operates nonlinearly. The Basilar membrane functions as a resonator, with its basal portion responsible for processing high-frequency signals and the apical portion responsible for low-frequency signals. This kind of frequency selectivity is due to the traveling wave generated along the Basilar membrane. For low-frequency sounds, the traveling wave peaks near the apex of the Cochlea, while for high-frequency sounds, the peak occurs near the base. The traveling wave causes displacement of the Basilar membrane, which is tuned to different locations along its length. The sharpness of the Basilar membrane's tuning resembles that of the Auditory nerve. The tuning curves are sharper for high frequencies and broader for low frequencies.

Non-linearity of the Cochlea

The cochlear system is completely non-linear in nature. In a linear system, there is a 1:1 ratio between the input and the output of the sound. In the linear system, if the input sound doubles, the output also doubles. However, in a non-linear system, there is no 1:1 ratio between the input and output of the sound. In the Cochlea, the relation between the input and the output sound is more complex, particularly at high and moderate intensity sound. The response of the Cochlea varies depending on the frequency and the intensity of the sound. The nonlinearity of the Cochlea is vital to the following mechanisms

(a) **Selective amplification by Outer hair cells:** The Outer hair cells have a special type of protein complex known as Prestin. Prestin is a voltage-dependent motor protein. Prestin is responsible for changing the shape of the Outer hair cells in response to signals, and thus, it helps in the amplification of the cochlear partition. At low sound levels, the Outer hair cells amplify the Basilar membrane vibration. Amplification of the Basilar membrane vibrations improves the detection of faint sounds. At high-intensity sound, the Outer hair cells reduce the amplification via gain compression to prevent overstimulation and damage to the Outer hair cells. This selective nonlinear amplification by the Outer hair cells allows the amplification of the faint sound, yet prevent damage from loud sound.

(b) **Compression of dynamic range:** The non-linearity of the Cochlea contributes to the compression of the dynamic range of the input sound. Dynamic range compression is important for the maintenance of comfortable hearing over a wide variety of sound inputs.

(c) **Generation of distortion products:** The Cochlea produces distortion products in response to two tones presented simultaneously. These emissions arise due to non-linear interactions in the Cochlea and can be used clinically to assess cochlear function.

References

Abnet, C. C., & Freeman, D. M. (2000). Deformations of the isolated mouse tectorial membrane produced by oscillatory forces. *Hearing Research, 144*(1–2), 29–46.

Allen, J. B. (1980). Cochlear micromechanics- A physical model of transduction. *Journal of Acoustical Society of America, 68*, 1660–1670.

Altschuler, R. A., Hoffman, D. W., & Wenthold, R. J. (1986). Neurotransmitters of the cochlea and cochlear nucleus: Immunocytochemical evidence. *American Journal of Otolaryngology, 7*(2), 100–106.

Ashmore, J. F. (1987). A fast motile response in Guinea-pig outer hair cells: The cellular basis of the cochlear amplifier. *The Journal of Physiology, 388*, 323–347.

Atturo, F., Schart-Morén, N., Larsson, S., Rask-Andersen, H., & Li, H. (2018). The human cochlear aqueduct and accessory canals: A micro-CT analysis using a 3D reconstruction paradigm. *Otology & Neurotology, 39*(6), e429–e435.

Axelsson, A. (1968). The vascular anatomy of the cochlea in the Guinea pig and in man. *Acta Oto-Laryngologica, 243*(suppl 3), 3+.

Bekesy, G. (1960). *Experiments in hearing*. McGraw-Hill.

Brodal, P. (2004). *Central nervous system: Structure and function*. Oxford University Press.

Brownell, W. E. (1983). *Mechanisms of hearing*. Monash University Press.

Brownell, W. E., Bader, C. R., Bertrand, D., & de Ribaupierre, Y. (1985). Evoked mechanical responses of isolated cochlear outer hair cells. *Science (New York, N.Y.), 227*(4683), 194–196.

Brugge, J. F., & Howard, M. A. (2002). *Encyclopedia of the human brain*. Academic.

Charachon, R. (1961). *Anatomie de l'artère auditive interne chez l'homme* (Doctoral dissertation, Faculté de médecine et de pharmacie de Lyon).

Cohen-Salmon, M., El-Amraoui, A., Leibovici, M., & Petit, C. (1997). Otogelin: A glycoprotein specific to the acellular membranes of the inner ear. *Proceedings of the National Academy of Sciences of the United States of America, 94*(26), 14450–14455.

Dallos, P., Evans, B. N., & Hallworth, R. (1991). Nature of the motor element in electrokinetic shape changes of cochlear outer hair cells. *Nature, 350*(6314), 155–157.

Doherty, J. K., & Linthicum, F. H., Jr. (2004). Spiral ligament and stria vascularis changes in cochlear otosclerosis: Effect on hearing level. *Otology & Neurotology, 25*(4), 457–464.

Dorland, W. (2011). *Dorland's illustrated medical dictionary* (32nd ed.). Elsevier Saunders.

Dos Santos, J. C., Musso, F., Mayer, W. P., & Baptista, J. D. S. (2020). Descriptive and topographical analysis of the labyrinthine artery in human fetuses. *Anatomical Science International, 95*(3), 374–380.

Duvall, A. J., & Rhodes, V. T. (1967). Ultrastructure of the organ of Corti following intermixing of cochlear fluids. *The Annals of Otology, Rhinology, and Laryngology, 76*(3), 688–708.

Flock, A. (1980). Contractile proteins in hair cells. *Hearing Research, 2*(3–4), 411–412.

Flock, Å., Flock, B., & Murray, E. (1977). Studies on the sensory hairs of receptor cells in the inner ear. *Acta Oto-Laryngologica, 83*(1–6), 85–91.

Flock, A., Bretscher, A., & Weber, K. (1982). Immunohistochemical localization of several cytoskeletal proteins in inner ear sensory and supporting cells. *Hearing Research, 7*(1), 75–89.

Flock, A., Flock, B., & Ulfendahl, M. (1986). Mechanisms of movement in outer hair cells and a possible structural basis. *Archives of Oto-Rhino-Laryngology, 243*(2), 83–90.

Geisler, C. D. (1998). *From sound to synapse: Physiology of the mammalian ear*. Oxford University Press.

Ghaffari, R., Aranyosi, A. J., & Freeman, D. M. (2007). Longitudinally propagating traveling waves of the mammalian tectorial membrane. *Proceedings of the National Academy of Sciences of the United States of America, 104*(42), 16510–16515.

Gray, H., & Carter, H. V. (2008). *Gray's anatomy: The anatomical basis of clinical practice*. Elsevier.

Gulley, R. L., & Reese, T. S. (1976). Intercellular junctions in the reticular lamina of the organ of Corti. *Journal of Neurocytology, 5*(4), 479–507.

Hardy, M. (1938). The length of the organ of Corti in man. *American Journal of Anatomy, 62*(2), 291–311.

Häusler, R., & Levine, R. A. (2000). Auditory dysfunction in stroke. *Acta Oto-Laryngologica, 120*(6), 689–703.

Hawkins, J. E. (2024, December 12). Cochlea. In *Anatomy of the human ear*. Britannica. https://www.britannica.com/science/ear/Cochlea#ref531831.

Howarth, A., & Shone, G. R. (2006). Ageing and the auditory system: This article is part of a series on ageing edited by Professor Chris Bulpitt. *Postgraduate Medical Journal, 82*(965), 166–171.

Huang, D., Chen, P., Chen, S., Nagura, M., Lim, D. J., & Lin, X. (2002). Expression patterns of aquaporins in the inner ear: Evidence for concerted actions of multiple types of aquaporins to facilitate water transport in the cochlea. *Hearing Research, 165*(1–2), 85–95.

Jasser, A., & Guth, P. S. (1973). The synthesis of acetylcholine by the olivocochlear bundle. *Journal of Neurochemistry, 20*, 45–50.

Johnstone, B. M., Patuzzi, R., Syka, J., & Sykova, E. (1989). Stimulus-related potassium changes in the organ of Corti of Guinea-pig. *The Journal of Physiology, 408*(1), 77–92.

Kitcher, S. R., Pederson, A. M., & Weisz, C. J. C. (2022). Diverse identities and sites of action of cochlear neurotransmitters. *Hearing Research, 419*, 108278.

Konishi, T., & Kelsey, E. (1973). Effect of potassium deficiency on cochlear potentials and cation contents of the endolymph. *Acta Oto-Laryngologica, 76*(6), 410–418.

Küçük, B., Abe, K., Ushiki, T., Inuyama, Y., Fukuda, S., & Ishikawa, K. (1991). Microstructures of the bony modiolus in the human cochlea: A scanning electron microscopic study. *Journal of Electron Microscopy, 40*(3), 193–197.

Legan, P. K., Rau, A., Keen, J. N., & Richardson, G. P. (1997). The mouse tectorins. Modular matrix proteins of the inner ear homologous to components of the sperm-egg adhesion system. *The Journal of Biological Chemistry, 272*(13), 8791–8801.

Liberman, M. C. (1982). Single-neuron labeling in the cat auditory nerve. *Science (New York, N.Y.), 216*(4551), 1239–1241.

Lim, R., & Brichta, A. M. (2016). Anatomical and physiological development of the human inner ear. *Hearing Research, 338*, 9–21.

Marcus, D. C., Marcus, N. Y., & Thalmann, R. (1981). Changes in cation contents of stria vascularis with ouabain and potassium-free perfusion. *Hearing Research, 4*(2), 149–160.

McGuirt, W. T., Prasad, S. D., Griffith, A. J., Kunst, H. P., Green, G. E., Shpargel, K. B., Runge, C., Huybrechts, C., Mueller, R. F., Lynch, E., King, M. C., Brunner, H. G., Cremers, C. W., Takanosu, M., Li, S. W., Arita, M., Mayne, R., Prockop, D. J., Van Camp, G., & Smith, R. J. (1999). Mutations in COL11A2 cause non-syndromic hearing loss (DFNA13). *Nature Genetics, 23*(4), 413–419.

Mei, X., Atturo, F., Wadin, K., Larsson, S., Agrawal, S., Ladak, H. M., Li, H., & Rask-Andersen, H. (2018). Human inner ear blood supply revisited: The Uppsala collection of temporal bone-an international resource of education and collaboration. *Upsala Journal of Medical Sciences, 123*(3), 131–142.

Mei, X., Glueckert, R., Schrott-Fischer, A., Li, H., Ladak, H. M., Agrawal, S. K., & Rask-Andersen, H. (2020). Vascular supply of the human spiral ganglion: Novel three-dimensional analysis using synchrotron phase-contrast imaging and histology. *Scientific Reports, 10*(1), 5877.

Moller, A. R. (2006). *Hearing: Anatomy, physiology and disorders of the auditory system* (2nd ed.). Academic.

Nabeya, D. (1923). A study in the comparative anatomy of the blood-vascular system of the internal ear in mammalia and in homo (Japanese), *16*, 1–120.

Neng, L., Zhang, J., Yang, J., Zhang, F., Lopez, I. A., Dong, M., & Shi, X. (2015). Structural changes in thestrial blood-labyrinth barrier of aged C57BL/6 mice. *Cell and Tissue Research, 361*(3), 685–696.

Nikolakopoulou, A. M., Montagne, A., Kisler, K., Dai, Z., Wang, Y., Huuskonen, M. T., Sagare, A. P., Lazic, D., Sweeney, M. D., Kong, P., Wang, M., Owens, N. C., Lawson, E. J., Xie, X., Zhao, Z., & Zlokovic, B. V. (2019). Pericyte loss leads to circulatory failure and pleiotrophin depletion causing neuron loss. *Nature Neuroscience, 22*(7), 1089–1098.

Norma, Slepecky Mats, Ulfendahl Åke, Flock (1988) Effects of caffeine and tetracaine on outer hair cell shortening suggest intracellular calcium involvement *Hearing Research 32*(1) 11-21 https://doi.org/10.1016/0378-5955(88)90143-8

Nunes, F. D., Lopez, L. N., Lin, H. W., Davies, C., Azevedo, R. B., Gow, A., & Kachar, B. (2006). Distinct subdomain organization and molecular composition of a tight junction with adherens junction features. *Journal of Cell Science, 119*(Pt 23), 4819–4827.

Oghalai, J. S. (2004). The cochlear amplifier: Augmentation of the traveling wave within the inner ear. *Current Opinion in Otolaryngology & Head and Neck Surgery, 12*(5), 431–438.

Pauna, H. F., Monsanto, R. C., Schachern, P. A., Costa, S. S., Kwon, G., Paparella, M. M., & Cureoglu, S. (2017). The surgical challenge of carotid artery and Fallopian canal dehiscence in chronic ear disease: A pitfall for endoscopic approach. *Clinical Otolaryngology, 42*(2), 268–274.

Perlman, H. B., & Kimura, R. (1957). XLIII experimental obstruction of venous drainage and arterial supply of the inner ear. *Annals of Otology, Rhinology & Laryngology, 66*(2), 537–546.

Pickles, J. (2013). *An introduction to the physiology of hearing* (4th ed.). BRILL.

Proctor, B., Bollobas, B., & Niparko, J. K. (1986). Anatomy of the round window niche. *The Annals of Otology, Rhinology, and Laryngology, 95*(5 Pt 1), 444–446.

Rask-Andersen, H., Schrott-Fischer, A., Pfaller, K., & Glueckert, R. (2006). Perilymph/modiolar communication routes in the human cochlea. *Ear and Hearing, 27*(5), 457–465.

Rask-Andersen, H., Liu, W., Erixon, E., Kinnefors, A., Pfaller, K., Schrott-Fischer, A., & Glueckert, R. (2012). Human cochlea: Anatomical characteristics and their relevance for cochlear implantation. *Anatomical Record (Hoboken, N.J.: 2007), 295*(11), 1791–1811.

Raufer, S., Guinan, J. J., Jr., & Nakajima, H. H. (2019). Cochlear partition anatomy and motion in humans differ from the classic view of mammals. *Proceedings of the National Academy of Sciences of the United States of America, 116*(28), 13977–13982.

Richardson, G. P., Russell, I. J., Duance, V. C., & Bailey, A. J. (1987). Polypeptide composition of the mammalian tectorial membrane. *Hearing Research, 25*(1), 45–60.

Richardson, G. P., Lukashkin, A. N., & Russell, I. J. (2008). The tectorial membrane: One slice of a complex cochlear sandwich. *Current Opinion in Otolaryngology & Head and Neck Surgery, 16*(5), 458–464.

Robertson, D. (1983). Functional significance of dendritic swelling after loud sounds in the Guinea pig cochlea. *Hearing Research, 9*(3), 263–278.

Robles, L., & Ruggero, M. A. (2001). Mechanics of the mammalian cochlea. *Physiological Reviews, 81*(3), 1305–1352.

Santos-Sacchi, J. (1992). On the frequency limit and phase of outer hair cell motility: Effects of the membrane filter. *The Journal of Neuroscience, 12*(5), 1906–1916.

Shpargel, K. B., Makishima, T., & Griffith, A. J. (2004). Col11a1 and Col11a2 mRNA expression in the developing mouse cochlea: Implications for the correlation of hearing loss phenotype with mutant type XI collagen genotype. *Acta Oto-Laryngologica, 124*(3), 242–248.

Siebenmann, F. (1894). *Die Blutgefässe im Labyrinthe des menschlichen Ohres*. JF Bergmann.

Spoendlin, H. (1966). The organization of the cochlear receptor. *Fortschritte der Hals-Nasen-Ohrenheilkunde, 13*, 1–227.

Spoendlin, H. (1969). Innervation patterns in the organ of corti of the cat. *Acta Oto-Laryngologica, 67*(2), 239–254.

Spoendlin, H. (1971). Primary structural changes in the organ of Corti after acoustic overstimulation. *Acta Oto-Laryngologica, 71*(2), 166–176.

Standring, S. (2016). *Gray's anatomy: The anatomical basis of clinical practice* (41st ed.). Elsevier Limited.

Thalmann, I. (1993). Collagen of accessory structures of organ of Corti. *Connective Tissue Research, 29*(3), 191–201.

Thalmann, I., Thallinger, G., Crouch, E. C., Comegys, T. H., Barrett, N., & Thalmann, R. (1987). Composition and supramolecular organization of the tectorial membrane. *The Laryngoscope, 97*(3 Pt 1), 357–367.

Toro, E. F., Borgioli, F., Zhang, Q., Contarino, C., Müller, L. O., & Bruno, A. (2018). Inner-ear circulation in humans is disrupted by extracranial venous outflow strictures: Implications for Ménière's Disease. *Veins and Lymphatics, 7*(1).

v. Békésy, G. (1949). The vibration of the cochlear partition in anatomical preparations and in models of the inner ear. *The Journal of the Acoustical Society of America, 21*(3), 233–245.

Watanabe, Y., Nakashima, T., & Yanagita, N. (1988). Venous communications of the cochlea after acute occlusion of the vein of the cochlear aqueduct. *Archives of Oto-Rhino-Laryngology, 245*(6), 340–343.

Weaver, S. P., & Schweitzer, L. (1994). A radial gradient of fibril density in the gerbil tectorial membrane. *Hearing Research, 76*(1–2), 1–6.

Wever, E. G. (1954). *Physiological acoustics*. Princeton University Press.

Yeh, T. H., Tsai, M. C., Lee, S. Y., Hsu, M. M., & Tran Ba Huy, P. (1997). Stretch-activated nonselective cation, Cl- and K+ channels in apical membrane of epithelial cells of Reissner's membrane. *Hearing Research, 109*(1–2), 1–10.

Zhang, K., Wang, F., Zhang, Y., Li, M., & Shi, X. (2002). [Anatomic investigation of the labyrinthine artery]. *Zhonghua Er Bi Yan Hou Ke Za Zhi, 37*(2), 103–105.

Zhong, S. X., & Liu, Z. H. (2003). Expression of aquaporins in the cochlea and endolymphatic sac of Guinea pig. *ORL: Journal for Oto-Rhino-Laryngology and Its Related Specialties, 65*(5), 284–289.

Chapter 2
Functional Organisation of the Afferent Auditory Pathway

Ajith Kumar Uppunda and Shezeen Abdul Gafoor

Abstract This chapter delves into the basic neuroanatomy and neurophysiology of hearing, with a focus on the functional organization of the central auditory pathway. It explores the journey of auditory signals from the cochlea to the auditory cortex, focusing on auditory relay nuclei such as the cochlear nucleus, superior olivary complex, lateral lemniscus, inferior colliculus and medial geniculate body. A comprehensive understanding of this pathway is crucial for understanding auditory signal processing, unraveling auditory disorders and advancing auditory (re) habilitation.

Keywords Auditory nerve · Afferent auditory pathway · Spiral ganglions · Frequency coding · Speech processing

Introduction

The afferent auditory pathway has specialized neural structures to process complex acoustic events such as speech, music or environmental sounds that contain highly dynamic information. The peripheral auditory system analyses spectro-temporal features of acoustic events, and these features are processed, and ecologically relevant information are decoded in the higher centres. The auditory afferent pathway comprises the auditory (VIII cranial nerve) nerve, cochlear nucleus, superior olivary complex, lateral lemniscus, inferior colliculus and the auditory cortex. Figure 2.1 shows the schematic diagram of the afferent auditory pathway.

A. K. Uppunda (✉)
Department of Audiology and Center for Hearing Sciences, All India Institute of Speech and Hearing (AIISH), Mysore, Karnataka, India

S. A. Gafoor
Department of Audiology and Speech-Language Pathology, Kasturba Medical College, Mangalore, Manipal Academy of Higher Education, Mangalore, Karnataka, India

P. Kumar et al. (eds.), *Advances in Implantation Otology*,
https://doi.org/10.1007/978-981-96-8671-1_2

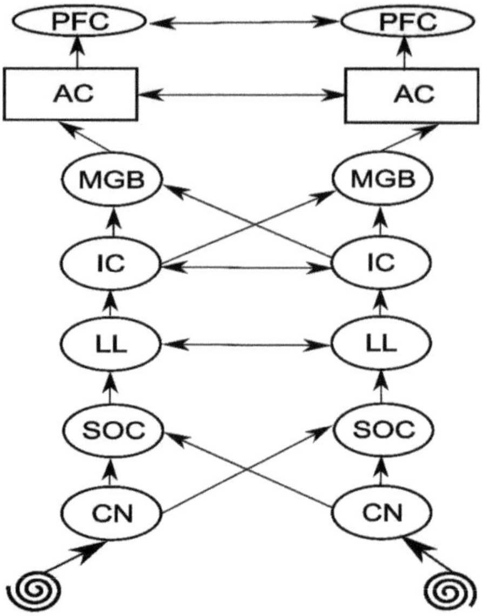

Fig. 2.1 Schematic representation of the afferent auditory pathway—the relay centres and the major connections (Hints: AC- auditory cortex, PFC- prefrontal cortex, MGB- medial geniculate body, IC- inferior colliculous, LL- lateral lemniscus, SOC- superiory olivary complex, CN- cochlear nucleus)

Auditory Nerve

In the inner ear, the auditory nerve's cell bodies (VIII cranial nerve) are situated in a canal formed by the bony spirals called Rosenthal's canal. Each cell body emits two processes—the peripheral and central process. The peripheral process enters the organ of Corti and innervate the cochlea's sensory cells. On the other hand, the central process projects to the cochlear nucleus via the internal auditory meatus. The internal auditory meatus is a bony canal that houses the central process of the VIII cranial nerve and facial nerve. The cell bodies of VIII cranial nerve is located in the spiral ganglion and forms the afferent innervation of the organ of Corti. Two sub-types of the spiral ganglion cells have been identified: Type I and Type II (Fig. 2.2). The type I spiral ganglion cells (representing 90–95% of the total spiral ganglion cells) are relatively larger and bipolar, and forms the primary sensory innervation in the auditory system (Rusznák & Szucs, 2009). A thick myelin sheath wraps the cell body and dendrites of the type I cells. The type I fibres innervate the inner hair cells (IHC). Activation of the IHC by the type I cells generates action potential. The type II spiral ganglion cells are relatively small, pseudo-bipolar or monopolar, representing 5–10% of the population (Malmierca & Hackett, 2012). The processes of type II fibres are unmyelinated and innervate the outer hair cells. The functions of the type II fibers are currently unclear. However, it has been hypothesized that the type II fibers monitor the activity of the outer hair cells and send this information to the central nervous system. The central nervous system fine-tunes the sensitivity of the outer hair cells

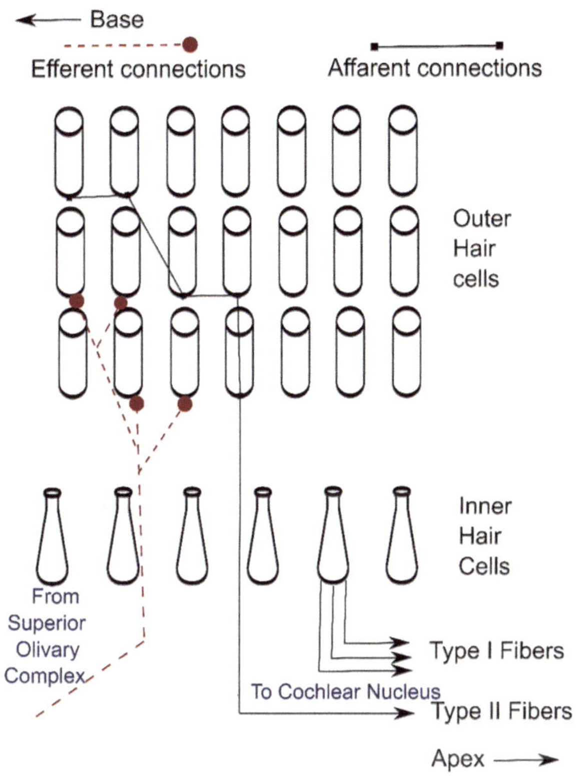

Fig. 2.2 Schematic diagram of innervation of type I and type II fibres in the organ of Corti

(via top-down modulations), which in turn ensures optimal functioning of the cochlea (Rusznák & Szucs, 2009).

Type I Spiral Ganglion Neurons

The Peripheral Process

The type I spiral ganglion neurons' peripheral processes pass through spiral lamina—a thin bony plate. Upon exiting from habenula perforata (opening in spiral lamina) into the organ of Corti, neurons shed their myelin sheath and innervate IHC. Each IHC receives about 15–20 different type I auditory nerve fibres (Fig. 2.2). The precise number of nerve fibres that innervate each IHC varies depending on the location of the IHCs on the basilar membrane. It has been shown that the number of synapses per IHCs is higher at functionally important frequency regions. For

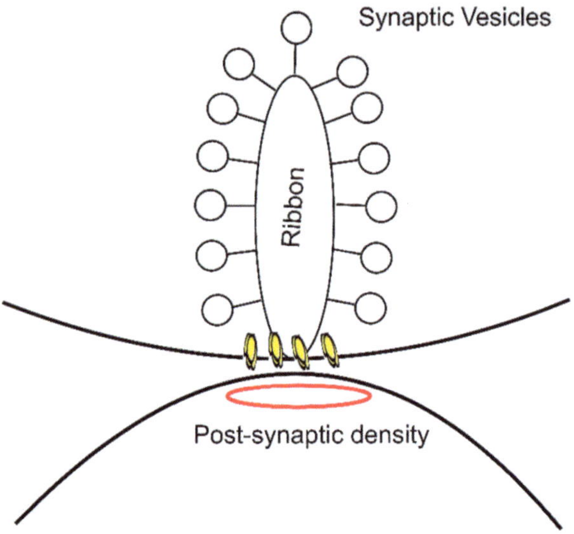

Fig. 2.3 Schematic representation of a ribbon synapse

example, in mice, the number of type I fibres innervating per single IHC peaks around the middle turn of the cochlea, which is sensitive to 12–16 Hz (Meyer et al., 2013). Furthermore, the location on the IHC where the type I neurons synapse depends on the spontaneous rate of the auditory nerve fibre. Low spontaneous rate auditory neurons are thinner and have synapses on the modular side of the IHC. In contrast, high spontaneous rate auditory neurons are thicker and synapses on the pillar side of the IHC (Liberman, 1982). The high spontaneous rate neurons have a low threshold and help code lower intensity sounds. The low spontaneous fibres have a higher threshold than the high spontaneous rate neurons; they help in encoding high intensity sounds. Hence, multiple type I afferent neurons innervating an IHC serve functionally distinct purposes (Winter et al., 1990).

The synapse between the IHC and type I afferent neurons is a ribbon synapse. The name ribbon synapse derives from its appearance. The ribbon is a spherical electron-dense body near the presynaptic membrane of the IHC (Fig. 2.3). Each ribbon is less than a micron, and approximately 100 synaptic vesicles are attached to it. The ribbon synapse helps release neurotransmitters at a very high rate, enabling high temporal precision essential for localisation and coding speech (Fuchs et al., 2003). These properties make the IHC-auditory neuron synapse a highly specialised, ultrafast rate synapse.

The Central Projections

The axons of the type I spiral ganglion cells via internal auditory meatus enter the brainstem at the Schwan-glial border—the point where individual nerve fibers (which are surrounded by Schwann cells), enter the cochlear nucleus (which contains glial cells). These axons ascend into the cochlear nucleus from the ventral aspect. All auditory nerve fibres terminate at the cochlear nucleus—the first relay station in the ascending auditory pathway. Individual axons bifurcate into ascending and descending branches as they enter the cochlear nucleus complex. The precise location of this bifurcation depends on the characteristic frequency of the auditory nerve fibres. The fibres that innervate the cochlea's basal regions, which are sensitive to high frequencies, bifurcate more dorsally in the cochlear nucleus. In contrast, the auditory nerve fibres that originate from the apical regions of the cochlea, which are sensitive to low frequencies, bifurcate more ventrally in the cochlear nucleus. Due to this, low frequencies are represented ventrally in the cochlear nucleus, and high frequencies are represented more dorsally (Nayagam et al., 2011). The terminal swelling of the ascending branch of the auditory nerve, which is formed by the synapse between auditory nerve fibre and cochlear nucleus neuron, is called the end bulb of Held. A single end bulb of Held can contain up to 2000 synaptic release sites. Such high density of synaptic release sites ensures high-fidelty transmission of the acoustic events to the cochlear nucleus neurons (Ryugo & Spirou, 2016).

Physiology of the Auditory Nerve

In the late 1970s, techniques were invented to record the responses from individual auditory neurons. Like any other neuron, the auditory nerve generates all or none electrical discharge upon stimulation called action potential. When action potentials are recorded with an electrode, they appear as spikes. The number of action potentials generated per second is known as spike rate, firing rate, or discharge rate. The number of action potentials generated per second by the nerve without any stimulus is called the spontaneous rate (Gelfand, 2010). Extracellular recordings of auditory neurons have shown some essential features of auditory nerve responses, which are discussed below.

Response Pattern

Each neuron responds to stimulus onset with an initial high rate. However, the high rate is not maintained, and the fibres adapt rapidly. Within a fraction of a millisecond, the discharge rate decreases to a lower rate, which is subsequently held for a sustained duration (Fig. 2.4). The lower rate is maintained until the stimulus is turned off. Following this, the rate falls sharply below the spontaneous rate for a few milliseconds, and then the spontaneous rate is gradually regained (Taberner & Charles Liberman, 2005).

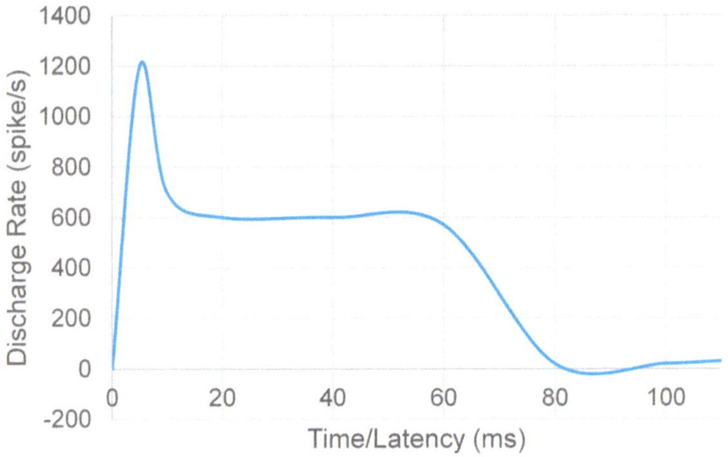

Fig. 2.4 Representation of the typical response pattern of an auditory nerve fibre for a pure tone. Note that initial high discharge rate falls quickly and is maintained at a lower level for the subsequent period of the signal

Frequency Coding

Each auditory neuron responds to a very narrow range of frequencies. The frequency with the greatest firing rate is called the characteristic frequency (CF) or best frequency of the fibre. This property is essentially determined by the cochlear mechanics and depends on site of innervation of the auditory nerve in the cochlea. Fibres that innervate the base of the cochlea are sensitive to high frequencies, whereas fibres that innervate the apical regions of the cochlea are sensitive to low frequencies. This anatomical arrangement is at times referred to as rate-place code for frequency processing. The response of the single auditory neuron as a function of frequency is called the tuning curve (Fig. 2.5). In the tuning curve, frequency is represented on the x-axis and the level needed to reach the neuron's threshold or discharge rate at a suprathreshold intensity is represented on the y-axis. The tip of the tuning curve represents the CF of the neuron. Notice in the Fig. 2.5 that neurons respond to a broad range of frequencies at higher intensities and are asymmetrical around the CF. A neuron responds to a wide frequency range at higher intensities below its CF but only to a restricted range above its CF. Therefore, the low-frequency slope of the tuning curves is shallow, while that of high-frequencies is very steep.

Neurons exhibit phase-locking to the stimulus, at least in low frequencies. Phase locking refers to the property of the auditory nerve fibre where the action potentials tend to fire at a particular phase of the stimulus. It has been shown that responses of the auditory nerve are phase-locked to the stimulus up to 4000 Hz to 5000 Hz (Oxenham, 2018). The strength of the phase-locking decreases steeply at higher frequencies. These findings suggest that timing information conveyed by the interval between action potentials is used to transmit the frequency information, at least

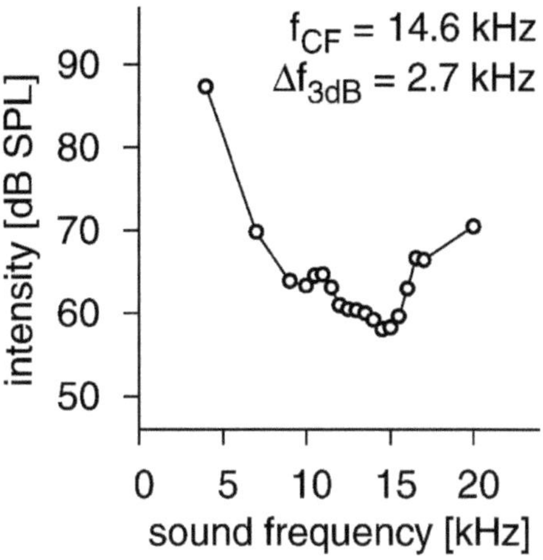

Fig. 2.5 Representation of a frequency tuning curve with a characteristic frequency of 14.6 kHz. Note that low frequency tails are shallow while high frequency tails are steep

for low-frequency pure tones—a process called temporal coding of frequency. The phase-locking results in the synchronised firing of action potentials.

Intensity Coding

The neuron's discharge rate increases with the stimulus intensity within the dynamic range of the neurons. The relationship between the intensity of the stimulus and a neuron's discharge rate is called rate-level function. The dynamic range of a single auditory nerve fibre is only about 20 dB to 40 dB. Within this narrow range, the nerve fibres increase the discharge rate with increase in intensity. For example, a fibre with a threshold of 10 dB SPL and a dynamic range of 40 dB will continue to increase the discharge rate up to 50 dB SPL. However, beyond this intensity, the discharge rate will saturate, and the neuron's firing rate stop increasing with increase in intensity of the stimulus. Therefore, a single fibre cannot accommodate the large dynamic range of hearing, which is about 120 dB. However, studies have shown that a single IHC receives multiple type I neurons, which differ in threshold and dynamic range. Liberman (1988) identified three distinct groups of auditory nerve fibres with respect to the spontaneous rate, threshold and shape of the rate level function. Auditory nerve fibres with high spontaneous rate have a low threshold and a saturating type of rate level function. It is believed that these fibres help in coding low-intensity sounds. Fibres with medium spontaneous rate have a medium threshold and a sloping-saturating type of rate level function. The dynamic range of medium spontaneous rate fibres is wider than that of low spontaneous rate fibres. It appears that these groups of fibres help code moderate intensities. The third group of nerve fibres have a lower spontaneous rate, higher threshold and wider dynamic range than the other two groups. The rate level function of these fibres is straight. These fibres code high-intensity sounds. These three groups of nerve fibres, in combination, are believed to help code the entire dynamic range of hearing. Furthermore, it is also shown that synchronisation of action potential increases with the increase in intensity.

Speech Processing

In everyday speech, vowels are relatively stable and periodic over a limited time interval. Therefore, it is easier to study the neural encoding of vowels compared to other classes of speech sounds. The frequency of the first and the second formants largely determines the identity of vowels. There is a clear rate-place representation of vowels at moderate sound pressure levels: the discharge rates are higher in fibres with characteristic frequency near the formants than in those with characteristic frequency remote from the formants. Nevertheless, at high intensity, the fibres with characteristic frequency between the formants increase their discharge. In contrast, fibres at the formant frequency reach saturation, causing formant-related peaks to lose differentiation and eventually to become obscured. However, human vowel identification is unchanged at the highest sound levels. Hence, the rate-place code is inadequate to represent vowels at all sound levels. Saturation of the discharge rate takes place only for high spontaneous fibres with narrow dynamic range. However, when the discharges from the low spontaneous fibres are included, the formant-related peaks in the discharge rate can be distinguished at the highest stimulus intensity. In the real world, there may be a contribution from the efferent system, which helps increase the auditory nerve's dynamic range. Since the spectra of the speech sounds are primarily restricted to frequencies below 5 kHz, individual nerve fibres are phase-locked to components of speech sounds. As a result, fibres which are phase-locked to formant frequencies dominate the responses and code the formant related information. In fact, it has been shown that at low intensities, it is the rate-place code, while at high intensities, it is both the rate-place and temporal (phase locking) code that helps in coding the spectral information of speech in the auditory nerve (Uysal et al., 2007).

Cochlear Nucleus Complex

The cochlear nucleus complex (CNC) is situated in the pons and is the first relay centre in the central auditory pathway. All auditory nerve fibres terminate in the CNC. Auditory nerve fibres synapse with the CNC neurons while maintaining the cochlea's tonotopic representation (discussed earlier). CNC is subdivided into anteroventral, posteroventral and dorsal cochlear nuclei. The ascending branch of the auditory nerve fibre supplies to the anteroventral, and descending branch of the auditory nerve fibre supplies to posteroventral and dorsal cochlear nuclei. Histopathological studies have identified several neuronal types in the CNC. These neurons are labelled based on their appearance as spherical bushy, stellate, octopus etc. (Nayagam et al., 2011; Palmer, 1987; Ryugo & Parks, 2003).

The Ventral Cochlear Nucleus

Ventral cochlear nucleus is subdivided into anteroventral and posteroventral cochlear nucleus each having specialized neurons. Spherical bushy cells are found in the anteroventral CNC; Octopus cells are found primarily in the posteroventral CNC and the globular bushy, multipolar, and small cells are found in both anteroventral and posteroventral CNC. The somatic surface of spherical and globular bushy cells is covered with the synaptic terminals to form end bulbs of Held. The responses of spherical and globular bushy cells are similar to auditory neurons and are called primary-like responses. Due to these features, spherical and globular bushy cells transmit temporal information with high fidelity. Tuning curve properties, rate-level functions and coding of speech-like stimuli in bushy cells are similar to that of the auditory nerve.

Synapses in the octopus cells are relatively small compared to spherical and globular bushy cells. Responses of the octopus cells are locked to the onset of the stimulus. Hence, it is hypothesised that these cells with onset-response play a major role in spatial hearing and coding pitch periods. Apart from these, two types of multipolar cells have been identified in ventral cochlear nucleus: T- stellate cells and D-stellate cells. The response pattern of T-stellate cells is called chopper type—a response pattern similar to the auditory nerve but with multiple peaks separated by regular intervals unrelated to the stimulus' frequency. The response pattern of the D-stellate cells is on-chop—a few onset spikes followed by no sustained response (Malmierca & Hackett, 2012).

The Dorsal Cochlear Nucleus

The dorsal cochlear nucleus has a laminar structure (Fig. 2.6). At least three superficial laminae have been identified in rodents. The primary cells of the dorsal cochlear nucleus are fusiform or pyramidal cells. The cell bodies of the pyramidal cells occupy layer II; spiny apical dendrites occupy layer I, and aspiny basal dendrites occupy layer III (as seen in Figure 2.6). The basal dendrites are supplied by auditory nerve fibres in a tonotopical manner. Layer I and layer III also contain several different types of interneurons that connect the dendrites of pyramidal cells. Primarily two types of interneuron systems have been identified: a basal tuberculoventral system and an apical granule system. The tuberculoventral system provides frequency-specific inhibitory inputs to ventral and dorsal cochlear nuclei neurons. Cells of the granule system provide inhibitory inputs to the pyramidal cells. The inhibitory inputs from the two interneuron systems influence the response patterns

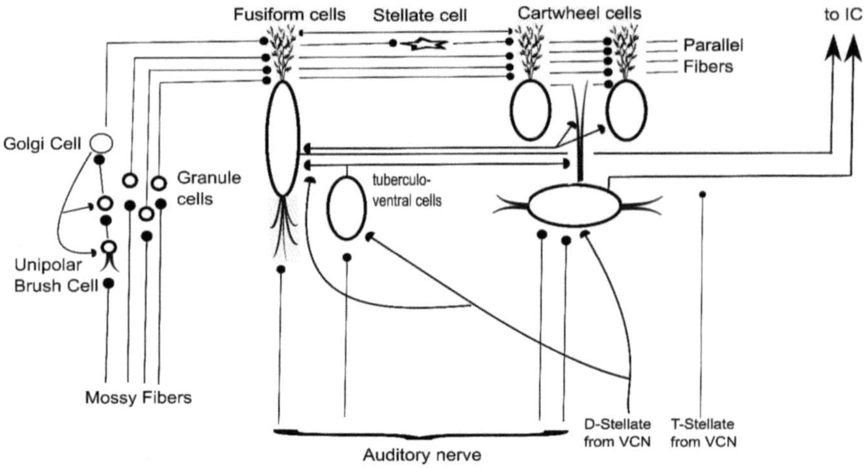

Fig. 2.6 Schematic representation of dorsal cochlear nucleus showing connections between various cell types (Hints: IC- inferior colliculus, VCN- ventral cochlear nucleus)

of the pyramidal cells. The response pattern of the pyramidal cells is termed as pauser—onset response followed by a pause and then the resumption of the response—and build-up—a slow increase in the discharge rate following the onset (Oertel & Young, 2004). Tuning curves of pyramidal cells are more complex, with a zone of activation surrounded by a zone of inhibition. Several studies have shown that the pyramidal cells are specialised in processing spectral cues that are important for localisation in the vertical plane.

Central Projections of CNC

The projections from spherical and globular bushy cells form ventral acoustic stria; the ventral acoustic stria is also known as the trapezoid body. The spherical bushy cells send projections to the bilateral medial superior olive and to the ipsilateral lateral superior olive. The globular bushy cells project to the contralateral nucleus of the trapezoid body. The octopus cells' axons project via intermediate acoustic stria to the bilateral superior paraolivary nucleus and contralateral lateral lemniscus. The axons of T-stellate cells via ventral acoustic stria innervate the periolivary region of the superior olivary complex and the nuclei of the lateral lemniscus. The D-stellate cells send projections to the contralateral CNC and interconnect the other neurons within the ipsilateral CNC. The axons of T- stellate cells are also called commissural neurons as they interconnect two CNCs. The pyramidal cells of dorsal cochlear nucleus project to the contralateral inferior colliculus (IC) through dorsal acoustic stria.

Superior Olivary Complex

The superior olivary complex (SOC) is a group of distinct nuclei located between the CNC and midline of the brainstem. Three prominent SOC nuclei can be identified in most mammalian species: lateral superior olive (LSO), medial superior olive (MSO), and medial nucleus of the trapezoid body (MNTB). The SOC nuclei receive input from bilateral CNC, representing the first stage of binaural information processing. The size and architecture of the SOC nuclei vary considerably across species. The LSO and MNTB are well developed in animals but are pretty small in humans. In contrast, MSO is well developed in humans but underrepresented in animals. The upper-frequency range of hearing is one of the factors contributing to the inter-species differences in the anatomical properties of the SOC. The two binaural cues, inter-aural time and intensity differences are encoded in the MSO and LSO, respectively. Predominantly, the LSO contains medium and high frequency fibers, while the LSO contains low frequency fibers (Ehret & Romand, 1997). The SOC neurons are also classified based on how they respond to stimuli from two ears, using a code of two letters: the first letter corresponds to stimulation from the contralateral ear and the second letter corresponds to stimulation from the ipsilateral ear. Among them, 'E' represents excitatory influence, 'I' shows inhibitory influence and 'O' represents no influence (Ehret & Romand, 1997). The Table 2.1 shows different SOC neurons and their responses to stimulation from two ears (to be inserted).

Medial Superior Olive

The MSO is located between LSO and MNTB. MSO receives excitatory inputs from bilateral spherical bushy cells. Lateral dendrites of MSO neurons receive excitatory inputs from ipsilateral CNC, whereas medial dendrites receive excitatory inputs from the contralateral side. In addition, the stomata (cell body) of the MSO receive inhibitory inputs from MNTB on both sides. Because of these arrangements, the MSO neurons are sensitive to the inter-aural time difference. However, despite many years of research, it remains unclear how MSO neuron integrates four different inputs to produce a well-defined inter-aural sensitivity. The major output from the MSO project to the inferior colliculus (Grothe et al., 2010).

Table 2.1 The responses observed in the various SOC nuclei

Nuclei	Response (Contralateral Ipsilateral)
MNTB	Predominantly EO
MSO	65% EE 25% EI/IE 10% EO
LSO	Majority IE A few OE

Note. *E* excitatory, *I* inhibitory, *O* no influence

Lateral Superior Olive

LSO of many mammals are typically S-shaped and tonotopically organised in a way that low frequencies are represented more laterally compared to the high frequencies. Most of the nucleus of LSO is devoted to higher frequencies than MSO. The LSO receives excitatory input from ipsilateral spherical bushy cells while it receives inhibitory inputs from contralateral MNTB. As LSO neurons receive information from both ears, it is considered the initial site for encoding the inter-aural level difference. A simple subtraction process (excitatory input from spherical bushy cells minus inhibitory input from MNTB) can encode inter-aural level difference at LSO neurons. The LSO projects bilaterally to the inferior colliculus.

Medial Nucleus of the Trapezoid Body

The principal cells of the MNTB resemble globular bushy cells and receive their input from the contralateral anteroventral cochlear nucleus. The MNTB neurons are inhibitory in nature (major inhibitory neurotransmitter in the auditory system—Glycine and Gamma Amino butyric acid are present here) and project widely within ipsilateral and contralateral SOC and to lateral lemniscus.

Lateral Lemniscus and Inferior Colliculus

Lateral Lemniscus

With respect to cytoarchitecture, the lateral lemniscus is divided into a dorsal nucleus and a ventral nucleus. The dorsal nucleus receives primary input from bilateral MSO and ipsilateral LSO, while the ventral nucleus receives its input primarily from the ventral cochlear nucleus. Accordingly, the dorsal nucleus processes binaural inputs, whereas the ventral nucleus primarily processes monoaural inputs. The neurons of the ventral lateral lemniscus are specialised in coding temporal events with very high precision. The dorsal nucleus plays a vital role in sound localisation. The main output projections from the lateral lemniscus are to the opposite lateral lemniscus via commissure of Probst and to the bilateral inferior colliculus. Some neurons from lower levels, however, bypass the lateral lemniscus and connect directly to the IC. The general connections and the physiologic properties of the lateral lemniscus are similar to that of the IC (Winer & Schreiner, 2005).

Inferior Colliculus

Almost all the input from the lower centre synapses at the inferior colliculus. Hence it is a very important convergence point. The inferior colliculus is formed by disk-shaped cells interconnected with the stellate cells. The IC consists of a central nucleus surrounded by the cortex, consisting of the pericentral and external nucleus of IC. Apart from auditory inputs from the lower centre, IC also receives inputs from visual and somatosensory systems. Response patterns of neurons in IC vary according to the intensity and frequency of the stimulus. Basically, all response types seen in CNC can also be seen in IC. A majority of the neurons of IC are sensitive to inter-aural level and time differences. Furthermore, 'type O' neurons of the central nucleus of IC receives direct input from pyramidal cells of the dorsal cochlear nucleus and form an important circuit responsible for vertical (monoaural) localisation. The central nucleus of IC projects to the ventral division of the medial geniculate body, which in turn projects to the auditory cortex.

Auditory Cortex

Large degrees of inter-species differences are reported in the auditory cortex. However, in most species, three areas have been identified: a central primary region designated as core, a surrounding secondary area called belt and a third region covering the belt area called para-belt (Fig. 2.7). The core includes a caudal primary auditory cortex (AI), a rostral core area and an even more rostral temporal area. These areas are distinguished from each other based on the tonotopic organisation. Tonotopic organisation of the rostral area is opposite from that of the primary auditory cortex. Cortical neurons in all three core areas respond to sound with short latencies and have narrowly tuned tuning curves. They receive input from the ventral nucleus of the medial geniculate body. Each core area is interconnected with other core areas. In addition, each core area projects to adjacent belt areas. The core areas also project to homologous core areas of the opposite hemisphere. A variety

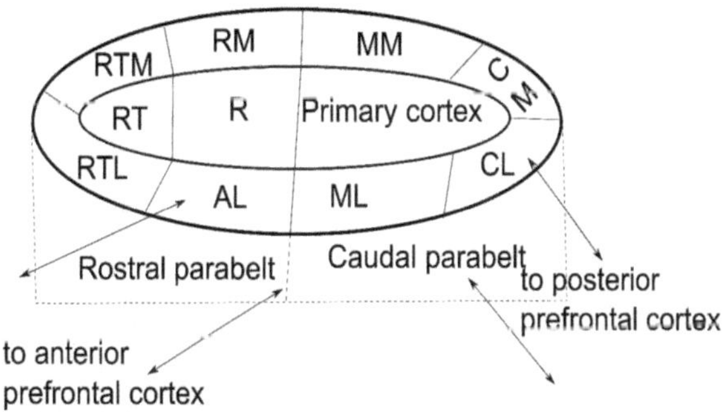

Fig. 2.7 Auditory cortical areas in core, belt and parabelt areas (schematic representation of the cross section) (Hints: RT- rostro temporal, R- rostral, M- medial, C- Caudal, L- lateral, AI- primary cortex)

of evidence has shown that in humans core auditory cortex is situated in the transverse temporal gyrus of Heschl (Kaas & Hackett, 2000).

The area lateral to core areas are often referred to as 'belt areas'. The Belt area surrounds the core area. The Belt area has strong connections with each of the core areas. It appears that the belt is an obligatory second stage of cortical processing, and the core inputs do not bypass the belt. The belt has been subdivided into many areas depending on the tonotopic organisation. The belt areas connect to both the adjoining core and the belt areas. In addition, belt areas also connect to distant belt areas, parabelt areas and the frontal cortex. The parabelt areas lie lateral to the belt area. Two distinct parabelt areas have been identified in the cortex of primates—caudal parabelt and rostral parabelt areas. Parabelt areas receive their inputs from belt areas. Both belt and parabelt connect to homotopic areas of the opposite hemisphere via callosal connections. The Parabelt area is also connected to adjacent temporal, parietal and frontal lobes (Kaas & Hackett, 2000).

It is belived that due to the interconnected areas, cortical processing of acoustic stimuli is hierarchical and involves different streams. Hickok and Poeppel (2007) proposed a dual-stream model of the cortical organisation of speech and language (Fig. 2.8). They proposed that after spectro-temporal analyses and phonological processing in the bilateral auditory cortices, the neural network divides into two streams: a ventral stream that maps phonological representation to lexical concepts and a dorsal stream converts phonological maps to articulatory-motor representation. They proposed that centres for processing spectro-temporal and phonological features are situated in the superior temporal gyrus and sulcus, respectively. The temporal-parietal junction (spt) is believed to be the sensory-motor interface.

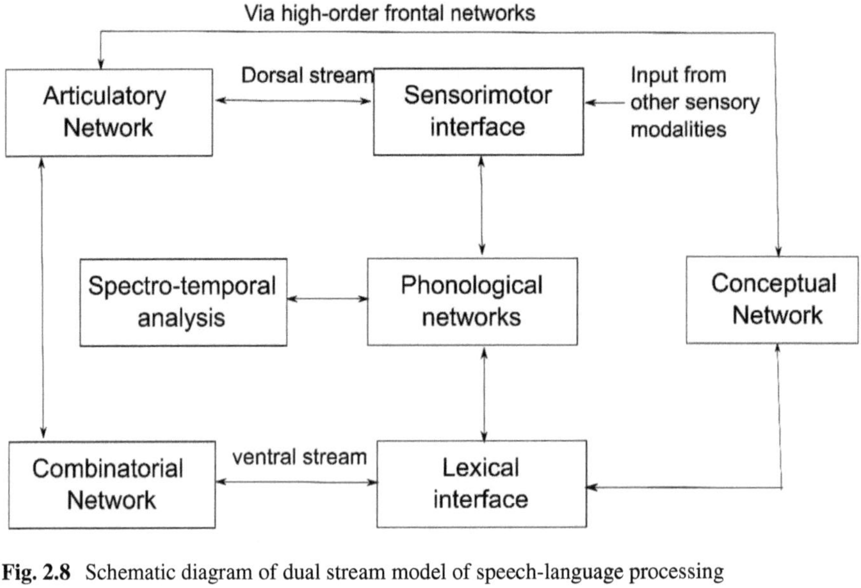

Fig. 2.8 Schematic diagram of dual stream model of speech-language processing

Conclusions

The ascending auditory pathway comprises of highly complex and interconnected neurons. The auditory neurons and synapses between the auditory neurons and IHC are specialised in encoding the acoustic events with high fidelity and temporal precision. Neurons of the CNC and SOC are specialised in analysing spectral cues, and inter-aural time and level difference cues to encode spatial hearing. IC is an important convergence point in the mid-brain and plays a vital role in coding spectral and temporal information in the acoustic stimulus. The auditory cortex integrates and analyses the information received from lower centres to detect and recognise sound in the auditory space.

References

Ehret, G., & Romand, R. (1997). *The central auditory system*. Oxford University Press.

Fuchs, P. A., Glowatzki, E., & Moser, T. (2003). The afferent synapse of cochlear hair cells. *Current Opinion in Neurobiology, 13*(4), 452–458.

Gelfand, S. A. (2010). *Hearing: An introduction to psychological and physiological acoustics* (5th ed.). Essex.

Grothe, B., Pecka, M., & McAlpine, D. (2010). Mechanisms of sound localization in mammals. *Physiological Reviews, 90*(3), 983–1012.

Hickok, G., & Poeppel, D. (2007). The cortical organization of speech processing. *Nature Reviews Neuroscience, 8*(May), 393–402.

Kaas, J. H., & Hackett, T. A. (2000). Subdivisions of auditory cortex and processing streams in primates. *Proceedings of the National Academy of Sciences of the United States of America, 97*(22), 11793–11799.

Liberman, M. C. (1982). Single-neuron labeling in the cat auditory nerve. *Science, 216*(4551), 1239–1241.

Liberman, M. C. (1988). Physiology of cochlear efferent and afferent neurons: Direct comparisons in the same animal. *Hearing Research, 34*(2), 179–191.

Malmierca, M. S., & Hackett, T. A. (2012). Structural Organization of the Ascending Auditory Pathway. In *The Oxford handbook of auditory science the auditory brain*. Oxford University Press.

Meyer, J., Dentel, L., & Meunier, F. (2013). Speech recognition in natural background noise. *PLoS One, 8*(11), e79279. https://doi.org/10.1371/journal.pone.0079279

Nayagam, B. A., Muniak, M. A., & Ryugo, D. K. (2011). The spiral ganglion: Connecting the peripheral and central auditory systems. *Hearing Research, 278*(1–2), 2–20.

Oertel, D., & Young, E. D. (2004). What's a cerebellar circuit doing in the auditory system? *Trends in Neurosciences, 27*(2), 104–110.

Oxenham, A. J. (2018). How we hear: The perception and neural coding of sound. *Annual Review of Psychology, 69*, 27–50.

Palmer, A. R. (1987). Physiology of the cochlear nerve and cochlear nucleus. *British Medical Bulletin, 43*(4), 838–855.

Rusznák, Z., & Szucs, G. (2009). Spiral ganglion neurones: An overview of morphology, firing behaviour, ionic channels and function. *Pflügers Archiv – European Journal of Physiology, 457*(6), 1303–1325.

Ryugo, D. K., & Parks, T. N. (2003). Primary innervation of the avian and mammalian cochlear nucleus. *Brain Research Bulletin, 60*(5–6), 435–456.

Ryugo, D. K., & Spirou, G. A. (2016). Giant synaptic terminals: Endbulbs and calyces of the auditory system. *The Curated Reference Collection in Neuroscience and Biobehavioral Psychology, 1*, 759–770.

Taberner, A. M., & Charles Liberman, M. (2005). Response properties of single auditory nerve fibers in the mouse. *Journal of Neurophysiology, 93*(1), 557–569.

Uysal, I., Sathyendra, H., & Harris, J. G. (2007). A duplex theory of spike coding in the early stages of the auditory system. In *2007 IEEE international conference on acoustics, speech and signal processing – ICASSP '07* (pp. IV-733–IV-736). IEEE.

Winer, J. A., & Schreiner, C. E. (2005). The central auditory system: A functional analysis. In *The Inferior Colliculus* (pp. 1–68). Springer New York.

Winter, I. M., Robertson, D., & Yates, G. K. (1990). Diversity of characteristic frequency rate-intensity functions in Guinea pig auditory nerve fibres. *Hearing Research, 45*(3), 191–202.

Chapter 3
Anatomy and Physiology of the Vestibular System

Kapil Sikka and Debadeep Bagchi

Abstract Humans are creatures of movement and locomotion. From our natural movements of walking, running and swimming, to the more vicarious activities of driving or riding, the act of balance is paramount to all. Once we realise how wonderfully stable our vision remains even on vigorous shaking of the head, something that is very difficult to mimic even with the most cutting edge cameras ever made by human minds, we realise how intricate and complex this act must be. In this chapter, we shall review the basic anatomy and physiology, including the embryological origins of the miraculous organ, the vestibular apparatus, that functions as the gyroscope to the biological machine, the human body.

Keywords Vestibular system · Utricle · Saccule · Semi-circular canal · Macula · Basilar artery

Embryology

To understand the anatomy and physiology of the vestibular system, it is first essential to understand its origins and embryology. The vestibular system starts its development by the fourth week of gestation and is complete by about 25 weeks (O'Rahilly, 1963). Initially starting in the surface ectoderm of the 22-day old embryo, a portion of the ectoderm over the first occipital somite thickens to form the otic placode. This otic placode eventually invaginates to form the otic pit, which then pinches off from the surface to form the otic vesicle or otocyst after about a week of its beginning as the otic placode (Paparella et al., 1991). At the same time, a portion of the neural crest migrates towards this structure, and eventually forms the acousticofacial ganglion. The geniculate ganglion drifts further away from this

K. Sikka (✉)
Department of ENT, All India Institute of Medical Sciences (AIIMS), New Delhi, India

D. Bagchi
State Cancer Institute, Guwahati, Assam, India

P. Kumar et al. (eds.), *Advances in Implantation Otology*,
https://doi.org/10.1007/978-981-96-8671-1_3

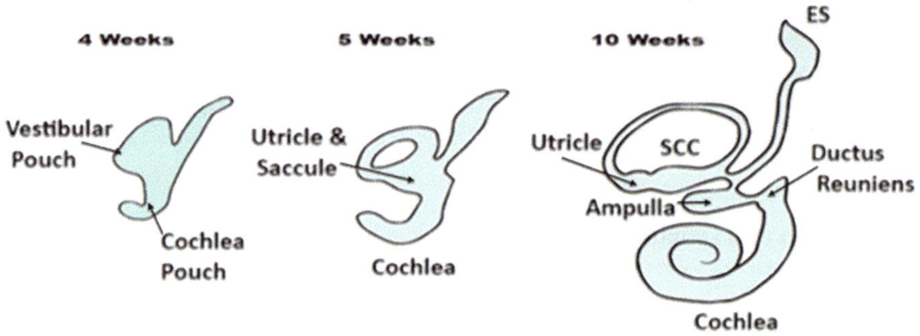

Fig. 3.1 Developmental stages of the membranous labyrinth

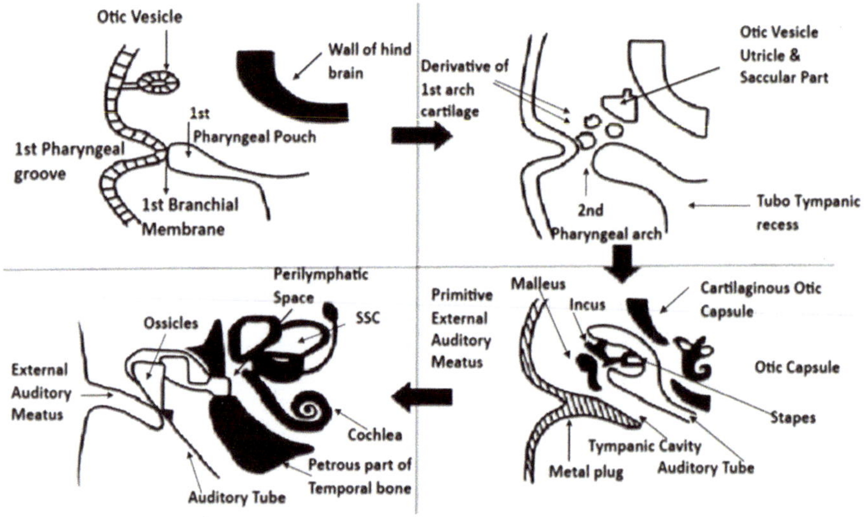

Fig. 3.2 Stages of embryological development of different parts of the ear

cluster, and only the vestibulocochlear ganglion remains in place. Following its development, the otic ganglion undergoes additional changes. Its medial segment evolves into the endolymphatic diverticulum, while the lateral segment gives rise to the utriculosaccular chamber. This chamber further differentiates through narrow constrictions into two distinct parts: the utricular chamber and the saccular chamber. The utricular chamber includes the utricle and semicircular ducts, whereas the saccular chamber leads to the formation of the saccule and cochlea. The mesoderm encasing the growing membranous labyrinth forms the bony otic capsule (Tsai et al., 2003) (Figs. 3.1 and 3.2).

The first to develop is the utricular chamber. It gives off three diverticula, which at about 35 days of gestation, fuse at the centre and break down. The superior semicircular canal develops first, followed by the posterior, and then the lateral, in that order, by the canalisation of the perimeter of the three diverticula. One end of each

Table 3.1 The timeline of development of major parts of the peripheral vestibular apparatus

Part of the vestibular apparatus	Gestational age of initiation of development	Gestational age of completion development
Hair cells	7–8 weeks	9 weeks
Maculae	6–7 weeks	14–16 weeks
Cristae ampularis	7–8 weeks	23 weeks

of the three canals widens to form the ampulla. The development of utricle and saccule begins approximately at 6 weeks of gestation. Within the saccular chamber, the cochlear segment forms as the cochlear duct coils. Although it detaches from the saccule, it stays connected through a small structure known as the ductus reuniens (Post, 2003).

As the structure of the vestibular system develops, the neural elements also infiltrate it and develop in tandem. Afferent nerve endings arrive at the end organ first, followed by the development of specialised neuroepithelium. A common neuroepithelium, called a macula, develops first at around the third week, followed by its division and specialisation. The superior portion leads to the formation of the crista ampullaris of the superior and lateral semicircular canals and the macula of the utricle, whereas the inferior portion yields the macula of the saccule as well as the crista ampullaris of the posterior semicircular canal. By 25 weeks of gestational age, the peripheral vestibular system achieves adult size and configuration. The timeline for the development of different major components are elucidated in Table 3.1.

Anatomy of the Vestibular System

Gross Anatomy

The vestibular apparatus is encased in a bony cavity called the vestibule, located within the petrous portion of the temporal bone. The whole system occupies the space between the internal auditory meatus medially, and the middle ear laterally. While the cochlea lies anterior to the vestibule, mastoid air cells lie at its posterior edge. The mastoid air cells continue to bound the lateral edge along with the aditus and antrum. The superior boundary of the vestibule is formed by the middle cranial fossa whereas the posterior cranial fossa lies medial to it (Kandel & Schwartz, 1985).

The vestibular system consists of three semicircular canals, which are arranged in an orthogonal plane (almost right angles) to each other. The vestibular apparatus also contains two otolith organs housing their respective maculae. Of the three semicircular canals, the two vertically oriented canals, anterior (superior) and posterior, form an angle of about 45° to the sagittal plane, whereas the horizontally oriented lateral canal has an anterior inclination of about 30° from the true horizontal plane. The two vertical canals share a common non-ampullary arm. Among the

Fig. 3.3 Orientation of the vestibular system

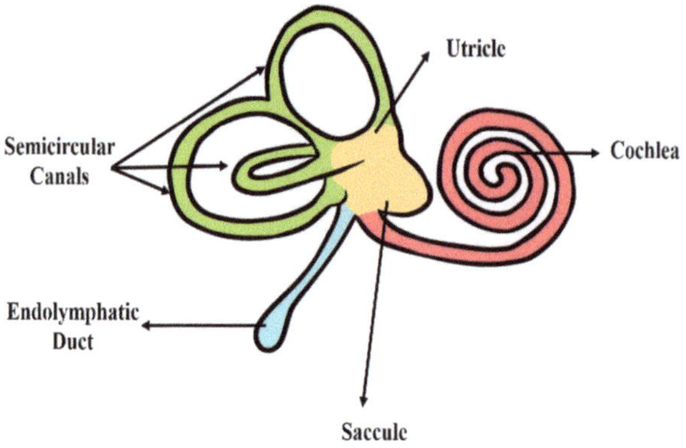

Fig. 3.4 Orientation of the vestibular system relative to the oval and round windows

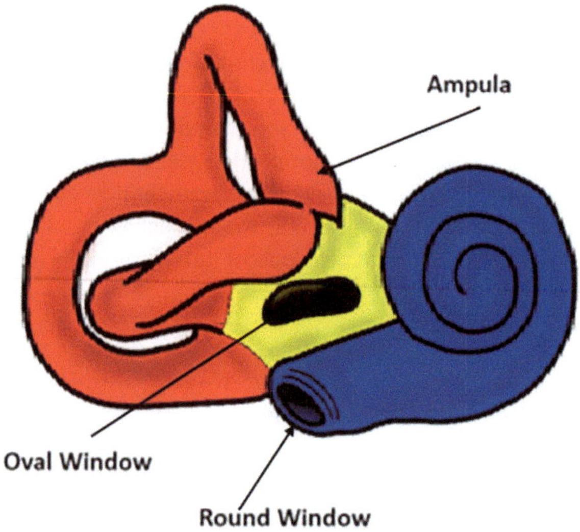

two maculae, the utricular macula is roughly horizontal whereas the saccular macula is almost vertically oriented. These sensory structures of the vestibular apparatus are contained in the membranous labyrinth, which contains endolymph. The membranous labyrinth is in turn housed within the bony labyrinth, which contains perilymph (Barber & Stockwell, 1976).

The vertical semicircular canals on either side are arranged in such a manner, that posterior semicircular canals form parallel pairs with the anterior semicircular canals of the opposite side. Among the maculae, the utricular macula lies superior and posterior to the saccular macula. The saccular macula is separated from the cochlea, which lies anteriorly, by the ductus reuniens (Barber & Stockwell, 1976). Figures 3.3 and 3.4 shows orientation of the vestibular system.

Nerve Supply

The vestibular system is supplied by the vestibular portion of the vestibulocochlear nerve (VIIIth cranial nerve) on each side. The VIIIth and VIIth cranial nerves both originate adjacent to each other from the brain stem at the cerebellopontine angle (Goldberg & Fernández, 1984). From there, they travel laterally to enter the internal auditory meatus. Here they are arranged such that the facial nerve lies anterior and superior to the vestibulocochlear nerve, eventually running in its own canal until it exits the canal lateral to the inner ear. The vestibulocochlear nerve itself separates into a vestibular division and a cochlear division. The cochlear division lies anteriorly to supply the cochlea, and the vestibular division lies posteriorly to supply the vestibule. The vestibular division is further subdivided into the superior (anterior) vestibular nerve and the inferior (posterior) vestibular nerve. The superior nerve is responsible for innervating the anterior and horizontal cristae, along with the utricular macula, and the inferior nerve innervates the posterior crista and the saccular macula (Goldberg & Fernández, 1984). There exist anastomoses between the various branches of the VIIIth cranial nerves. The two major anastomoses are Voit's anastomosis, which connects the superior vestibular nerve to the anterosuperior part of the sulcus, and Oort's anastomosis, which links the inferior vestibular nerve to the cochlear nerve. These anastomoses are theorised to carry parasympathetic innervation to the vestibular labyrinth.

The vestibular division contains the Scarpa's ganglia, which is positioned at the base of the internal auditory meatus. The ganglia has two parts, the superior vestibular ganglion and the inferior vestibular ganglion. Large cells from the ganglia innervate the central regions of the cristae and maculae, whereas the peripheral regions of these structures are innervated by the small ganglionic cells. These cells are responsible for the afferent input from these end organs. The efferent supply to the vestibular system begins with the group of around 200 neurons, which are lying lateral to the abducens nucleus and the genu of the facial nerve. The pathway that these nerve fibres follow is explained in Fig. 3.5.

The efferent fibres synapse with the hair cells and the afferent fibres by the way of bouton nerve endings. Post-ganglionic sympathetic nerve fibres also reach here, and are of two types, nonvascular and perivascular. The nonvascular fibres have free nerve endings near the Scarpa's ganglion and sensory epithelium, but do not seem to penetrate their basement membrane. The functional role of these fibres remains unknown (Wersäll & Bagger-Sjöback, 1974).

Blood Supply

The blood supply of the vestibular system comes from the internal auditory (labyrinthine) artery. The branches and subdivisions of this artery is given in the flowchart below. This artery arises from either anterior cerebellar artery, superior cerebellar artery, or the basilar artery (Nabeya, 1923) (Figs. 3.6 and 3.7).

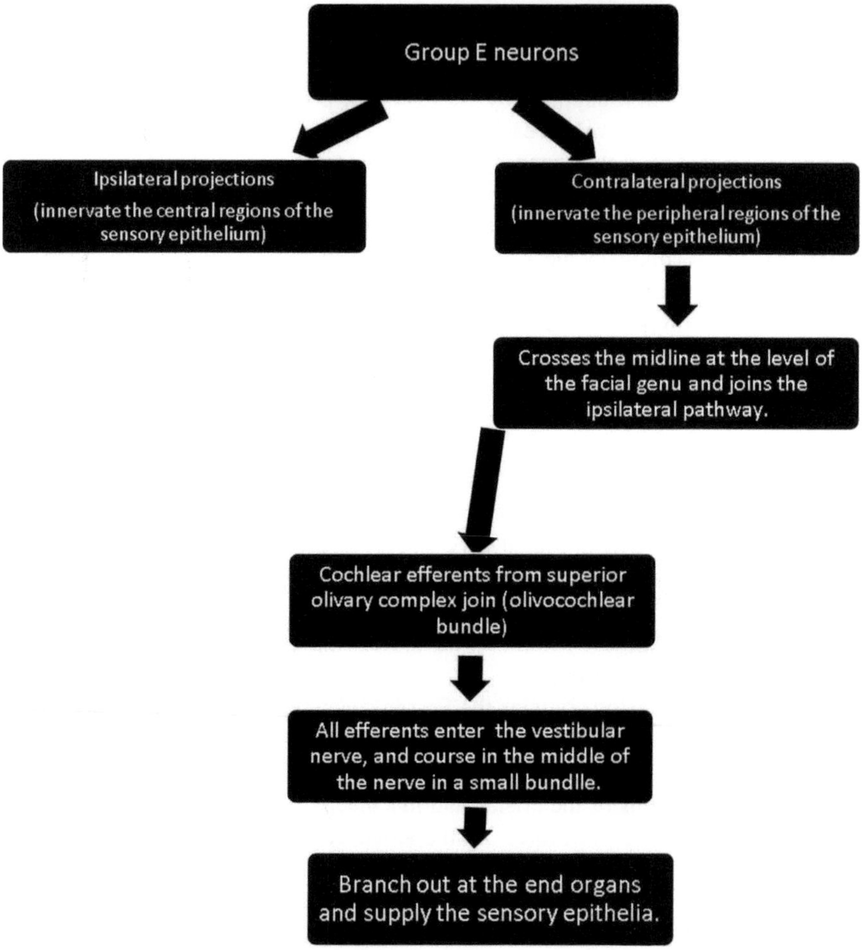

Fig. 3.5 Schematic representation of the efferent supply of the vestibular system

Ultrastructure

Semi-circular Canals

The end of each semicircular canal is dilated to form the ampulla, which contains the neuroepithelium of the respective canal. The neuroepithelium, crista ampullaris, is a saddle shaped raised area of the ampullary wall, which extends along the ampullary floor at a right angle to the long axis of the tube. It is divided into two main areas- the central area, which lies near the apex, and the peripheral slope (Paparella et al., 1991).

The hair cells in the crista ampullaris are modified columnar cells, which are coated with microvilli on their superior surface, many of which are elongated to

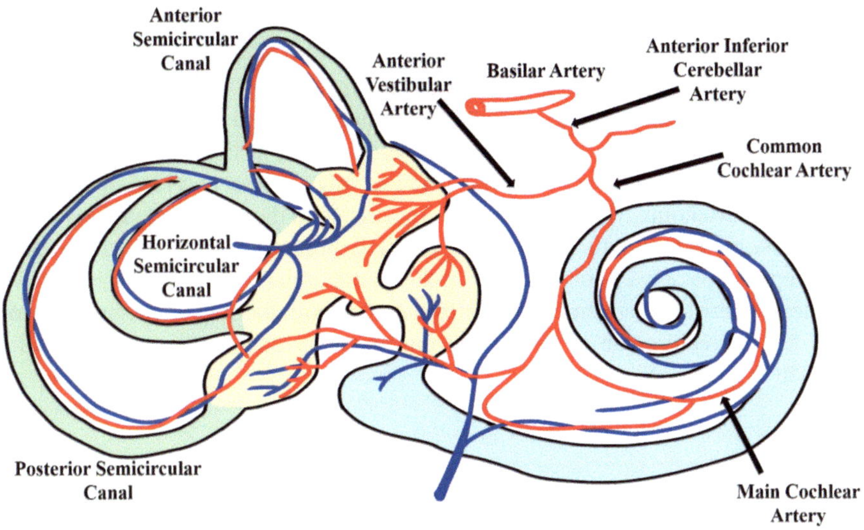

Fig. 3.6 Blood supply to the vestibular system : Aterial supply (red) and venous drainage (blue)

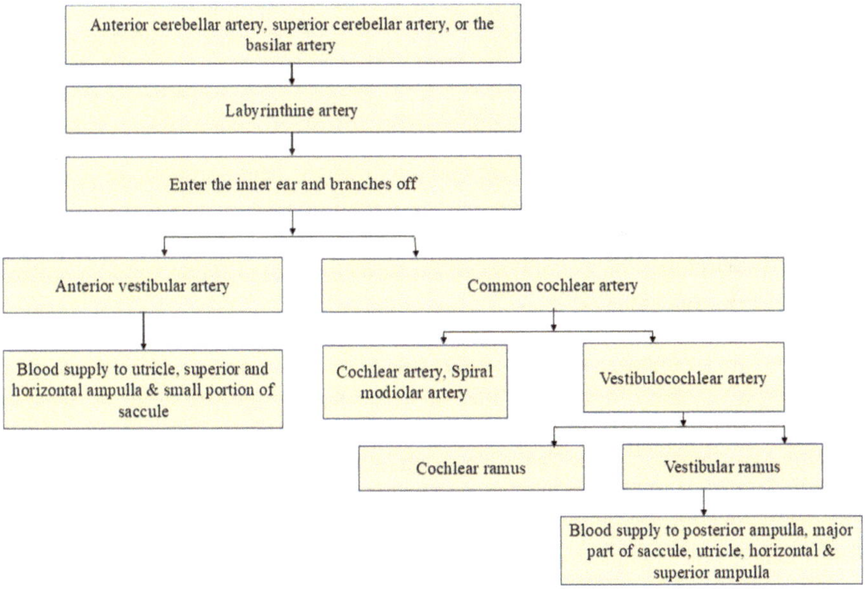

Fig. 3.7 Schematic representation of the blood supply to the vestibular system

form stereocilia. A single kinocilium is also present in each hair cell, which is a true cilium showing a 9 + 1 arrangement of microtubules. These are longer than the stereo cilia, and are placed eccentrically, imparting a polarity to the cell (Wersäll & Bagger-Sjöback, 1974). The position of the kinocilia differs in the cristae of the three canals. It lies closer to the side closest to the utricle in the horizontal semicircular canal's cristae, whereas and the cristae in the verical semicircular canals have them located on the side farthest to the utricle (Lindeman, 1969). This has a significance in the way the haircells respond to the head movement in different planes. This concept has been discussed in greater detail in the physiology section.

The cupula is a gelatinous matrix, made of mucopolysachharides in a keratin meshwork, extending from the surface of the cristae to the roof and lateral walls of the membranous labyrinth. This creates a watertight partition in the labyrinth, with a subcupular space overlying the apex of the centre of the crista. The hair cells have bundles of fibres that are embedded in this cupula, with the subcupular space theorised to be giving some space for the movement of endolymph and stereocilia (Wersäll & Bagger-Sjöback, 1974).

Otolith Organs

The macula of the utricle is oriented largely in the horizontal plane, and that of the saccule is oriented majorly in a vertical plane (Paparella et al., 1991). Just as the semicircular canals have the cupula, the utricle and saccule have the otolithic membrane, which is an analogous gelatinous structure. The otoliths (otoconia), which are calcium carbonate or calcite crystals varying in size from 0.5 to 30 micrometers, lie atop the otolithic membrane in a way that they are partially embedded in it. The macular hair cells' cilia are also embedded in the otolithic membrane, analogous to the semicircular canals. The central region of this otolithic membrane is called the striola, which appears as a thin stripe running down the centre of both the maculae. The otoliths contained in this zone are very small (approximately 1 micrometer). The thickness of the membrane itself is reduced in the utricle and increased in the saccule. The afferent fibres supplying these zones are also different from the rest of the macula (Lindeman, 1969).

The direction of polarisation of the hair cells is such that the longest steriocila (kinocilia) are facing each other on either side of striola in the utricle, whereas they are facing away from from each other on either side of the striola in the saccule (Igarashi, 1966). The maculae and striola of both otolith organs are curved, almost forming a straightish s-shape, in the horizontal plane in the utricle and in the verticle plane in the saccule. The pattern of excitation and inhibition of the maculae are complex, and all head movements lead to excitation of some haircells and simultaneous inhibition of others in the same macula.

Hair cells can be either type I or type II, depending on whether or not they have a calyx (chalice). The calyx/chalice is a type of afferent ending which has specialised to completely surround the hair cell except at the apical surface (Barber & Stockwell, 1976). The presence of a calyx around the flask-shaped hair cells define it as a type I hair cell, which can be further grouped as either a simple calyceal ending (calyx surrounding a single type I hair cell) or as a complex calyceal ending (single calyx surrounding multiple type I hair cells). Complex calyceal endings are found more commonly in the striola than in the periphery. On the other hand, type

II hair cells are cylindrical in shape, with bouton endings of the nerves terminating at their basal surfaces. These boutons can be afferent or efferent in nature (Wersäll & Bagger-Sjöback, 1974).

Another way to classify the hair cells in the otolith organs is based on their firing pattern. The striolar region is comprised majorly of irregularly firing hair cells and the shortness in their height ensures that the steriocilia of these hair cells are not embedded in the gelatinous matrix above (in a way similar to the inner hair cells of the cochlea). They respond only to high frequency vibrations, such as those produced by intense sounds used to obtain vestibular-evoked myogenic potentials. The rest of the macula has abundance of regularly firing hair cells, which respond to low frequency vibrations, tilts and translations. The function of regularly firing hair cells is typically assessed using subjective visual vertical/horizontal tests (Igarashi, 1966).

Physiology of the Vestibular System

The purpose of the vestibular organs is to impart the sense of balance and orientation in our day-to-day movements. They accomplish this by an intricate and finely balanced interplay between the organs on both sides, as well as with other parts and systems of our body, such as the eyes, the spine, and the muscle spindles in our limbs. In this interplay, the output from both balance organs are vital for the brain to create an accurate understanding of its surroundings (Goldberg & Fernández, 1984). The utricle and saccule are sensitive to linear acceleration, such as for forward motion, gravity, and bobbing movements of the head. Similarly, the semicircular canals encode for the angular acceleration of the head, such as during head turns and nodding.

The hair cells of the semicircular canal and the otolith organs are responsible for the detection of acceleration in their respective planes and axes, and form the vestibular afferent signal by modulating the discharge rate from the organs. As seen in the section on the ultrastructure of the sensory epithelium above, the cells constituting the sensory epithelium have a polarity imparted to them by virtue of the arrangement of the sterocilia and kinocilia (Wersäll & Bagger-Sjöback, 1974). As the head of a person moves through space, inertia causes the cilia to bend in the opposite direction of movement. If this displacement is towards the kinocilum, it causes potassium channels to open along the cilia, which leads to depolarisation of the hair cell. This depolarisation can be a graded response, with more ciliary displacement leading to a greater degree of depolarisation. Post depolarisation, there is an increase in the inflow of calcium at the basal end, which leads to the release of neurotransmitters in the synaptic junction just deep to the neuroepithelium. Likewise, movement of the cilia in the opposite direction leads to hyperpolarisation, and a consequent decrease in the neurotransmitter release (Precht, 1979). Depending on the orientation of the kinocilia in the hair cells, the polarity is different among the semicircular canals and the otolithic organs.

Among the semicircular canals, the horizontal canal is excited when the head rotates to the same side, and inhibited by a movement to the opposite direction. The superior canal shows maximum excitation when the movement is a downward rotation to the same side in the plane of the canal, whereas for the posterior canal, it is seen on an upward rotation to the side, in the plane of the canal. Anomalous excitation of the semicircular canals can lead to the expression of characteristic nystagmus, which can be used to localise the source of pathology to the responsible canal. Table 3.2 shows a simplified version of the complex nystagmus patterns arising from anomalous excitation in various semicircular canals. An easy way to remember these emanates from the Ewald's first law, which states that the nystagmus direction duplicates the orientation of the semicircular canal whose stimulation produces it.

The maculae of the otolithic organs are responsible for detecting linear acceleration, with the utricle responsible for detecting lateral tilt and translational movements, and the saccule detecting back to front tilt, translational movements, as well as motion along the line of gravitational pull (Precht, 1979).

Nerve Discharge According to Stimulus

The afferent nerve fibres run in the vestibular nerve to the brain stem, where they relay to the vestibular nuclei. These neurons are bipolar, with a resting/spontaneous discharge rate of around 100 spikes per second. The presence of these resting spikes mean that the organs can detect both excitatory as well as inhibitory impulses (Park et al., 2001). As the maximum possible excitation, which can go up to 350/s is greater than the maximum possible inhibition, which can only fall up to 0/s-, the response of the vestibular organs is greater to excitatory stimuli than to inhibitory stimuli, popularly referred as the Ewald's second law (Baird et al., 1988). Three groups of neurons can be found in the vestibular nerves. The core characteristics of these neuron types are described in Table 3.3.

Table 3.2 A simplified version of the complex nystagmus patterns arising from anomalous excitation in various semicircular canals

Canal responsible	Nystagmus produced
Horizontal SCC	Horizontal nystagmus, with slow phase towards the opposite canal, and resetting saccade towards the canal being excited.
Superior SCC	Vertical torsional nystagmus, with slow phase of the vertical component of the eye movement directed upwards, and resetting saccade downwards. The tortional component's slow phase is directed towards the canal in question and the resetting saccade away from it.
Posterior SCC	Vertical torsional nystagmus, with slow phase of the vertical component of the eye movement directed downwards, and resetting saccade upwards. The tortional component of the eye movement has a slow phase of rotation away from the side of the posterior canal in question and the resetting saccade towards it.

Table 3.3 Types of neurons found in the vestibular nerve, their innervation and characteristics

Neuron	Innervating	Characteristic
Bouton only afferents	Terminate exclusively on type II hair cells (Park et al., 2001).	Regularly discharging with low rotational sensitivity (Baird et al., 1988).
Dimorphic afferents	Calyx endings terminating on type I hair cells. Bouton endings terminating on type II hair cells (Hullar et al., 2005).	Peripheral zone- regularly discharging. Central zone- irregularly discharging with greater rotational sensitivity (Baird et al., 1988).
Calyx only afferents	Terminate exclusively on type I hair cells (Highstein & Baker, 1985).	Irregularly discharging with low sensitivity at low stimulus frequency, and high sensitivity at high stimulus frequency (Hullar et al., 2005).

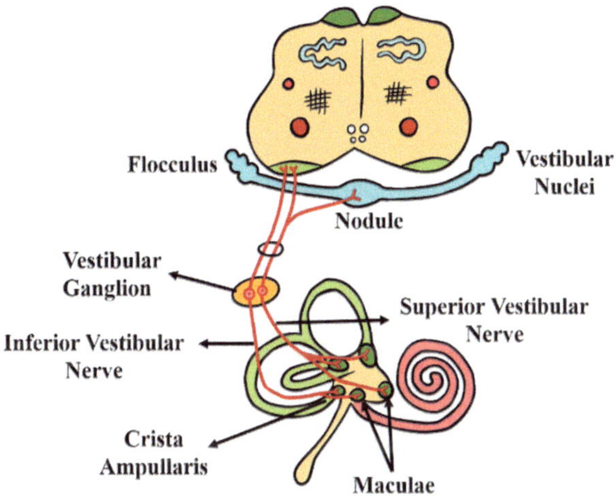

Fig. 3.8 Vestibulo-occular reflex pathway

Central Control

The vestibular nuclei located in the brainstem are responsible for the integration of signals from not only the two vestibular organs, but also from other pathways, such as vision and proprioception (Ewald, 1892). These nuclei project to multiple other organs, such as the eyes, the muscles of the neck and spine, the cerebellum, the cerebral cortex, and the thalamus. These projections to other systems play an integral role in the stabilisation of multiple movements, such as the vestibulo-ocular reflex (responsible for maintaining a stable object-image on the retina during head movements by counter-rolling of the eye opposite to the direction of movement), vestibulo-collic reflex, and vestibulo-spinal reflex (responsible for righting reflex of the body in response to movement of the body through space) (Tabak et al., 1997). The cerebellum is also included in the central circuit, which helps in fine tuning various movements and bring smoothness and grace (Fig. 3.8).

References

Baird, R. A., Desmadryl, G., Fernández, C., & Goldberg, J. M. (1988). The vestibular nerve of the chinchilla. II. Relation between afferent response properties and peripheral innervation patterns in the semicircular canals. *Journal of Neurophysiology, 60*(1), 182–203. https://doi.org/10.1152/jn.1988.60.1.182

Barber, H. O., & Stockwell, C. W. (1976). *Manual of electronystagmography*. Mosby, St. Louis.

Ewald, J. R. (1892). *Physiologische Untersuchungen über das Endorgan des Nervus Octavus*. Bergmann.

Goldberg, J. M., & Fernández, C. (1984). The vestibular system. In I. Darian-Smith (Ed.), *Handbook of physiology: The nervous system* (pp. 977–1031). American Physiological Society.

Highstein, S. M., & Baker, R. (1985). Action of the efferent vestibular system on primary afferents in the toadfish, Opsanus tau. *Journal of Neurophysiology, 54*(2), 370–384. https://doi.org/10.1152/jn.1985.54.2.370

Hullar, T.E., Della, S. C. C., Hirvonen, T., Lasker, D. M., Carey, J. P., & Minor, L. B. (2005). Responses of irregularly discharging chinchilla semicircular canal vestibular-nerve afferents during high-frequency head rotations. *Journal of Neurophysiology, 93*, 2777–2786.

Igarashi, M. (1966). Dimensional study of the vestibular end organ apparatus. In A. Graybiel (Ed.), *Second symposium on the role of vestibular organs in space exploration* (pp. 33–46). NASA SP-115. U.S. Government Printing Office.

Kandel, E. R., & Schwartz, J. W. (1985). *Principles of neural science* (2nd ed.). Elsevier.

Lindeman, H. H. (1969). Studies on the morphology of the sensory regions of the vestibular apparatus with 45 figures. *Ergebnisse der Anatomie und Entwicklungsgeschichte, 42*(1), 1–113.

Nabeya, D. (1923). A study of the comparative anatomy of the blood-vascular system of the internal ear in Mammalia and in Homo [in Japanese]. *Acta Schol Med Imp Kioto, 6*(1), en1–en120.

O'Rahilly, R. (1963). The early development of the otic vesicle in staged human embryos. *Journal of Embryology and Experimental Morphology, 11*, 741–755.

Paparella, M. M., Shumrick, D. A., Gluckman, J. L., & Meyerhoff, W. L. (Eds.). (1991). *Otolaryngology* (3rd ed., pp. 3–21). Saunders.

Park, J. J., Tang, Y., Lopez, I., & Ishiyama, A. (2001). Age-related change in the number of neurons in the human vestibular ganglion. *The Journal of Comparative Neurology, 431*(4), 437–443. https://doi.org/10.1002/1096-9861(20010319)431:4<437::aid-cne1081>3.0.co;2-p

Post, J. C. (2003). Molecular biology in pediatric otolaryngology. In C. D. Bluestone, S. E. Stool, C. M. Alper, et al. (Eds.), *Pediatric otolaryngology* (pp. 66–81). Saunders.

Precht, W. (1979). Vestibular mechanisms. *Annual Review of Neuroscience, 2*, 265–289. https://doi.org/10.1146/annurev.ne.02.030179.001405

Tabak, S., Collewijn, H., Boumans, L. J., & Van der Steen, J. (1997). Gain and delay of human vestibulo-ocular reflexes to oscillation and steps of the head by a reactive torque helmet. I. Normal subjects. *Acta Oto-Laryngologica, 117*(6), 785–795. https://doi.org/10.3109/00016489709114203

Tsai, A.-H., Stool, S. E., & Post, J. C. (2003). Phylogenetic aspects and embryology. In C. D. Bluestone, S. E. Stool, C. M. Alper, et al. (Eds.), *Pediatric otolaryngology* (pp. 1–21). Saunders.

Wersäll, J., & Bagger-Sjöback, D. (1974). Morphology of the vestibular sense organ. In H. H. Kornhuber (Ed.), *Handbook of sensory physiology* (pp. 124–170). Springer.

Chapter 4
Radiology from the Perspective of Implantable Hearing Devices: Normal Anatomy

Gaurav Medikeri and Shankar Medikeri

Abstract The present chapter is an attempt to simplify the whole process of being able to read a scan and presume that the reader already possesses sufficient anatomical knowledge of the temporal bone. This chapter is discussed under various segments which include definition, history and development, different planes of computed tomography, and magnetic resonance imaging.

Keywords HRCT · CT scan · MRI · Temporal bone · DICOM · Internal auditory canal

Introduction

The temporal bone is a complex one and its radiological anatomy is equally complicated. The temporal bone is a paired bone located on the sides and base of the skull, playing a critical role in protecting the brain and supporting sensory organs. It is highly complex, consisting of four main parts:

1. *Squamous part*: The thin, flat portion forming part of the lateral skull wall. It includes the zygomatic process, which articulates with the zygomatic bone to form the zygomatic arch.
2. *Tympanic part*: A small, curved portion surrounding the external acoustic meatus, contributing to the external ear canal.
3. *Mastoid part*: Located posteriorly, this portion contains the mastoid process, a bony prominence that serves as an attachment point for neck muscles. Internally, it houses air cells connected to the middle ear.
4. *Petrous part*: The densest part of the temporal bone, housing the structures of the inner ear (cochlea, vestibule, and semicircular canals) responsible for hearing

G. Medikeri (✉) · S. Medikeri
Medikeri Super Speciality ENT Centre, Bangalore, India

P. Kumar et al. (eds.), *Advances in Implantation Otology*,
https://doi.org/10.1007/978-981-96-8671-1_4

and balance. It also contains the internal acoustic meatus, through which the facial and vestibulocochlear nerves pass.

Additionally, the temporal bone contains key foramina such as the stylomastoid foramen, which transmits the facial nerve, and the carotid canal, allowing passage of the internal carotid artery. Its intricate anatomy underscores its critical functions in protection, sensory processing, and structural support.

The present chapter is an attempt to simplify the whole process of being able to read a scan and presume that the reader already possesses sufficient anatomical knowledge of the temporal bone (Refer to Chap. 1 for detail anatomy). This chapter is discussed under various segments which include definition, history and development, different planes of the computed tomography, and magnetic resonance imaging.

1. Computed tomography
   (a) History and development
   (b) Definitions
   (c) Planes of Imaging of the temporal bone
   (d) Normal Anatomy of the Temporal Bone

Since the chapter relates to the normal anatomy, we will not be discussing anomalies which will be covered in the forthcoming chapters. Before we jump into these details, let us study a little bit about the basics of radiology, of imaging the temporal bone. There are two main modalities of imaging of the temporal bone-

A. Computed tomography—which involves radiation exposure.
B. Magnetic resonance imaging—by means of ionization.

Computed Tomography (CT)

History and Development

Historically X-rays were used to study the anatomy of the temporal bone. The use of **X-rays for imaging the temporal bone** has a rich history dating back to the early twentieth century, shortly after Wilhelm Röntgen discovered X-rays in 1895. Physicians quickly realized the potential of X-rays for visualizing bony structures, including the complex anatomy of the temporal bone. In the 1920s and 1930s, **Schüller and Stenters views** were developed to image the mastoid air cells and petrous portions of the temporal bone, respectively. These views became standard techniques for evaluating mastoiditis, cholesteatoma, fractures, and other pathologies. The imaging relied heavily on the experience of radiologists to interpret the intricate details of overlapping structures.

By the mid-twentieth century, the use of plain film X-rays began to decline as Computed tomography emerged, offering greater detail of the temporal bone. In the

1970s, the introduction of computed tomography (CT) revolutionized temporal bone imaging by providing highly detailed, three-dimensional representations of bony anatomy, rendering X-ray techniques largely obsolete for detailed diagnostics.

Today, X-rays are rarely used for temporal bone imaging, reserved mainly for specific conditions like mastoiditis or in settings where advanced imaging modalities are unavailable.

Commonly employed views include:

1. ***Lateral oblique view (Stenvers or Schüller view):*** Highlights the mastoid air cells and middle ear anatomy, often used for evaluating mastoiditis or fractures.
2. ***Towne's view:*** Provides a comprehensive view of the temporal bone, including the petrous ridges.
3. ***Modified Waters view:*** Assesses the petrous part and inner ear structures.
4. ***Trans-orbital view:*** This View is extensively used even today, to ascertain the position of the electrode array after a successful cochlear implant surgery.

X-ray imaging of the temporal bone is generally limited by its low sensitivity in detecting soft tissue abnormalities. It has largely been supplanted by advanced imaging techniques like CT (for detailed bony anatomy) and MRI (for soft tissue and neurovascular evaluation). However, it remains useful in specific cases, such as mastoid pathology, bony fractures, or surgical planning for otologic conditions. Proper positioning is crucial for clear visualization of the complex anatomy.

Computed tomography has overtaken the use of X-rays for a multitude of reasons (Goldman, 2007).

1. Poor X ray absorption—The rate of X-ray absorption is only about 25%, which means that 75% of the data, which is available, is missing from our purview.
2. High amount of X-ray scatter—more than 50% of the photons are scattered during an X ray, therefore creating poor image contrast.
3. Inconspicuous images due to superimposition of anatomical structures—There is significant overlap of anatomical structures making it difficult to see specific anatomical structures like the cochlea or the internal auditory canal, quite difficult.
4. Limited range of exposures—This drawback makes X-Ray images less useful clinically.

The invention of computed tomography was predominantly the work of Mr. Godfrey Hounsfield in 1967, who was an engineer at Electric and Musical Industries (EMI) Corp. in Great Britain. The first functional, clinically accepted CT machine was installed at the Atkinson Morley Hospital in Southwest London in September 1971 (Hounsfield, 1976). We have come a long way since then and presently modern CT scanners are of the fourth generation bearing some improvements thereafter. The most standard CT scanners used now, and known as Multislice CT scanners. This involves continuous rotation and data acquisition as the patient table is moved through the gantry.

Cone beam CT scans are another development in making the whole contraption of CT imaging compact. It involves a rotating gantry around a patient who is seated.

Within a span of about 15 seconds, complete imaging can be obtained. The advantage is it requires a very small amount of space to install, has lesser radiation exposure with more or less the same resolution of a multi-slice scanner, and is overall quite cheaper. One of the disadvantages of this technique is excessive motion artifact since the patient is sitting (Aschendorff et al., 2005; Bremke et al., 2013; Guyader et al., 2018; Zou et al., 2015).

Definitions

1. *Hounsfield units (HU)*—Also referred to as the CT unit, is a measure of the radio density of tissues on a CT image. Arbitrarily distilled water at standard temperature and pressure is considered to have a HU of zero; Air as HU of −1000 and bone is considered as HU of +1000. Certain dense bones, such as the cochlea, have a HU of +2000 (DenOtter & Schubert, 2023).
2. *Image Windowing*—One of the advantages of a CT scan image is that, one can increase or decrease the number of Hounsfield units (HU) which have been included in that scan. This is done merely by manually adjusting the settings, to change the Hounsfield unit value that is set as the central value. This phenomenon is called as windowing or changing the window. There are different types of windows, such as bone window, soft tissue window, etc. (Kimpe & Tuytschaever, 2007).
3. *Multiplanar reformatting (MPR)*—Although the transverse or axial scans are one of the most commonly used methods of viewing a CT scan, today's software has the ability to reconstruct this data into coronal and sagittal images as well. The resolution of the reconstruction depends entirely on the slice thickness and the amount of data, which has been extracted. MPR, however, requires large volumes of space to store these reconstructed images.
4. *Slice thickness*—It is the distance between the two slices of a CT scan. The lesser the number, the better the spatial and contrast resolution of the scan. High resolution CT scan involves a slice thickness of 0.625 millimeters (mm).
5. *Voxel*—Each CT image is composed of multiple pixels. The volume element of each pixel is a Voxel. The size of each voxel depends on three parameters- section thickness, field of view and matrix size (Prokop & Galanski, 2003; Perandini et al., 2010).
6. *Image rendering*—It is the process of altering the number of voxels to represent the imaged tissue in different resolutions. The resolution is directly proportional to the number of voxels involved. 3D Volume Rendering (3DVR), Shaded Surface Display (SSD), Maximum and Minimum Intensity Projection (MIP), Sliding Thin Slab Reconstruction (STS Reconstruction) are all different types of Image Rendering (Rubin et al., 1996; Dalrymple et al., 2005).
7. *Contrast media*—Is a dye, which is injected intravascularly to identify structures based on the vascular supply, predominantly in the evaluation of tumors and infections. Intravenous contrast media can be broadly classified into ionic and

non-ionic monomers and dimers (Hermena, 2023). In temporal bone imaging, contrast media is specifically used for vascular tumors, such as Glomus Tympanicum, Glomus Jugulare etc.

8. *Scout film*—It is an image representing a broad survey of the region being studied, which also includes the structures around the area of anatomical interest. This image is then used to identify the area of definite interest and acquire detailed images. The Scout film gives us an idea about the area of interest, the slice thickness and the number of slices taken through the area of interest (Albano et al., 2020; Makker & Mukherjee, 2013).
9. *DICOM*—DICOM stands for Digital Imaging and Communications in Medicine, which is a standard protocol for image storage, exchange, image related information and file structure. DICOM applications include management of network images, image interpretation, image printing and imaging procedure along with offline storage of the data (Bidgood Jr et al., 1997). This data can be retrieved, viewed, interpreted, reported and modified with the help of a DICOM viewer which is a computer-based software.

Planes of Imaging of the Temporal Bone

The temporal bone is usually scanned in four different planes- Axial, Coronal, Sagittal and oblique. Each of these allows distinct anatomical structures to be seen clearly. However, for beginners, the axial plane is one of the best to study the temporal bone with relative ease. It is prudent that prior to studying radiological anatomy, the surgeon has an in-depth knowledge of normal anatomy of the temporal bone. A detailed description of the normal anatomy of the temporal bone is beyond the scope of this chapter (Refer to Chap. 1). However, we shall discuss the radiological anatomy of the temporal bone.

Imaging Parameters for HRCT

0.75-mm collimation, 0.625-mm section thickness, 140 kVp, 120 mAs, pitch of 0.8, a 15-cm Field of View (FOV), and a 512 × 512 matrix.

Classically, the temporal bone is divided into five distinct embryological components—the petrous, mastoid, tympanic, squamous, and styloid parts.

Normal Radiological Anatomy of the Temporal Bone

One of the best ways to study temporal bone scans is from above downwards. Figures 4.1, 4.2, 4.3, 4.4, 4.5, 4.6, 4.7, 4.8, 4.9, 4.10, 4.11, 4.12, 4.13, 4.14, 4.15, 4.16, 4.17, 4.18, 4.19, 4.20, 4.21, 4.22, 4.23, 4.24, and 4.25 demonstrate the normal anatomy of the temporal bone in a sequential manner, in the axial plane from above downwards.

Earlier, physicians would use CT films to study scans, but nowadays it is prudent that one uses a DICOM viewer to study DICOM images. CT Films have grossed limitation in terms of their ability to provide a magnified view, their longevity, and inability to bear exposure to sunlight. Whereas digital data on the other hand lasts forever and can be easily transferred from one place to another without the need for physical films. They also provide a magnified view and the ability for Multiplanar reconstruction and the ability to render the images in 3D. This helps the surgeon in understanding the anatomy in a much better manner. Not to mention that this form of data acquisition is much cheaper in the long run.

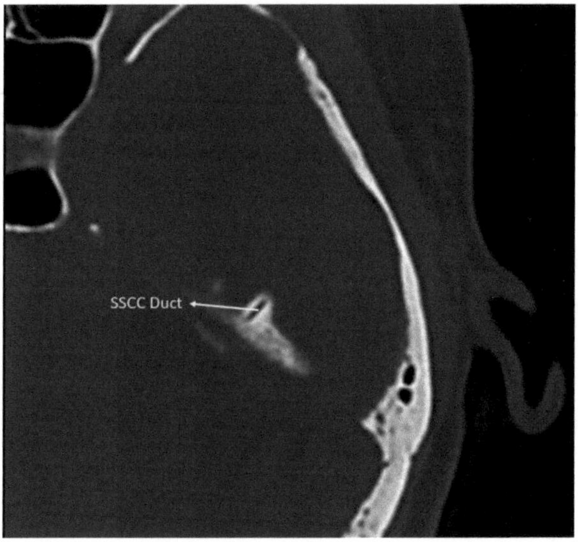

Fig. 4.1 As we scan through the images from above downwards, the first structure is that of the dome of the superior semicircular canal (SSCC). This appears a nubbin of hyperdense bone around the membranous semicircular canal duct whereas the duct itself appears hypodense. The arrangement of the cochleovestibular apparatus is such that the semicircular canals are at a higher level as compared to the cochlea. This is why the cochlea appears in the sections lower down. (Hints: SSCC Superior Semi Circular Canal)

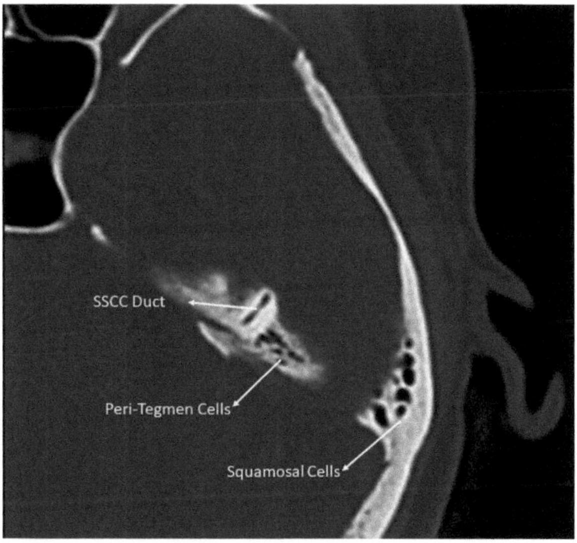

Fig. 4.2 In this section, if the mastoid is well pneumatized, you will see peri-tegmen cells lateral to the SSCC and the squamosal cells far laterally. The duct of the SSCC appears more elongated. (Hints: SSCC Superior Semi Circular Canal)

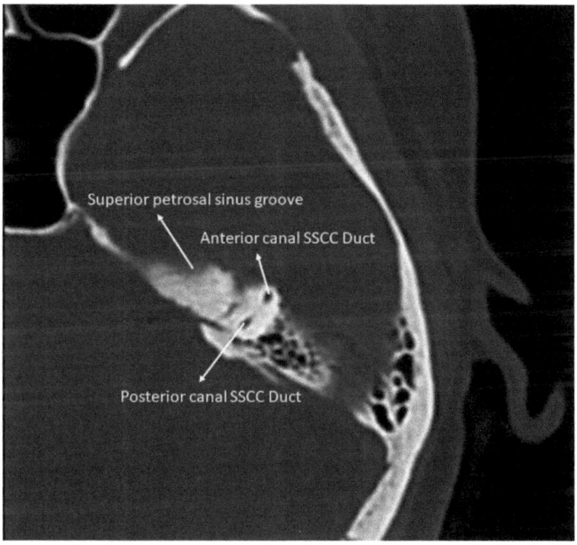

Fig. 4.3 The next cut shows the anterior and posterior limb of the SSCC as two distinct entities. Medial to the SSCC you will find the groove for the superior petrosal sinus, which communicates with the cavernous sinus. (Hints: SSCC Superior Semi Circular Canal)

As the facial nerve turns laterally and proceeds downwards to form the tympanic segment, the epitympanum and their contents come into view- body of incus laterally and head of malleus medially. A bony projection is seen lateral to them which is the scutum which usually gets eroded in cases with cholesteatoma. In this section, the vestibule and the lateral semi-circular canal together form the signet ring appearance.

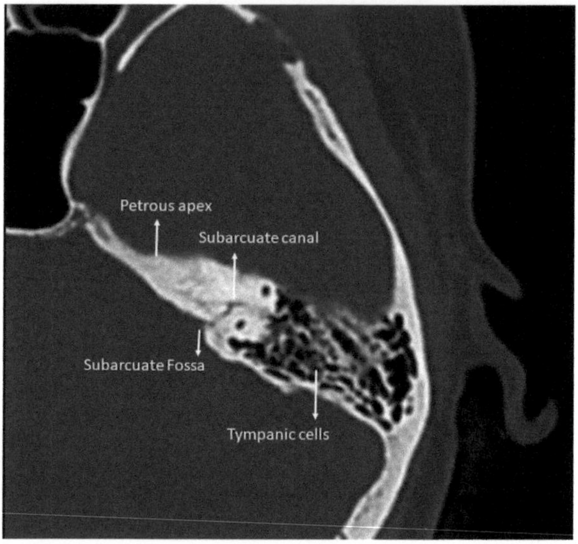

Fig. 4.4 Lower down, the petrous apex starts to appear medial to the SSCC. Between the two limbs of the SSCC, one can find a hypodense line like structure called the Petromastoid or Subarcuate canal which houses the Subarcuate vessels. This is an important landmark for the Internal auditory canal (IAC) which lies roughly 4 mm below the canal. The Subarcuate canal traverses medially to reach a concave depression on the postero-medial petrous apex called as the Subarcuate fossa

Basics of Magnetic Resonance Imaging (MRI)

MRI uses powerful magnets to align the protons in an excited state in the tissues, which contain water. When these protons de-excite, and give up energy detected by scanners, which is captured in the form of an image. Since bones do not contain fluid, MRI is blind when it comes to visualising bone or osseous pathologies such as Osteoma. However, MRI can visualise bone marrow since it contains fat. There are different modalities of imaging within MRI and it would be beyond the scope of this chapter to go into details of the same. However, before we embark on the journey of studying MRI for implantation otology, the reader must understand that T1 sequences show fat more prominently and T2 sequences show fluid like CSF, Aqueous and Vitreous humour.

Imaging Sequences for MR Imaging of the Temporal Bone

There are two main sequences, which are important in imaging for implantation

(a) ***3D CISS***—Continuous interface in steady state **OR 3D FIESTA**—Fast Imaging Employing Steady-state Acquisition—Both these sequences are used to visual-

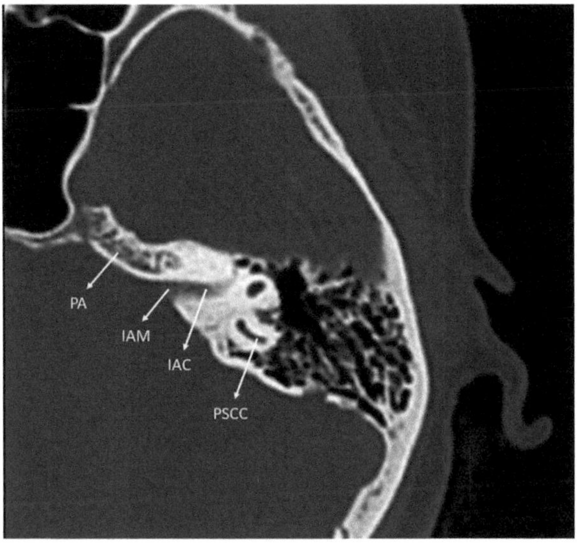

Fig. 4.5 The Petrous apex is bound by the petro-occipital fissure medially, inner ear structures laterally, petrosphenoidal fissure and Internal carotid artery anteriorly and the posterior cranial fossa posteriorly. Between the Subarcuate fossa and the petrous apex is where the IAC will appear as we proceed lower down. Due to the presence of bone marrow in the petrous apex, it usually appears hypodense or grey in color in majority of the patients. (Hints: PA Petrous Apex, IAM Internal Auditory Meatus, IAC Internal Auditory Canal, PSCC Posterior Semi-Circular canal)

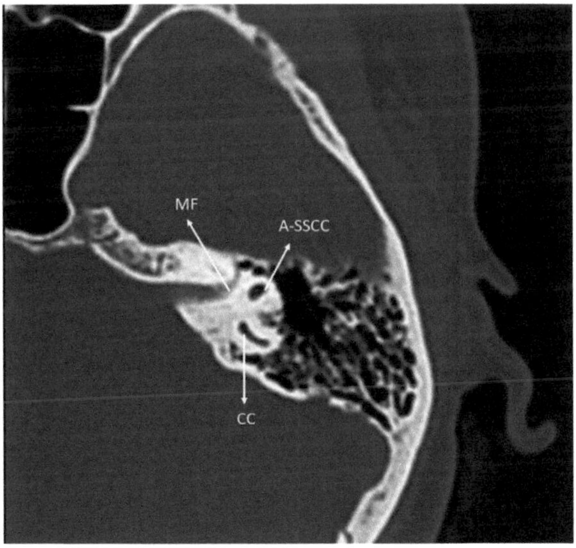

Fig. 4.6 In the next sections, we can find that the posterior limb of the superior semi-circular canal, along with the superior limb of the posterior semicircular canal (Both non-ampullary ends), form the crus commune and share a common opening into the vestibule lower down. (Hints: MF Meatal Foramen, FC-L Facial Canal (Labyrinthine segment), A-SSCC Ampullated End Superior Semi-Circular Canal, CC Crus Commune)

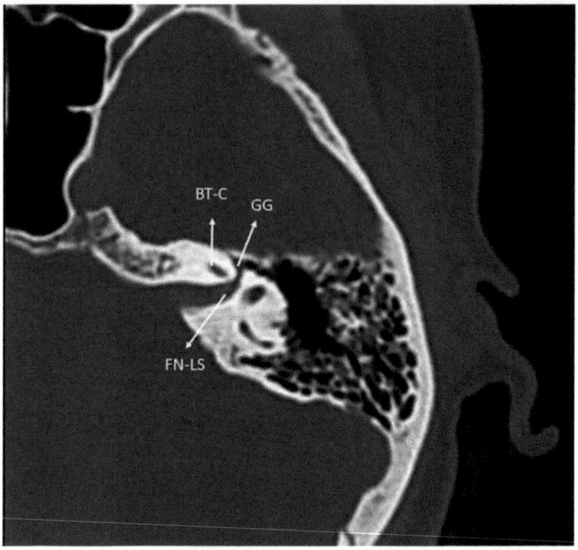

Fig. 4.7 Just lateral to the petrous apex, the IAC starts to appear and the first structure within the IAC you see is the facial canal, which is present antero-superiorly. This is the labyrinthine segment of the facial nerve. The narrowest part of the labyrinthine segment is known as the meatal foramen. Beyond it is the geniculate ganglion where the facial nerve takes its first turn—the first genu which signifies the end of the labyrinthine segment. This segment is the shortest part of the intra-temporal part of the facial nerve. Medial to the facial canal is the appearance of the Basal Turn of the Cochlea. (Hints: BT-C Basal Turn of Cochlea, GG Geniculate Ganglion, FN-LS Facial Nerve Labyrinthine Segment)

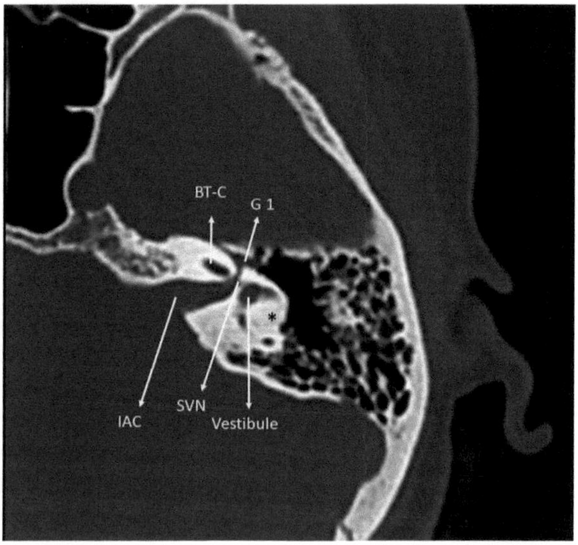

Fig. 4.8 One can also appreciate the appearance of thick bone laterally prior to the appearance of the lateral semicircular canal (LSCC). From the IAC, we can see a thin nerve making its way to the vestibule—the Superior vestibular nerve. (Hints: G 1 1st Genu of Facial nerve, BT-C Basal Turn of Cochlea, SVN Superior Vestibular Nerve, IAC Internal Auditory Canal, - Thick Bone Prior to appearance of Lateral Semi Circular Canal)

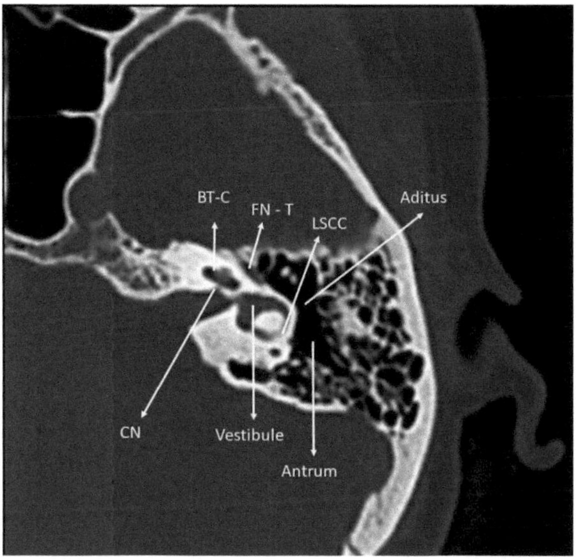

Fig. 4.9 The basal turn of Cochlea is clearly seen, with its communication with the IAC through which the Cochlear nerve can be visualized. Antero-Lateral to the Cochlea, the facial nerve is seen coursing to form the tympanic segment of the Facial Nerve. The vestibule then comes into view, into which the semicircular canals are opening. The Lateral Semi Circular Canal is seen making an appearance lateral to the vestibule. The Vestibule and the LSCC together form the "Signet Ring appearance". Lateral to the LSCC, the Antrum and Aditus are visualized. Anterior to the Aditus, one can see the appearance of the Epitympanum and its contents. (Hints: G 1 1st Genu of Facial nerve, BT-C Basal Turn of Cochlea, SVN Superior Vestibular Nerve, CN Cochlear Nerve, LSCC Lateral Semi Circular Canal)

Fig. 4.10 The 2nd turn of cochlea is making an appearance lower down with the cochlear nerve. The Malleus head and body of Incus are seen in the Epitympanum and can be clearly distinguished from each other as distinct entities. The Sigmoid sinus can be seen far laterally. (Hints: CT2 2nd Turn of Cochlea, SS Sigmoid sinus, CN Cochlear Nerve)

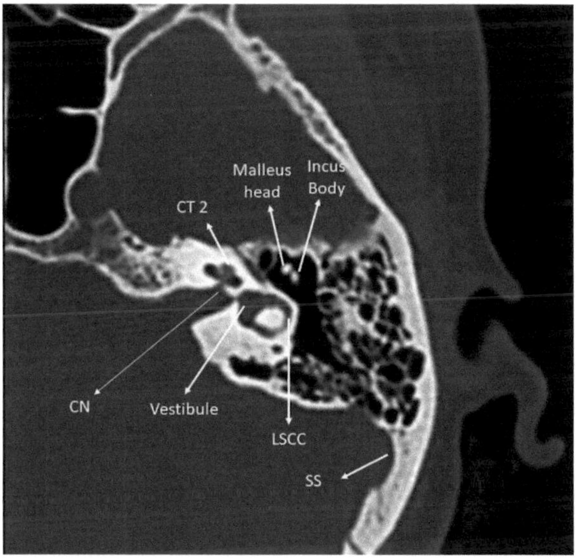

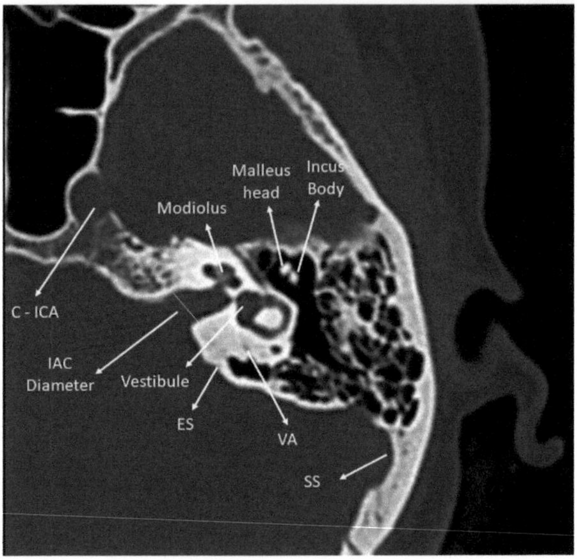

Fig. 4.11 From the posterior end of the vestibule, we can see the vestibular aqueduct (VA) appearing and moving backwards towards the endolymphatic sac. Normally, the vestibular aqueduct should be less than 0.5 mm in width. If it is more than 2 mm, it is considered as an enlarged vestibular aqueduct and is the most common radiological anomaly known in the temporal bone. The 2nd turn of Cochlea is now more prominent. The modiolus is the point of entry of the Cochlear Nerve into the Cochlea. The diameter of the IAC is measured at this level as it is the widest here. A narrow IAC would hint towards thin or absent Cochlear Nerve. Normal IAC diameter is said to be between 2 to 8 mm with an average of about 4 mm. Cavernous segment of the Internal Carotid Artery (C-ICA) can be seen

ise, the cochlea, the Internal Auditory canal (IAC) and the cochlear nerve. Of the two, CISS sequence has better Contrast to noise ratio making it the choice for imaging the IAC and cochlear nerve. This is significant in decision making in a patient with thin cochlear nerves. The plane of imaging is in the oblique parasagittal view, perpendicular to the plane of the internal auditory canal.

(b) ***T2 weighted images*** are used for screening the brain, more specifically the auditory and speech cortex by imaging in the axial plane.

Role of Magnetic Resonance Imaging (MRI) in Temporal Bone Imaging for Implantation

Although majority of the temporal bone has a bony framework and can be imaged with computed tomography, Magnetic resonance imaging (MRI) is crucial in implantation otology to identify the membranous anatomy of the cochlea and Vestibule, Internal Auditory meatus and the auditory cortex. The main goals of MR imaging in the evaluation of a patient considered for an implant would be (Al-Rawy et al., 2017).

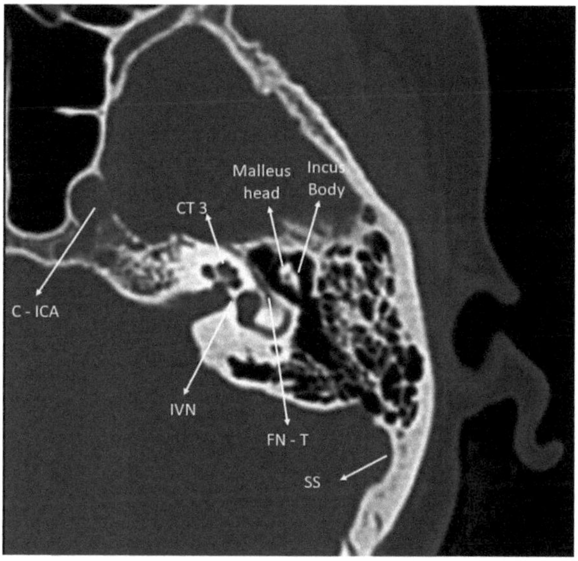

Fig. 4.12 The 3rd turn of the Cochlea is starting to show and the Inferior vestibular Nerve is seen going to the Saccule. The Tympanic segment of the facial nerve it travelling laterally and downwards. Ossicles are appearing much clearer. This arrangement of the Incus and Malleus is known as the "Ice cream cone appearance". This implies that the cuts have been taken through the Mesotympanum. (Hints: CT 3 3rd Cochlear Turn, C-ICA Cavernous Internal Carotid Artery, SS Sigmoid sinus, FN-T Facial Nerve Tympanic Segment, IVN Inferior Vestibular Nerve)

1. To determine if an implant is contraindicated.
2. Identify radiological anomalies that might make implantation difficult, such as round window, niche access, degree of mastoid aeration, course of the facial nerve, cochlear patency etc.
3. To identify the type of implant best suited for a patient.
4. Prognosis in terms of hearing and speech and language development after implantation.
5. To identify the side that is better suited for implantation in terms of ease of surgery and prognosis.
6. To ascertain the timing of surgery.
7. To counsel the parents or the patient about the outcomes and possible complications of surgery.

MRI fares better than CT to identify the presence or absence of cochlear nerve, to identify the caliber of the nerve and to assess higher auditory pathway pathologies.

Disadvantages of MRI include:

1. Added cost, as it cannot replace a CT scan.
2. May need sedation in children.
3. Motion artefacts are higher, as the hearing-impaired patient may not remain still, due to lack of communication and comprehension.

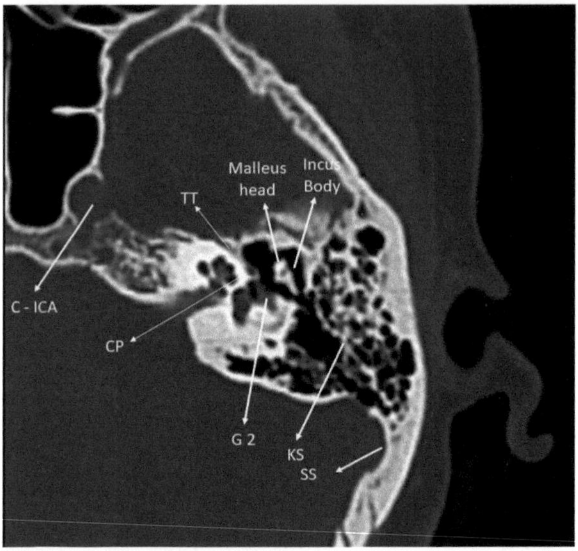

Fig. 4.13 The cavernous segment of the Internal carotid artery can be seen appearing adjacent to the Sphenoid sinus. Tensor Tympani Muscle is seen in close proximity to where the Eustachian Tube will appear lower down. The Facial Nerve is taking it's 2nd turn (2nd Genu—G2) to become the mastoid segment lower down. The Koerner's septum is a bony partition between the Squamous and Petrous portion of the Mastoid air cells. The Cochleariform Process is seen as a partition between the Tensor Tympani and the Eustachian Tube. (Hints: TT Tensor Tympani, KS Koerner's septum, CP Cochleariform Process, G2 2nd Genu)

Fig. 4.14 The Singular Nerve is entering the ampullated end of the Posterior Semi-Circular Canal (PSCC - A). This can be distinguished from the IVN, which supplied the Saccule in the previous cuts

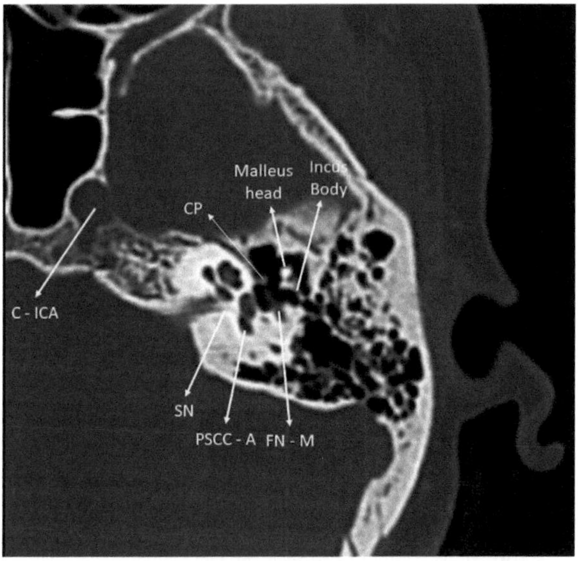

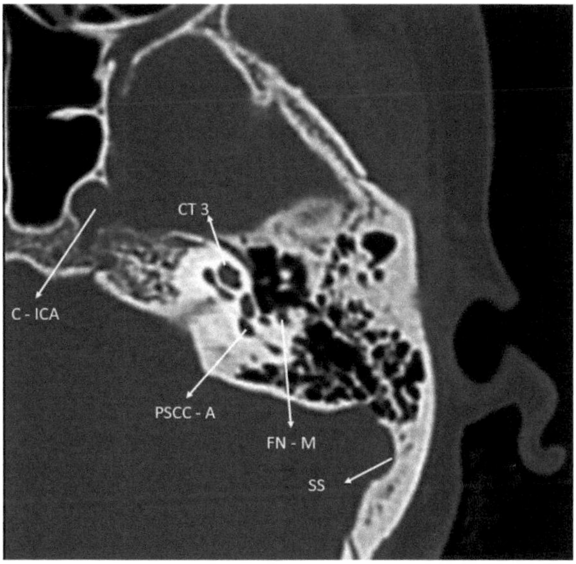

Fig. 4.15 The Mastoid segment of the Facial Nerve is seen as a dot since it is now vertical and the cuts taken through the temporal bone are Axial. The IAC is almost coming to an end depicted by the appearance of bone in the same place

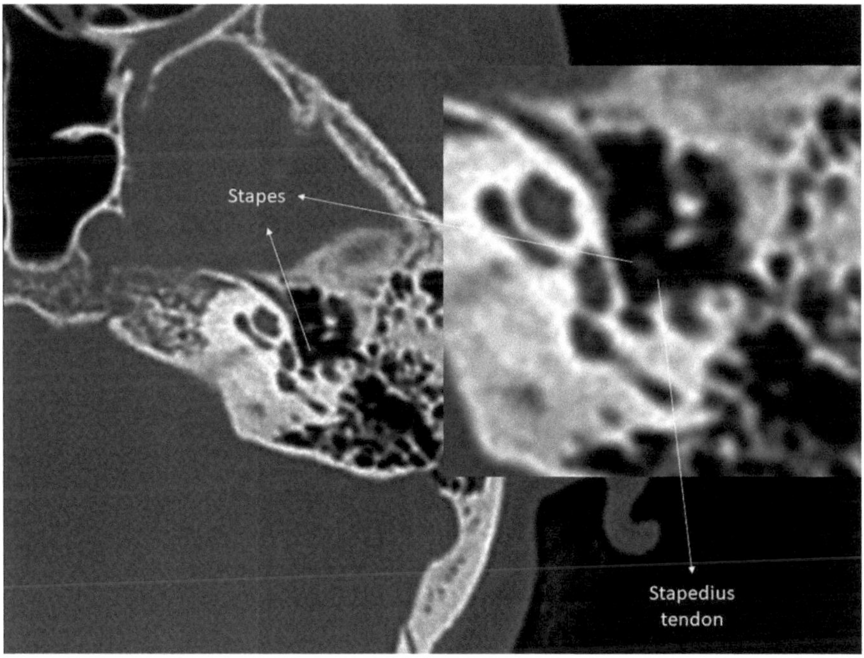

Fig. 4.16 The stapes can be seen in a zoomed in view along with the Stapedius tendon arising from the Pyramidal process underneath which the Mastoid segment of the facial nerve travels

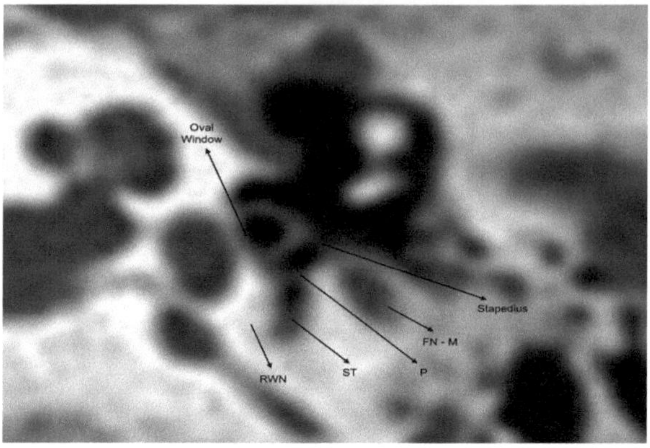

Fig. 4.17 Zoomed in. The sinus tympani is separated from the oval window by the ponticulus & from the RW by the subiculum. The Round window niche is seen here lateral to which is the sinus tympani, which is a depression between the pyramidal process and the RWN. (Hints: FN - M Facial Nerve Mastoid segment, P Ponticulus, ST Sinus Tympani, RWN Round Window Niche)

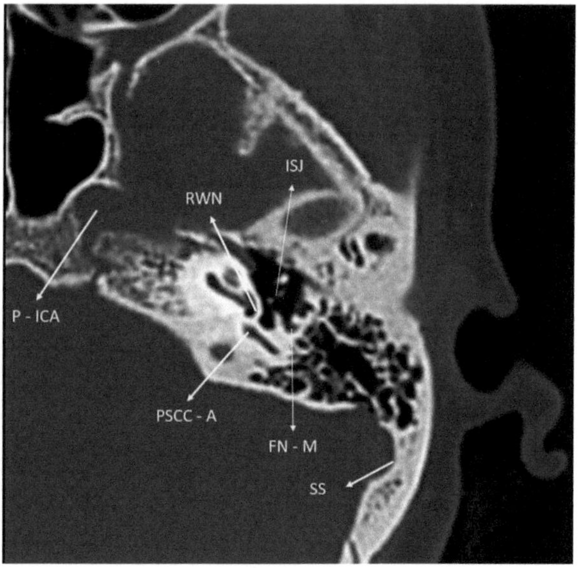

Fig. 4.18 The ICA has become horizontal to form the Petrous segment of ICA. The Incudo-stapedial joint can be seen as a faint line

Anatomy of the Internal Auditory Canal (IAC)

The anatomy of the IAC is best studied on a 3 T MRI with reformatted T2 images in the Oblique Parasagittal plane, which is perpendicular to the plane of the IAC (Fig. 4.26). The Internal auditory canal contains five nerves—The facial, Cochlear, Superior and Inferior Vestibular and Singular nerves. The anatomy of the IAC is such that, the Facial Nerve appears antero-superiorly while the Cochlear Nerve

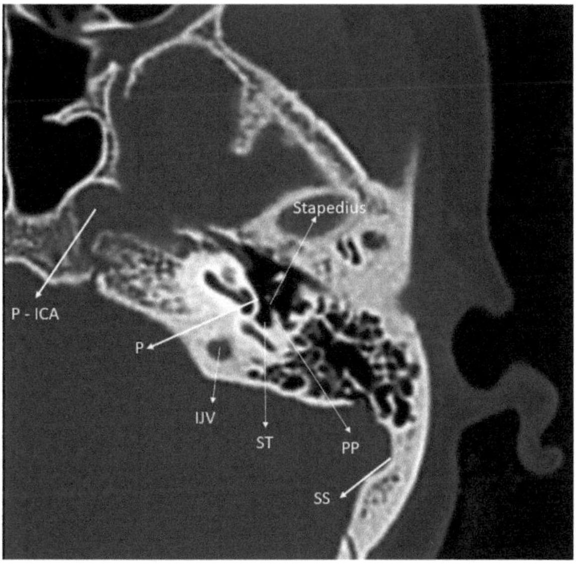

Fig. 4.19 The Promontory and Internal Jugular Vein have started to make an appearance. Labels point to the stapedius muscle, P-ICA (presumably the internal carotid artery), P (possibly petrous part), IJV (internal jugular vein), ST (stapes), PP (possibly petrous part of the temporal bone), and SS (sigmoid sinus)

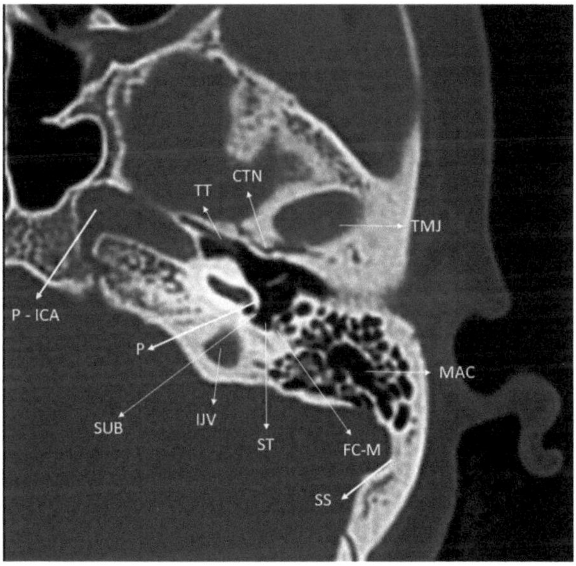

Fig. 4.20 The Tensor tympani Muscle is seen appearing anterior to the horizontal ICA. Antero-lateral to that is the Chorda tympani Nerve behind the Temporo-mandibular Joint (TMJ). (Hints: MAC Mastoid air cells, TMJ Temporomandibular joint, TT Tensor Tympani, P-ICA Petrous Internal Carotid Artery, ST Sinus Tympani, PP Pyramidal process, SUB Subiculum, P Promontory, CTN Chorda Tympani Nerve)

appears antero-inferiorly. The Superior and Inferior Vestibular Nerves appear postero-superiorly and postero-inferiorly respectively. In this oblique view, the thickness of the facial nerve and the Cochlear nerve can be compared.

There are five nerves that run through the IAM:

1. Nervus intermedius (sensory component of CN VII)
2. Facial motor root (motor component of CN VII)
3. Cochlear nerve (component of CN VIII)

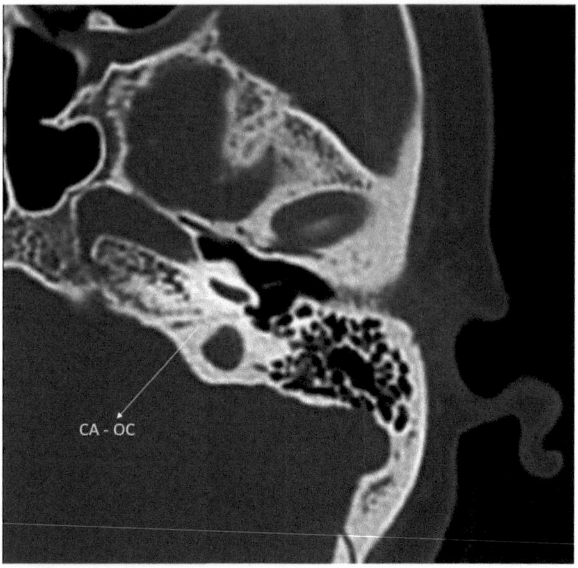

Fig. 4.21 The Cochlear Aqueduct can be seen appearing from the Basal Turn of Cochlea and moving towards the Posterior cranial fossa. (Hints: CA-OC Cochlear Aqueduct – Otic Capsule segment)

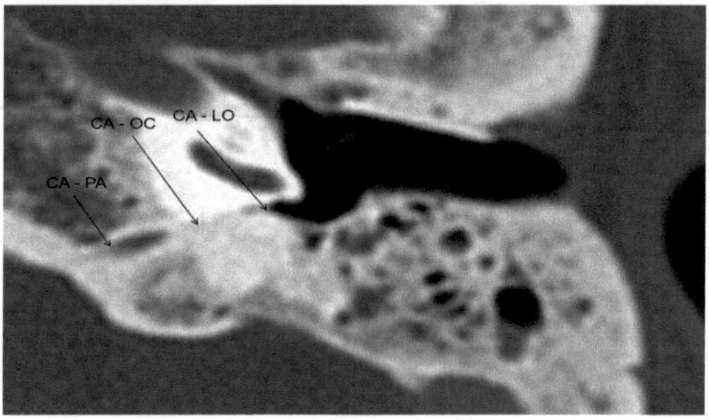

Fig. 4.22 The Cochlear Aqueduct has 4 parts. (Hints: This image shows 3 of the 4—CA-LO Cochlear Aqueduct Lateral Orifice, CA-PA Cochlear Aqueduct Petrous Apex segment, CA-OC Cochlear Aqueduct Otic Capsule Segment)

4. Inferior vestibular nerve (component of CN VIII)
5. Superior vestibular nerve (component of CN VIII)

The Nerves passing through the Internal Auditory Meatus can present through a variation in the number of nerve bundles. Figure 4.26 shows 4 variations ranging from a single bundle to 5 separate bundles through which the nerves can emerge through the IAM.

Anatomy of the Cochlear Nerve

3D Continuous interface in Steady State (CISS) sequence is the best way to produce high-resolution images of the Cochlear Nerve within the IAC. This is achieved because of better flow compensation in the Cerebrospinal Fluid (CSF) and provision

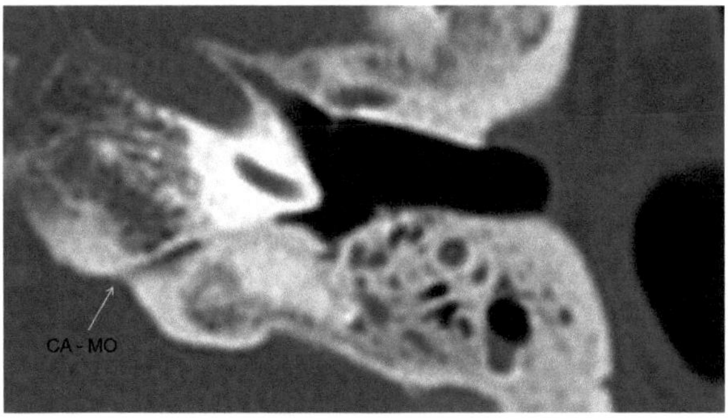

Fig. 4.23 The last part of the Cochlear Aqueduct is the Medial orifice through which it opens into the cranial cavity. (Hints: CA- MO Cochlear Aqueduct Medial Orifice)

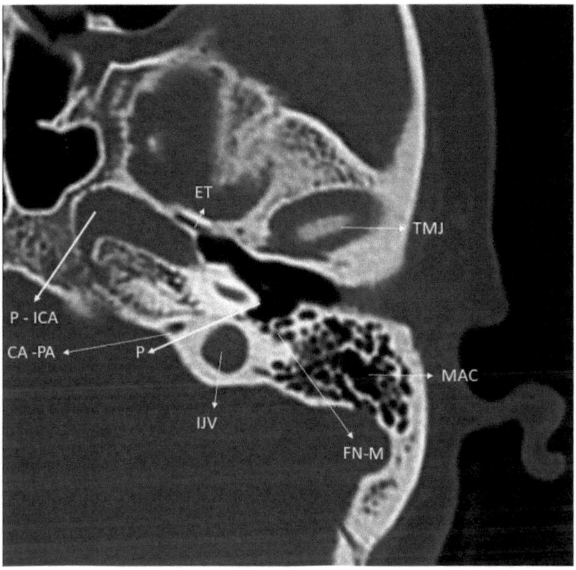

Fig. 4.24 The appearance of air anterior to the Pertous ICA denotes the beginning of the Eustachian Tube. Internal Jugular Vein will be seen becoming more prominent as the slices proceed downwards. (Hints: CA-PA Cochlear aqueduct – Petrous Apex Segment, MAC Mastoid air cells, TMJ Temporomandibular joint, ET Eustachian Tube, P-ICA Petrous Internal Carotid Artery, P Promontory, IJV Internal Jugular Vein, FN –M Facial Nerve Mastoid Segment)

of homogenous image in CSF resulting in high contrast images with better geometrical resolution which allows better image reconstruction (Özdemir & Kavak, 2019). There is statistical evidence that the horizontal and vertical diameters along with the cross-sectional area of the cochlear nerve, reduce with age (Özdemir & Kavak, 2019).

Concerning implantation, identifying the presence of the Cochlear nerve and its size are the two most crucial aspects of studying the IAC. For a rough reference point on the MRI, the Cochlear Nerve should be at least the same size of the Facial Nerve if not larger. A Cochlear nerve with a vertical diameter of less than 1.4 mm (± 0.21 mm), horizontal diameter of less than 1.0 mm (± 0.15 mm), or a cross-sectional area of less than 1.1 mm^2 (± 0.26 mm^2) can be considered as hypoplastic as per a study of normal Cochlear nerve parameters in 45 ears using high resolution MRI (Figs. 4.27 and 4.28) (Jaryszak et al., 2009). It is also important to compare the thickness and functionality of the cochlear nerve on both sides. If the audiological parameters of both the ears are more or less similar, then the side with the thicker cochlear nerve can be chosen for implantation (Fig. 4.29).

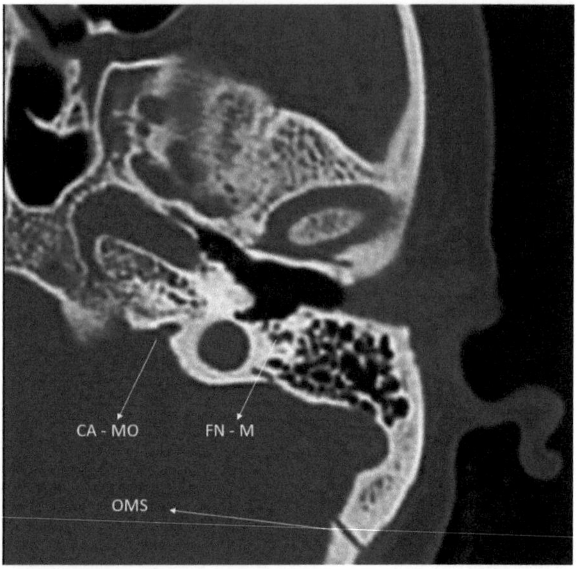

Fig. 4.25 The Medial orifice of the Cochlear Aqueduct is seen as we proceed downwards. The Occipitomastoid suture line can be visualised as well. (Hints: CA – MO Cochlear Aqueduct Medial Orifice, FN-M Facial Nerve Mastoid segment, OMS Occipito-Mastoid Suture line)

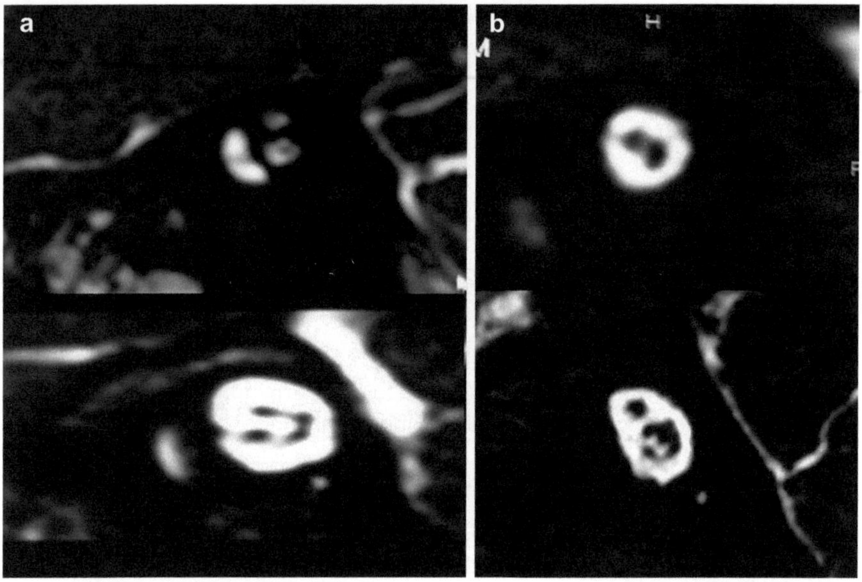

Fig. 4.26 (**a**) Single nerve bundle in IAM; (**b**) Two nerve bundles in IAM; (**c**) Four nerve bundles in IAM; (**d**) Five nerve bundles in IAM

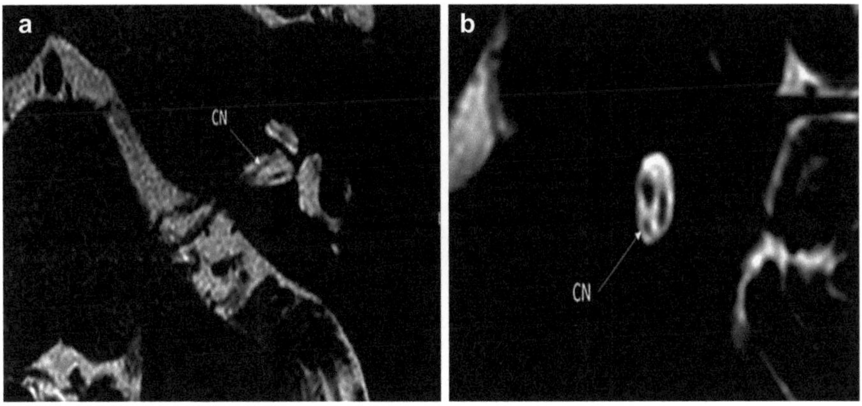

Fig. 4.27 (**a**) Hypo-plastic cochlear nerve (CN), axial view. (**b**) Hypo-plastic cochlear nerve (CN), Sagittal oblique view. Cochlear aplasia is usually accompanied by cochlear nerve aplasia. Cochlear nerve (CN) may be hypoplastic or aplastic, when Cochlea is hypoplastic. Cochlear nerve hypoplasia and aplasia can also be observed in a normal cochlea

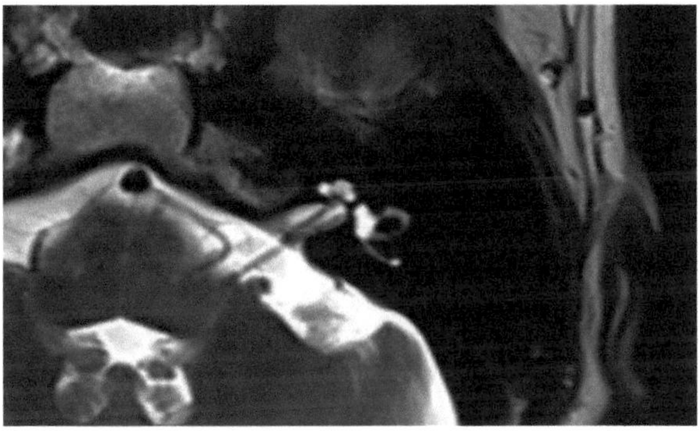

Fig. 4.28 Axial T2 MRI of the Left Inner ear showing the turns of the Cochlea, Modiolus and the entry point of the Cochlear Nerve. The cochlear nerve can be seen coming from the cerebellopontine angle. The nerve going to the vestibule alongside the cochlear nerve is the Inferior vestibular nerve

Anatomy of the Labyrinth

The inner ear is studied in detail using heavy T2W images, which can delineate all of the 2.75 turns of the membranous labyrinth. In some cases, pre and post Gadolinium images may be used. An MR Vestibulo-Cochleogram show us the Cochlea and the Semi-Circular canals so as to assess the anatomical configuration and presence of any anomalies of the cochlea or vestibule (Fig. 4.30).

The length of insertion of the electrode can be calculated prior to surgery on the MRI using rendering along with placement of multiple reference points along the

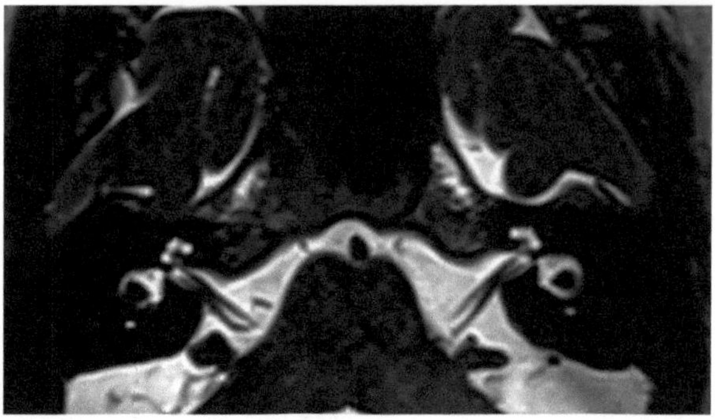

Fig. 4.29 Bilateral view of the Cochlear and Inferior Vestibular nerve arising from the Cerebellopontine junction. It is important to compare both the nerves simultaneously to decide the side of implantation in cases of Bilateral hearing loss

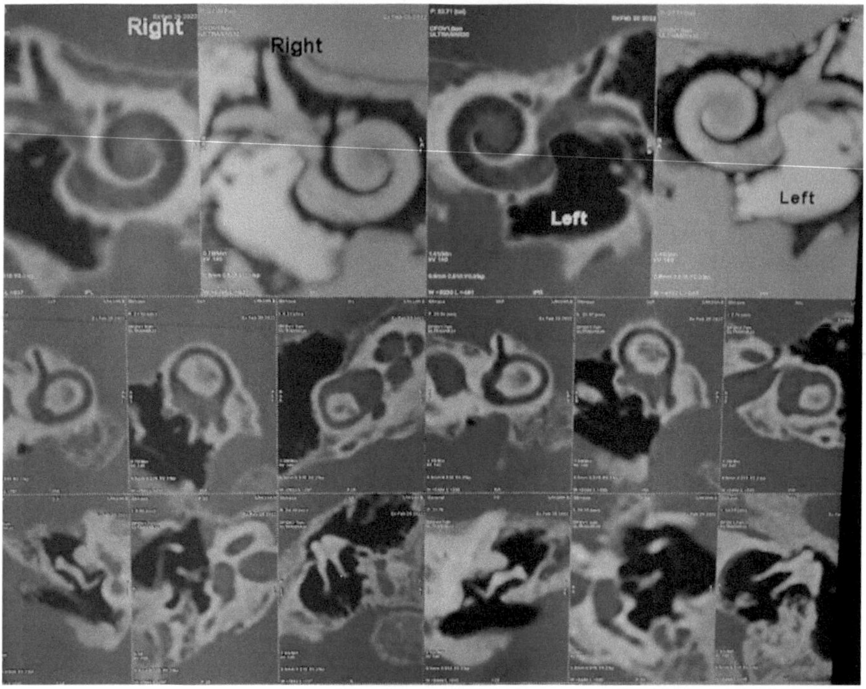

Fig. 4.30 MR Vestibulo-Cochleogram showing the normal anatomy of the Cochlea and Vestibule

lateral wall of the cochlear duct starting from the mid-round window. MRI is superior to CT in its ability to identify fibrosis in the Cochlear Duct, specially near the round window or lateral cochlear duct. The most accurate method of measuring the Cochlear length is by means of 3D reconstruction. The average length of the Cochlear duct is about 35.04 mm when measured at the level of the Organ of Corti and is 37.07 mm, when measured at the level of the lateral wall of Cochlea (Figs. 4.31 and 4.32) (Koch et al., 2017; Sato et al., 1991; Singh et al., 2020; Kawano et al., 1996; Meng et al., 2016).

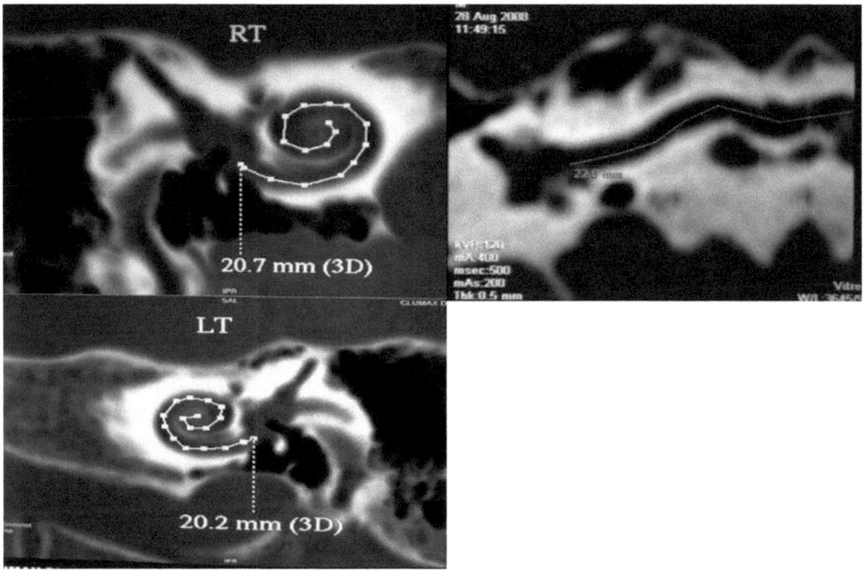

Fig. 4.31 CT scan of a hypoplastic Cochlear duct with measurements made with the help of 3D Reconstruction. This is the most accurate way of measuring the length of the cochlear duct

Fig. 4.32 MR Cochleogram showing the Cochlear turns and Semi-circular canals on either side

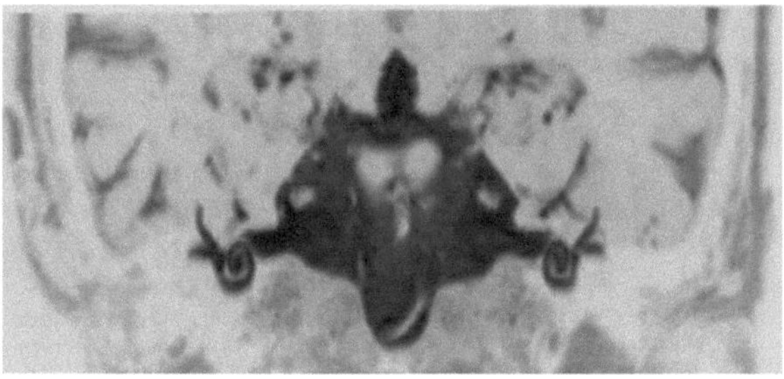

Anatomy of the Auditory Pathway

T2W images of the brain should be used to get high-definition images delineating the complete auditory pathway from the Cochlear nuclei to the Superior temporal gyrus. The left side is more dominant in cases of right-handed individuals in majority of the cases. There are 6 areas beyond the cochlear nerve that one should pay attention to while tracing the Auditory pathway.

1. Cochlear nucleus at the Ponto-medullary junction
2. Superior Olivary complex at the lower pons
3. Lateral lemniscus at the pons
4. Inferior colliculus at the Tectum

5. Medial Geniculate body at the thalamus
6. Primary auditory cortex or Broadmann areas 41 and 42 at the Superior Temporal Gyrus.

Pathologies in these areas must be duly identified and confirmed with a neuroradiologist and correlated clinically with a Pediatric or adult neurologist. Such pathologies might mitigate the outcome of cochlear implantation.

References

Albano, S., Ramnot, A., Siddiqi, J., & Mahato, D. (2020). Medical and legal implications of MRI scout imaging in a surgical patient with case presentation. *Cureus, 12*(1), e6833.

Al-Rawy, A. S., al-Shatouri, M., El Tabbakh, M., & Gad, A. A. (2017). Systematic approach by computed tomography and magnetic resonance imaging in cochlear implantation candidates in Suez Canal University Hospital. *The Egyptian Journal of Radiology and Nuclear Medicine, 48*(4), 877–884.

Aschendorff, A., Kubalek, R., Turowski, B., Zanella, F., Hochmuth, A., Schumacher, M., Klenzner, T., & Laszig, R. (2005). Quality control after cochlear implant surgery by means of rotational tomography. *Otology and Neurotology, 26*(1), 34–37.

Bidgood, W. D., Jr., Horii, S. C., Prior, F. W., & Van Syckle, D. E. (1997). Understanding and using DICOM, the data interchange standard for biomedical imaging. *Journal of the American Medical Informatics Association: JAMIA, 4*(3), 199–212.

Bremke, M., Lüers, J. C., Stenner, M., Bovenschulte, H., Dorn, F., Unkel, C., Höllering, J., & Beutner, D. (2013). Radiologic examinations in human temporal bone specimens using digital volume tomography and high-resolution computed tomography after implantation of middle ear prosthesis and cochlear implant electrode array. *Otology and Neurotology, 34*(7), 1321–1328.

Dalrymple, N. C., Prasad, S. R., Freckleton, M. W., & Chintapalli, K. N. (2005). Informatics in radiology (infoRAD): Introduction to the language of three-dimensional imaging with multidetector CT. *Radiographics: A Review Publication of the Radiological Society of North America, Inc, 25*(5), 1409–1428.

DenOtter, T. D., & Schubert, J. (2025, January). Hounsfield Unit. [Updated 2023 Mar 6]. In *StatPearls [Internet]*. StatPearls Publishing. Available from: https://www.ncbi.nlm.nih.gov/books/NBK547721/

Goldman, L. W. (2007). Principles of CT and CT technology. *Journal of Nuclear Medicine Technology, 35*(3), 115–130.

Guyader, E., Savéan, J., Clodic, C., Letellier, P., Meriot, P., & Marianowski, R. (2018). Three-dimensional reconstruction of the temporal bone: Comparison of in situ, CT, and CBCT measurements. *European Annals of Otorhinolaryngology, Head and Neck Diseases, 135*(6), 393–398.

Hermena, S. (2023, August 8). *CT-scan image production procedures*. StatPearls [Internet]. https://www.ncbi.nlm.nih.gov/books/NBK574548/

Hounsfield, G. N. (1976). Historical notes on computerized axial tomography. *Journal of the Canadian Association of Radiologists, 27*(3), 135–142.

Jaryszak, E. M., Patel, N. A., Camp, M., Mancuso, A. A., & Antonelli, P. J. (2009). Cochlear nerve diameter in normal hearing ears using high-resolution magnetic resonance imaging. *The Laryngoscope, 119*(10), 2042–2045.

Kawano, A., Seldon, H. L., & Clark, G. M. (1996). Computer-aided three-dimensional reconstruction in human cochlear maps: Measurement of the lengths of organ of Corti, outer wall, inner wall, and Rosenthal's canal. *The Annals of Otology, Rhinology, and Laryngology, 105*(9), 701–709.

Kimpe, T., & Tuytschaever, T. (2007). Increasing the number of gray shades in medical display systems – how much is enough? *Journal of Digital Imaging, 20*(4), 422–432.

Koch, R. W., Ladak, H. M., Elfarnawany, M., & Agrawal, S. K. (2017). Measuring Cochlear Duct Length – a historical analysis of methods and results. *Journal of Otolaryngology – Head & Neck Surgery, 46*(1), 19.

Makker, R., & Mukherjee, P. (2013). The importance of scout films. *BJA: British Journal of Anaesthesia, 111*(eLetters).

Meng, J., Li, S., Zhang, F., Li, Q., & Qin, Z. (2016). Cochlear size and shape variability and implications in cochlear implantation surgery. *Otology and Neurotology, 37*(9), 1307–1313.

Özdemir, M., & Kavak, R. P. (2019). Morphometric analysis of facial and cochlear nerves in normal-hearing ears using 3D-CISS. *Journal of Otology, 14*(4), 136–140.

Perandini, S., Faccioli, N., Zaccarella, A., Re, T., & Mucelli, R. P. (2010). The diagnostic contribution of CT volumetric rendering techniques in routine practice. *The Indian Journal of Radiology & Imaging, 20*(2), 92–97.

Prokop, M., & Galanski, M. (2003). *Spiral and multislice computed tomography of the body*. Thieme.

Rubin, G. D., Napel, S., & Leung, A. N. (1996). Volumetric analysis of volumetric data: Achieving a paradigm shift. *Radiology, 200*(2), 312–317.

Sato, H., Sando, I., & Takahashi, H. (1991). Sexual dimorphism and development of the human cochlea. Computer 3-D measurement. *Acta Oto-Laryngologica, 111*(6), 1037–1040.

Singh, A., Kumar, R., Manchanda, S., Bhalla, A. S., Sagar, P., & Irugu, D. V. K. (2020). Radiographic measurement of cochlear duct length in an Indian cadaveric population – importance of custom fit cochlear implant electrodes. *International Archives of Otorhinolaryngology, 24*(4), e492–e495.

Zou, J., Lähelmä, J., Koivisto, J., Dhanasingh, A., Jolly, C., Aarnisalo, A., Wolff, J., & Pyykkö, I. (2015). Imaging cochlear implantation with round window insertion in human temporal bones and cochlear morphological variation using high-resolution cone beam CT. *Acta Oto-Laryngologica, 135*(5), 466–472.

Chapter 5
Radiology from the Perspective of Implantable Hearing Devices: Abnormal Auditory System

Gyanaranjan Nayak and Naresh Panda

Abstract This chapter examines the role of radiology in evaluating the abnormal auditory system, particularly in the context of implantable hearing devices such as cochlear implants and bone-anchored hearing systems. It discusses various congenital and acquired auditory anomalies, including cochlear malformations, auditory nerve abnormalities, and external ear defects. The chapter highlights how advanced imaging techniques like high-resolution CT and MRI are essential for identifying these abnormalities and guiding surgical planning. Emphasis is placed on how radiological findings impact the selection and success of implantable hearing devices, providing critical insights for optimizing outcomes in patients with complex auditory conditions.

Implantable hearing devices are the devices that carry the sound energy and deliver it directly to the cochlear perilymph or stimulate the cochlear nerve and ganglion and nuclei. These devices are different from other passive devices and hearing aid devices. The indications of its usage are beyond the scope of the chapter and will be discussed elsewhere.

Keywords Radiological imaging · CT · MRI · Inner ear anomalies · Cochlear nerve deficiency · Labyrinthitis ossificans

Introduction

Radiological imaging of auditory pathway plays a crucial role in implantation otology to screen for various conditions that will guide the surgeon to implement the process successfully. Imaging also plays an integral part in gauging preoperative surgical candidacy, intraoperative monitoring and postoperative position of the implant. Advances in resolution of Computed tomography (CT) and Magnetic

G. Nayak (✉) · N. Panda
Department of Otolaryngology-Head and Neck Surgery, Post Graduate Institute of Medical Education and Research (PGIMER), Chandigarh, India

P. Kumar et al. (eds.), *Advances in Implantation Otology*,
https://doi.org/10.1007/978-981-96-8671-1_5

resonance imaging (MRI) has given the clinician detailed information of external, middle and inner ear and identification of abnormal auditory pathway.

Aural Atresia

Congenital aural atresia (CAA) is characterized by absence or partial formation of external auditory canal. CAA can be unilateral or bilateral and can occur in isolation or present as a part of syndromic association. Bilateral presentation is seen in approximately one third of patients with CAA (Kösling et al., 2009).

The internal auditory canal and inner ear structures are mostly normal in view of their earlier and different embryologic origin. The middle ear structure findings are variable with a wide range of spectrum (Gassner et al., 2004). The malleus and incus may be rudimentary and/or fused to each other.

HRCT is the imaging modality of choice for CAA (Fig. 5.1). Detection of ossicular malformations warrant good resolution of CT with a small slice thickness bony algorithm (0.5–1 mm). The CT grading given by Jahrsdoerfer et al. is specifically done to assess the outcomes of surgery (Jahrsdoerfer et al., 1992; Shonka Jr et al., 2008). The presence of normal stapes is given maximum weightage in preoperative CT scan which determines the hearing outcome of surgery. The course of facial nerve may be more anteriorly placed or in some instances bifid around the stapes footplate. The internal carotid artery may have an anomalous course which can further complicate the surgery. Although the aberrant course of facial nerve and internal carotid artery do not exclude the possibility of surgery completely, but the risk of increase of complication is increased. Patients with severe malformed ossicles with low scores on Jahrsdoerfer grading (<5) are considered as contraindication of atresioplasty.

The auditory rehabilitation in CAA can be provided by:

1. External auditory canal atresioplasty
2. Atresioplasty with hearing aids

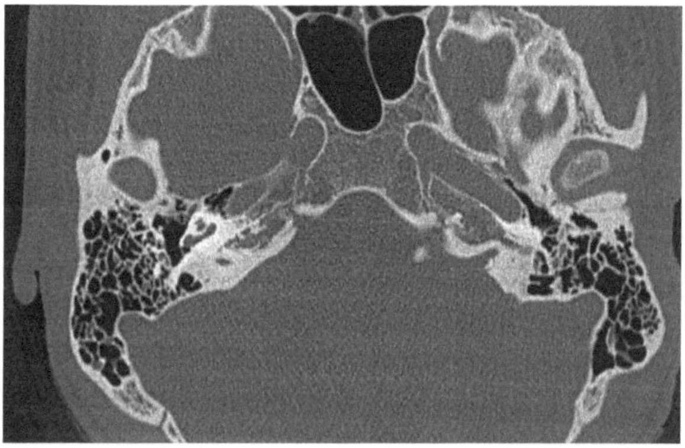

Fig. 5.1 HRCT temporal bone showing Bilateral Congenital Aural Atresia

3. Bone anchored hearing devices
4. Conventional bone conduction hearing aids

The patients who are poor candidates for atresioplasty or those who have not achieved satisfactory hearing gain on EAC reconstruction can be considered for Bone conduction implants. With the current literature it will not be prudent to compare EAC atresioplasty with Bone anchored implants because the majority of patients who are taken for reconstruction have good CT score. With the advent of osseointegrated implant systems for direct bone conduction stimulating the cochlea and bypassing the external and middle ear has led to a revolutionary change in auditory rehabilitation for patients with conductive and mixed hearing loss (Håkansson et al., 1984; Tjellström et al., 1981). The candidacy and details of implant will be discussed elsewhere in the following chapters.

Radiology consideration for Bone anchored implant:

1. Grade of atresia (HRCT)
2. Thickness of calvaria for adequate bed drilling for implant (CT)
3. Associated Inner anomaly (MRI)

Although the development of external, middle and inner ear are from different anlages, the congenital malformation of external and middle ear can coexist with inner ear malformations with reported frequencies ranging from 10% to 47% (Ishimoto et al., 2005; Swartz & Faerber, 1985; Weidenbecher, 1988).

The radiological anatomy of the temporal bone is essential for planning of tissue integrated implant in the calvarium. CT gives a complete information not only about the external and middle ear status but also suggests appropriate site for placement of implant (Casselman et al., 1995; Takumi et al., 2008). The site of placement of implant should be in such a place to avoid encountering the dura, sigmoid sinus and any mastoid air cell. Thin calvarium over these sites can increase the risk of bleeding and any abutment entering the mastoid air cells can impede the adequate bone transmission. Minimum thickness of bone should be more than 4 mm to accommodate the abutment. Smaller fixtures of 3 mm can be used but they tend to loosen overtime with longer use (Takumi et al., 2008). The semi-implantable system Bonebridge™ has a Floating mass transducer (FMT) of thickness 4.5 mm with anchoring screws of 4 mm. The implant bed should be adequately prepared for holding the FMT and the screws. The use of 3D simulation software along with CT scan to accurately establish the site of implantation can avoid a potential complication (Law et al., 2016). (Fig. 5.2).

Inner Ear Anomalies

Inner ear malformations constitute approximately 20% of cases of congenital sensorineural hearing loss on the basis of radiology (Sennaroglu, 2010). The morphological of inner ear during the embryologic development will provide major clues to

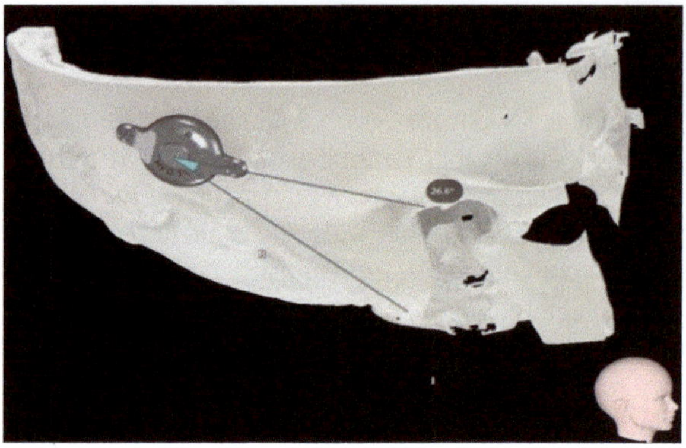

Fig. 5.2 The tentative positioning and planning of Bonebridge (MED-EL) placement in Congenital Aural Atresia

Table 5.1 The summary of inner ear development

Gestational age	Inner ear development
Week 3	Otic placode and otic pits
Week 4	Otocyst and utriculo-saccular division
Week 6	Utricular division to vestibule and utricle formation and saccular division to Cochlea and saccule formation.
Week 8	Membranous cochlea 2.5 turns complete
Week 12	Completion of membranous labyrinth
Week 24	Ossification of cochlea complete

our understanding. Hence it will be pertinent to discuss the brief embryology of inner ear which will provide relevant understanding of the inner ear malformation (Table 5.1).

The arrested development at different stages of formation of inner ear leads to various types of cochlea-vestibular anomalies. Earlier the arrest more severe is the malformation. Italian anatomist Carlo Mondini in his monograph in 1791 described an abnormality of inner ear associated with bilateral congenital hearing loss in an 8 year old child (Mondini, 1997). His original description included three classical features: (1) one and half turns of cochlea with normal basal turn and cystic apex; (2) enlarged vestibule with normal semicircular canals; (3) enlarged vestibular aqueduct. For a long time the term Mondini's dysplasia was used for virtually all the types of cochlea-vestibular anomalies until Jackler et al. classified the cochleovestibular anomalies on the basis of radiological findings (Jackler et al., 1987a). They classified cochleovestibular malformation on the basis of abnormal cochlea and normal cochlea (Table 5.2).

Since multiple malformations can coexist together the recent literature classifies the inner ear malformation into following types (Fig. 5.3a-c).

Table 5.2 The sequence of arrest during gestational growth and the associated abnormality

Arrested development during gestation	Cochlear Malformation
3rd week	Complete labyrinthine aplasia (Michel's aplasia)
4th week	Common Cavity
5th week	Cochlear aplasia
6th week	Cochlear Hypoplasia (Varying degree)
7th week	Incomplete partition

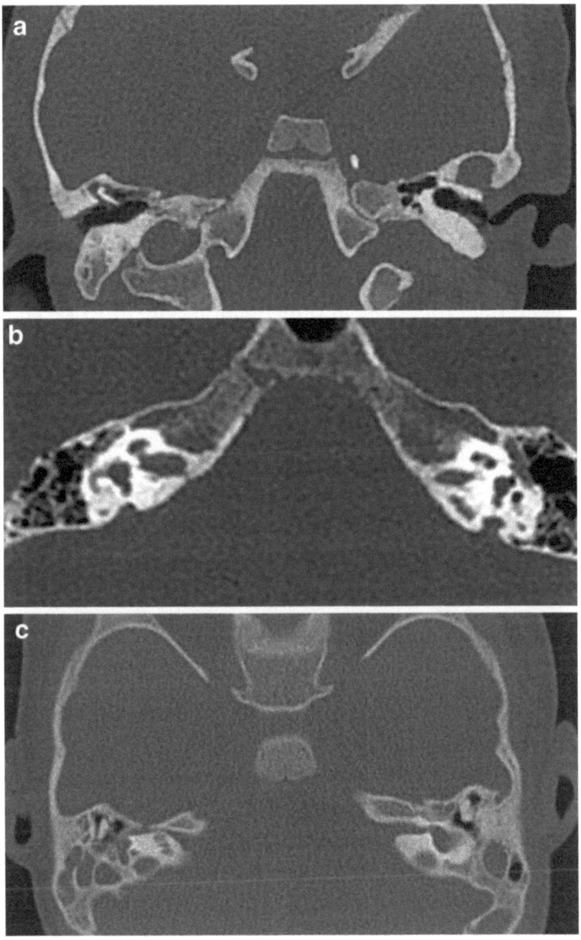

Fig. 5.3 HRCT temporal bone showing (**a**) Bilateral Michel's Aplasia, (**b**) Incomplete Partition Type 2 IEM on right side, (**c**) Cochlear Aplasia with Dilated Vestibule (CADV)

1. Complete labyrinthine aplasia (Michel's Aplasia)
   (i) CLA with hypoplastic or aplastic petrous bone
   (ii) CLA without otic capsule
   (iii) CLA with otic capsule

2. Rudimentary Otocyst
3. Common cavity
4. Cochlear Aplasia
5. Cochlear Hypoplasia
6. Incomplete partition
    (i) Incomplete Partition type I
    (ii) Incomplete Partition type II
    (iii) Incomplete Partition type III

Labyrinthitis Ossificans

Labyrinthitis ossificans is progressive ossification of membranous labyrinth leading to SNHL and is usually in response to an inflammatory or infective condition. The multitude of causes include meningitis, labyrinthitis, inflammatory or autoimmune conditions, trauma, prior surgical trauma etc. The reported incidence of labyrinthitis ossificans is 2%. However, the incidence of labyrinthitis ossificans in patients undergoing for cochlear implantation is up to 13%. The hearing loss following meningitis range from 6% to 37% and approximately 5% of patients being profoundly deaf.

Labyrinthitis Ossificans pathophysiology involves the following phases

1. Acute stage
2. Fibrotic stage
3. Ossification stage

Radiology in Labyrinthitis Ossificans

Radiological imaging in the form of MRI and HRCT temporal bone provides key information about labyrinthitis ossificans (Figs. 5.4 and 5.5). The accurate degree of ossification on radiology prior to surgery can alert a surgeon for potential challenges to be faced during the surgery. It also helps in prior arrangement of the appropriate electrode like double electrode array or compressed array to be used in case of drill out procedures. The limitations of HRCT are inability to detect Labyrinthitis ossificans in early stages, partial volume averaging and poor intercompartmental visualization of cochlea. However, MRI overcomes these shortcomings in assessing the status of inner ear in greater detail (Isaacson et al., 2009).

Initial efforts were to identify cochlear patency on CT in apical, middle and basal turn of cochlea along with round and oval window (Frau et al., 1994; Jackler et al., 1987b). Later, many investigators have suggested detailed radiological analysis of semicircular canals, as their involvement may prelude cochlear ossification (Muren & Bredberg, 1997; Buch et al., 2019). The literature lacks in an uniform

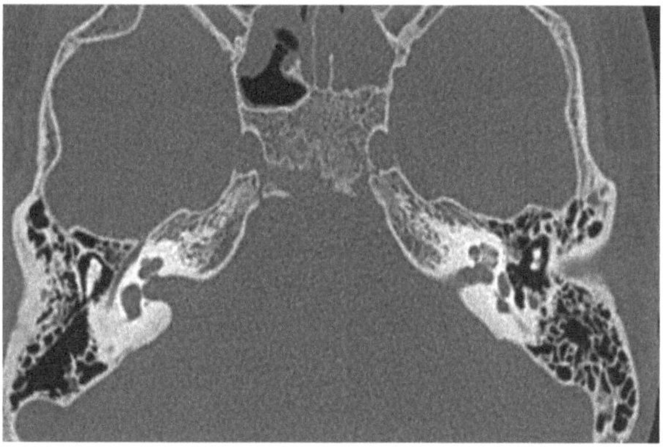

Fig. 5.4 HRCT temporal bone showing Labyrinthitis Ossificans in left cochlea post-pneumococcal meningitis

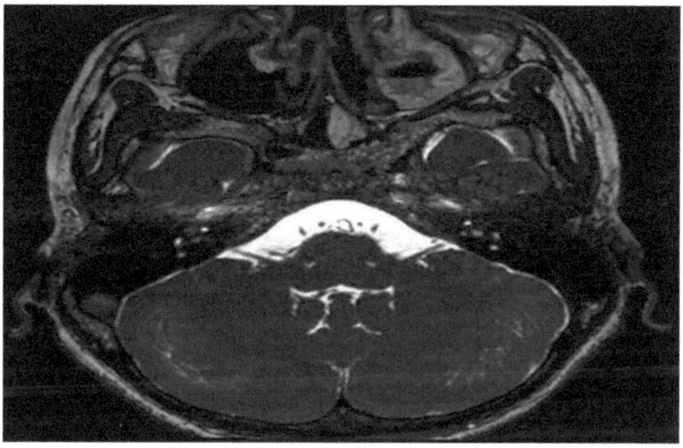

Fig. 5.5 Labyrinthitis Ossificans on MRI temporal bone image

radiological grading system of labyrinthitis ossificans (Seidman et al., 1994; Buch et al., 2019).

Seidman et al. proposed a grading system based on amount of cochlear ossification. Class 1, no ossification noted; class 2, round window membrane ossified; class 3, ossification of the round window extending 0 to 2 mm into the scala tympani but coils patent; class 4, ossification at the round window extending 3 to 8 mm into the scala tympani with patent coils; class 6, diffuse cochlear ossification (Seidman et al., 1994).

Cochlear Nerve Deficiency

Cochlear nerve deficiency (CND) was first described on MRI in 1997 (Casselman et al., 1997). It is defined as thin or absent nerve on radiological imaging. The definition includes the absent or thinned out nerve as well as its bony conduit. The bony conduit includes both internal auditory canal (IAC) and bony cochlear nerve canal. The approximate estimate of CND is around 1% of paediatric bilateral sensorineural hearing loss (Parry et al., 2005; Roland et al., 2012; Wu et al., 2009). The incidence of CND among cochlear implant recipients ranges from 2.5% to 11% (Buchman et al., 2011; Valero et al., 2012).

Radiological Imaging in CND

The diagnosis of CND is established on radiological imaging. High resolution 3D MRI is the most sensitive imaging modality to identify the CND (Adunka et al., 2007; Parry et al., 2005). However, HRCT temporal bone cuts <1 mm give intricate anatomical detail of the labyrinth and the osseous conduit i.e. IAC and bony cochlear nerve canal (Buchman et al., 2011; Parry et al., 2005). HRCT also gives better detail of mastoid air cell system, fallopian canal and bony labyrinth which might be abnormal in CND (Fig. 5.6). Approximately 50% of patients with CND can have normal IAC, hence, the presence of normal internal auditory canal does not preclude the possibility of CND (Adunka et al., 2007; Buchman et al., 2011; Carner et al., 2009).

The 3D MRI techniques including constructive interface steady state(CISS) and fast imaging employing steady state acquisition (FIESTA) in axial and oblique sagittal cuts perpendicular to IAC gives exquisite detail of nerve in IAC (Buchman et al., 2011; Casselman et al., 1997; Valero et al., 2012).

Casselman et al. in 1997 and later on modified by Govaerts et al. in 2003 described the classification of cochlear nerve deficiency in relation to labyrinth (Casselman et al., 1997; Govaerts et al., 2003) (Table 5.3).

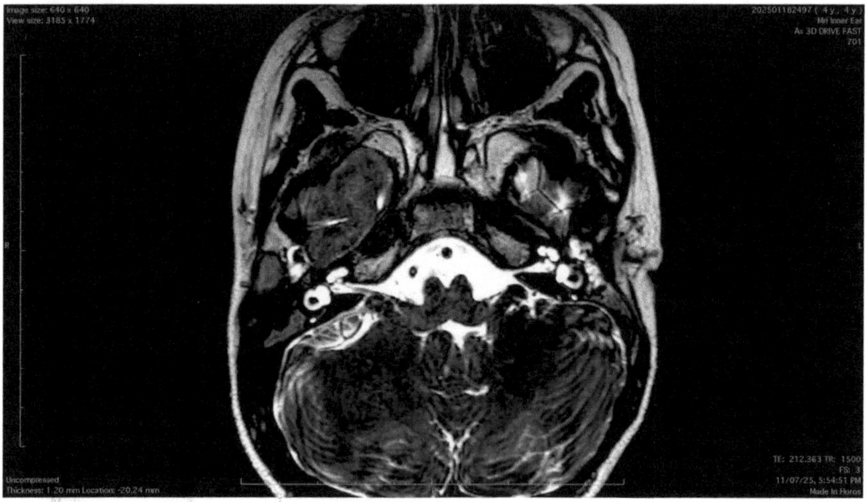

Fig. 5.6 HRCT temporal bone showing cochlear nerve aplasia on the right Side with thin nerve on the left side

Table 5.3 The classification of cochlear nerve deficiency in relation to labyrinth

Type	Description
Type I	Absent cochleovestibular nerve with normal/abnormal labyrinth
Type IIa	Present common cochleovestibular nerve with no cochlear branch along with labyrinthine dysplasia
Type IIb	Present common cochleovestibular nerve with no cochlear branch along with normal labyrinth
Type III	Present common cochleovestibular nerve with no vestibular branch (Theoretical possibility; not proven)

References

Adunka, O. F., Jewells, V., & Buchman, C. A. (2007). Value of computed tomography in the evaluation of children with cochlear nerve deficiency. *Otology & neurotology: Official publication of the American Otological Society, American Neurotology Society [and] European Academy of Otology and Neurotology, 28*(5), 597–604. https://doi.org/10.1097/01.mao.0000281804.36574.72

Buch, K., Baylosis, B., Fujita, A., Qureshi, M. M., Takumi, K., Weber, P. C., & Sakai, O. (2019). Etiology-specific mineralization patterns in patients with labyrinthitis ossificans. *AJNR. American Journal of Neuroradiology, 40*(3), 551–557. https://doi.org/10.3174/ajnr.A5985

Buchman, C. A., Teagle, H. F., Roush, P. A., Park, L. R., Hatch, D., Woodard, J., Zdanski, C., & Adunka, O. F. (2011). Cochlear implantation in children with labyrinthine anomalies and cochlear nerve deficiency: Implications for auditory brainstem implantation. *The Laryngoscope, 121*(9), 1979–1988. https://doi.org/10.1002/lary.22032

Carner, M., Colletti, L., Shannon, R., Cerini, R., Barillari, M., Mucelli, R. P., & Colletti, V. (2009). Imaging in 28 children with cochlear nerve aplasia. *Acta Oto-Laryngologica, 129*(4), 458–461. https://doi.org/10.1080/00016480902737978

Casselman, J. W., Ars, B., Van de Heyning, P., & Koekelkoren, E. (1995). Preoperative computed tomography in patients requiring a bone-anchored hearing aid. *European Archives of Oto-Rhino-Laryngology: Official Journal of the European Federation of Oto-Rhino-Laryngological Societies (EUFOS): Affiliated with the German Society for Oto-Rhino-Laryngology – Head and Neck Surgery, 252*(7), 401–404. https://doi.org/10.1007/BF00167309

Casselman, J. W., Offeciers, F. E., Govaerts, P. J., Kuhweide, R., Geldof, H., Somers, T., & D'Hont, G. (1997). Aplasia and hypoplasia of the vestibulocochlear nerve: Diagnosis with MR imaging. *Radiology, 202*(3), 773–781. https://doi.org/10.1148/radiology.202.3.9051033

Frau, G. N., Luxford, W. M., Lo, W. W., Berliner, K. I., & Telischi, F. F. (1994). High-resolution computed tomography in evaluation of cochlear patency in implant candidates: A comparison with surgical findings. *The Journal of Laryngology and Otology, 108*(9), 743–748. https://doi.org/10.1017/s0022215100128002

Gassner, E. M., Mallouhi, A., & Jaschke, W. R. (2004). Preoperative evaluation of external auditory canal atresia on high-resolution CT. *AJR. American Journal of Roentgenology, 182*(5), 1305–1312. https://doi.org/10.2214/ajr.182.5.1821305

Govaerts, P. J., Casselman, J., Daemers, K., De Beukelaer, C., Yperman, M., & De Ceulaer, G. (2003). Cochlear implants in aplasia and hypoplasia of the cochleovestibular nerve. *Otology & Neurotology: Official publication of the American Otological Society, American Neurotology Society [and] European Academy of Otology and Neurotology, 24*(6), 887–891. https://doi.org/10.1097/00129492-200311000-00011

Håkansson, B., Tjellström, A., & Rosenhall, U. (1984). Hearing thresholds with direct bone conduction versus conventional bone conduction. *Scandinavian Audiology, 13*(1), 3–13. https://doi.org/10.3109/01050398409076252

Isaacson, B., Booth, T., Kutz, J. W., Jr., Lee, K. H., & Roland, P. S. (2009). Labyrinthitis ossificans: How accurate is MRI in predicting cochlear obstruction? *Otolaryngology – Head and Neck Surgery: Official journal of American Academy of Otolaryngology-Head and Neck Surgery, 140*(5), 692–696. https://doi.org/10.1016/j.otohns.2008.12.029

Ishimoto, S., Ito, K., Yamasoba, T., Kondo, K., Karino, S., Takegoshi, H., & Kaga, K. (2005). Correlation between microtia and temporal bone malformation evaluated using grading systems. *Archives of Otolaryngology – Head & Neck Surgery, 131*(4), 326–329. https://doi.org/10.1001/archotol.131.4.326

Jackler, R. K., Luxford, W. M., & House, W. F. (1987a). Congenital malformations of the inner ear: A classification based on embryogenesis. *The Laryngoscope, 97*(3 Pt 2 Suppl 40), 2–14. https://doi.org/10.1002/lary.5540971301

Jackler, R. K., Luxford, W. M., Schindler, R. A., & McKerrow, W. S. (1987b). Cochlear patency problems in cochlear implantation. *The Laryngoscope, 97*(7 Pt 1), 801–805.

Jahrsdoerfer, R. A., Yeakley, J. W., Aguilar, E. A., Cole, R. R., & Gray, L. C. (1992). Grading system for the selection of patients with congenital aural atresia. *The American Journal of Otology, 13*(1), 6–12.

Kösling, S., Omenzetter, M., & Bartel-Friedrich, S. (2009). Congenital malformations of the external and middle ear. *European Journal of Radiology, 69*(2), 269–279. https://doi.org/10.1016/j.ejrad.2007.10.019

Sennaroglu, L. (2010). Cochlear implantation in inner ear malformations – a review article. *Cochlear Implants International, 11*(1), 4–41. https://doi.org/10.1002/cii.416

Law, E. K., Bhatia, K. S., Tsang, W. S., Tong, M. C., & Shi, L. (2016). CT pre-operative planning of a new semi-implantable bone conduction hearing device. *European Radiology, 26*(6), 1686–1695. https://doi.org/10.1007/s00330-015-3983-x

Mondini, C. (1997). Minor works of Carlo Mondini: The anatomical section of a boy born deaf. *The American Journal of Otology, 18*(3), 288–293.

Muren, C., & Bredberg, G. (1997). Postmeningitic labyrinthine ossification primarily affecting the semicircular canals. *European Radiology, 7*(2), 208–213. https://doi.org/10.1007/s003300050137

Parry, D. A., Booth, T., & Roland, P. S. (2005). Advantages of magnetic resonance imaging over computed tomography in preoperative evaluation of pediatric cochlear implant candidates. *Otology & Neurotology: Official publication of the American Otological Society, American Neurotology Society [and] European Academy of Otology and Neurotology, 26*(5), 976–982. https://doi.org/10.1097/01.mao.0000185049.61770.da

Roland, P., Henion, K., Booth, T., Campbell, J. D., & Sharma, A. (2012). Assessment of cochlear implant candidacy in patients with cochlear nerve deficiency using the P1 CAEP biomarker. *Cochlear Implants International, 13*(1), 16–25. https://doi.org/10.1179/146701011X12962268235869

Seidman, D. A., Chute, P. M., & Parisier, S. (1994). Temporal bone imaging for cochlear implantation. *The Laryngoscope, 104*(5 Pt 1), 562–565. https://doi.org/10.1002/lary.5541040510

Shonka, D. C., Jr., Livingston, W. J., 3rd, & Kesser, B. W. (2008). The Jahrsdoerfer grading scale in surgery to repair congenital aural atresia. *Archives of Otolaryngology – Head & Neck Surgery, 134*(8), 873–877. https://doi.org/10.1001/archotol.134.8.873

Swartz, J. D., & Faerber, E. N. (1985). Congenital malformations of the external and middle ear: High-resolution CT findings of surgical import. *AJR. American Journal of Roentgenology, 144*(3), 501–506. https://doi.org/10.2214/ajr.144.3.501

Takumi, Y., Suzuki, N., Moteki, H., Kobayashi, K., & Usami, S. (2008). Pre-Baha operation three dimensional computed tomography with markers for determining optimal implant site. *The Laryngoscope, 118*(10), 1824–1826. https://doi.org/10.1097/MLG.0b013e31817f4cf6

Tjellström, A., Lindström, J., Hallén, O., Albrektsson, T., & Brånemark, P. I. (1981). Osseointegrated titanium implants in the temporal bone. A clinical study on bone-anchored hearing aids. *The American Journal of Otology, 2*(4), 304–310.

Valero, J., Blaser, S., Papsin, B. C., James, A. L., & Gordon, K. A. (2012). Electrophysiologic and behavioral outcomes of cochlear implantation in children with auditory nerve hypoplasia. *Ear and Hearing, 33*(1), 3–18. https://doi.org/10.1097/AUD.0b013e3182263460

Weidenbecher, M. (1988). Missbildungen des Felsenbeins und der angrenzenden Schädelbasis [Abnormalities of the petrous bone and the adjacent base of the skull]. *Archives of Oto-Rhino-Laryngology. Supplement = Archiv fur Ohren-, Nasen- und Kehlkopfheilkunde. Supplement, 1*, 1–62.

Wu, C. M., Ng, S. H., Wang, J. J., & Liu, T. C. (2009). Diffusion tensor imaging of the subcortical auditory tract in subjects with congenital cochlear nerve deficiency. *AJNR. American Journal of Neuroradiology, 30*(9), 1773–1777. https://doi.org/10.3174/ajnr.A1681

Chapter 6
Bone Conduction Implants: Audiological Perspectives

Prawin Kumar, Prabuddha Bhatarai, Apurva Kumar, Kumari Apeksha, and Niraj Kumar Singh

Abstract Bone conduction implants (BCIs) are advanced hearing solutions designed for individuals with conductive or mixed hearing loss, and for those unable to benefit from conventional hearing aids. BCIs offer a low-risk surgical solution that enhances hearing ability and sound quality. Used for decades in hearing rehabilitation, the first BCI was implanted in 1977 in Gothenburg, Sweden. Over 100,000 BCIs have since been implanted with various devices and external processors. A BCI includes an external processor that amplifies sound and an internal component that sends vibratory energy directly to the temporal bone, bypassing damaged air conduction pathways to stimulate the cochlea. BCIs are particularly beneficial for patients with chronic ear conditions, congenital malformations, and single-sided deafness, offering a safe and reliable rehabilitation option.

Keywords Bone conduction implants · Hearing loss · Deafness · Bone anchored hearing aids · Transcutaneous device · Conductive hearing loss

P. Kumar (✉) · N. K. Singh
Department of Audiology, All India Institute of Speech and Hearing, University of Mysore, Mysore, India

P. Bhatarai
Department of Audiology, All India Institute of Speech and Hearing, University of Mysore, Mysore, India

The University of Texas at Dallas, Dallas, TX, USA

A. Kumar
Ashadeep ENT Centre & Apollo Hospital, Bangalore, India

K. Apeksha
MarThoma College of Special Education, Kerala University of Health Sciences, Kasaragod, Kerala, India

P. Kumar et al. (eds.), *Advances in Implantation Otology*,
https://doi.org/10.1007/978-981-96-8671-1_6

Introduction

Hearing loss significantly impacts communication, social interaction, educational opportunities, and quality of life. Even when fitted appropriately, many hearing-impaired individuals may have limited benefits with conventional hearing aids. This is more relevant for individuals with unilateral deafness and conductive pathologies where traditional hearing aids are not viable. For these individuals, bone conduction implants (BCI) constitute a relatively low-risk surgical option that can improve aided hearing ability and sound quality. BCIs have been widely used for decades in the field of hearing rehabilitation. Anders Tjellstrom implanted first BCI in 1977 in Gothenburg, Sweden (Iseri et al., 2015). Since then, more than 100,000 BCIs have been implanted using various implants and external processors (Iseri et al., 2015). Basic BCI parts include an external processor that detects and amplifies sound and an internal component that sends sound energy directly to the temporal bone, stimulating the cochlea by transmitting vibratory energy. The bone conduction device bypasses defective air conduction pathways and stimulate intact cochlea directly through the bone conduction mode. BCIs are most useful for single-sided deafness and conductive hearing loss where air-conduction hearing aids are not an appropriate option (for example auditory atresia, chronically discharging middle ear etc.). Furthermore, in single-sided deafness, BCIs are reliable options for providing binaural cues to those individuals (den Besten et al., 2019; Hampton et al., 2022; Kruyt et al., 2020; Mylanus et al., 2020; Pai et al., 2012).

History

The concept of bone conduction hearing is old and is known since at least as early as the first century AD. However, the application of the concept to hearing devices took several centuries. Girolamo Cardano, an Italian physicist in the early sixteenth century, was among the earliest to demonstrate how sound may be transmitted to the ear by means of a rod or shaft of a spear held between one's teeth. These experiments were described as a curiosity rather than having practical value. It was in the seventeenth and eighteenth centuries that these experiments were applied clinically as aids in the form of teeth stimulators to the hearing impaired. This was also the birth of the functional diagnosis of hearing disorders; the patients benefitting from the teeth stimulators were believed to have a disease of the tympanic membrane, and those who did not benefit were believed to have a lesion in the auditory nerve. In the late nineteenth century, various devices like the Fonifero, the Audiophone, and the Dentaphone were developed and gained popularity. At the start of the twentieth century, the advancement of carbon microphone made it possible to create the bone vibrator that could be placed on the mastoid. Initially, the vibrator was held by a lorgnette handle. Soon, the vibrator was mounted onto a headband, and later onto eyeglasses (Berger, 1976).

First Bone Conduction Implant: Bone-Anchored Hearing Aid (BAHA)

Eventually, as the problem of loss of sound through the soft tissues of the mastoid was understood, the idea to implant the vibrator into the mastoid was developed and the first BAHA was implanted by Anders Tjellström in 1977 (Mudry & Tjellstrom, 2011). Initially, the surgical procedure was a two-step process to allow osseointegration of the implant into the mastoid bone. This still remains the procedure in young children; however, in adults, a one-stage procedure is recommended. Soft tissue reduction was later added to the procedure to reduce soft tissue complications. Passive and active transcutaneous devices were later introduced where the internal component is fixed to the skull, and the external component is attached to it through intact skin via a magnet. The surgical procedure about the bone anchored hearing aids is discussed in detail in Chapter. 7.

Classification of Bone Conduction Implants and Their Components

The Food and Drug Administration (FDA) has approved three types of bone conduction implants to date. These include Percutaneous BCI (pBCI), Transcutaneous BCI (tBCI) and Active BCI (aBCI). Figure 6.1 shows schematic representation of

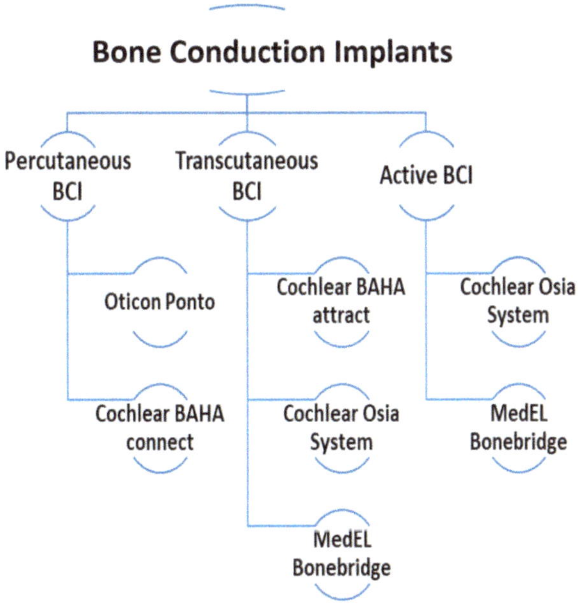

Fig. 6.1 Types of bone conduction implants and the models available from various manufacturers under the umbrella of each type

the types of bone conduction implants. Each of the BCIs has its own advantages and limitations.

Percutaneous BCI (pBCI)

These devices involve a titanium implant that penetrates the skin to transmit vibrations directly to the skull. The examples include devices like Cochlear Baha, and Oticon Ponto. Three major parts make up a percutaneous bone conduction implants: an abutment, a titanium screw, and a processor (Fig. 6.2).

The patient must undergo temporal bone surgery to fit the titanium screw under general or local anaesthesia (more details in Chap. 7). After implantation, the screw needs roughly 3 months for adults and 6 months for children for osseointegration. Osseointegration is the process by which an implant, typically made of titanium or a similar material, fuses directly with the bone. This allows the implant to become securely anchored in the bone, providing stability and support for the bone conduction hearing devices. Once osseointegration has taken place, an enduring skin-penetrating abutment can affix the external receiver to the implant.

Compared to other BCIs, percutaneous BCIs offer several advantages and a few drawbacks. Percutaneous BCI's strength is direct bone coupling which provides efficient sound transmission. The risk of skin infections or irritation at the implant site is one of the challenges. The other practical advantage is the possibility of implant placement under local anesthesia, which lowers patient anesthesia risk and expensive operating room time. Most patients have improved hearing thresholds irrespective of unilateral or bilateral implantation. Additionally, since the abutment does not produce a significant artifact like the magnets from the percutaneous and active BCIs, pBCIs is the best choice for patients needing repeated Magnetic resonance imaging (MRI). The primary drawback is caused by the abutment's close proximity to the skin. A study has found that about 14% of patients have skin overgrowth, granulation tissue development, keloids, infections, and other soft

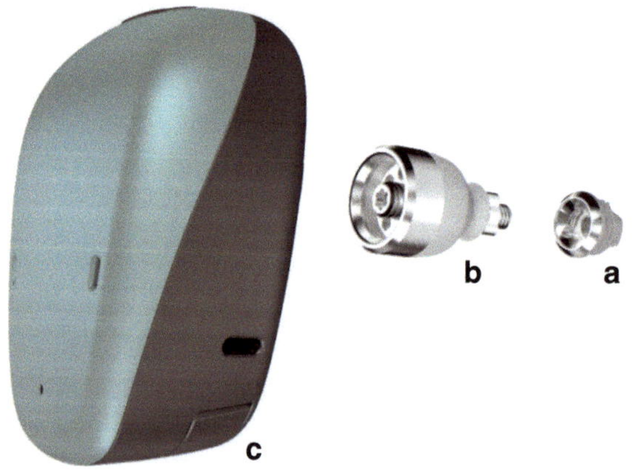

Fig. 6.2 A percutaneous bone conduction implant Cochlear™ Baha® 6 Max Connect System with its components (**a**) implant (**b**) abutment (**c**) sound processor

tissue problems post implantation (Iseri et al., 2015). The bone conduction implant surgery, and risk and complications associated with it are discussed in Chapter. 7. Most of these consequences can be adequately handled by modifying daily hygiene, receiving outpatient antibiotic medication, or undergoing clinic procedures like debridement or cautery of granulation tissue (Richards et al., 2020). Children and patients with a history of implant trauma are more likely to experience complications, which may call for additional medications or treatments (Dun et al., 2012; Iseri et al., 2015). Additionally, many patients may have significant aesthetic concerns since the transcutaneous abutment always protrudes from the post-auricular skin, whether or not the processor is in place (Iseri et al., 2015).

Transcutaneous BCI (tBCI)

Transcutaneous BCI uses an intact skin interface, with external and internal components connected magnetically. Examples include devices like Cochlear Baha Attract and MED-EL Bonebridge. A titanium screw placed into the mastoid bone, a subcutaneous magnet, and an external processor make up the fundamental elements of these implants, which are comparable to those found in pBCIs. The main distinction is the method by which the processor is connected to the implant. Transcutaneous BCIs employ magnets to attach the processor to a totally subcutaneous abutment and transmit the sound to an internal transducer. The external processor may be set up and configured around a month after implantation.

Compared to other BCIs, the transcutaneous BCIs provide several advantages, but also have some disadvantages. The tBCI is more aesthetically preferable because no external component is visible when the processor is taken out, with only an outline of the subdermal magnet. Patients may feel that tBCIs are simple for use and maintenance of hygiene is less complicated. However, the powerful magnet's continual pressure, which is necessary for this design to transfer vibrations to the internal magnet, may reduce patient pleasure (Richards et al., 2020). Over the magnet site, patients may experience erythema, discomfort, and even skin necrosis. The internal tBCI components must be implanted under general anesthesia or closely controlled sedation since doing so involves more extensive dissection. The surgery, risk and complications details about the transcutaneous BCI is mentioned in Chapter. 7. Finally, since the Baha Attract, which is 11 cm in diameter, creates a strong artifact, it should not be utilized on patients who may eventually require an MRI of the internal auditory canal (IAC) (Jansson et al., 2015; Kohan & Ghossaini, 2019).

The major drawbacks of transcutaneous BCIs are their audiological restrictions. In contrast to pBCIs, tBCIs have increased acoustic signal attenuation due to the presence of soft tissue between the implant and processor. Experimental simulations suggest that a percutaneous device may produce sound input that is at least 10 dB louder than a comparable transcutaneous device (Hol et al., 2013), with the discrepancy growing at higher frequencies. Because of this, the tBCI's hearing advantages are most significant at lower speech frequencies, but effectiveness decreases over 3000 Hz (Magele et al., 2019). In the presence of noise, this high-frequency roll-off is particularly detrimental to speech comprehension. A few studies directly examining audiometric results show that transcutaneous devices perform worse than percutaneous devices in improving speech reception threshold (Iseri et al., 2015) and poorer improvement at high frequencies (Hol et al., 2013; Iseri et al., 2015).

Active Bone Conduction Implants (aBCI)

Active bone conduction implants feature an actuator surgically implanted to stimulate the bone directly. These systems bypass the skin's barrier to improve sound transmission and reduce complications associated with external interfaces. The examples of the device include MED-EL Bonebridge (Fig. 6.3) and Cochlear Osia system (Fig. 6.4). The MEDEL Bonebridge and Cochlear Osia BCIs are programmed using SYMFIT and Osia fitting software, respectively.

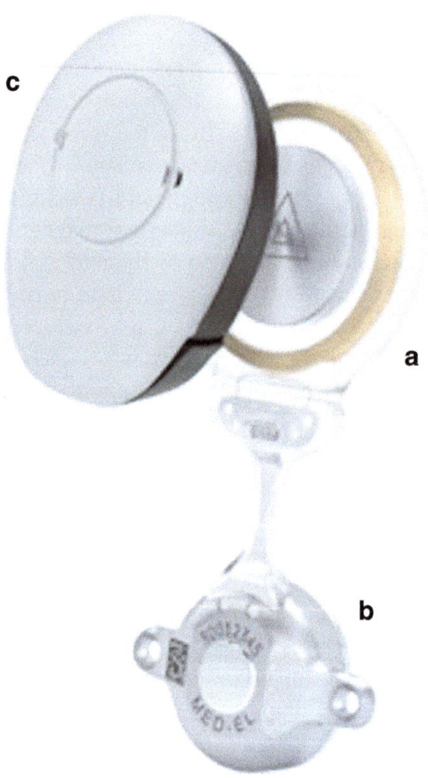

Fig. 6.3 An active bone conduction implant BoneBridge™ having (**a**) BCI602 implant (**b**) Bone conduction floating mass transducer (BC-FMT) (**c**) Samba sound processor

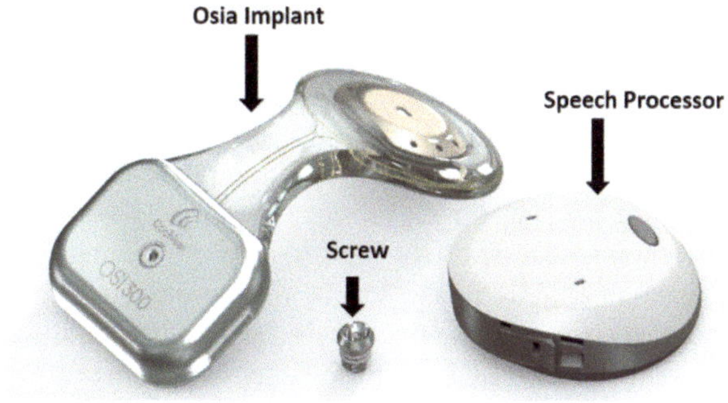

Fig. 6.4 An active bone conduction implant Cochlear™ Osia300® System. consisting of Implant, Screw, and Sound processor

The MED-EL bonebridge is an active transcutaneous implant using a bone conduction floating mass transducer (BC-FMT) placed within the skull. The Cochlear Osia System is a piezoelectric implant system that combines an implantable actuator (Osia OSI200 Implant) with an external sound processor (Osia 2). The piezoelectric stimulation mechanism ensures efficient vibration transmission to the cochlea.

In 2018, the FDA gave approval to a new category of bone conduction implants called active BCIs. Currently, the MED-EL Bonebridge and the Cochlear Osia are the two aBCIs available for commercial use. These implants consist of both external and internal parts. The external components include a sound processor with microphone, a magnet, and a coil for transmitting the signal through the skin. The internal components, which consist of a magnet and receiver coil, work together to directly stimulate an implant placed on the mastoid.

The MED-EL Bonebridge is kept in place by two titanium screws that transmit sound vibrations to the bone, and it employs a floating mass transducer to convert electrical impulses into mechanical vibrations (Schmerber et al., 2017). Piezoelectric material is put in place with a single screw mechanism in the Cochlear Osia to generate broad mechanical stress and vibrations in response to an electric charge (Goycoolea et al., 2020).

The patient receives several advantages from the active BCI. Since there is no visible abutment, the active BCI system offers the same advantages as the transcutaneous BCI system by using a magnet to link the internal and exterior components. Similar aesthetic and hygiene-related advantages to transcutaneous BCI systems are provided by the absence of an external abutment, with a low incidence of unfavourable soft tissue responses and skin problems (Goycoolea et al., 2020). Additionally, compared to those used in tBCIs, transcutaneous magnets utilized in aBCIs might be of lesser strength since the vibrator in these devices is not connected to the processor, and is in direct contact with the temporal bone. Compared to the tBCI and pBCI, this leads to fewer skin problems and greater patient comfort (Goycoolea et al., 2020). The major advantages of the active BCIs are associated with improvement of sound quality due to direct stimulation of the bone, lower risk of skin infections as compared to percutaneous devices and better aesthetics and patient comfort. The major challenges with aBCI are increased surgical complexity and dependence on compatibility between internal and external components for optimal function. The surgery, risk and complications associated with the a BCI is mentioned in Chapter. 7.

The active BCI may be activated 2–4 weeks after surgical implantation and does not require a lengthy osseointegration phase. aBCIs enhance output from 2500 to 6500 Hz and offer a high-frequency hearing boost, in contrast to the soft tissue attenuation that restricts high-frequency hearing gains in transcutaneous BCIs (Rigato et al., 2016). The Profile of Hearing Aid Benefit, which measures communication ease, communication in favourable conditions, and reverberations, also found that active BCIs perform better overall in real-world scenarios (Rigato et al., 2016). Additionally, patients claim to use their hearing implants more frequently than those who use similar equipment throughout the day (Goycoolea et al., 2020). There are certain drawbacks with aBCI systems as well. People with bone conduction thresholds (sensorineural hearing loss levels) no higher than 55 dBHL are recommended for these devices. As a result, individuals with more severe sensorineural loss (above 55 dBHL to up to 65 dBHL) would require a tBCI or pBCI. Additionally, the implant has a significant MRI artifact due to the internal magnet, which, like the pBCI, might impede the view of important structures (Jansson et al., 2015).

Those individuals who are reluctant to undergo surgical procedures for bone conduction implantation, have options for other non-surgical bone conduction devices such as SoundArc, ADHEAR and SoundBite. Non-surgical devices can be worn on a headband, soft band, or eyeglasses, or can be attached directly to the skin with an adhesive (Wazen et al., 2003). This option is best suited for children who are not old enough for the surgical procedure or adults whose hearing loss is mild or who cannot/do not want to have surgery. It may be used for trial which allows the patients to take an informed decision about proceeding with the surgery and gives them an insight into the quality of hearing they can expect post-operatively. The non-surgical bone conduction device worn on a Softband or a SoundArc is now described by the Cochlear™ Corporation as Baha® Start (Verstraeten et al., 2009) (Fig. 6.5).

In non-surgical devices, the external device remains in contact with the skin and vibrates in response to sound. These vibratory signals are then transmitted through the intact skin and soft tissue to the skull, eventually leading to bone conduction hearing. However, with these devices, higher frequency sounds tend to be

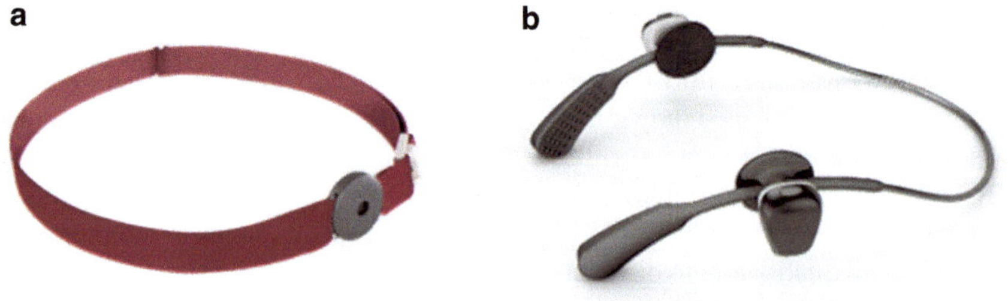

Fig. 6.5 Non-surgical bone conduction devices with (**a**) Baha Soft band (**b**) SoundArc™ (Cochlear™ Baha® Start)

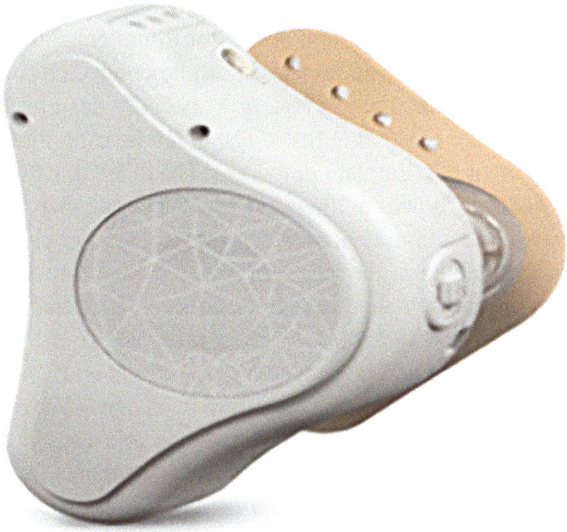

Fig. 6.6 Non-surgical bone conduction device with an adhesive option: ADHEAR by MED-EL®

attenuated by transmission as the signal travels through soft tissue and unpleasant levels of feedback can occur which can affect the device wearing time (Skarzynski et al., 2019). An adhesive option, the ADHEAR from MED-EL is also commercially available (Fig. 6.6).

In ADHEAR, an adhesive is applied to the skin over the mastoid bone and the sound processor is attached to it. The processor vibrates in response to sound and drives the vibratory signals through the skin and soft tissue to the underlying bone (Sprinzl & Wolf-Magele, 2016). Another non-surgical device is the SoundBite™ (Sonitus Technologies, San Mateo, CA, USA), which is a dental appliance that transmits vibratory signals to the skull via the teeth (Gurgel & Shelton, 2013). The SoundBite™ consists of a piezoelectric transducer placed on the maxillary molars on their buccal surface and a microphone is placed in the hearing-impaired individual's ear.

Candidacy Evaluation of Bone Conduction Implants

The candidacy evaluation for implanted bone conduction devices is done through an audiometric examination. In particular, bone conduction pure tone thresholds at 250, 500, 1000, 1500, 2000, 3000, and 4000 Hz should be measured. Furthermore, masked bone conduction thresholds should be measured for each ear. In addition, air conduction pure tone thresholds at cotave frequencies (and if needed, at mid-octave frequencies) between 250 and 8000 Hz for each ear must also be examined. In non-cooperative or difficult to test cases, bone conduction auditory brainstem responses can be useful. Measuring speech recognition scores can help predict post-implant performance. Further, adults and older children should be tested with a bone-conduction sound processor to understand bone-conduction devices viability better. The sound processor can be connected to a soft headband, a metal headband, a test band, a test rod, or a specially designed head-worn coupler to conduct pre-operative listening tests. The aided hearing thresholds are likely excellent predictors of post-implant outcomes. The aided thresholds acquired with a test band or test rod are, however, likely to be less accurate than that with percutaneous implanted bone conduction devices. According to Kurz et al. (2014), percutaneous implanted bone conduction devices had warbled tone thresholds of 5 to 10 dB higher than those of transcutaneous devices between 1000 and 2000 Hz and 10 to 25 dB higher between 4000 and 8000 Hz (Kurz et al., 2014). In speech audiometry, word recognition scores should be carried out for people with conductive and mixed hearing loss in the sound field at a presentation level consistent with typical conversational level speech (60 dBA/65 dB SPL) and also at a presentation level consistent with soft speech (i.e., 50 dBA/45 dB SPL). Performance levels attained in the unaided and aided situations and in the air conduction hearing aid and bone conduction conditions should be compared. An additional test, speech recognition in noise, might help the audiologist understand individuals' ability in the presence of noise and gather information to decide about the BCIs.

A candidate with single sided deafness should undergo a modified version of a usual listening test. Word recognition score in quiet is unlikely to alter between unaided and aided circumstances since the better-hearing ear has a normal auditory function. Consequently, words/sentence recognition in noise [for example, Bamford-Kowal-Bench Speech-in-Noise (BKB-SIN) test, Quick Speech in Noise (QuickSIN) test, Hearing in Noise Test (HINT)] should be performed with and without the bone conduction sound processor. Loudspeakers should be positioned at 90° azimuth and 270° azimuth of the listener, respectively. The loudspeaker next to the ear with poorer hearing should play the target signal, while the loudspeaker next to the ear with better hearing should play the unwanted noise signal. Using adaptive speech recognition in noise is the simplest approach to show how a bone conduction device helps a listener with single sided deafness (SSD). The benefits a bone conduction device may offer for a candidate with SSD when the signal of interest arrives at the side of the poorer ear in a noisy environment should be predicted by the difference in the signal-to-noise ratio (SNR) required for 50% correct performance between the unaided and aided conditions. To estimate the presentation level required for 50% accurate performance in the unaided condition, the audiologist may also alter the level of the competing noise signal. The testing can then be performed in both the unaided and aided situations at the same fixed SNR. The improvement in the SNR in the aided condition once again serves as a predictor of potential benefits in noise. In addition to audiological evaluation, the complete evaluation for the candidacy of bone conduction implants may entail speech and language testing, psychological tests, and any other additional evaluation from other professionals that may be felt necessay on a case-to-case basis. Although not always applicable, it may specifically be helpful to predict speech, language, and functional outcomes post-implantation.

Furthermore, it may also help to provide reasonable expectations for the parents of children with multiple problems regarding speech and language development.

Outcomes of Bone Conduction Implants

The post-implantation prognosis of bone conduction devices depends on the audiometric characteristics and expectations of the client. The benefit may differ based on the type and degree of hearing loss. In patients with conductive / mixed hearing loss, who have bone conduction thresholds in the normal to mild hearing loss range, an implanted bone conduction device will often produce a significant increase in audibility. Poorer outcomes in implanted bone conduction devices are more likely in patients with poorer bone conduction thresholds. The preoperative assessment with a bone conduction sound processor on a test band or soft band can better predict post-implantation outcomes with those with poorer BC thresholds.

Unilateral Conductive Hearing Loss/ Mixed Hearing Loss

People with unilateral conductive hearing loss may hear conversational speech via their normal-hearing side. When the target signal is towards the poorer ear, the head shadow effect may make it challenging to hear high-frequency (>1500 Hz) speech sounds. So, when the target signal comes from the side of the poorer ear, unilateral conductive hearing loss patients will see an improvement in speech recognition in quiet when using a BCI. A study by Snik and colleagues found that 4 out of the 8 subjects had a statistically significant improvement in their SRT in quiet when speech stimuli were presented via a loudspeaker situated at 0° azimuth while using the bone conduction implant (Snik et al., 2002). Similarly, Kunst et al. (2008) found that using a bone conduction sound processor improves the SRT in some patients with unilateral conductive hearing loss compared to the unaided condition (Kunst et al., 2008). However, there was no statistically significant improvement in speech recognition in the presence of noise between the groups; though most participants had better speech perception scores when noise was presented towards the better-hearing ear. Studies evaluating the possible improvement in speech recognition in noise offered by implantable bone conduction implants for those with unilateral conductive hearing loss show mixed success. A review indicated a dearth of compelling data supporting the audiological advantages of BCI for people with unilateral conductive hearing loss (Danhauer et al., 2010). Studies done by Hol et al. (2005) and Priwin et al. (2007) concluded that BC devices are helpful for unilateral conductive hearing loss (CHL), especially when the air-bone gap is 50 dB or more. To sum up, a bone conduction implant is expected to enhance speech recognition in noise when the target signal comes from the side of the worse ear for those with unilateral conductive hearing loss. Similarly, a bone conduction implant may help with speech recognition when the noise is towards the better-hearing ear.

The outcomes concerning the localization in unilateral CHL also inconsistent. Five out of the eight individuals in the Snik et al. (2002) study had a considerable improvement in localization (Snik et al., 2002), while 20 subjects did not show a statistically significant increase in their mean localization ability in a study by Kunst and colleagues (Kunst et al., 2008). In conclusion, some patients with unilateral conductive hearing loss may benefit (show improved localization) from a bone conduction implant, but not all. More studies are needed to evaluate the prognosis of BCI concerning localization.

Bilateral Conductive Hearing Loss/ Mixed Hearing Loss

An implanted bone conduction device can significantly enhance audibility for people with bilateral conductive hearing loss. Implantable bone conduction devices have been proven to substantially increase speech recognition in quiet and warbled tone sound-field thresholds compared to the unaided situation. Speech recognition in quiet should improve with a bone conduction implant due to the improvement in audibility, especially when the speech is towards the front or the side of the implanted ear. When the speech is towards the side of the non-implanted ear, the head shadow effect may make it difficult for recipients of unilateral implantable bone conduction device to recognize speech. Therefore, bone conduction implantation is a viable option for people with bilateral conductive hearing loss. An implantable bone conduction device will also almost certainly improve speech recognition in noise for people with significant conductive or mixed hearing loss due to improved audibility. The SRT is improved with bilateral BCI as compared to unilateral. A study by Priwin and colleagues observed a 5.8 dB improvement in the SRT in quiet with bilateral implantable bone conduction device over the unaided condition (Priwin et al., 2004). The use of bilateral implantable bone conduction devices has been shown to improve speech recognition in noise compared to the use of a unilateral implantable bone conduction device (Bosman et al., 2001; Colquitt et al., 2011; Janssen et al., 2012; Priwin et al., 2004). A study reported that the bilateral bone conduction devices resulted in a 2.8 dB increase in the SNR for 50% accurate performance in noise compared to unilateral usage (Priwin et al., 2004). However, studies have also shown that when competing noise is towards the side of the better-hearing ear, bilateral BCI might cause a slight decline in speech recognition in the presence of noise (compared to the unilateral condition) (Janssen et al., 2012; Priwin et al., 2004). The use of bilateral implantable bone conduction devices significantly improves spatial hearing ability compared to unilateral implantation in people with bilateral conductive hearing loss (Bosman et al., 2001; Colquitt et al., 2011; Janssen et al., 2012; Priwin et al., 2004). Overall, using a BCI will probably improve speech recognition in quiet and noisy environments for people with bilateral conductive hearing loss. Additionally, compared to a unilateral BCI, using bilateral BCI offers greater audibility, speech recognition in quiet and noise, and localization.

Single-Sided Deafness (SSD)

The reduction of the head shadow effect is the main advantage of an implanted bone conduction device for those with single-sided sensorineural deafness. The bone conduction device will probably improve speech recognition in quiet and in noise when speech originates from the side of hearing loss (Bosman et al., 2003; Hol et al., 2004; Lin et al., 2006; Wazen et al., 2003). However, using a BCI does not increase speech recognition of noise when speech is coming from the front, and the noise is diffused. Additionally, using a BCI may reduce speech recognition in noise when the speech signal is towards the front or the side of the ear with better hearing and the competing noise primarily comes from the side of the ear with poorer hearing (Bosman et al., 2003; Hol et al., 2004; Lin et al., 2006; Wazen et al., 2003). Studies on localization have typically demonstrated that using an implanted bone conduction device does not improve a single-sided deaf person's spatial hearing (Bosman et al., 2003; Hol et al., 2004; Lin et al., 2006; Nicolas et al., 2013). Nicolas et al. (2013) studied 36 people with single-sided deafness with BCI and looked at long-term satisfaction and performance. Findings suggested that 82% of individuals used their bone conduction sound processor for more than 4 hours per day, while 64% used it for more than 8 hours per day. Additionally, the subjects generally stated that their bone conduction implants were helpful in everyday life usage, even though localization did not improve and only slight gains were detected in speech recognition in noise (Nicolas et al., 2013). In brief, using an implanted bone conduction device will help people with single-sided deafness avoid the head shadow effect, but it is unlikely to significantly enhance speech recognition in noisy environments or spatial hearing abilities significantly. However, patients who do well in a preoperative trial with a bone conduction sound processor worn on a test band or soft band are more likely to benefit from using an implanted bone conduction device in a real-world setting. Overall, bone conduction implants are reported to have mixed finding in terms of audiological outcome, yet they may be useful for several patients with unilateral/bilateral conductive hearing loss as well as in single sided deafness.

References

Berger, K. W. (1976). Early bone conduction hearing aid devices. *Archives of Otolaryngology, 102*(5), 315–318.

Bosman, A. J., Snik, A. M., van der Pouw, C. T. M., Mylanus, E. A. M., & Cremers, C. W. R. J. (2001). Audiometric evaluation of bilaterally fitted bone-anchored hearing aids. *International Journal of Audiology, 40*(3), 158–167.

Bosman, A. J., Hol, M. K., Snik, A. F., Mylanus, E. A., & Cremers, C. W. (2003). Bone-anchored hearing aids in unilateral inner ear deafness. *Acta Oto-Laryngologica, 123*(2), 258–260.

Colquitt, J. L., Loveman, E., Baguley, D. M., Mitchell, T. E., Sheehan, P. Z., Harris, P., et al. (2011). Bone-anchored hearing aids for people with bilateral hearing impairment: A systematic review. *Clinical Otolaryngology, 36*(5), 419–441.

Danhauer, J. L., Johnson, C. E., & Mixon, M. (2010). Does the evidence support use of the Baha implant system (Baha) in patients with congenital unilateral aural atresia? *Journal of the American Academy of Audiology, 21*(4), 274–286.

den Besten, C. A., Monksfield, P., Bosman, A., Skarzynski, P. H., Green, K., Runge, C., Wigren, S., Blechert, J. I., Flynn, M. C., Mylanus, E. A. M., & Hol, M. K. S. (2019). Audiological and clinical outcomes of a transcutaneous bone conduction hearing implant: Six-month results from a multicentre study. *Clinical Otolaryngology, 44*(2), 144–157.

Dun, C. A. J., Faber, H. T., De Wolf, M. J. F., Mylanus, E. A. M., Cremers, C. W. R. J., & Hol, M. K. S. (2012). Assessment of more than 1,000 implanted percutaneous bone conduction devices: Skin reactions and implant survival. *Otology and Neurotology, 33*(2), 192–198.

Goycoolea, M., Ribalta, G., Tocornal, F., Levy, R., Alarcón, P., Bryman, M., Cagnacci, B., Catenacci, C., Oyanguren, V., Vilches, I., Briones, V., & García, R. (2020). Clinical performance of the OsiaTM system, a new active osseointegrated implant system. Results from a prospective clinical investigation. *Acta Oto-Laryngologica, 140*(3), 212–219.

Gurgel, R. K., & Shelton, C. (2013). The SoundBite hearing system: Patient-assessed safety and benefit study. *The Laryngoscope, 123*(11), 2807–2812.

Hampton, T., Milinis, K., Whitehall, E., & Sharma, S. (2022). Association of bone conduction devices for single-sided sensorineural deafness with quality of life: A systematic review and meta-analysis. *JAMA Otolaryngology–Head & Neck Surgery, 148*(1), 35–42.

Hol, M. K. S., Bosman, A. J., Snik, A. F. M., Mylanus, E. A. M., & Cremers, C. W. R. J. (2004). Bone-anchored hearing aid in unilateral inner ear deafness: A study of 20 patients. *Audiology and Neuro-Otology, 9*(5), 274–281.

Hol, M. K. S., Snik, A. F. M., Mylanus, E. A. M., & Cremers, C. W. R. J. (2005). Does the bone-anchored hearing aid have a complementary effect on audiological and subjective outcomes in patients with unilateral conductive hearing loss? *Audiology and Neurotology, 10*(3), 159–168.

Hol, M. K. S., Nelissen, R. C., Agterberg, M. J. H., Cremers, C. W. R. J., & Snik, A. F. M. (2013). Comparison between a new implantable transcutaneous bone conductor and percutaneous bone-conduction hearing implant. *Otology and Neurotology, 34*(6), 1071–1075.

Iseri, M., Orhan, K. S., Tuncer, U., Kara, A., Durgut, M., Guldiken, Y., & Surmelioglu, O. (2015). Transcutaneous bone-anchored hearing aids versus percutaneous ones: Multicenter comparative clinical study. *Otology and Neurotology, 36*(5), 849–853.

Janssen, R. M., Hong, P., & Chadha, N. K. (2012). Bilateral bone-anchored hearing aids for bilateral permanent conductive hearing loss: A systematic review. *Otolaryngology – Head and Neck Surgery, 147*(3), 412–422.

Jansson, K. J. F., Håkansson, B., Reinfeldt, S., Rigato, C., & Eeg-Olofsson, M. (2015). Magnetic resonance imaging investigation of the bone conduction implant—A pilot study at 1.5 tesla. *Medical Devices: Evidence and Research, 8*, 413–423.

Kohan, D., & Ghossaini, S. N. (2019). Osseointegrated auditory devices-transcutaneous: Sophono and Baha attract. *Otolaryngologic Clinics of North America, 52*(2), 253–263.

Kruyt, I. J., Monksfield, P., Skarzynski, P. H., Green, K., Runge, C., Bosman, A., Blechert, J. I., Wigren, S., Mylanus, E. A. M., & Hol, M. K. S. (2020). Results of a 2-year prospective multicenter study evaluating long-term audiological and clinical outcomes of a transcutaneous implant for bone conduction hearing. *Otology and Neurotology, 41*(7), 901–911.

Kunst, S. J. W., Hol, M. K. S., Mylanus, E. A. M., Leijendeckers, J. M., Snik, A. F. M., & Cremers, C. W. R. J. (2008). Subjective benefit after BAHA system application in patients with congenital unilateral conductive hearing impairment. *Otology and Neurotology, 29*(3), 353–358.

Kurz, A., Flynn, M., Caversaccio, M., & Kompis, M. (2014). Speech understanding with a new implant technology: A comparative study with a new nonskin penetrating Baha system. *BioMed Research International, 2014*(1), 416205.

Lin, L. M., Bowditch, S., Anderson, M. J., May, B., Cox, K. M., & Niparko, J. K. (2006). Amplification in the rehabilitation of unilateral deafness: Speech in noise and directional hearing effects with bone-anchored hearing and contralateral routing of signal amplification. *Otology and Neurotology, 27*(2), 172–182.

Magele, A., Schoerg, P., Stanek, B., Gradl, B., & Sprinzl, G. M. (2019). Active transcutaneous bone conduction hearing implants: Systematic review and meta-analysis. *PLoS One, 14*(9), e0221484.

Mudry, A., & Tjellström, A. (2011). Historical background of bone conduction hearing devices and bone conduction hearing aids. In *Implantable bone conduction hearing aids* (Vol. 71, pp. 1–9). Karger Publishers.

Mylanus, E. A. M., Hua, H., Wigren, S., Arndt, S., Skarzynski, P. H., Telian, S. A., & Briggs, R. J. S. (2020). Multicenter clinical investigation of a new active osseointegrated steady-state implant system. *Otology & Neurotology, 41*(9), 1249–1257.

Nicolas, S., Mohamed, A., Yoann, P., Laurent, G., & Thierry, M. (2013). Long-term benefit and sound localization in patients with single-sided deafness rehabilitated with an osseointegrated bone-conduction device. *Otology and Neurotology, 34*(1), 111–114.

Pai, I., Kelleher, C., Nunn, T., Pathak, N., Jindal, M., O'Connor, A. F., & Jiang, D. (2012). Outcome of bone-anchored hearing aids for single-sided deafness: A prospective study. *Acta Oto-Laryngologica, 132*(7), 751–755.

Priwin, C., Stenfelt, S., Granström, G., Tjellström, A., & Håkansson, B. (2004). Bilateral Bone-Anchored Hearing Aids (BAHAs): An audiometric evaluation. *Laryngoscope, 114*(1), 77–84.

Priwin, C., Jönsson, R., Hultcrantz, M., & Granström, G. (2007). BAHA in children and adolescents with unilateral or bilateral conductive hearing loss: A study of outcome. *International Journal of Pediatric Otorhinolaryngology, 71*(1), 135–145.

Richards, J. P., Symms, J. T., Beasley, K., & Coffman, H. M. (2020). Bone conduction implants. *Current Opinion in Otolaryngology & Head and Neck Surgery, 28*(5), 308–313.

Rigato, C., Reinfeldt, S., Hakansson, B., Freden Jansson, K. J., Hol, M. K. S., & Eeg-Olofsson, M. (2016). Audiometric comparison between the first patients with the transcutaneous bone conduction implant and matched percutaneous bone anchored hearing device users. *Otology and Neurotology, 37*(9), 1381–1387.

Schmerber, S., Deguine, O., Marx, M., Van de Heyning, P., Sterkers, O., Mosnier, I., Garin, P., Godey, B., Vincent, C., Venail, F., Mondain, M., Deveze, A., Lavieille, J. P., & Karkas, A. (2017). Safety and effectiveness of the Bonebridge transcutaneous active direct-drive bone-conduction hearing implant at 1-year device use. *European Archives of Oto-Rhino-Laryngology, 274*(4), 1835–1851.

Skarzynski, P. H., Ratuszniak, A., Osinska, K., Koziel, M., Krol, B., Cywka, K. B., & Skarzynski, H. (2019). A comparative study of a novel adhesive bone conduction device and conventional treatment options for conductive hearing loss. *Otology & Neurotology, 40*(7), 858–864.

Snik, A. F. M., Mylanus, E. A. M., & Cremers, C. W. R. J. (2002). The bone-anchored hearing aid in patients with a unilateral air-bone gap. *Otology and Neurotology, 23*(1), 61–66.

Sprinzl, G. M., & Wolf-Magele, A. (2016). The Bonebridge bone conduction hearing implant: Indication criteria, surgery and a systematic review of the literature. *Clinical Otolaryngology, 41*(2), 131–143.

Verstraeten, N., Zarowski, A. J., Somers, T., Riff, D., & Offeciers, E. F. (2009). Comparison of the audiologic results obtained with the bone-anchored hearing aid attached to the headband, the testband, and to the "snap" abutment. *Otology & Neurotology, 30*(1), 70–75.

Wazen, J. J., Spitzer, J. B., Ghossaini, S. N., Fayad, J. N., Niparko, J. K., Cox, K., Brackmann, D. E., & Soli, S. D. (2003). Transcranial contralateral cochlear stimulation in unilateral deafness. *Otolaryngology – Head and Neck Surgery, 129*(3), 248–254.

Chapter 7
Bone Conduction Implants: Surgical Perspectives

Sunil Narayan Dutt, Swathi Vadlamani, Aanchal Aggarwal Mittal, and Sumit Kumar Gaur

Abstract Bone conduction devices work by the principle of bone conduction hearing which works through the intact cochlear function regardless of the status of the external and middle ear function. The surgically implanted devices are classified as percutaneous and transcutaneous devices, and the transcutaneous devices include 'active' and 'passive'. Active transcutaneous devices are the newest bone conduction devices and have several advantages over their predecessors owing to their audiological benefits and reduced complications. Complications that may be encountered with surgical devices range from minor skin infections to severe necrosis sometimes requiring removal of the device. When done with meticulous techniques, surgical complications are rare and can be managed well. Bone conduction devices, when used for appropriate indications have proven to be extremely beneficial with significant improvement in patient satisfaction and audiological outcomes.

Keywords Bone conduction devices · Bone anchored hearing aids · Conductive hearing loss · Abutment · Osseointegration

Introduction

Bone Anchored Hearing Aid (BAHA) is a well-established device used in the field of otology and audiology. Owing to its improving technology over the past few decades, the term "Bone Conduction Device (BCD)/Bone Conduction Implants (BCI)" is being increasingly used instead of BAHA (Ellsperman et al., 2021). So, BCDs/BCIs and BAHAs are essentially the same, albeit BAHA is the device's brand name manufactured by the Cochlear™ Corporation. Bone conduction devices are used for hearing rehabilitation of patients who cannot be fitted with conventional hearing aids (Håkansson et al., 1990, 2019; Tjellström & Håkansson, 1995;

S. N. Dutt (✉) · S. Vadlamani · A. A. Mittal · S. K. Gaur
Department of ENT, Apollo Hospital, Bengaluru, India

P. Kumar et al. (eds.), *Advances in Implantation Otology*,
https://doi.org/10.1007/978-981-96-8671-1_7

McDermott et al., 2002). With a BCD, the sound is transmitted directly to the cochlea, bypassing the external and middle ears.

Principle of Bone Conduction Devices

Bone conduction devices, in general, work by the principle of bone conduction hearing, which is unique and works through the intact cochlear function regardless of the status of the external and middle ear function. Tjellström and Granström (1994) demonstrated that bone conduction hearing occurs by three mechanisms: (1) Inertial movement of middle ear ossicles and inner ear fluids, (2) Direct compression of the cochlea and (3) Sound vibrations in the skull coming from the external and middle ear spaces. The same mechanism was described later in detail by Stenfelt and Goode (2005), who added pressure transmission from the cerebrospinal fluid also as a contributor to bone conduction hearing. Using this principle of the natural form of hearing, bone conduction devices have been designed and are widely available today in various forms. Some of the surgically fitted bone conduction devices work on the principle of osseointegration, which is an interaction that occurs at the dynamic bone conduction implant-tissue interface (Stenfelt & Goode, 2005). A direct structural and functional connection is formed between the implant and the living bone, which is essential for implant stability and is a pre-requisite for implant loading and hence the long-term success of the implant. Osseointegration is a dynamic process that takes about 6–12 weeks to develop following implantation. The implant has to be completely immobile during this process, which is essential for its successful integration and function (Branemark, 1985).

Indications for Bone Conduction Devices

The indications for BCDs may be classified into clinical and audiological indications. As the audiological indications have been mentioned in the previous chapter (Chap. 6), only the clinical indications will be discussed in this chapter. Worldwide, the most common indication for placement of BCD is in patients with microtia and congenital aural atresia who have maximum conductive hearing loss but intact cochlear function (D'Editità et al., 2012). They are also advised in chronic mastoiditis, discharging ears, and otosclerosis (conductive hearing loss or mixed hearing loss) where conventional hearing aids cannot be used (Snik et al., 2005). Another important indication for BCD is single-sided deafness. In single-sided deafness, the BCD is placed on the diseased side, which utilizes the transcranial conduction property of the skull and is used to stimulate the intact cochlea on the normal hearing side (Macnamara et al., 1996; Schrøder et al., 2010). The clinical indications for BCD are illustrated in Table 7.1.

Table 7.1 Clinical indications for bone conduction devices/implants

Conductive hearing loss	**Ear pinna and canal:** Congenital aural atresia and microtia, Chronic eczema, Chronic discharging ears, acquired closure of the external auditory canal
	Middle ear: Chronic otitis media / Cholesteatoma /otosclerosis/ ossicular dislocation / discharging mastoid cavities/syndromic congenital ear malformations
Single sided deafness	Eighth nerve tumors (Ex: Acoustic neuroma), Idiopathic sudden unilateral SNHL, SNHL secondary to trauma or surgery of the middle ear, Meniere's disease, Congenital unilateral SNHL

Note: *SNHL* Sensorineural hearing loss

Bone conduction implant surgery is currently FDA-approved for children 5 years of age or older (Kulasegarah et al., 2018). Children too young for implantation or adult patients for whom surgery is contraindicated may use non-surgical bone conduction devices until they are old enough or allow the surgical procedure. Surgical procedures of four commonly used bone conduction devices/implants will be discussed. They are:

1. Cochlear™ Baha® Connect System (Percutaneous BCI)
2. Cochlear™ Baha® Attract System (Transcutaneous passive BCI)
3. Bonebridge™ (MED-EL) (Transcutaneous Active BCI)
4. Cochlear™ Osia® System (Transcutaneous Active BCI)

Cochlear Baha® Connect

Cochlear™ Baha® Connect is a percutaneous BCD made by the Cochlear™ Corporation. The system consists of an implant, a small abutment that connects the implant with the sound processor, and a sound processor, which is shown in Fig. 7.1. The sound vibrations from the sound processor are directly transmitted to the inner ear. Functionally, Cochlear™ Baha® Connect performs better when compared to the transcutaneous Cochlear™ Baha® Attract as the sound is directly transmitted without any attenuation from the skin. However, cosmetic troubles and maintenance of the device is a challenge owing to which, transcutaneous devices have been developed.

Single-Stage Surgery

The surgery can be done as a single or two-stage surgery. The implant site is marked around 50–70 mm behind the external auditory canal ensuring that the superior edge of the processor is in line with the top of the pinna. A linear incision is marked in the direction of the hairline at least 10 mm anterior to the implant site. The skin flap

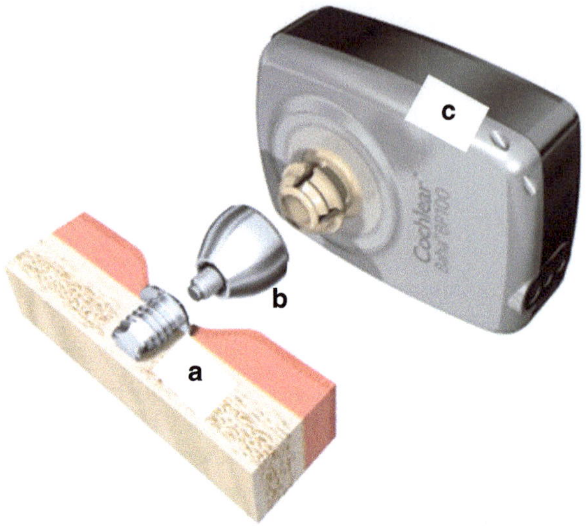

Fig. 7.1 Cochlear™ Baha® Connect System: Consists of (**a**) Implant (**b**) The abutment (**c**) Sound processor (BP100). (Image Courtesy of Cochlear Limited)

thickness can be measured at this point with the help of a hypodermic needle and a ruler. The local anesthesia is injected around the implant site. According to the measured skin thickness, an appropriate length of the abutment is chosen based on the suggested guidelines by the company. If the soft tissue flap is over thick (more than 14 mm), fat tissue is removed to achieve a thickness of around 11 mm (Ricci et al., 2011). Figure 7.2 A to I represents the different steps involved in the single or two-stage surgery.

A linear incision is made along the marked line down to the periosteum. A cruciate incision is then made in the periosteum to expose the bone just enough for the implant. A guide drill with a 3 mm spacer is used to drill a burr hole in the bone. The drilling has to be done at a perpendicular angle to the bone surface. The bottom of the hole needs to be checked regularly for bone and if there is adequate bone thickness, a depth of 4 mm can be achieved. Next, a widening drill is used to widen the previous burr hole to create a countersink in the bone. It is important to ensure that adequate coolant is used during the drilling. This is to preserve the osteocytes for osseointegration. The implant is then placed using the implant inserter using a torque setting at 40–50 Ncm. A punch hole is made in the skin next to the incision exactly where the abutment is placed. Skin edges have to be sharp and should not create an unwanted pocket around the abutment. The incision is then sutured. A healing cap with a plug is placed over the abutment. The dressing is to be applied beneath the healing cap to ensure a good seal between the hydroxyapatite coating and the full thickness of the surrounding tissue. Dressing can be removed around 2–3 weeks post-operatively.

The same surgery can be done in two stages in recommended cases where the bone thickness is less than 3 mm or where there is compromised or soft bone. The

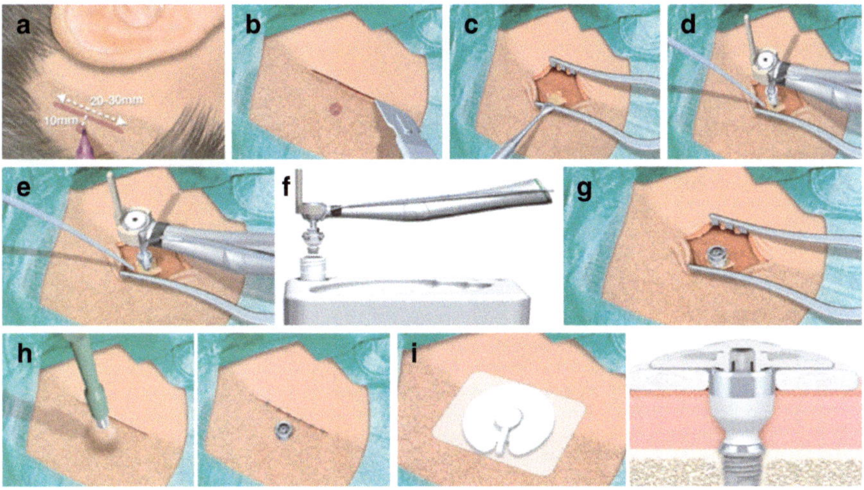

Fig. 7.2 (**a**) Marking of skin incision and the point of the abutment; (**b**) Incision; (**c**) Elevation of skin flap and incision of the periosteum; (**d**) Drill with guide drill; (**e**) Drill with widening drill; (**f**) Implant along with the abutment is lifted; (**g**) Implant is placed; (**h**) Skin is punched at the level of the abutment so that the abutment is exposed to the outside and the incision is sutured; (**i**) Healing cap is placed, and non-adherent dressing is done around the abutment

surgical steps are similar to that of one-stage surgery but the abutment is disconnected from the implant and only the implant is placed in the first stage. Placing a sleeper implant is recommended as there is a higher rate of implant loss in children. In such cases, a gap of at least 10 mm is maintained between the two implants. Next, a cover screw is inserted over the implant to protect the internal threads of the implant from bone and tissue overgrowth.

Two-Stage Surgery

In the second stage, the implant position is located and a skin incision is made at the same location as the first stage. Before making the incision, soft tissue thickness is measured with the help of a needle. Soft tissue reduction is done if the thickness is more than 14 mm. Periosteum is then exposed, and the implant with the cover screw is identified. The cover screw is removed with the help of a unigrip screwdriver. The abutment is then connected at a torque set to 25 Ncm. Using a biopsy punch, a skin hole is made at the level of the implant and the abutment, ensuring that the skin edges don't create an unwanted pocket around the abutment. The skin incision is sutured and the appropriate dressing is done in such a way that there is a good seal between the dressing and the healing cap. Dressing and the healing cap are removed 14 days post-operatively and the device is switched on.

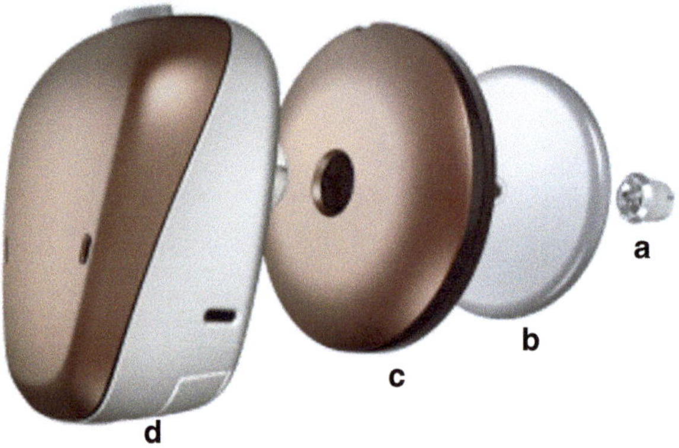

Fig. 7.3 Cochlear™ Baha Attract® System: Consists of (**a**) Implant (**b**) Internal Magnet (**c**) External Magnet (**d**) Sound processor. (Image Courtesy of Cochlear Limited)

Cochlear Baha® Attract

Cochlear™ Baha® Attract system is a transcutaneous bone conduction hearing device system that consists of a small titanium implant, an internal magnet, an external magnet, and a sound processor. The sound processor is attached to the external magnet, which attracts the internal magnet. The internal magnet is connected to the implant. Parts of the Cochlear™ Baha Attract System are given in Fig. 7.3. The sound vibrations from the processor are transmitted to the implant through the external magnet, skin and soft tissue of the skull, and the internal magnet. The implant vibrations then stimulate the intact cochlea, leading to bone conduction hearing. The implant and the internal magnet are surgically placed behind the ear (Ricci et al., 2011) (Fig. 7.4).

Preparation and Marking

The implant is placed around 50–70 mm postero-superior to the ear canal in line with the temporal line. A "C" shaped incision is marked anterior to the position of the magnet, ensuring that the sound processor and the sound processor magnet do not touch the pinna. Skin flap thickness is measured, and soft tissue reduction is done at a later stage if it is more than 6 mm.

Incision

The incision is given along the marked area, and a posteriorly based flap is raised at the level of the temporalis fascia. Then, an anterior inferiorly-based muscular flap is raised in such a way that the periosteum is still intact. Any soft tissue reduction of

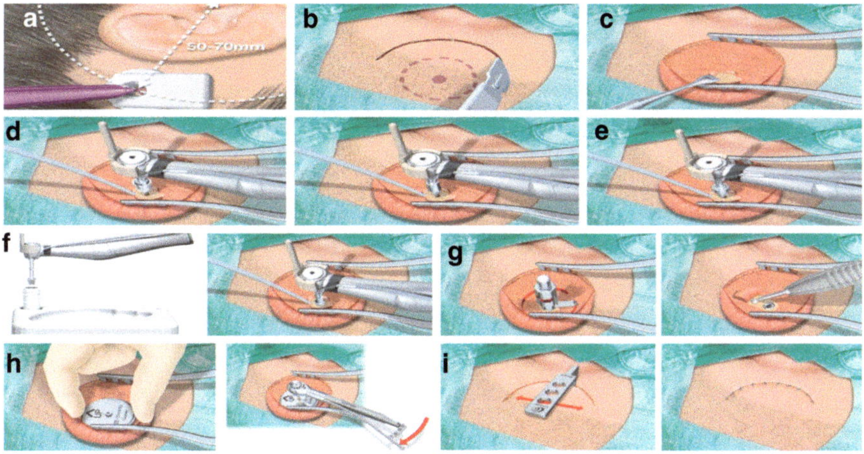

Fig. 7.4 (**a**) Marking of the skin incision; (**b**) Incision; (**c**) Raising of skin flap and incision of the periosteum; (**d**) Drill with guide drill with and without spacer; (**e**) Drilling with widening drill; (**f**) The implant is picked up using the implant inserter and placed; (**g**) Bone bed indicator is placed to check for the smooth bone surface and the excessive bone is drilled; (**h**) The implant magnet is attached and tightened to 25 Ncm torque; (**i**) Thickness of the flap is evaluated using a soft tissue gauge and the skin is sutured. **If the surgery is planned in two stages after the implant is placed, it is covered with the help of a cover screw, and the rest of the surgery is done in the second stage*

the flap can be done at this point. Bone bed indicator is used to ensure that the surface of the cranium is flat in the implant area. The incision is given on the periosteum at the point where marking has been previously done for the implant, and the periosteum is raised.

Placement of the Implant

There are two drills used: first, the guide drill is used to identify the depth of the cranium, and second, the counter sink drill is used to widen the well. The inserter is used to pick up the implant, and the implant is inserted with slow torque in such a way that it sits flush on the bone. The bone flatness identifier is hand screwed and encircled around to ensure that the surface of the cranium is flat around the implant. The internal magnet is then inserted over the screw, and low-power torque is used to fix it to the screw. The wound is then closed in layers. A pressure dressing is applied which is removed after a week. The implant is switched on with the speech processor after 3–4 weeks, allowing for osseointegration to happen.

MED-EL Bonebridge™

The Bonebridge™ (MED-EL, Innsbruck, Austria) consists of an external part, the audio processor, and an implanted part, the Bone Conduction Implant (BCI). BCI consists of a receiver coil, a demodulator, and a Bone Conduction Floating Mass Transducer (BC-FMT) (Fig. 7.5).

Bonebridge was first introduced in 2012 as BCI601, and in 2019, a newer internal part named BCI602 was launched. The difference between BCI601 and BCI602 is that the size of the BC-FMT has been narrowed down from 8.7 mm to 4.5 mm. So, the newer generation Bonebridge™ (BCI602) can be used with ease in limited anatomical conditions.

BC-FMT is implanted into the temporal bone with appropriate screws, and the receiver coil is secured under the postauricular periosteal pocket (Fig. 7.6). Bonebridge™ does not require osseointegration for its audiological performance. However, the BC-FMT with its screws needs to be osseointegrated for better fixation and prevention of complications. Typically, Bonebridge™ is switched on around 4 weeks after the surgery.

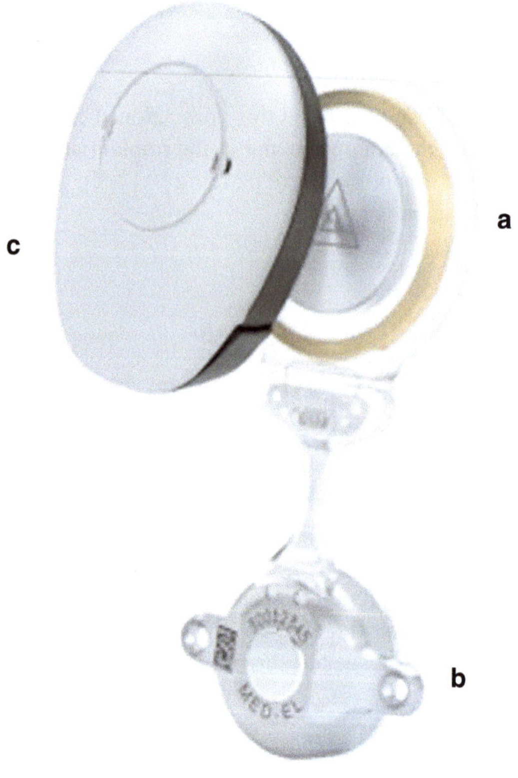

Fig. 7.5 The BoneBridge™ (**a**) BCI602 Implant; (**b**) BC-FMT (Bone Conduction-Floating Mass Transducer); (**c**) Samba Sound processor. (Image Courtesy of MED-EL Company)

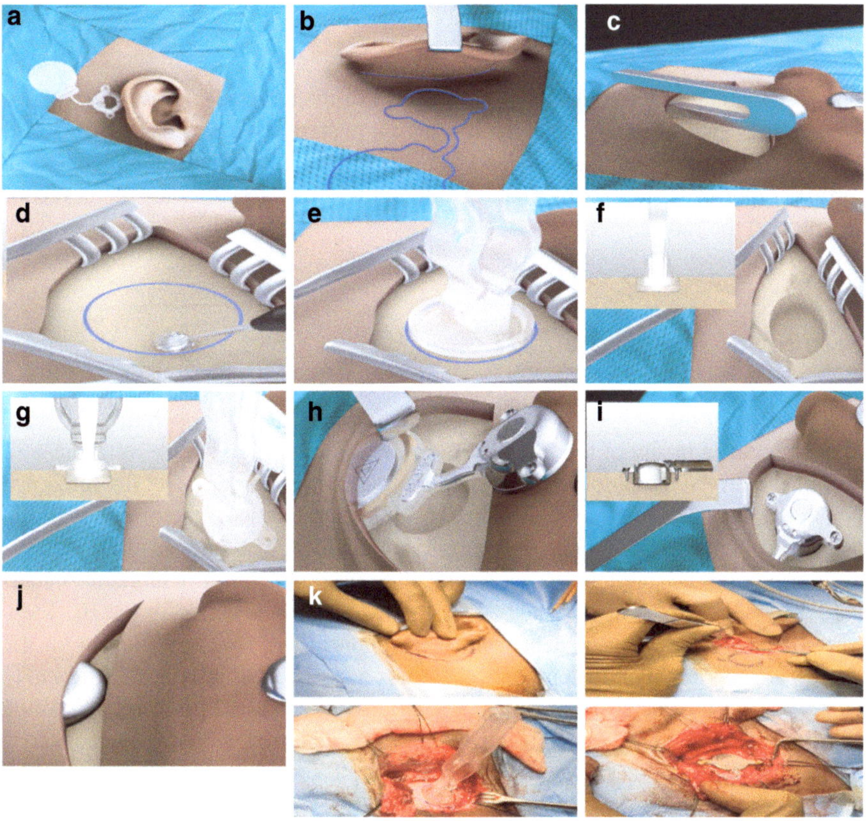

Fig. 7.6 (**a**) Position of the bonebridge implant; (**b**) Marking of skin incision and the implant; (**c**) Incision, periosteal pocket and measurement of thickness of the skin flap (to be <7 mm); (**d**) Position of BC-FMT is marked with the help of Transducer-sizer and drilling of the well for BC-FMT is done; (**e**) Checking the depth of the well with the help of Transducer-sizer; (**f**) The size of the well should be in flush with the size of the BC-FMT; (**g**) Flatness of the skull for the screws is checked; (**h**) Placement of the receiver coil in the periosteal pocket; (**i**) Fixation of BC-FMT in the bone well with screws; (**j**) Incision is closed in layers; (**k**) Intra-operative pictures of Bonebridge Implantation. (Image: MED-EL Company)

Preparation for Bonebridge Surgery

The procedure is usually done under general anesthesia, although it can be done under local anesthesia also. Preparation of the site starts with shaving the hair for at least 2 cm beyond the intended incision. The incision is marked 5 mm behind the post-auricular groove, leaving at least a 5 mm gap from the edge of the template. This is to minimize the risk of device extrusion and postoperative infections.

Incision

The incision is given and deepened to the level of the temporalis fascia. Skin flaps are elevated anteriorly and posteriorly. Next, a posteriorly-based or an anteriorly-based musculoperiosteal flap is raised and secured. The skin incision may be given further posteriorly in cases of microtia and aural atresia to allow for pinna reconstruction in the future.

Creation of Bed for BC-FMT

The position of the BC-FMT depends on the findings of the preoperative CT scan. It can be placed in any of the three locations, i.e., the sinodural angle, retromastoid portion, or on the temporal line. If it is placed at the sinodural angle, the reference points are the spine of Henley, the temporal line, and the tip of the mastoid. If it is placed in the retrosigmoid area, the digastric attachment and the mastoid tip are the reference points. Using the T-sizer, the position of the BC-FMT is marked. A standard drill is used to create a bone bed for the BC-FMT. The depth for the BC-FMT is verified with the help of depth-gauge assembly. If no line can be seen on the depth-gauge assembly, the depth of the bone is adequate. Otherwise, BCI lifts may be needed for the accurate placement of the BC-FMT. Next, a periosteal pocket is made to accommodate the coil and the demodulator of the BCI. The pocket is checked with the C-sizer in combination with the T-sizer. The thickness of the skin flap over the receiving coil should not exceed 7 mm. The thickness can be measured with the help of a skin flap gauge, and the flap can be thinned accordingly.

BCI Fixation

The holes for BCI fixation are made using the supplied drill bit and the stopper. Either the T-sizer or the Depth-gauge assembly is used as a guide for this process. The diameter of the drill bit is 1.5 mm. Next, the implant coil and the demodulator are placed in the periosteal pocket, and the BC-FMT is placed in the well. With the help of a screwdriver, an appropriate screw is placed in each anchor hole of the BC-FMT and secured tightly with the help of a torque wrench. The maximum torque that can be used is 32 Ncm.

Closure

The BC-FMT is palpated to make sure it is secure, and the incision is closed in layers. Only bipolar cautery should be used to achieve hemostasis, and a pressure dressing is applied. Since osseointegration of the screws is not needed, the audio processor can be activated as soon as the post-auricular wound has healed.

Cochlear Osia®

Cochlear™ Osia® System is an active transcutaneous bone conduction implant system. Components of the system include the external audio processor and the internal implant system. The implant system consists of OSI200 and BI300 implants. The OSI200 contains the receiver coil with the magnet, which continues into the transducer that vibrates in response to the sound. The transducer is attached to the BI300 implant, which osseointegrates into the skull (Fig. 7.7). The sound collected by the audio processor is transmitted to the internal implant system, which vibrates the skull and activates the bone-conduction hearing mechanism (Cywka et al., 2021).

Preparation is similar to that of any craniofacial procedure (Fig. 7.8). Template marking is done in the correct position in such a way that the sound processor does not interfere with the pinna. The position of the osseointegrated screw is marked at the level of the external auditory meatus. An incision is marked around 5 mm-1 cm behind the post-auricular groove. Local anesthetic is injected in the post-auricular area at the site of the incision.

Incision and Creation of Posterior Pocket

A "C" shaped or lazy "S" shaped incision is given in the post-auricular area. A posterior subperiosteal pocket is created to place the implant. The depth of the pocket can be tested using the implant template provided. If the thickness of the skin flap is

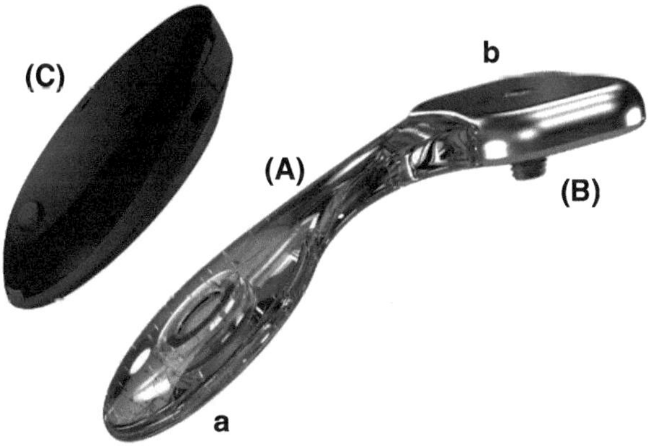

Fig. 7.7 OSIA System: (**A**) OSI200 implant, which consists of (**a**) Receiver-stimulator coil with the magnet (**b**) Actuator; (**B**) BI300 Implant; (**C**) Sound processor. (Image Courtesy of Cochlear Limited)

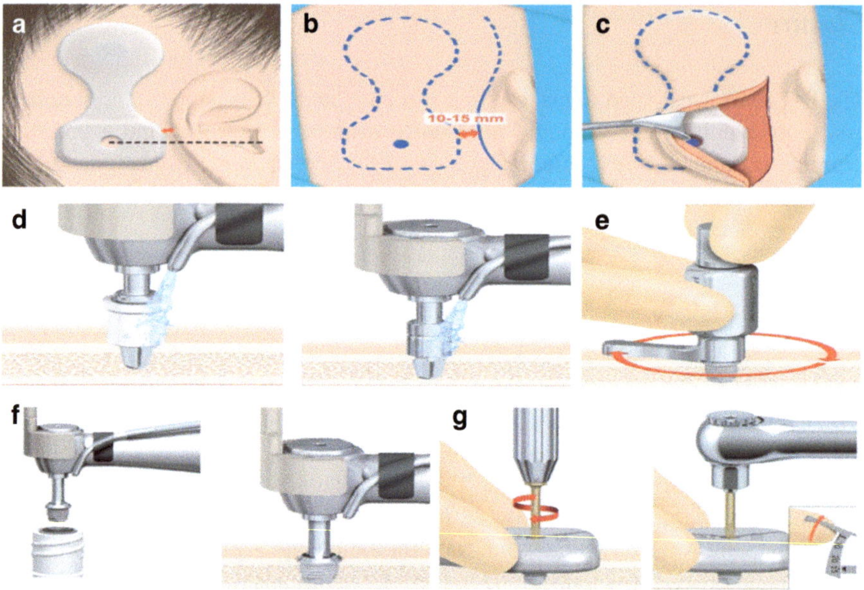

Fig. 7.8 (**a**) Marking of the position of the OSIA implant; (**b**) Marking of skin incision 10–15 mm away from the position of the implant; (**c**) Incision and periosteal pocket for the implant; (**d**) Drill with a guide and widening drill; (**e**) Checking for bone flatness; (**f**) Picking up of the BI200 implant and placement; (**g**) Attachment of the actuator to the implant. (Image Courtesy of Cochlear Limited)

outside the surgical recommendations, the skin flap is made thinner by placing the implant lateral to the periosteum. However, if the skin flap is adequate, it is always advisable to place the implant medial to the periosteum to achieve a tighter fit.

Placement of BI300 Implant

The site of the implant placement must be devoid of the periosteum, and the bone should be even. The location of the BI300 implant is marked, and the guide drill is used to make a hole in the skull. Drilling is done at a speed of 2000 rpm, and the drill is placed perpendicular to the bone surface. Generous irrigation is needed to avoid heat trauma, which can affect the osseointegration later. The drilling site is regularly inspected for the bone to avoid penetration of the sigmoid sinus or the dura. The minimum depth required is 3 mm. If there is adequate space, a depth of 4 mm can also be done. Then, a widening drill is used to widen the site. Once an adequate drill hole is achieved, the BI300 implant is placed using the implant inserter perpendicular to the bone surface. The implant inserter is used to drill the implant into the hole made earlier. For this, the drill unit is set to a torque setting, which is suggested by the company to be 40–50 Ncm for a compact skull bone and

20–30 Ncm for a soft skull bone. Once the implant is in place, the implant inserter is removed vertically from the implant.

OSI200 Implant Placement

Before the placement of the OSI200 implant, it is essential to check that the surface of the bone is flat. This is done using a bone bed indicator, which is placed on the BI300 implant and rotated clockwise. Any interfering bone is drilled, and then, using the implant template, a final check is made of the bone surface to see if the implant fits well into the periosteal pocket. Using the screwdriver unigrip 95 mm, the fixation screw is picked up and screwed on the actuator. The implant is then taken out of the package and placed, coil first in the periosteal pocket, and then the center of the actuator is placed on the top of the BI200 implant and hand-tightened with the screwdriver (Torque 25 Ncm). This ensures the complete fixture of the implant. The skin flap over the implant is then placed, and the skin is sutured, and a pressure dressing is applied. The sound processor is fitted around 4 weeks after the surgery.

Assessment of Benefits After BCI Surgery

The benefits of a bone anchored hearing devices can be assessed in two ways:

Subjective patient satisfaction: Various questionnaires are available to assess the quality of life of the patients fitted with BCD, including:

(a) APHAB (Abbreviated Profile of Hearing Aid Benefit) (de Wolf et al., 2011).
(b) GBI (Glasgow Benefit Inventory) (Cox & Alexander, 1995).
(c) Glasgow Hearing Aid Benefit and Differences Profile (GHABP & GHADP)
(d) Hearing Device Satisfaction Scale (HDSS) (Robinson et al., 1996).
(e) Health Utilities Index Mark 3 (Gatehouse, 1999).

Several studies have used the questionnaires to evaluate the change in the quality of life after using a BCD and have found that BCD reduced the level of disability and provided more patient satisfaction when compared to air-conduction hearing devices when used for appropriate indications.

Audiological Evaluation

This provides objective evidence of the benefit of using BCD

(a) Pure Tone Audiometry (PTA); aided and unaided

(b) Speech Audiometry

(i) Speech perception in noise
(ii) Word recognition in quiet

BCDs have shown gains in both PTA and Speech audiometry. However, when compared to air-conduction hearing aids, the benefit of BCD is more in patients with pure conductive hearing loss than in patients with mixed hearing loss. With the advent of active transcutaneous BCDs, the benefits of the devices have been maximized while avoiding the problems of skin attenuation (Feeny et al., 2002). The electronic signal transmission, strong bone conduction efficiency, and reduction of skin complications make them the most efficient devices available today.

Complications

The complications associated with surgery of the BCDs may be classified into intra-operative and post-operative complications (Horsman et al., 2003; Oh et al., 2019; Shirazi et al., 2006) (Fig. 7.9). For the purpose of ease, the complications are

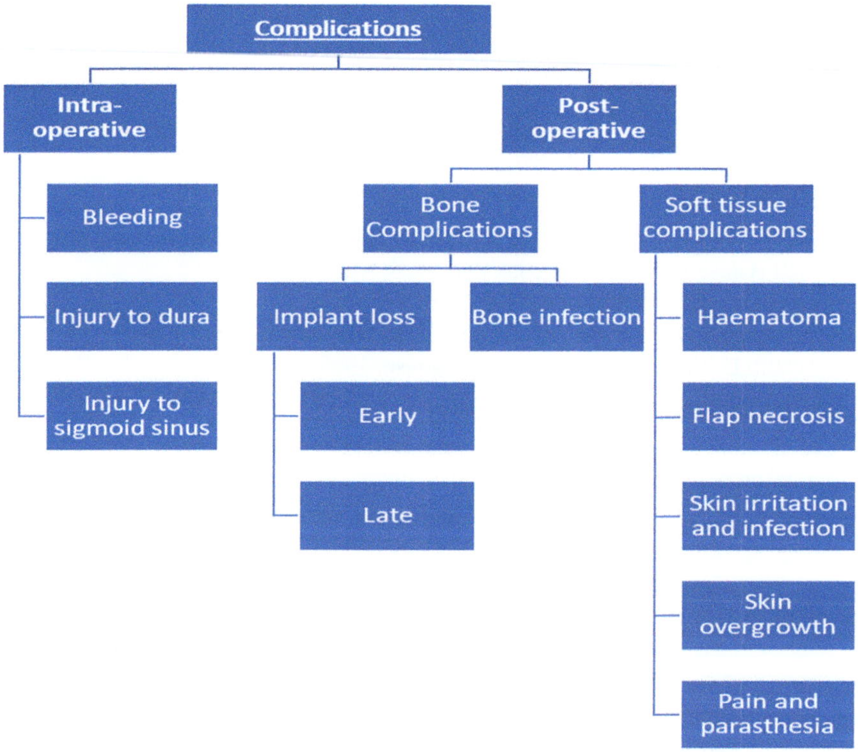

Fig. 7.9 Complications of placement of surgical bone conduction devices

discussed in general and apply to all surgical BCDs. However, skin complications can be ignored for transcutaneous devices.

Intra-operative Complications

(a) *Bleeding*: This can happen from emissary veins, scalp, and muscles, which can be easily controlled using bipolar cautery.
(b) *Injury to the dura*: This can occur while drilling the bone well for the bone bridge or while placing the implant of Baha Connect, or Baha Attract, or OSIA.
(c) *Injury to the sigmoid sinus:* This can be controlled by inserting bone wax or muscle into the site of penetration into the sinus.

Post-operative Complications

1. Bone complications:

(a) Implant loss: Complications leading to implant loss can be categorized as early, i.e., failure to osseointegrate; and late, i.e., loss of osseointegration or disintegration.

The osseointegration process is necessary for both stability of the implant and audiological outcome in Baha® Connect and Baha® Attract whereas in transcutaneous active implants, osseointegration is essential for the stability of the implant only.

Children have a higher risk of implant loss as they have a thinner skull bone and lesser mineral content than adult skull bones. Other factors that affect osseointegration include diabetes and radiation therapy, which impede osseointegration and increase the risk of bone complications. The following steps must be done in order to promote osseointegration.

- Proper selection of the implant site, preferably along the temporalis line where the bone is thicker with smaller air cells.
- Fastidious surgical technique with constant cooling irrigation of the implant site and proper handling of the implant.
- Uninterrupted connection between the bone and the implant.
- Adequate healing time.
- Even distribution of stress over the implant.

(b) Bone infection: Bone is relatively resistant to infection, and hence, osteitis is rare even in patients with prolonged soft tissue infections.

2. *Soft tissue complications* include the following (Holgers et al., 1988): Table 7.2 mentions the details about Holger's classification related to the soft tissue complications and possible solutions.

Table 7.2 Holger's classification of skin complications following placement of percutaneous bone conduction devices and their recommended treatment strategy

Grade	Description	Management
0	No irritation	Remove epithelial debris if present
1	Slight redness	Local treatment
2	Red and slightly moist tissue (no granuloma)	Local treatment
3	Reddish and moist (may have granulation tissue)	Revision surgery indicated
4	Infection	Removal of skin penetrating the implant

(a) Haematoma: It is a rare complication. However, if a hematoma occurs, it must be evacuated promptly to reduce the risk of flap necrosis from devascularisation.
(b) Flap necrosis: Partial or total flap necrosis occurs in about 10% of the patients. It usually occurs in areas of inadequate blood supply. Excessive pressure over the flap can also cause necrosis.
(c) Skin irritation and infection: This is the most common skin complication.
(d) Skin overgrowth-this is rarely seen now because of the advent of transcutaneous devices.
(e) Pain and Paraesthesia: The patients must be informed about the possibility of a small area of numbness around the surgical site. This area, however, reduces over the next 4–6 months. Persistent pain at the implant site may be seen in about 4% of the patients and may even require explanation.

Skin complications have been classified by Holgers et al. (1988) into different grades, as mentioned below and in Table 7.2.

Minor complications (erythema = Holgers grade 1, maceration or minimal infection = Holgers grade 2, hypertrophic scar) require regular wound care, antisepsis, application of eosin to dry the lesion in the case of maceration, and sometimes the application of topical antibiotics. Corticosteroid ointment or silver nitrate cauterization is sometimes necessary to treat granulation tissue. Local corticosteroid injections are sometimes effective in treating hypertrophic scar nodules.

Treatment of major complications (granulomas = Holgers grade 3, primary or secondary defect of osseointegration = Holgers grade 4, hypertrophic scar refractory to conservative treatment) ranges from simple excision under local anesthesia to removal of the abutment under general anesthesia.

Steps to be taken to minimize soft tissue complications:

- The skin around the abutment must be as thin as possible, with the removal of all hair follicles.
- Resection of subcutaneous tissue must be extended 1 to 2 cm beyond the limits of the flap to ensure a gently sloping junction between the adjacent skin and the zone of implantation.
- The periosteum must be thoroughly dissected to avoid any residual tissue between the skin graft and the periosteum.

- Skin margins must be immobilized by suturing them to the periosteum before placement of the flap or skin graft.
- Resection of the subcutaneous tissue around the implant site must be even more extensive in obese patients or patients with a thick scalp.
- At the end of the procedure, the skin graft must be firmly maintained in place: some authors prefer to use a bolster dressing as an alternative to the healing cap provided by the manufacturer.

References

Branemark, P. I. (1985). Introduction to osseointegration. In P.-I. Branemark, C. Zarb, & T. Albrektsson (Eds.), *Tissue-integrated prostheses. Osseointegration in clinical dentistry* (pp. 11–76). Quintessence Publishing.

Cox, R. M., & Alexander, G. C. (1995). The abbreviated profile of hearing aid benefit. *Ear and Hearing, 16*(2), 176–186.

Cywka, K. B., Skarzynski, H., Król, B., & Skarzynski, P. H. (2021). The Bonebridge BCI 602 active transcutaneous bone conduction implant in children: Objective and subjective benefits. *Journal of Clinical Medicine, 10*(24), 5916.

de Wolf, M. J., Hol, M. K., Mylanus, E. A., Snik, A. F., & Cremers, C. W. (2011). Benefit and quality of life after bone-anchored hearing aid fitting in children with unilateral or bilateral hearing impairment. *Archives of Otolaryngology – Head & Neck Surgery, 137*(2), 130–138.

D'Eredità, R., Caroncini, M., & Saetti, R. (2012). The new Baha implant: A prospective osseointegration study. *Otolaryngology-Head and Neck Surgery, 146*(6), 979–983.

Ellsperman, S. E., Nairn, E. M., & Stucken, E. Z. (2021). Review of bone conduction hearing devices. *Audiology Research, 11*(2), 207–219.

Feeny, D., Furlong, W., Torrance, G. W., Goldsmith, C. H., Zhu, Z., DePauw, S., Denton, M., & Boyle, M. (2002). Multiattribute and single-attribute utility functions for the health utilities index mark 3 system. *Medical Care, 40*(2), 113–128.

Gatehouse, S. (1999). Glasgow hearing aid benefit profile: Derivation and validation of a client-centered outcome measure for hearing aid services. *Journal of the American Academy of Audiology, 10*(02), 80–103.

Håkansson, B., Lidén, G., Tjellström, A., Ringdahl, A., Jacobsson, M., Carlsson, P., & Erlandson, B. E. (1990). Ten years of experience with the Swedish bone-anchored hearing system. *The Annals of Otology, Rhinology & Laryngology, 151*, 1–16.

Håkansson, B., Reinfeldt, S., Persson, A. C., Jansson, K. F., Rigato, C., Hultcrantz, M., & Eeg-Olofsson, M. (2019). The bone conduction implant – A review and 1-year follow-up. *International Journal of Audiology, 58*(12), 945–955.

Holgers, K. M., Tjellström, A., Bjursten, L. M., & Erlandsson, B. E. (1988). Soft tissue reactions around percutaneous implants: A clinical study of soft tissue conditions around skin-penetrating titanium implants for bone-anchored hearing aids. *The American Journal of Otology, 9*(1), 56–59.

Horsman, J., Furlong, W., Feeny, D., & Torrance, G. (2003). The Health Utilities Index (HUI): Concepts, measurement properties and applications. *Health and Quality of Life Outcomes, 1*, 54.

Kulasegarah, J., Burgess, H., Neeff, M., & Brown, C. R. S. (2018). Comparing audiological outcomes between the Bonebridge and bone conduction hearing aid on a hard test band: Our experience in children with atresia and microtia. *International Journal of Pediatric Otorhinolaryngology, 107*, 176–182.

Macnamara, M., Phillips, D., & Proops, D. W. (1996). The bone anchored hearing aid (BAHA) in chronic suppurative otitis media (CSOM). *The Journal of Laryngology & Otology, 110*(21), 38–40.

McDermott, A. L., Dutt, S. N., Reid, A. P., & Proops, D. W. (2002). An intra-individual comparison of the previous conventional hearing aid with the bone-anchored hearing aid: The Nijmegen group questionnaire. *The Journal of Laryngology & Otology, 116*(S28), 15–19.

Oh, S. J., Goh, E. K., Choi, S. W., Lee, S., Lee, H. M., Lee, I. W., & Kong, S. K. (2019). Audiologic, surgical and subjective outcomes of active transcutaneous bone conduction implant system (Bonebridge). *International Journal of Audiology, 58*(12), 956–963.

Ricci, G., Volpe, A. D., Faralli, M., Longari, F., Lancione, C., Varricchio, A. M., & Frenguelli, A. (2011). Bone-anchored hearing aids (Baha) in congenital aural atresia: Personal experience. *International Journal of Pediatric Otorhinolaryngology, 75*(3), 342–346.

Robinson, K., Gatehouse, S., & Browning, G. G. (1996). Measuring patient benefit from otorhinolaryngological surgery and therapy. *The Annals of Otology, Rhinology, and Laryngology, 105*(6), 415–422.

Schrøder, S. A., Ravn, T., & Bonding, P. (2010). BAHA in single-sided deafness: Patient compliance and subjective benefit. *Otology & Neurotology, 31*(3), 404–408.

Shirazi, M. A., Marzo, S. J., & Leonetti, J. P. (2006). Perioperative complications with the bone-anchored hearing aid. *Otolaryngology – Head and Neck Surgery, 134*(2), 236–239.

Snik, A. F., Mylanus, E. A., Proops, D. W., Wolfaardt, J. F., Hodgetts, W. E., Somers, T., Niparko, J. K., Wazen, J. J., Sterkers, O., Cremers, C. W., & Tjellström, A. (2005). Consensus statements on the BAHA system: Where do we stand at present? *Annals of Otology, Rhinology & Laryngology, 114*(12), 2–12.

Stenfelt, S., & Goode, R. L. (2005). Bone-conducted sound: Physiological and clinical aspects. *Otology & Neurotology, 26*(6), 1245–1261.

Tjellström, A., & Granström, G. (1994). Long-term follow-up with the bone-anchored hearing aid: A review of the first 100 patients between 1977 and 1985. *Ear, Nose & Throat Journal, 73*(2), 112–114.

Tjellström, A., & Håkansson, B. (1995). The bone-anchored hearing aid. Design principles, indications, and long-term clinical results. *Otolaryngologic Clinics of North America, 28*(1), 53–72.

Chapter 8
Middle Ear Implants: Audiological Perspectives

Chandrakant Vishwakarma and Prem Ranjan

Abstract Middle Ear Implants (MEI) have emerged as a viable alternative for individuals who gain minimal benefit from traditional amplification and are not candidates for cochlear implantation. Through a historical lens, the development of MEIs has evolved from early experiments in the 1930s. MEIs function by converting acoustic energy into vibrations that stimulate the ossicles, overcoming impedance mismatch challenges. The Vibrant Sound Bridge (VSB) and Esteem are currently notable active MEIs in the market, each with distinct mechanisms and candidacy criteria. Selection for these devices requires thorough audiological and radiological evaluations, ensuring appropriateness for conductive, mixed, or sensorineural hearing loss.

Keywords Vibrant Sound Bridge · Floating mass transducer · Percutaneous MEI · Transcutaneous MEI

Introduction

Hearing loss is an invisible disability. Unless you face the situation, you would not know the amount of information missed due to hearing loss. As per World Health Organization (WHO) report 2021, almost 5% of world's population (430 million) has disabling hearing loss, and it is estimated that by 2050 over 700 million people will have disabling hearing loss.

There are different types and degree of hearing loss, of which sensorineural hearing loss often requires amplification, whereas the conductive hearing loss is invariably treated by medication or surgery. With the aid from technology sophistication and miniaturization, hearing aids continue to be the first choice for helping

C. Vishwakarma (✉)
Shabda-Brahma Speech, Hearing & Vertigo Clinic, Ahmedabad, India

P. Ranjan
MEDEL Pvt Ltd, Innsbruck, Austria

P. Kumar et al. (eds.), *Advances in Implantation Otology*,
https://doi.org/10.1007/978-981-96-8671-1_8

individuals with sensorineural hearing loss. While 20% of the population with hearing impairment seek assistance from amplification, nearly 15% of them discontinue using the device for various reasons (Kochkin, 2005). Despite having sophistication in digital signal processing of hearing aids there remains some limitations which could not give comfort and satisfaction to the user. The reasons could be acoustic feedback, occlusion effect, recurrent infection, skin irritation, frequent battery change/maintenance etc. In the modern world, looks have become as important as anything else. Hence, the social stigma of wearing a visible hearing aid is among the leading causes behind denial to use hearing aids. If the amplification devices were surgically placed within the ear, several such concerns could be resolved. This inspired the emergence of an implantable hearing device in the middle ear, called the 'Middle Ear Implant' (MEI). Among the several degrees of hearing loss, MEI as an alternative was developed for a group that receive minimal benefit with conventional amplification and are not severe enough to undergo cochlear implantation. However, it has been used for milder hearing loss (Leysieffer et al., 1998) and people having conductive hearing loss (Kartush & Tos, 1995). MEI is not advisable for persons with recurrent otitis media as it can hamper the functioning of the device to its full potential and may lead to further complications.

Brief History

Looking back at the early days of research, one can say that credit for the inception of thought and making middle ear implants goes to Alvar (Wilska's, 1935) experiment. Wilska placed iron particles over the tympanic membrane and made the tympanic membrane vibrate by generating an electromagnetic field using an electromagnetic coil placed in the earphone. The vibration from tympanic membrane to ossicles and sound to inner ear was perceived. With this experiment, she demonstrated that puretone could be perceived by mechanical stimulation of ossicles. Later (Rutschmann, 1959) successfully reported stimulation of ossicles by keeping a magnet of 10 mg at the umbo of the tympanic membrane and applying an alternating magnetic field by an electromagnetic coil.

A patented design of an implantable hearing aid was made by the University of Pittsburgh's, Department of Electrical Engineering in 1967 but was never put to test (Goode, 1970). Animal experiments made things better, and finally, the first device for humans was made in Japan in 1980s (Suzuki, 1988). In these experiments, the piezoelectric-type devices were attached to the ossicles, and an external microphone coupled to the sound processor were used in them.

In 1986 researchers at Case Western-reserve University created a device where a magnetic implant was placed on the incus and was separated from the induction coil driving the implant. This was called a semi-implantable middle ear electromagnetic hearing device system (SIMEHD). It was granted FDA approval in 1996 but there is no further data on this device (Bankaitis & Fredrickson, 2002). Later, Michigan Ear Institute along with Smith & Nephew Richards company created another device over three phases. In phase 1, the electromagnetic ossicular augmentation device (EOAD) involved temporarily fixing a small target magnet onto the lateral surface of the tympanic membrane in patients with sensorineural hearing loss. In phase 2 the target magnet was incorporated into an ossicular prosthesis and used in patients with mixed hearing loss. In phase 3, the EOAD was fixed onto the lateral surface of the eardrum and sensorineural hearing loss patients. An electromagnetic coil in a customised mould drove these devices. While initial results seemed promising this device is no longer in use (Chasin, 2001; Ball, 2010; Dumon et al., 1995).

The Direct Acoustic Cochlear Stimulator (DACS) was developed by Cochlear and Phonak acoustics. It has an electromechanical transducer attached to a stapes prosthesis and is driven by an external auditory processor. This was designed primarily for patients with advanced otosclerosis and moderate to severe mixed hearing losses. Limited studies have shown benefit in patients with moderate to severe mixed hearing losses (Fisch et al., 2001). The middle ear transducer (MET) developed by Otologics was a semi-implantable device. The electromagnetic transducer was mounted on a titanium bracket and fixed to the mastoid. The transducer was coupled to the body of the incus by a laser drilled hole to accommodate the tip of the actuator. The external component of the microphone, processor and battery was attached transcutaneously by magnet. The fully implantable device was called the Carina wherein all the components were implanted. It received European union CE mark for moderate to severe sensorineural hearing loss in 2006 and mixed hearing loss in 2007. The Carina was subsequently acquired by Cochlear corporation but is no longer available (Goode et al., 1995; Gyo et al., 1984). In Japan, workers developed a piezoelectric middle ear implant in the 1970s called the RION. Partially implantable version one approved for use in 1993 but was subsequently discontinued (Kartush & Tos, 1995; Ball, 2010). Efforts by different groups of scientists and engineers have contributed immensely to the development of middle ear implants. Today there are various middle ear devices available in the market worldwide, broadly categorized into partially or totally implantable devices.

Types of Middle Ear Implants

Middle ear Implant transform acoustic energy to stimulate the ossicles of the middle ear. Some MEIs stimulate the tympanic membrane or even the cochlear fluids. As the outer ear is bypassed, the impedance mismatch between the air in the external ear and fluid in the cochlea is drastically reduced/eliminated, and greater amount of energy is transferred to the inner ear. Generally, a MEI has two parts- an external wearable processor and an internal implantable part which is fixed to the ossicles. The external processor has a microphone that picks the sound, processes it, and delivers the energy to the middle ear as mechanical vibration. There are three types of middle ear implants based on transduction mode used. They could be piezoelectric, electromagnetic, or electromechanical. Each device has its advantages and limitations based on frequency response, power, reliability, and maintenance of the device.

The Piezoelectric MEIs are made up of monomorphic or bimorphic piezoelectric material. These types work on the principle that the application of voltage to a piezoelectric material leads to a change in the shape of the material. The change in shape acts as a mechanical stimulator to drive the ossicles. There are three major sub-types of Piezoelectric MEIs- Partially Implantable Hearing Aid (PIHA), Totally Implanted Cochlear Amplifier (TICA), and Fully Implantable devices (e.g. St. Croix Envoy). A PIHA is implanted in ears having a mixed hearing loss due to chronic otitis media without an active infection and with a bone conduction pure tone average of less than 40 dB HL (Yanagihara et al., 1997). A TICA is a fully implantable device which is intended for patients having moderate to severe degrees of sensorineural hearing loss. The microphone in this type of device is implanted under the skin in the external auditory canal, whereas the processor is placed subcutaneously over the mastoid bone. The processor contains a battery which can be charged using a transcutaneous inductive link. The St. Croix Envoy is also a fully implantable device having two transducers. One transducer takes the acoustic signal from the malleus. This signal is processed and given to stapes via the second transducer. When using this type of device, the incus is removed to make the ossicular chain discontinuous. It is intended for patients having moderate to severe hearing loss. The major limitations of piezoelectric devices are the limited power output, restricted frequency response, intentional damage to middle ear ossicle, and acoustic feedback in some cases.

The Electromagnetic MEIs are made up of magnet and energizing coil. The material of the magnet is either samarium cobalt or neodymium iron boron. The acoustic input leads to generation of fluctuating magnetic field by the coil which helps the magnet to vibrate. This further leads to ossicular chain and/or cochlear fluids movements. There are three major sub-types of Electromagnetic MEIs- the electromagnetic device developed by the group of Case Western Reserve University researchers (Maniglia et al., 1988) Total Ossicular Replacement Prosthesis (TORP) or Partial Ossicular Replacement prosthesis (PORP) (Kartush et al., 1991; Kartush & Tos, 1995) where magnet is encapsulated in the TORP or PORP, and Direct Drive Hearing System (DDHS) from SoundTec which has an energizing coil and a magnet. The Electromagnetic MEI developed by Case Western Reserve University has a magnet attached to the ossicles. An electromagnetic coil is placed in attic area of the middle ear. A radio frequency receiver is placed behind the ear subcutaneously which is used for receiving acoustic input. This device is intended for patients having symmetrical moderate to severe cochlear hearing loss and word recognition scores of 60% or better. In TORP or PORP the electromagnetic coil for stimulation is placed in a custom ear mould. The use of such device on humans is not reported. In the DDHS, the energizing coil is placed in the ear canal with magnet placed on the ossicular chain. The major limitations of these devices are occlusion of ear canal due to placement of the energizing coil, the coil and the magnet must be close for better transmission of sound, and more distance results in changed frequency response and output.

The Electromechanical MEIs have energizing coil and magnet which are placed together as closed magnetic circuit. This helps with issues related with the frequency response and the output. In this type, the mechanical energy is supplied directly to the electromechanical transducer. The energy is further passed on to the ossicular chain to which the transducer is directly attached. There are two major sub-types of Electromechanical MEIs- Otologics Middle Ear Transducer (MET) developed by (Fredrickson et al., 1973, 1995) at Washington University Medical School at St.Louis, and Symphonix Vibrant developed by. The MET has the receiver-stimulator in silastic casing which is placed subcutaneously in mastoid recess behind the ear. There is a drive rod and probe tip which attaches the transducer further to the incus. The indication includes patients with bilateral moderately-severe to severe sloping sensorineural hearing loss. Vibrant has an electromagnetic Floating Mass Transducer (FMT) which is used to move the ossicular chain. The FMT has an assembly where a coil is wound around the magnet. The FMT is placed on the long process of the incus so that its axis of motion is parallel to the axis of the lenticular process (Arnold et al., 2010). An external unit is worn over the head which is magnetically attached to implanted demodulator. The major limitations of Electromechanical devices are the requirement of a surgery under general anaesthesia followed by a few days of stay in the hospital, and considerations before doing MRI because of a magnet in the implanted part.

Vibrant Sound Bridge

Vibrant Sound Bridge (VSB) was invented by (Geoff Ball, 2010) who is also a bilateral VSB user (Fig. 8.1). It consists of two parts- the Vibrating Ossicular Prosthesis (VORP) and the Audio Processor. The VORP, which is surgically implanted, contains a receiving coil, a demodulator package, a conductor link, and the FMT. The Audio Processor is worn externally on the head, posterosuperior to the pinna. The Audio Processor is fixed with magnetic attraction between the implanted magnet in the VORP and the magnet in the Audio Processor. The Audio Processor houses a microphone, electronics for sound processing with multichannel automatic gain compressor, and a battery. The signal from the Audio Processor is transmitted across the skin to the internal receiver in the VORP. The signal is then sent through the demodulator via the conductor link to the FMT, which is fixed to the long process of the incus. The FMT component of the VSB that makes the system unique. The VSB directly drives the ossicular chain to provide louder perception of sound by the user.

The FMT is 2.3 mm in length, has a diameter of 1.8 mm and weight of 25 mg. The conductor link further has diameter of 0.6 mm. The Samba 2 sound processor picks up the sound and converts it into a digital signal, this signal is sent to the internal implant using radio frequency. The internal Implant decodes it and converts it into electrical signal. This signal is then transferred to the FMT which further converts the signal to mechanical energy and vibrates the ossicles to which it is attached.

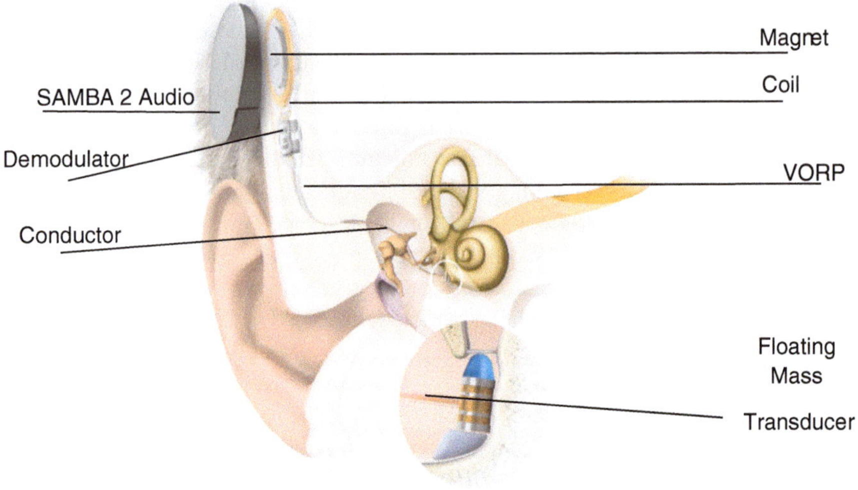

Fig. 8.1 Vibrant Sound Bridge (VSB) system with the round window soft coupler. (Image Courtesy of MED-EL Company)

The Samba 2 processor has undergone multiple developments over the years. The current audio processor generation has adaptive directional microphones for better beam forming and noise suppression, speech tracking for directionality towards source of speech, intelligent sound adapter which is a self-learning algorithm which learns the user's preferences, Samba 2 remote app to control the audio processor via smart phone, streaming possibilities among many other features. A very important feature is the low pressure on the skin of the user which is important for daily use. The programming could be done by Symfit 8.0 software which is compatible with the latest Noah 8.0.

Till the time of writing this chapter, this is the only MEI to have a single point attachment which makes it independent of skull growth. Compared to a hearing aid which gives acoustic amplification, the VSB directly drives the ossicles. The "direct drive" technology of the FMT gives natural sound quality without obstructing the ear canal.

Audiological Candidacy Criteria

Candidacy criteria are crucial for the outcomes, and it should be done by a team of surgeon and audiologist. Detailed audiological and radiological work-up is required. VSB can be used with patients of all types of hearing losses viz., sensorineural, conductive, and mixed hearing losses. Middle ear surgery sometimes doesn't give optimal outcomes due to many factors like anatomical, pathological, and physiological. In such conditions hearing aids may not be the best solution. A preserved anatomy of the inner ear, despite a hearing loss, makes it stimulable with the available technology. The FMT can be coupled directly to the round window or the existing part of stapes (Fig. 8.2).

The bone conduction hearing thresholds decide which device to choose for best outcome for an individual. Figure 8.3 depicts the clear-cut demarcation who can consider either for VSB or a bone conduction device, Bonebridge (BB), or only a VSB. The description of bone conduction devices separately is beyond the scope of this chapter 6.

Over time, several developments were done to the VSB. Vibrating Ossicular Prosthesis (VORP) 501 was the first-generation device. This was indicated only for

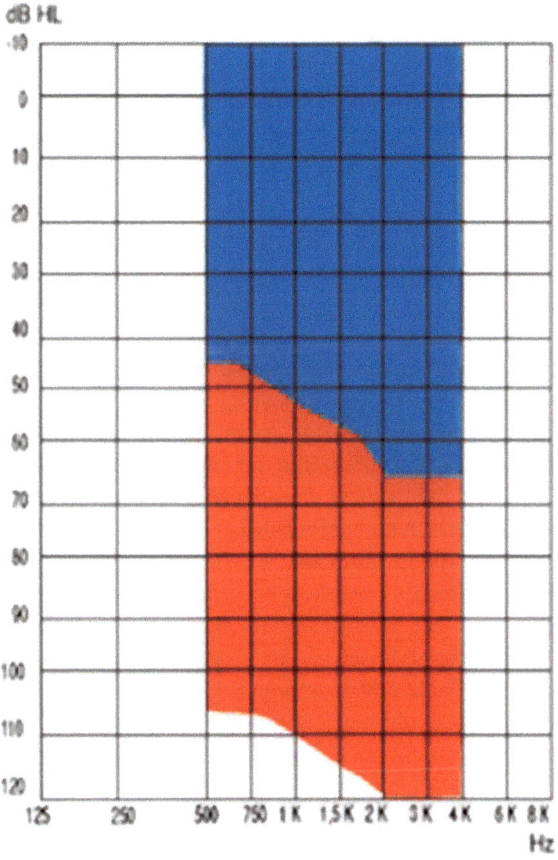

Fig. 8.2 Candidacy criteria to be considered for Vibrant Sound Bridge. The bone conduction thresholds should remain within the darker region whereas the air conduction thresholds could remain anywhere within the lighter shaded region. Among individuals with a sensorineural hearing loss, the best candidates for MEI are ones with a stable hearing loss falling within the shaded region in the audiogram (Fig. 8.2), provided there are no signs of a retro-cochlear pathology

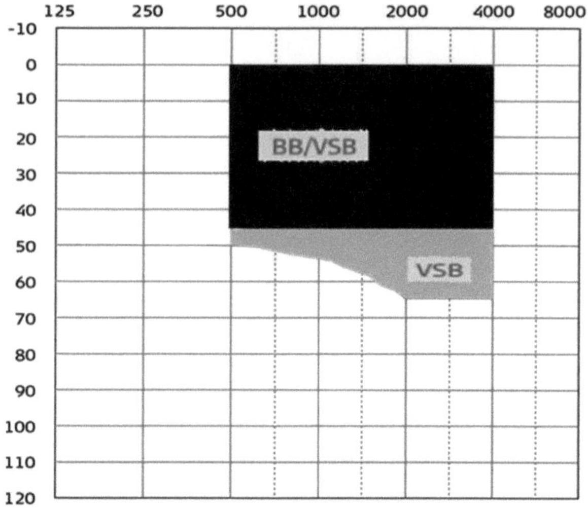

Fig. 8.3 Candidacy criteria for VSB and bone conduction device. If the bone conduction thresholds fall within the light shaded region, the candidacy holds good for bone conduction device as well as VSB. In case, the bone conduction thresholds fall within the dark shaded region, the candidacy criteria are met exclusively for the VSB

patients with sensorineural hearing loss. It was discontinued in 1997. This marked the introduction of VORP 502 in 1998 in Europe and in 2000 in the USA. This was indicated in the USA for patients with sensorineural hearing loss only. In Europe, the indication included all types of hearing loss, viz., conductive, sensorineural, and mixed. In 2014, VORP 3 was introduced which featured conditional MRI at 1.5 T. It was thinner than the previous devices. The indication included all types of hearing loss, viz., conductive, sensorineural, and mixed. The Vibrant Soundbridge represents a significant advancement in hearing restoration technology, offering benefits that extend beyond those of traditional hearing aids and bone conduction systems. Its ability to provide enhanced hearing performance, high user satisfaction, and long-term reliability makes it a compelling option for individuals with specific types of hearing loss. As with any medical device, candidacy for the Middle Ear Implant should be determined through comprehensive audiological and medical evaluations. Finally to conclude ,Middle Ear Implants are the device which drive the middle ear ossicles into vibration. Middle ear implants are better choice than hearing aids as it reduces the occlusion effect, skin irritation , feedback problem etc. The only big limitation at times the cost of device and involvement of surgical procedure. Reader should know all the available device options which can be discussed further in one of the couselling session as and when required for further management.

References

Arnold, A., Kompis, M., Candreia, C., Pfiffner, F., Häusler, R., & Stieger, C. (2010). The floating mass transducer at the round window: Direct transmission or bone conduction? *Hearing Research, 263*(1–2), 120–127.

Ball, G. R. (2010). The vibrant soundbridge: Design and development. *Advances in Oto-rhino-laryngology, 69*, 1–13.

Bankaitis, A. U., & Fredrickson, J. M. (2002). Otologics Middle Ear Transducer™ (MET™) implantable hearing device: Rationale, technology, and design strategies. *Trends in Amplification, 6*(2), 53–60.

Chasin, M. (2001). The ins and outs of middle ear implants. *The Hearing Journal, 54*, 34–35.

Dumon, T., Zennaro, O., Aran, J. M., & Bébéar, J. P. (1995). Piezoelectric middle ear implant preserving the ossicular chain. *Otolaryngologic Clinics of North America, 28*(1), 173–187.

Fisch, U., Cremers, C. W., Lenarz, T., Weber, B., Babighian, G., Uziel, A. S., Proops, D. W., O'Connor, A. F., Charachon, R., Helms, J., & Fraysse, B. (2001). Clinical experience with the vibrant Soundbridge implant device. *Otology and Neurotology, 22*(6), 962–972.

Fredrickson, J. M., Tomlinson, D. R., Davis, E. R., & Odkuist, L. M. (1973). Evaluation of an electromagnetic implantable hearing aid. *Canadian Journal of Otolaryngology, 2*(1), 53–62.

Fredrickson, J., Cotcchia, J., & Kohosla, S. (1995). Investigations into an implantable electromagnetic hearing device for moderate to severe sensorineural loss. *Otolargologic Clinics of North America, 28*(1), 107–120.

Goode, R. L. (1970). An implantable hearing aid. State of the art. *American Academy of Ophthalmology and Otolaryngology, 74*(1), 128–139.

Goode, R. L., Rosenbaum, M. L., & Maniglia, A. J. (1995). The history and development of the implantable hearing aid. *Otolaryngologic Clinics of North America, 28*(1), 1–16.

Gyo, K., Yanagihara, N., & Araki, H. (1984). Sound pickup utilizing an implantable piezoelectric ceramic bimorph element: Application to the cochlear implant. *The American Journal of Otology, 5*(4), 273–276.

Kartush, J. M., & Tos, M. (1995). Electromagnetic ossicular augmentation device. *Otolaryngologic Clinics of North America, 28*(1), 155–172.

Kartush, J. M., LaRouere, M. J., Graham, M. D., Bouchard, K. R., & Audet, B. V. (1991). Intraoperative cranial nerve monitoring during posterior skull base surgery. *Skull Base Surgery, 1*(02), 85–92.

Kochkin, S. (2005). MarkeTrak VII: Customer satisfaction with hearing instruments in the digital age. *The Hearing Journal, 58*, 30, 32–34, 38–40, 42–43, 30.

Leysieffer, H., et al. (1998). A totally implantable hearing aid for inner ear deafness: TICA LZ 3001. *HNO, 46*(10), 853–863.

Maniglia, A. J., Ko, W. H., Zhang, R. X., Dolgin, S. R., Rosenbaum, M. L., & Montague, F. W., Jr. (1988). Electromagnetic implantable middle ear hearing device of the ossicular-stimulating type: Principles, designs, and experiments. *The Annals of Otology, Rhinology & Laryngology. Supplement, 136*, 3–16.

Rutschmann, J. (1959). Magnetic audition: Auditory stimulation by means of alternating magnetic fields acting on a permanent magnet fixed to the eardrum. *IRE Transactions on Medical Electronics, 6*(1), 22–23.

Suzuki, J. (1988). *Middle ear implant: Implantable hearing aids*. Adv Audiol Karger.

Wilska A. (1935). *A method of identification of hearing threshold amplitudes of the ear drum at various frequencies*. Scandinavian Archives of Physiology. 72;161–165.

Yanagihara, N., Hinohira, Y., & Gyo, K. (1997). Surgical rehabilitation of deafness with partially implantable hearing aid using piezoelectric ceramic bimorpli ossicular vibrator. *Auris Nasus Larynx, 24*(1), 91–98.

Chapter 9
Middle Ear Implants: Surgical Perspectives

Ameet Kishore and Sunil Narayan Dutt

Abstract Middle ear implant (MEI) was developed over time with the idea that they would overcome some of the limitations encountered by conventional hearing aids. These concerns have included but are not limited to sub-optimal acoustics, occlusion effect, chronic ear discharge due to chronic otitis media or mastoid cavities and inability to tolerate healing aids due to chronic otitis externa. The Vibrant Sound Bridge (VSB), is a semi-implantable device designed by Geoffrey Ball. It was originally designed to be coupled to the incus long process in patients with sensorineural hearing loss. Of all the active middle ear implants, the maximum experience worldwide has probably been with the Vibrant Sound Bridge (VSB). For this reason, the surgical considerations for the vibrant sound bridge middle ear implant will be discussed in detail in this chapter.

Keywords Sensorineural hearing loss · Middle ear implant · Floating mass transducer · Vibrant Sound bridge · Vibrating ossicular replacement prosthesis

Introduction

Active middle ear implants (MEI) were developed over time with the idea that they would overcome some of the limitations encountered by conventional hearing aids. These concerns have included but are not limited to sub-optimal acoustics, occlusion effect, chronic ear discharge due to chronic otitis media or mastoid cavities and inability to tolerate healing aids due to chronic otitis externa. In middle ear implant, the broad components include a microphone, a processor with its power source and a transducer coupled to the middle ear. The surgically implanted coupler which is

A. Kishore (✉)
Department of ENT, Indraprastha Apollo Hospital, Sarita Vihar, New Delhi, Delhi, India

S. N. Dutt
Department of ENT, Apollo Hospital, Bengaluru, India

P. Kumar et al. (eds.), *Advances in Implantation Otology*,
https://doi.org/10.1007/978-981-96-8671-1_9

attached to either the ossicles or the round window membrane transmits energy directly to the endo-cochlear fluid and thus bypasses the external ear canal. These transducers can either be piezoelectric or electromagnetic-based actuators. By directly driving the ossicular chain, active middle ear implants can overcome the limitation and gain and potentially reduce the issues of distortion or feedback (Banakis Hartl & Jenkins, 2020). In Piezoelectric transducers, when an electric current is passed into a piezoceramic crystal, this changes its volume and thereby produces a vibratory signal which is transferred to the ossicular chain. As these transducers are inert in a magnetic field, they are MRI compatible (Suzuki et al., 1995). Whereas in electromagnetic transducers, passing an electric current into a coil creates a magnetic flux that drives an adjacent magnet. That small magnet is attached to one of the vibratory structures of the middle ear and vibrations are thus delivered to the ossicular chain. Currently there are the following three Active middle ear implants approved for use by the U. S. Food and Drug Administration (FDA): the Envoy Esteem (St. Paul, MN, USA), the Ototronix Maxum (formerly SOUNDTEC Direct; Houston, TX, USA), and the MED-EL Vibrant Sound Bridge (Innsbruck, Austria). Patients being considered for active middle implants should have used conventional hearing aids where possible. They need to be motivated and counselled regarding the possible limitations and complications of that particular device. Their audiological findings must fit the fitting criteria for that particular device.

Vibrant Sound Bridge (VSB)

The Vibrant Sound Bridge (VSB), is a semi-implantable device designed by Geoffrey Ball. It was originally designed to be coupled to the incus long process in patients with sensorineural hearing loss. It was the first middle ear implant to be approved for use by the US FDA in the year 2000. Since then, the device has been modified for coupling on other middle ear structures, such as the stapes, round window and oval window, thus expanding the potential indications to include conductive and mixed hearing losses (Ball, 2010; Lenarz et al., 1998). The VSB comprises an internal implant called the vibrating ossicular replacement prosthesis (VORP), and an external component, or audio processor. The VORP is composed of a receiving coil, a magnet, a demodulator, a conductor link, and a floating mass transducer (FMT). The external audio processor includes a microphone, a processor, battery, transmitter coil and a retention magnet (Fig. 9.1). The microphone receives the sound which is processed by the audio processor and the signal is transmitted across the skin by the transmitting coil. The internal coil receives the signal which is then sent to the floating mass transducer. The FMT which is made up of two electromagnetic coils around a magnet within a titanium housing converts the electric signal to mechanical vibrations via electromagnetic induction. It is the displacement of the FMT that drives the ossicles or the round window membrane. The frequency response of the VSB ranges from 100 to 10,000 Hz, maximally around 2000 Hz

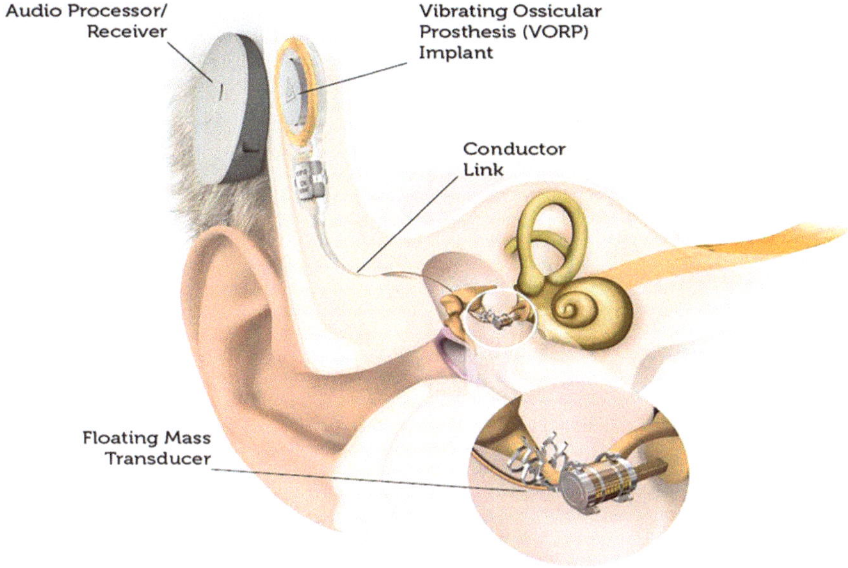

Fig. 9.1 Med-El Vibrant Sound bridge. (Image courtesy of Med-EL company)

with a coupling-dependent average gain of 30 to 55 dB. Several different couplers have been produced specific to various middle ear structures in order to optimize FMT coupling. The internal magnet on the newest generation of the VORP is MRI-compatible up to 1.5 Tesla (Labassi et al., 2017).

In a typical sensorineural hearing loss, the hearing thresholds are based on the fitting graph (Fig. 9.2a). A maximum of 65 dB HL hearing loss at 500 Hz with normal tympanometry. A Word recognition score of 50% or better at 65 dB for word lists, with amplification or at the most comfortable level under earphones ensures cochlear integrity. The middle ear anatomy should be normal and allow for coupling of the FMT at an appropriate site, usually the Incus (Fig. 9.2b).

In the cases of acquired conductive and mixed hearing losses, the Bone Conduction thresholds must be within the fitting range (Fig. 9.2c). Indications may be in ears with a radical stable mastoidectomy, failed ossiculoplasty, adhesive otitis media etc. There should be absence of active middle ear infections and the middle ear anatomy should allow the FMT to be positioned on a suitable vibratory structure—either a remnant ossicle or the round window. There must be an absence of retrocochlear & central auditory disorders.

The Vibrant Sound Bridge middle ear implant has also been used to treat conductive and mixed hearing losses in congenital ear atresia. The FMT can be coupled at different locations in the middle year such as the incus, stapes or the round window membrane. A pre-operative CT scan of the temporal bone is mandatory to assess the severity of the condition of the middle ear, ossicle chain and the position of the facial nerve (Thurnheer et al., 2023).

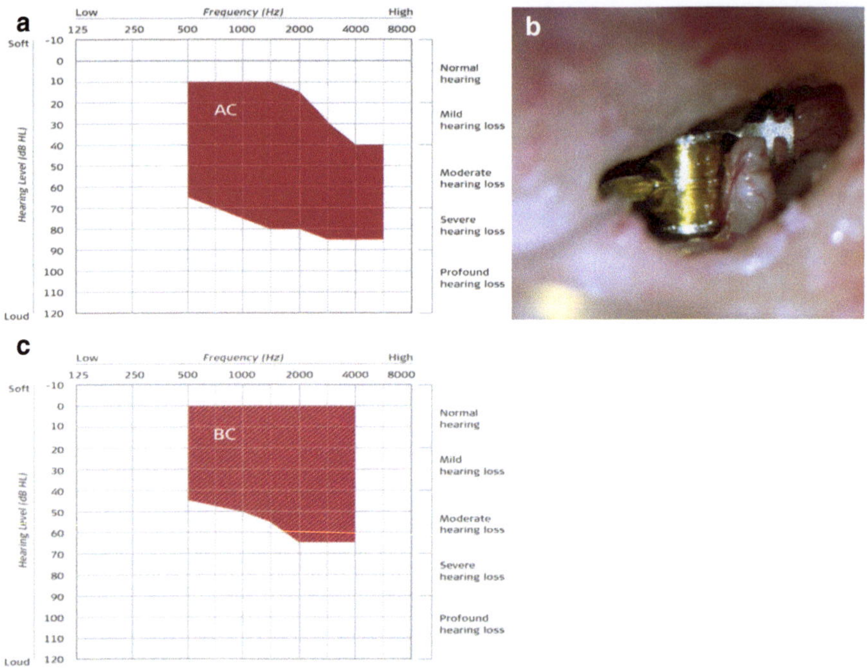

Fig. 9.2 (**a**) Fitting criteria for SNHL. Stable AC thresholds in the shaded area. (**b**) FMT fitted onto the Long process of the incus (left ear). (**c**) Fitting criteria for Conductive and Mixed Hearing Losses. Stable BC thresholds in the shaded area

Maxum

The Maxum System was formally the Soundtec direct drive hearing system developed by the Hough Institute in Oklahoma in the 1980s. It received US FDA approval in 2001. The device had a magnetic implant, a processor behind the ear and an ear mould coil assembly. In the current Maxum system by Ototronix, a magnet is surgically implanted and an integrated processor coil (IPC) unit is worn in the external ear canal. Sound received by the microphone within the IPC, is processed and amplified. The electric signal thus generated passes through the magnetic coil thus creating an electromagnetic field. This oscillates the implanted magnet thereby transmitting vibrations to the inner ear (Fig. 9.3) (Carlson et al., 2014; Pelosi et al., 2014; Matthews, 2002). The procedure is carried out via a trans-canal approach. The incudostapedial joint is visualized and the magnetic implant which is encased in a titanium cylinder is coupled to the stapes using a heat-sensitive nitinol clip (Pelosi et al., 2014).

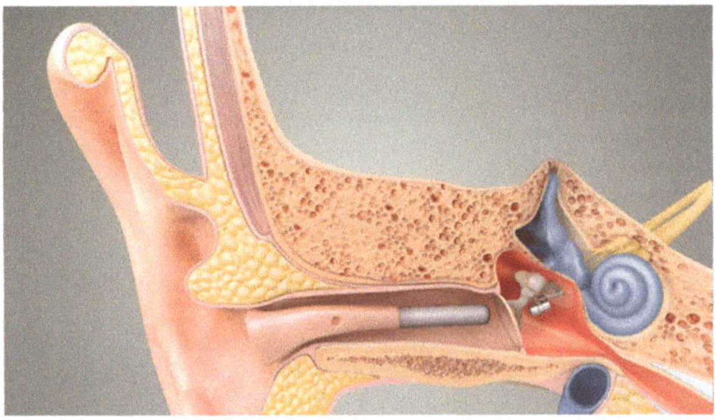

Fig. 9.3 Ototronix Maxum Middle Ear Implant. (Figure adapted from: Tisch (2017), licensed under Creative Commons Attribution 4.0 License. (*See license information at* http://creativecommons.org/licenses/by/4.0/))

Esteem

The Envoy Esteem is a totally-implantable non-rechargeable battery-powered hearing device comprising of a sensor, sound processor and driver. The company was founded in 1995 and the device received US FDA approval in 2010. The device utilizes two piezoelectric transducers—one is coupled to the incus and serves as a sensor by converting the tympanic membrane and ossicular chain vibration into an electric signal. The signal is received by the implanted sound processor which in turn filters, amplifies and sends the signal to the second transducer. The second transducer is coupled to the stapes and serves as a driver by converting the electrical signal into mechanical vibration. The device thus utilizes the tympanic membrane as the microphone for the system. This however firstly requires a healthy tympanic membrane and ossicular chain but also unfortunately necessitates disarticulation of the incudo-stapedial joint to prevent feedback (Marzo et al., 2014; Seidman et al., 2019). The implanted battery is non-rechargeable and needs to be replaced at regular intervals the suggested battery life is between 5 and 9 years (Fig. 9.4). (Chen et al., 2004; Barbara et al., 2009).

This device can be used in moderate to severe SNHL (Fig. 9.5) with a speech discrimination score of greater than 40%. The Middle ear anatomy must be normal.

Surgical Considerations

Of all the active middle ear implants, the maximum experience worldwide has probably been with the Vibrant Sound Bridge (VSB). The same is true in India, as well as with the author. For this reason, the surgical considerations for the vibrant sound bridge middle ear implant will be discussed in detail. The VSB comprises an internal implant called the Vibrating Ossicular Replacement Prosthesis (VORP), and an external component, or audio processor. The VORP is composed of a receiving coil, a magnet, a demodulator, a conductor cable, and a Floating Mass Transducer (FMT) (Fig. 9.6a).

Surgical implantation of the VSB has been termed as “Vibroplasty”.

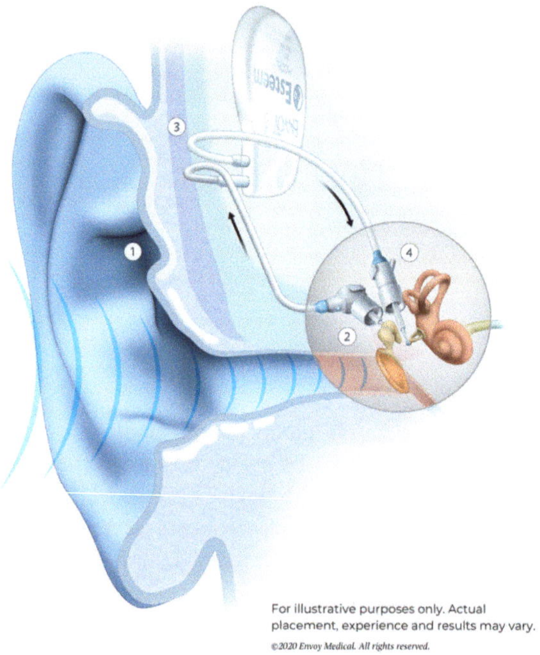

Fig. 9.4 Envoy Esteem. (Image courtesy Envoy Medical) [1-Tympanic membrane; 2-Sensor; 3-Sound processor; 4-Driver]

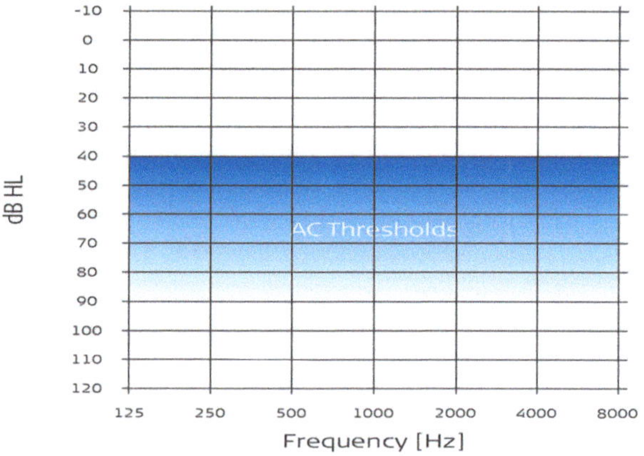

Fig. 9.5 Fitting criteria for SNHL. Stable AC thresholds in the shaded area

Preoperative Preparation

One needs to conduct audiological and otological assessments to confirm suitability for VSB implantation. It is important to obtain High-Resolution Computed Tomography (HRCT) to evaluate middle ear and mastoid anatomy. This helps the surgeon plan the procedure, assess the anatomy and determine the optimal

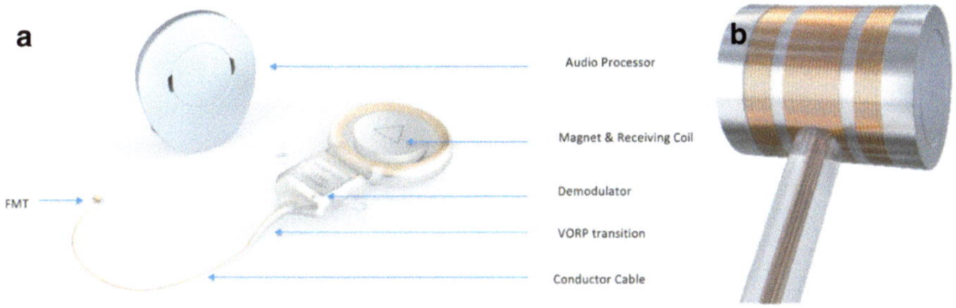

Fig. 9.6 (**a**) Vibrant Sound Bridge. (Image Courtesy of MED-EL Company). (**b**) Floating Mass Transducer (FMT). (Image Courtesy of MED-EL Company)

placement of the Floating Mass Transducer (FMT) based on individual anatomical considerations. Magnetic Resonance Imaging (MRI) may be indicated when evaluating for the sensorineural hearing loss. The patient's medical condition is assessed for fitness for general anaesthesia. Patients must be counselled and advised of potential risks such as hearing loss, dizziness, facial nerve trauma or infection.

Surgical Approaches

The procedure is usually carried out under general anaesthesia. The patient is positioned supine with the head turned to expose the surgical ear. An appropriate amount of hair is shaved and the surgical field is prepped and draped under sterile conditions. There are two primary surgical techniques for implantation: the traditional transmastoid/posterior tympanotomy approach and the alternative transcanal/transmeatal method.

The Transmastoid/Posterior Tympanotomy Approach

This is the more acceptable and commonly used method for Vibrant Soundbridge implantation. A postauricular approach is typically used, and may often follow existing surgical scars of an earlier mastoidectomy. The position of the VORP is marked using a template and this is usually placed at an angle of 45 degrees to the horizontal and at least 2 cm behind the proposed incision line (Fig. 9.7a). A C-shaped or curvilinear incision is made behind the pinna (Fig. 9.7b). A separate musculo-periosteal flap is elevated and a pocket is created under the periosteum to hold the implant. The thickness of the skin flap is checked using the skin flap gauge and should not exceed 7 mm to ensure good attachment of the audio processor later. The implant bed is drilled into the mastoid bone to secure the body of the VORP and the VORP transition and checked using the template. This ensures it does not shift

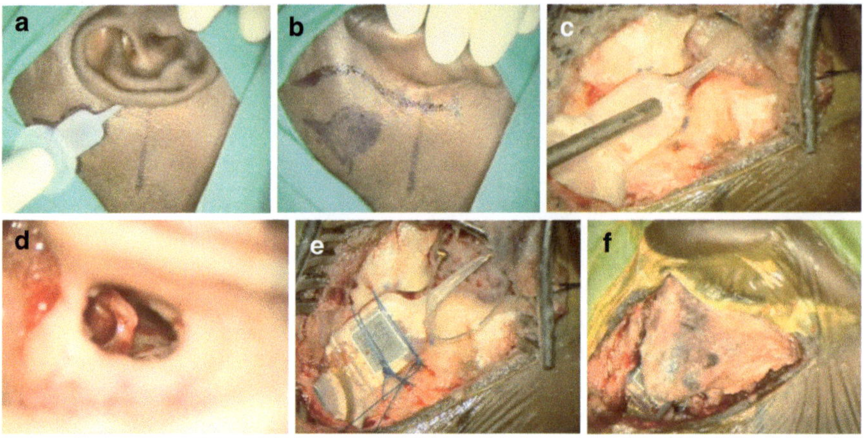

Fig. 9.7 (**a**) Marking the position of the VORP. (**b**) Marking the incision. (**c**) Body of the VORP placed in the bed drilled onto the mastoid cortex. (**d**) Posterior tympanotomy and identification of Incus long process and Stapes. (**e**) Body of the VORP and the VORP transition in position (This being an earlier version, was secured using tie-down sutures). (**f**) Musculo-periosteal flap replaced over the VORP

postoperatively and also prevents damage to the conductor cable (Fig. 9.7c). A cortical mastoidectomy is made preserving key structures such as the facial nerve, sigmoid sinus, and dura. Through a posterior tympanotomy, the facial recess is identified and adequately widened for access to the middle ear. Care is taken to preserve the chorda tympani nerve. One needs to Identify the incus and stapes and assess the condition of the middle ear and plan how the FMT is going to be attached to either one of the ossicles or the round window membrane (Fig. 9.7d). The body of the VORP consisting of the coil and demodulator is placed and fixed in its bed using the self-tapping screws that go through the two titanium flanges. The VORP transition is carefully placed in its groove leading to the edge of the cortical mastoidectomy (Fig. 9.7e). The conductor cable is carefully coiled and placed in the mastoid cavity. It is important to avoid kinking or damage of this lead. The FMT is attached in one of the methods described in the next section. The periosteal flap is replaced (Fig. 9.7f), the wound is closed in layers and a pressure dressing is applied for a couple of days.

Attachment of the FMT

Depending on the indication and situation, the FMT may be attached using one of the appropriate couplers to the Incus (short process or long process), Stapes or Round window. It can also be combined with a Partial Ossicular Replacement Prostheses (PORP), Total Ossicular Replacement Prostheses (TORP) or Stapes prosthesis depending on the need (Fig. 9.8).

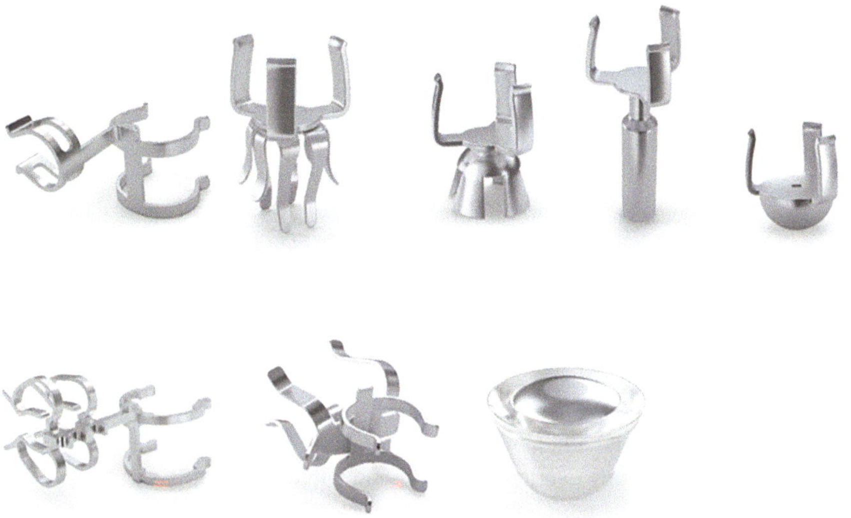

Fig. 9.8 Variety of Couplers for FMT attachment. (Image Courtesy of MED-EL Company)

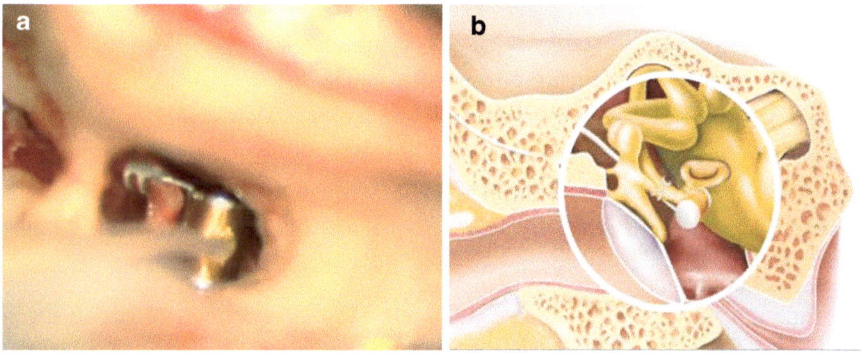

Fig. 9.9 (**a**) FMT fitted onto the Long process of the incus (right ear). (**b**) FMT fitted onto the Long process of the incus (schematic). (Image Courtesy of MED-EL Company)

Incus Attachment

The FMT can be attached to the long process of the incus using the LP coupler. The FMT is placed along the Stapes superstructure and the coupler is crimped onto the long process of the incus (Fig. 9.9a). The FMT may also be attached to the short process of the incus using the SP coupler.

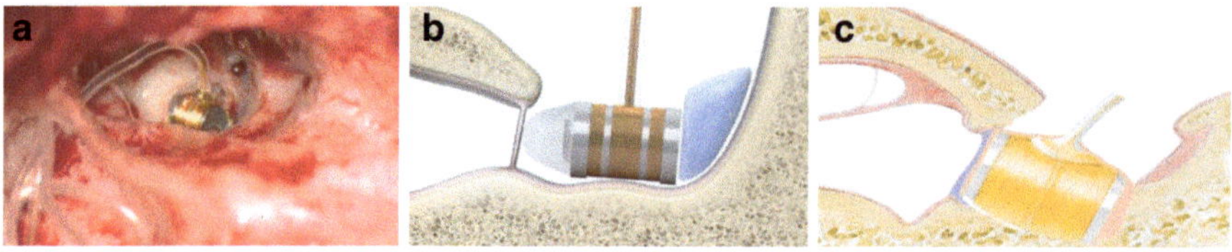

Fig.9.10 (**a**) FMT placed onto the Round Window (right ear). (**b**) FMT placed onto the Round Window using RW coupler (schematic). (Image Courtesy of MED-EL Company). (**c**) FMT placed onto the Round Window directly (schematic). (Image Courtesy of MED-EL Company)

Application to the Round Window

In situations where the ossicles are absent, the FMT may be placed directly over the round window. The round window membrane must be exposed by carefully removing excess tissue and bony overhang of the round window niche.

A layer of autologous perichondrium (harvested from the patient) is positioned between the FMT and the round window membrane to ensure hydromechanical coupling and reduce the risk of long-term complications. Alternatively, a round window coupler may be used. The FMT is placed perpendicular to the round window membrane and secured with cartilage to optimize vibration transfer (Fig. 9.10a).

FMT with Ossicular Replacement Prostheses

In cases where an ossicular replacement prosthesis is used, the FMT can be combined with it. If the stapes superstructure is intact, the FMT can be combined with a Partial Ossicular Replacement Prosthesis (PORP). The PORP is interposed between the tympanic membrane reconstruction and the stapes head, ensuring stable sound transmission. Alternatively, a Stapes coupler or a Clip coupler may be used to attach the FMT onto the head of the stapes. If the stapes superstructure is absent, FMT can be combined with a Total Ossicular Replacement Prosthesis (TORP). The combined unit is placed between the footplate of the stapes and the tympanic membrane reconstruction.

FMT with Stapes Prostheses

In cases of otosclerosis with mixed losses, the FMT is secured to the long process of the incus and connected to a stapes prosthesis. Proper alignment is required to ensure optimal sound transmission (Mlynski et al., 2010).

The Transcanal/Transmeatal Approach

The transcanal or transmeatal method is an alternative approach. Instead of accessing the middle ear through the mastoid and posterior tympanotomy, access is obtained through the ear canal. The bed is created for the VORP in the normal fashion. A shallow mastoidectomy is performed to accommodate the conductor cable. The tympanomeatal flap with annulus is elevated to expose the middle ear structures. The scutum is drilled to expose the ossicular chain and accommodate the FMT. A groove for the conductor cable is drilled in the bony canal terminating laterally at the edge of the mastoidectomy. Once the FMT is crimped onto the incus, the conductor cable is then covered in the groove of the bony ear canal with bone pate and fascia, before repositioning the tympanomeatal flap (McKinnon, 2010).

VSB in Congenital Aural Atresia

The Vibrant Sound Bridge Middle Ear implant has also been used to treat conductive and mixed hearing losses in congenital aural atresia. This is an established alternative to atresioplasty or use of a Bone Conduction Implant. A pre-operative CT scan of the temporal bone is mandatory to assess the severity of the condition of the middle ear, ossicle chain and the position of the facial nerve. The Jahrsdoerfer Score is commonly used to assess the condition of the middle ear. The FMT can be coupled at different locations in the middle ear such as the incus, stapes superstructure, oval window or the round window membrane. Systematic reviews suggest that recipients obtain a significant benefit following VSB implantation in congenital aural atresia in their pure tone auditory thresholds, speech recognition scores as well as quality of life measures (Alshalan & Alzhrani, 2024; McKinnon et al., 2014).

Postoperative Care

It is important to monitor the patient for facial nerve function, dizziness, and pain. Antibiotics and analgesics as needed are prescribed. About 4–6 weeks are allowed for healing before activating the device. An audiological programming and fine-tuning of the implant is conducted at the time of activation. It is mandatory to regularly monitor the implant's performance and address any complications (Pegan et al., 2019).

Complications

Similar to middle ear surgeries, complications include labyrinthine injury, worsening of hearing loss, facial nerve damage, wound breakdown or infection. The device may be damaged such as the conductor cable during handling or postoperative movement. Improper fixation of the VORP may lead to displacement or functional failure. In cases of a suboptimal hearing outcome, the programming parameters may need to be adjusted. In some situations one may need to consider revision surgery to reposition the FMT (Mlynski et al., 2010).

Outcomes

Several studies have been published evaluating the benefits of implantable hearing aids. While only a few provide direct comparison between performance with conventional hearing aids, most have demonstrated improvement in hearing performance over the unaided condition, low complication rates and high subjective satisfaction scores. Despite the consistent report of high patient satisfaction and subjective preference over conventional hearing aids in many cases, implantable hearing aids have not gained significant market penetrance. While some patients may prefer conventional aids over an implantable device requiring surgery and associated risks of anaesthesia and manipulation of the middle ear, additional factors may contribute to lack of widespread adoption.

A major concern in MEI surgery is the risk of hearing loss during ossicular loading and device coupling. Overall, studies evaluated for air and/or bone conduction threshold changes after surgery did not find statistically significant loss in air or bone conduction after surgery. All studies that compared the preoperative unaided condition and postoperative MEI assisted hearing demonstrated improvement of varying levels (mean of 25.2 dB improvement; range reported between 15.6 and 48.2 dB). However, when comparing the best aided preoperative condition with post-implantation performance, three-fourths of the studies demonstrated less than a 10-dB difference (weighted mean, 8.1 dB improvement; range reported between j8.4 and +13 dB) in functional gain, and only 1 reported a statistically significant improvement over optimally fitted hearing aids.

Hearing Aid Benefit Profiles demonstrated improvement in ease of communication, hearing in background noise, hearing in reverberant backgrounds, and decreased aversion to sound. Additional perceived benefits included improved quality of sound, elimination of occlusive effect, and an improved ability to lead an active lifestyle when compared with conventional hearing aid use (Kahue et al., 2014).

Regarding objective hearing outcomes, all 3 MEIs provided significant increases in functional gain over unaided hearing; however, only 1 of 12 studies demonstrated a statistically significant improvement over optimally fitted hearing aids. Similarly, regarding speech recognition performance, 7 of 12 studies revealed no statistically significant advantage of MEIs over optimally fitted hearing aids. When examining the results of patient-reported outcome measures, most studies demonstrated improvements with regard to sound clarity, occlusion effect, and feedback. Taken together, the objective audiometric benefits derived from MEIs are comparable to those received from conventional hearing aids, whereas patient-reported outcome measures demonstrate several potential advantages (Kahue et al., 2014). Complications that have been reported include infections, skin defects, pain, changes in taste, facial paresis and device failure. Device failure and revision surgery may be required for situations such as incus erosion, ossification, poor coupling of the transducer, middle ear adhesions (Zwartenkot et al., 2016).

The desire for the development of implantable hearing aids was to improve upon limitations of conventional hearing aids, including acoustics distortion, feedback and high output levels, gain limitations, removal of canal occlusion for patients with chronic otitis, and lifestyle limitations due to the need for an externally worn device. While some of these goals have been addressed, particularly related to perceived subjective benefit, data regarding acoustic performance improvement is mixed and a clear objective performance benefit remains elusive. Additionally, the advantage of removal of canal occlusion and externally worn aids remains incompletely realized as only one of the currently available devices is completely implantable and many patients must still wear external processors. Because MEI do not use acoustic speakers, the ear canal is left open. This leads to decreased acoustic feedback and occlusion, common complaints among conventional hearing aid users. Many conventional hearing aids are limited in their ability to deliver understandable speech at high frequencies because of a maximal degree of attainable amplification before feedback occurs. At sound levels beyond this point, sound escapes from around the hearing aid within the canal and is reamplified by the device, producing feedback. This phenomenon in conventional hearing aids is due to the juxtaposition of the microphone and receiver, a problem resolved by the design of MEI. Tight-fitting conventional hearing aid earmolds are used to dampen feedback at high frequencies but inherently carry occlusive effects. Removal of the occlusion sensation by MEIs results in sound that is subjectively clearer than the acoustic quality offered by conventional hearing aids. MEI are valuable treatment options for patients with disorders of the ear canal including eczema and resistant chronic otitis externa. Pain, itching, and poor sound quality contribute to poor tolerance and non-use of conventional hearing aids in patients with chronic otitis externa.

Candidacy for an active middle ear implant should be well considered, both audiological and medical. Possible complications concerning the surgical procedure and the follow-up period should be counseled. MRI compatibility will remain a challenge with an increasing frequency in MRI diagnostics and possible increase in field strength.

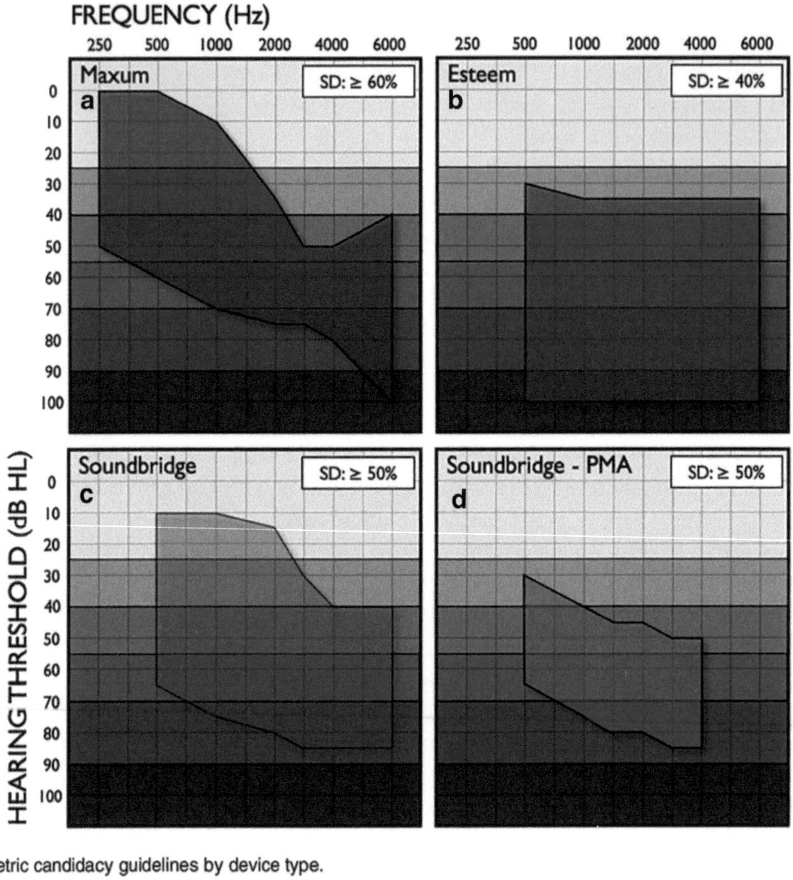

Fig. 9.11 Audiometric guidelines for the three different devices (Kahue et al., 2014)

The fitting ranges for the different Devices is shown in Fig. 9.11

The early data reported seems to support the use of MEI because, in general, they do not decrease residual hearing and result in a functional gain in hearing comparable with conventional hearing aids. The studies seem to indicate that perception of speech in noise may actually be better with MEI than conventional hearing aids, and that patients reported better sound quality with the MEI (Tysome et al., 2010).

References

Alshalan, A., & Alzhrani, F. (2024). Efficacy of vibrant sound bridge in congenital aural atresia: An updated systematic review. *European Archives of Oto-Rhino-Laryngology, 281*(6), 2849–2859. https://doi.org/10.1007/s00405-024-08629-6

Ball, G. R. (2010). The vibrant soundbridge: Design and development. *Advances in Oto-Rhino-Laryngology, 69*, 1–13. https://doi.org/10.1159/000318516

Banakis Hartl, R. M., & Jenkins, H. A. (2020). Implantable hearing aids: Where are we in 2020? *Laryngoscope Investigative Otolaryngology, 5*(6), 1184–1191. https://doi.org/10.1002/lio2.495

Barbara, M., Manni, V., & Monini, S. (2009). Totally implantable middle ear device for rehabilitation of sensorineural hearing loss: Preliminary experience with the Esteem, Envoy. *Acta Otolaryngologica, 129*(4), 429–432. https://doi.org/10.1080/00016480802593505

Carlson, M. L., Pelosi, S., & Haynes, D. S. (2014). Historical development of active middle ear implants. *Otolaryngologic Clinics of North America, 47*(6), 893–914. https://doi.org/10.1016/j.otc.2014.08.004

Chen, D. A., Backous, D. D., Arriaga, M. A., Garvin, R., Kobylek, D., Littman, T., Walgren, S., & Lura, D. (2004). Phase 1 clinical trial results of the envoy system: A totally implantable middle ear device for sensorineural hearing loss. *Otolaryngology--Head and Neck Surgery, 131*(6), 904–916. https://doi.org/10.1016/j.otohns.2004.05.027

Kahue, C. N., Carlson, M. L., Daugherty, J. A., Haynes, D. S., & Glasscock, M. E., 3rd. (2014). Middle ear implants for rehabilitation of sensorineural hearing loss: A systematic review of FDA approved devices. *Otology & Neurotology, 35*(7), 1228–1237. https://doi.org/10.1097/MAO.0000000000000341

Labassi, S., Beliaeff, M., Péan, V., & Van de Heyning, P. (2017). The vibrant Soundbridge® middle ear implant: A historical overview. *Cochlear Implants International, 18*(6), 314–323. https://doi.org/10.1080/14670100.2017.1358913

Lenarz, T., Weber, B. P., Mack, K. F., Battmer, R. D., & Gnadeberg, D. (1998). Vibrant Soundbridge System: Ein neuartiges Hörimplantat für Innenohrschwerhörige. Teil 1: Funktionsweise und erste klinische Erfahrungen [The Vibrant Soundbridge System: a new kind of hearing aid for sensorineural hearing loss. 1: Function and initial clinical experiences]. *Laryngo- Rhino-Otologie, 77*(5), 247–255. https://doi.org/10.1055/s-2007-996970

Marzo, S. J., Sappington, J. M., & Shohet, J. A. (2014). The envoy esteem implantable hearing system. *Otolaryngologic Clinics of North America, 47*(6), 941–952. https://doi.org/10.1016/j.otc.2014.08.006

Matthews, P. (2002). The SOUNDTEC direct system. *Trends in Amplification, 6*(2), 61–65. https://doi.org/10.1177/108471380200600206 5

McKinnon, B. J. (2010). Vibrant Soundbridge implantation: The transmastoid/posterior tympanotomy and transcanal approaches. *Operative Techniques in Otolaryngology-Head and Neck Surgery, 21*(3), 189–193.

McKinnon, B. J., Dumon, T., Hagen, R., Lesinskas, E., Mlynski, R., Profant, M., Spindel, J., Van Beek-King, J., & Zernotti, M. (2014). Vibrant soundbridge in aural atresia: Does severity matter? *European Archives of Oto-rhino-laryngology, 271*(7), 1917–1921. https://doi.org/10.1007/s00405-013-2680-0

Mlynski, R., Mueller, J., & Hagen, R. (2010). Surgical approaches to position the vibrant soundbridge in conductive and mixed hearing loss. *Operative Techniques in Otolaryngology-Head and Neck Surgery, 21*(4), 272–277.

Pegan, A., Ries, M., Ajduk, J., Bedeković, V., Ivkić, M., & Trotić, R. (2019). Active middle ear vibrant soundbridge sound implant. *Acta Clinica Croatica, 58*(2), 348–353. https://doi.org/10.20471/acc.2019.58.02.20

Pelosi, S., Carlson, M. L., & Glasscock, M. E., 3rd. (2014). Implantable hearing devices: The Ototronix MAXUM system. *Otolaryngologic Clinics of North America, 47*(6), 953–965. https://doi.org/10.1016/j.otc.2014.08.003

Seidman, M. D., Janz, T. A., & Shohet, J. A. (2019). Totally implantable active middle ear implants. *Otolaryngologic Clinics of North America, 52*(2), 297–309. https://doi.org/10.1016/j.otc.2018.11.011

Suzuki, J., Kodera, K., Nagai, K., & Yabe, T. (1995). Partially implantable piezoelectric middle ear hearing device. Long-term results. *Otolaryngologic Clinics of North America, 28*(1), 99–106.

Tisch, M. (2017). Implantable hearing devices. *GMS Current Topics Otorhinolaryngology Head and Neck Surgery, 16*, Doc06.

Thurnheer, S., Müller, T., Linder, T., Simmen, D., & Harder, M. (2023). Congenital aural atresia: Hearing rehabilitation using active middle-ear implants. *The Journal of Laryngology and Otology, 137*(8), 851–865. https://doi.org/10.1017/S0022215122002183

Tysome, J. R., Moorthy, R., Lee, A., Jiang, D., & O'Connor, A. F. (2010). Systematic review of middle ear implants: Do they improve hearing as much as conventional hearing AIDS? *Otology & Neurotology, 31*(9), 1369–1375. https://doi.org/10.1097/MAO.0b013e3181db716c

Zwartenkot, J. W., Mulder, J. J., Snik, A. F., Cremers, C. W., & Mylanus, E. A. (2016). Active middle ear implantation: Long-term medical and technical follow-up, implant survival, and complications. *Otology & Neurotology, 37*(5), 513–519. https://doi.org/10.1097/MAO.0000000000001015

Chapter 10
Cochlear Implants: History and Basic Concepts

Prawin Kumar, Priyanjali Harit, Prabhash Kumar, Niraj Kumar Singh, and Kumari Apeksha

Abstract About 1.5 billion people worldwide are affected by various degrees of hearing loss, out of which 430 million have moderate or higher degree of hearing loss as per the World hearing report of the World Health Organisation. The above data highlights the need for meaningful rehabilitation for huge chunk of the world's population. Cochlear implant innovation has been playing a pivotal role for such people, who would be otherwise lost in the world of deafness. The present chapter highlights the innovation of the cochlear implant, initial experiments that led to this present day marvel, and its basic functioning.

Keywords Cochlear implant · Speech processor · Cochlea · Receiver stimulator · Electrode array

Introduction

Today 1.5 billion people worldwide are affected by various degrees of hearing loss, out of which 430 million have moderate or higher degree of hearing loss in the better hearing ear, and as per the World hearing report (WHO, 2021), if this issue is not addressed in a timely manner, its adverse effects could lead to irreversible consequences. For several years during the era of hearing device development,

P. Kumar (✉) · N. K. Singh
Department of Audiology, All India Institute of Speech and Hearing, University of Mysore, Mysore, India

P. Harit
Army Hospital Research & Referral, New Delhi, Delhi, India

P. Kumar
Brahmnaad Speech and Hearing Clinic, New Delhi, Delhi, India

K. Apeksha
MarThoma College of Special Education, Kerala University of Health Sciences, Kasaragod, Kerala, India

P. Kumar et al. (eds.), *Advances in Implantation Otology*,
https://doi.org/10.1007/978-981-96-8671-1_10

individuals with severe to profound degrees of hearing impairment had very limited rehabilitation options, and despite being fitted with high-gain hearing aids, the outcomes were not appreciable in a vast majority of them. In late 1980's, the revolutionary change brought about by the invention of cochlear implant changed the landscape of treatment outcomes in people with severe to profound sensorineural hearing loss. Today many of the cochlear implant recipients enjoy ease of listening, and those affected by it congenitally are able to develop age appropriate communication skills.

The main function of a normal cochlea is to analyze and convert the sound vibration into a pattern of electrical signals that can be transmitted through the auditory nervous system to the brain. This process involves three major steps: sensory transduction, processing of the signals, and neurotransmission (For more details, refer to the Chapter 1). In the case of poorly functioning or non-functioning cochlea, various components of cochlear implant perform the function of the cochlea and stimulate the spiral ganglions of the cochlear nerve directly. A cochlear implant is, therefore, an electronic device that contains a current source and an implanted electrode array into the cochlea which stimulates the surviving auditory nerve fibers (Wilson, 2000).

In the initial days of their invention, the cochlear implants were single-channel devices, which have evolved over time in a way that the modern era boasts of several commercially available multichannel cochlear implant systems. Multichannel cochlear implants are the most successful sensory prosthetic device in the history of medicine technology in the area of deafness. Cochlear implant has not only resulted in providing hearing solution to those with severe to profound hearing loss but has also helped improve the overall quality of life of millions of such people. What was only a thought of the dreams a few decades ago has turned into a reality with children with severe to profound hearing loss now developing age appropriate speech and language skills when implanted at an early enough age (Geers, 2004; Geers et al., 2003, 2009). Among the several testimonies to this claim is a study by Dettman and colleagues, which evaluated speech and language skills of 403 children using cochlear implants and found that almost 81% of those implanted before 12 months of age had normal vocabulary development (Dettman et al., 2016). Hence, early cochlear implantation, especially during the critical period of development, shows promising outcomes.

Many clinical trials and patient feedback confirm that cochlear implantation also yields optimal benefits in adults with post-lingual hearing impairment. The far-reaching benefits of cochlear implantation also benefits those with pathological conditions related to the inner ear or auditory nerve, such as auditory neuropathy spectrum disorder (ANSD), some structural cochlear deformities (like incomplete partition & large vestibular aqueduct), hypoplastic auditory nerve and fairly significant degeneration of spiral ganglion fibers (Rance & Barker, 2008). The success of cochlear implantation is influenced by many factors, such as age of implantation, period of auditory deprivation, inner ear/cochlear/auditory nerve structure, co-morbidity, post-surgery residual hearing preservation, electrode positioning within the cochlea, quality of speech and language therapy, quality of the mapping/

program created by an Audiologist, client/parents' motivation and intelligence level of the recipient, etc.

The steady development in the technology of cochlear implants over the last three decades has led to the development of the modern-day masterpiece in the treatment of hearing impairment. Today's implants are not only highly reliable but also durable enough to last the lifetime of a patient. The evolution of technology and design over the years has led to the development of different types and various lengths of arrays to stimulate more than one site in the cochlea, and progressive improvements in sound processing strategies to provide the best possible inputs to brain. In this chapter, we describe how this modern day wonder saw the day light, and trace the path to its modern day glory.

The Evidence for the Very First Attempt

Though the cochlear implant as a device was invented only a few decades ago, the research and experiments that led to the final invention began centuries ago. The idea of using electrical stimulation of the auditory nerve fibers in individuals with severe to profound hearing loss dates back to 1800's, when an Italian physicist Alessandro Volta (Fig. 10.1), from the University of Padua, invented the battery cell (Volta, 1800). In his experiment in which he inserted metal rods into each of his own ears and connected them to a circuit of approximately 50 Volts, he described his experience as having a sensation of "*a shock within the head*", which was not pleasant at all. Alessandro Volta stated that he did not repeat this experiment as he believed that this displeasing sensation might be dangerous on clinical population as it created shock in the brain.

First Electrical Stimulation to Auditory System

The first attempt of developing a prosthetic device to stimulate the auditory nerve fibers dates back to 1957, when Andre Djourno, an electrophysiologist, and Charles Eyries, an otolaryngologist, used the principles of electromagnetic induction to stimulate the auditory nerve electrically through their newly designed implantable prosthesis. Andre Djourno's work was majorly focused on delivering the electromagnetic stimulation transcutaneously (across the skin) to the implantable induction coils to deliver electrical current to peripheral nerves or muscles, whereas Charles Eyrie's expertise was in facial nerve reconstruction. Both of them (Fig. 10.2), while working together at the same place, decided to implant Djourno's device, an induction stimulator, in order to provide electrical stimulation to the auditory nerve on a 57-year-old man. This man had previously gone for temporal bone resection in both ears sequentially due to bilateral cholesteatomas, and was left with bilateral deafness and bilateral facial nerve paralysis after the cholesteatoma removal

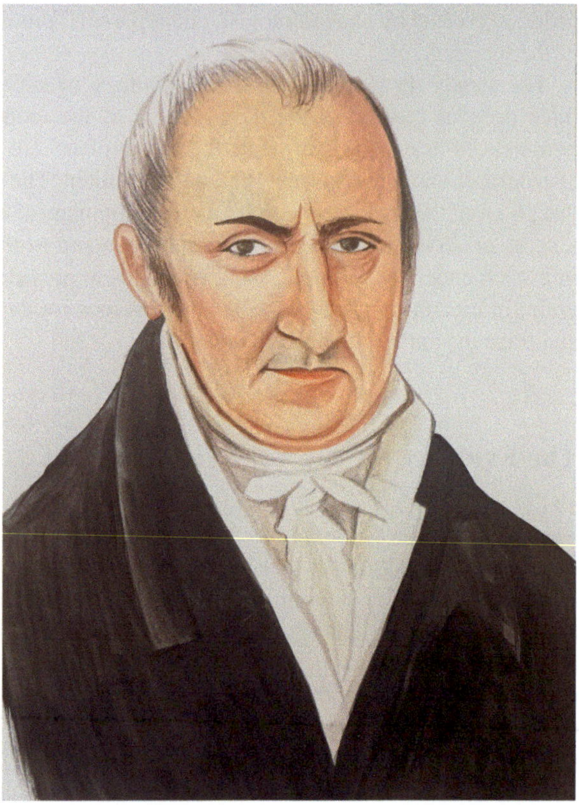

Fig. 10.1 Alessandro Volta, the first person to show that electricity can produce a hearing sensation

surgeries. This patient was taken up primarily for the facial nerve repair surgery by Charles Eyries, and later Eyries and Djourno decided to consider him for their first attempt to provide electrical stimulation to the auditory system.

The procedure was carried out on February 25, 1957, while Charles Eyries performed the right-sided facial nerve graft, Djourno and Eyries decided to place the active electrode into the remaining stump of the cochlear nerve and the induction coil into the temporalis muscle (Djourno & Eyries, 1957). The intraoperative testing included the presentation of a burst of 100 Hz impulse signal (low frequency alternating current) 15–20 times per minute, and words spoken into the microphone. The patient was able to distinguish changes in the intensity of stimulation but the frequency discrimination was poor. He reported his experience of hearing a sound like 'crickets or a roulette wheel". After the surgery, the patient underwent extensive rehabilitation with the implant under the guidance of a speech-language pathologist. Over the next few months, the patient's performance with this implant was evaluated with more complex stimuli; the patient was never able to develop good listening skills and could not develop the ability to understand speech, but he could differentiate between high and low frequencies and appreciated environmental noises and a few words. Before Djourno and Eyries could perform more experiments on their first implanted device, it malfunctioned after a short period of use.

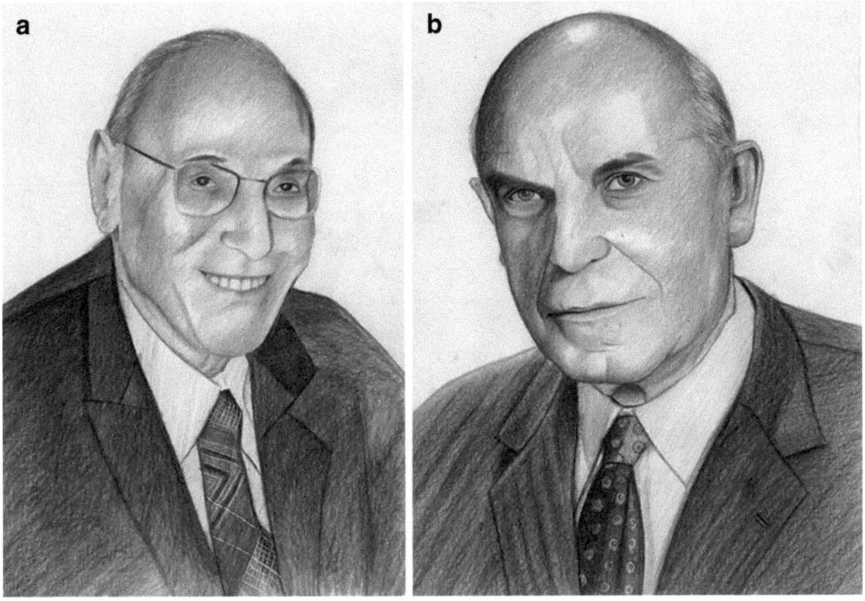

Fig. 10.2 The pioneers of electrical stimulation to the auditory nerve fibers that eventually led to the development of cochlear implant: (**a**) Andre Djourno; (**b**) Charles Eyries

Charles Eyries implanted a second device, but unfortunately, this device too malfunctioned. The Djourno's device was not considered as a true cochlear implant as it was not inserted in the cochlea and did not stimulate the auditory nerve as it was already damaged by the previous temporal bone surgery. Two years later, Djourno and Eyries parted ways due to personal and professional differences, leading to a pre-mature end to a wonderfully innovative work on the direct electrical stimulation of the auditory nerve.

First Single-Channel Cochlear Implant

In the year 1959, 2 years after the separation of Djourno and Eyries, William F. House (Fig. 10.3), an Otologist who was working at Otologic Medical Group in Los Angeles with his brother Howard House, was inspired by the summary of the research work by Djourno and Eyries on electric stimulation to replace hearing (House, 1976). Interestingly, this piece of article was brought to his notice by one of his patients. House, with his neurosurgeon colleague John Doyle, attempted electrical stimulation of cochlea using square wave stimuli to elicit hearing by placing needle electrode on the promontory or into the open oval window while conducting stapes surgery. They used ear speculum placed in the external auditory canal as a ground electrode. After observing that their patients were comfortable hearing the stimuli, and did not report dizziness and facial nerve stimulation upon activation of

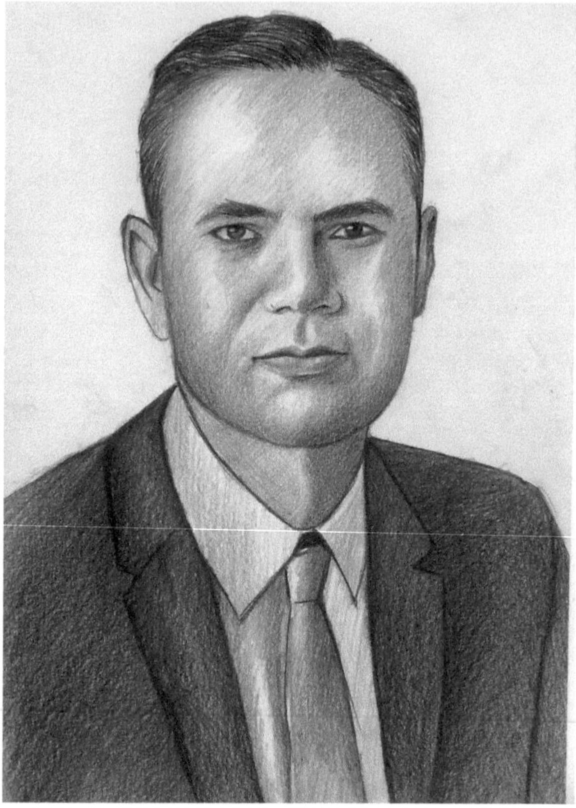

Fig. 10.3 William F. House

the device, House and Doyle were motivated to implant a patient with a hard-wire device.

On January 9, 1961, William House, used the post-auricular approach under local anaesthesia to insert a gold wire electrode into the round window of a 40-year old patient with severe hearing loss due to otosclerosis (House, 1974). The other end of the wire was taken out through the skin overlying the post-auricular region. Though the patient reported hearing the electrical stimuli, the wire was removed after a few days of the surgery due to poor loudness tolerance. Not discouraged by this somewhat failed attempt, William House made another attempt in the same month. This time, the patient had profound hearing loss and tinnitus due to congenital syphilis and was undergoing vestibular neurectomy using the middle fossa approach to seek relief from dizziness. The single gold wire electrode was into scala tympani at the basal part of the cochlea, whereas the one end of the wire was taken out through the skin incision. The patient reported hearing sensation when the electrode was stimulated; however, the fear of complications, such as infection or edema, was the reason for the removal of the wire, which led to a pre-mature cessation of the experiment on this patient. In February 1961, House and Doyle re-implanted their first patient (the one who had otosclerosis and was previously implanted in January 1961) with a five-wire implant, placed in scala tympani with varying depths in the cochlea, and the induction coil was placed in the post-auricular region in the skull. The patient could discriminate different frequencies with stimulation of different electrodes, which was highly encouraging for the researchers. However, this experiment too was short-lived and the device needed excision a few weeks later due to swelling in the post-auricular region.

William House and John Doyle took the help of Jim Doyle (John Doyle's brother and an electrical engineer) to develop instruments required for electrical stimulation of the inner ear (Mudry & Mills, 2013). After working in collaboration with each other on a few projects, their association came to an abrupt end as apparently, House was upset that the Doyle brothers prematurely released the information about their experiment on electrical stimulation of the cochlea in the media. This led to differences between them, which culminated in the end of their collaboration. Undeterred by the turn of events, the Doyle brothers continued implanting patients with their manufactured implants till 1968 but were forced into ceasing their investigations due to a lack of research funding. On the other side, till 1967, William House did not perform implant surgeries in the realization that cochlear implant material should be biocompatible and the method of implantation should be such that the device should last a long time (House, 2011). He was inspired by and appreciated the invention of other biomedical devices, such as pacemaker, which had hermetic sealing technology to prevent the contact of the electronic components with body fluid in order to keep these components protected over a long period of time.

In a period between 1969 and 1973, William House along with Jack Urban, an electric engineer, implanted patients with single-channel cochlear implants with a percutaneous plug, which was implanted within the skull and protruded through the skin. This time their focus was also on the durability and safety of the device and they published their single-case experience with cochlear implantation in the journal Annals of Otology, Rhinology, and Laryngology (1973). In 1972, one of Dr. House's patients received the first wearable sound processor that allowed the patients to use it outside the clinical settings. Dr. House was the first surgeon to implant electrodes into the cochlea and develop the first wearable sound processor. Therefore, to honour his incomparable contribution to the field of implantation otology, he is often remarked as ***'the Father of cochlear implantation'*** (Eshraghi et al., 2012).

During an experiment, when an amplitude-modulated signal with a 16,000-Hz carrier frequency was presented, a cochlear implant recipient reported better appreciation of higher frequencies than with unmodulated signals and also rated the hearing with the modulated signal higher than other signals. Dr. House made this a signal-processing strategy for his House/3M cochlear implant. By this time, cochlear implantation had great interest among otologists, audiologists, scientists, researchers, and many other clinicians, but many of them were doubtful of the extent of benefits in achieving open-set speech recognition with such an implantable device.

Robin Michelson, an Otolaryngologist from California, too showed great interest in cochlear implants and performed experiments while using a high-gain amplifier with an ear piece. Michelson placed the gold wire electrode against the round window and observed that the feedback from the amplifier could elicit the sensation of sound. Michelson's first clinical trial was on a woman with congenital severe to profound hearing loss, with a single-channel cochlear implant. Post-implantation, Michelson discovered that the patient could not only differentiate the two different stimuli (square wave & sine wave), but also perceive the pitch of less than 600 Hz with this implant. Following this successful experimentation, several other patients received the single channel cochlear implant, and the outcomes of this preliminary work was presented at the convention of the American Academy of Ophthalmology and Otolaryngology in 1971. Francis Sooy, the chairman of the Nascent department of otolaryngology, at the University of California San Francisco (UCSF), was inspired by the work of Robin Michelson and believed that University-based scientific foundation is a must for the successful development of cochlear implant. He invited Robin Michelson to join the team at his institute as a faculty. Soon after the joining of Michelson, and Merzenich, a neurophysiologist, too joined UCSF as faculty. Merzenich was also convinced of the success of the ongoing research trials on cochlear implants and believed in the positive outcomes from them (Merzenich, 2015). Michelson, Merzenich and Sooy joined hands for the development of the UCSF cochlear implant program. With their many trials, they concluded that a cochlear implant consisting of multiple electrodes would be necessary for the perception of complex sound signals. During this time, researchers were actively involved, more than ever before, in experimenting and developing a multichannel cochlear implant. By 1973, the only clinicians performing cochlear implants were House and Michelson, and significant work by these two surgeons made it clear that the direct stimulation of the auditory nerve was possible.

In the early 1980's Dr. House modified his single channel implant and was busy implanting several patients. Meanwhile, the other centres still believed in performing more and more research and developing a multichannel implant system. A 3-year old child became the youngest recipient, who was implanted with Dr. House's single-channel cochlear implant in 1981 (Eisenberg & House, 1982). Dr. House performed several trials to evaluate the efficacy of cochlear implantation in both children and adults, and later in the year 1982, the collaborative work of House, Urban and 3M Company developed the first commercial cochlear implant- the House/3M cochlear implant. The House/3M cochlear implant was evaluated for clinical trial by the U.S. Food and Drug Administration (FDA) (Eisenberg, 2015). In 1984, the FDA approved House/3M cochlear implants for commercial use in the United States, making it the first FDA approved device for commercial use (Eisenberg, 2015). By 1985, 164 children with an average age of 8 years were implanted with the House/3M cochlear implant and the findings were suggestive of modest outcomes post-implantation due to the higher upper age selected for the study. Investigators realized that many factors such as age of implantation, motivation level of family, mode of communication, and other factors specifically related to children such as their neurocognitive levels, cochlear structure, and co-morbidity, have a great impact on the post-implantation outcomes. A total of 265 children were implanted with House/3M cochlear implants by 1987 (Berliner et al., 1990), and in the same year, FDA recommended commercial approval of the device for implanting children after reviewing the data from many centers (Eisenberg, 2015).

Multichannel Cochlear Implant

In mid 1980's researchers like Merzenich, Michelson, and Robert Schindler among others at UCSF and Graeme Clark at the University of Melbourne in Australia were in a race to develop a multichannel cochlear implant. Graeme Clark, an otolaryngologist (Fig. 10.4) had a systematic scientific approach to developing a multichannel device. His work was focused on developing speech coding strategies, optimizing the electrode array, and developing a safe, reliable implantable receiver-stimulator. Graeme Clark implanted the first human subject in 1978, and with his research and clinical trials, he was the first to conclude that multiple channel cochlear implants would be required to achieve adequate speech recognition in open set tasks (Clark et al., 1977, 1978). Dr. Clark's work emphasized on many other important findings such as the dynamic range of electrical hearing was much lesser than that of acoustic hearing (Clark et al., 1978). His work also concluded that the insertion length of a minimum of 20 to 25 mm is required for systematic representation of spectral range across the cochlea. Dr. Clark and his colleagues reported that cochlear structures are less prone to damage if the electrode insertion is made in an anterograde

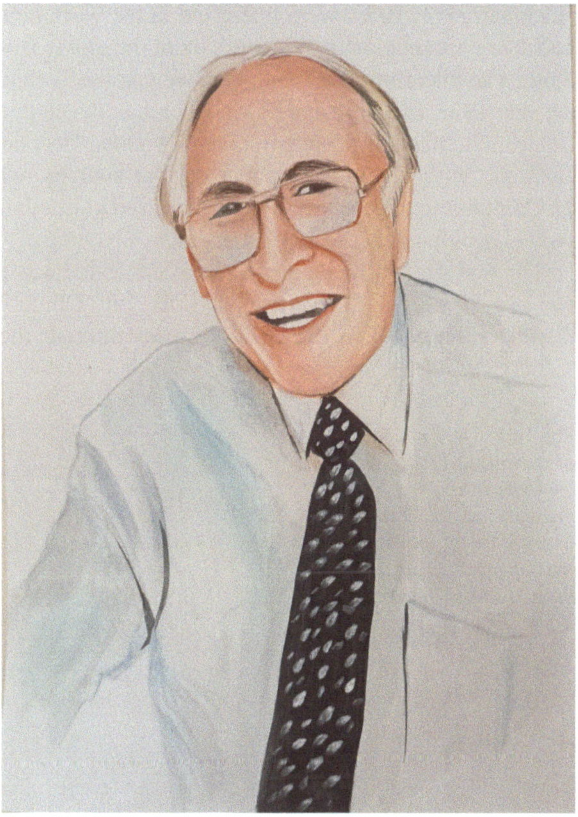

Fig. 10.4 Graeme Clark, the scientist behind the development of first multi-channel cochlear implant

direction through a single cochleostomy at a round window niche into scala tympani. Over the past decades, it has been proved by many clinical researchers that for better outcomes with cochlear implantation, preserving residual hearing during cochlear implantation should be the target. Dr. Clark's clinical work, which was funded jointly by Australian national telethons and government grants, culminated into the development of the first successfully commercialized multichannel cochlear implant under the name of Cochlear/Nucleus (Clark, 2003).

In 1985, Nucleus multichannel implant received FDA approval for adults and in 1990 for children under 2 years of age. Since then multichannel cochlear implants have become a safe option for both adults and children with profound hearing loss.

Cochlear Implant Development by Other Manufacturers

MED-EL

In the year 1975, Ingeborg Desoyer (better known as Ingeborg Hochmair or Ingebog Hochmair-Desoyer after she adopted her husband's family name) and Erwin Hochmair (Fig. 10.5), were interested in the work being carried out in the area of cochlear implantation in other corners of the globe. Both of them worked on developing a cochlear implant while they were at the Technical University of Vienna. In the year 1977, Ingeborg and Erwin Hochmair developed the world's first microelectronic multichannel cochlear implant in Vienna. They developed a flexible 8-channel electrode with eight independent current sources, which can be inserted up to 22–25 mm into the cochlea. This device used a stimulation rate of 10,000 pulses per second per channel. The Hochmairs' start-up company was named MED-EL.

The first surgery using this 8-electrode device was performed on December 16, 1977 by Prof. Kurt Burian at ENT University Clinic in Vienna, who inserted this flexible electrode into the scala tympani through the round window. Extensive

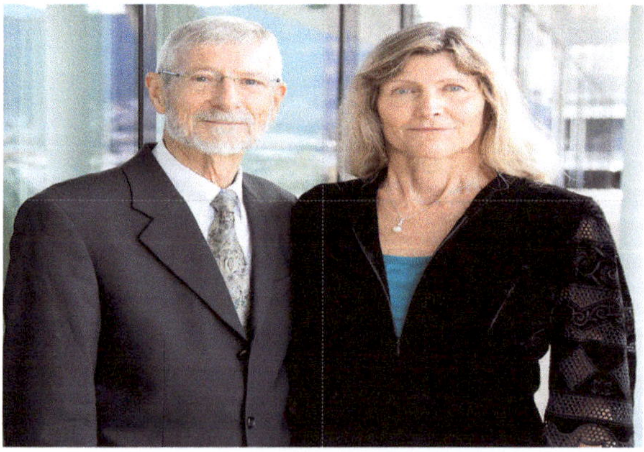

Fig. 10.5 The developers of the world's first micro-electric multichannel cochlear implant: Erwin Hochmair (left) Ingeborg Desoyer (later known as Ingeborg Hochmair) (right)

research work was carried out from 1978 to 1979 during which they developed a 6-channel and a 4-channel implant variant. One patient was implanted with a 4-channel cochlear implant in August 1979 and she received a portable sound processor after a few weeks of surgery. Many clinical evaluations were being carried out to assess speech coding strategies, stimulation field configuration, and adjustment of parameters in the speech processor as required for the optimal speech comprehension. During that period, various speech perception tests were also carried out to optimize the settings.

Later at the end of 1979, they developed the smallest body-worn speech processor and modified it further in March 1980. In 1986, the Hochmairs and their start-up company MED-EL moved to Innsbruck. In 1991, MED-EL launched the world's first behind-the-ear speech processor. The world's first bilateral implantation was also carried out using the MED-EL implants by Prof. Jan Helms and Joachim Muller. Prof. Jan Helms and Joachim Muller performed a sequential cochlear implant in the second ear after a gap of 2 years of the first implantation. The world's first electro-acoustic stimulation (EAS) developed in the year 2005 was also credited to MED-EL, as they launched the first duet speech processor where both acoustic and electrical stimulation is achievable in one compact device.

Advanced Bionics

Advanced Bionics (AB) was founded in 1993 by Alfred E. Mann, an entrepreneur from the United States of America, to provide good listening to those with hearing impairment. The technology behind AB's first cochlear implant system came from pioneering research at the University of California, San Francisco. However, the development of Clarion implant began in 1987 with congregated efforts of three groups: Advance Bionics (Sylmar, California), University of California, San Francisco (UCSF) and Research Triangle Institute (RTI), North California. The clinical trial for adults were started in 1991. The cochlear implantation began in Europe for children in 1993 and in the United States in 1995. In August 1996, Advanced Bionics received FDA approval to use their first cochlear implant Clarion with pre-formed electrodes for adults. FDA approval for the paediatric population was received in June 1997 (Eshraghi et al., 2012; Merzenich, 2015; Wilson & Dorman, 2008).

In 2001, the **Bionic Ear Association** was formed by Advanced Bionics to build a support network for cochlear implant candidates and their recipients. In the same year, they launched a CII Bionic ear implant and HiFocus electrode. With their steep development in the technology, in 2006 Advanced Bionics developed Harmony HiResolution Bionic ear & HiRes Fidelity 120 sound processing technology with current steering technology. HiRes Fidelity 120 technology provides five times more sound resolution with 120 spectral bands.

In 2009, Advanced Bionics joined hands with Phonak under the Sonova group by merging the hearing aid technology with the cochlear implant sound processor to provide the best hearing solutions to individuals with hearing impairment, and launched the Clear Voice sound technology, a revolutionary sound processing strategy in 2010. Clear Voice automatically analyzes and adapts to every listening situation and separates speech from distracting noise for improved understanding and comfortable listening.

In 2014, Advanced Bionics became the first company to develop a waterproof case for cochlear implant recipients to be worn in water and provide protection against sweating-related corrosion. In 2015, they launched another new-age sound processor, Naida CI Q series sound processors after receiving the approval from Technical Inspection Association (TUV). In 2016, the Phonak Naida Link Hearing aid was designed by the joint work of Advanced Bionics and Phonak specifically to work parallel with cochlear implants in bimodal stimulation. Naida Link CROS (contralateral routing of signal), a wireless audio transmitter with a concept of contralateral routing of signals, was launched in 2017, which allows unilateral cochlear implant recipients with no hearing in their opposite ear to hear from both sides. In 2018, they developed the HiRes Ultra 3D cochlear implant, which allows MRI compatibility without interrupting hearing.

The most recent development by Advanced Bionics is Naida CI Connect in 2019. It is a wireless receiver streaming accessory and Active Insertion Monitoring (AIM) system, the world's first commercially available monitoring and objective measurement tool for use during intra-operative testing and post-operatively. AIM uses the implant to measure real-time electrocochleography (ECochG) potentials generated by the inner ear and the auditory nerve in response to acoustic stimuli, which gives feedback to the cochlear implant surgeon regarding the insertion depth and basilar membrane damage during the surgery.

Cochlear Implants: Basic Concepts

As mentioned before, the cochlear implant is the most successful sensory prosthesis in the history of medicine. Although not in terms of the time, it feels no less than magic to note that children with severe to profound hearing loss, who receive cochlear implants by the time they reach 1 year of age develop spoken language skills akin their normal hearing peers, albeit after rigorous training (Ching et al., 2013; Dettman et al., 2016; Geers, 2004; Geers et al., 2003). In this section, we will describe the basic components of the modern day's cochlear implant technology that help initiate the "magic".

There are many differences in the hardware of cochlear implant systems produced by different manufacturers, but all cochlear implant systems possess some basic components that are common across manufacturers. The cochlear implant comprises of two general components: an external sound processor and the internal implant system.

External Part of the Cochlear Implant

The external part, also called the external sound processor, consists of five basic components: a microphone, a digital sound processor, a power source, an external transmitting coil, and an external magnet. The sound processors are available in different configurations; behind-the-ear (BTE), body-worn, and off-the-ear (OTE) sound processors. BTE (Fig. 10.6) and body-worn sound processors contain cable and coil to transmit the signal while off-the-ear sound processors do not contain a transmitting cable, because the microphone, digital signal processor, power source, and transmitting coil are housed in a single unit. Sound processors are operated by lithium-ion rechargeable batteries. This type of battery has the advantage of a flat voltage curve. The other option for power supply is a zinc-air 675 alkaline disposable battery.

Internal Part of the Cochlear Implant

The internal part of the cochlear implant consists of six basic components: internal transmitting coil, internal magnet, digital signal processor, stimulator for electric pulse generator, electrode leads, and electrode array (Fig. 10.7). The internal coil, digital signal processor, and stimulator are together called receiver-stimulator. The receiver-stimulator is housed in a biocompatible titanium case. The electrode leads

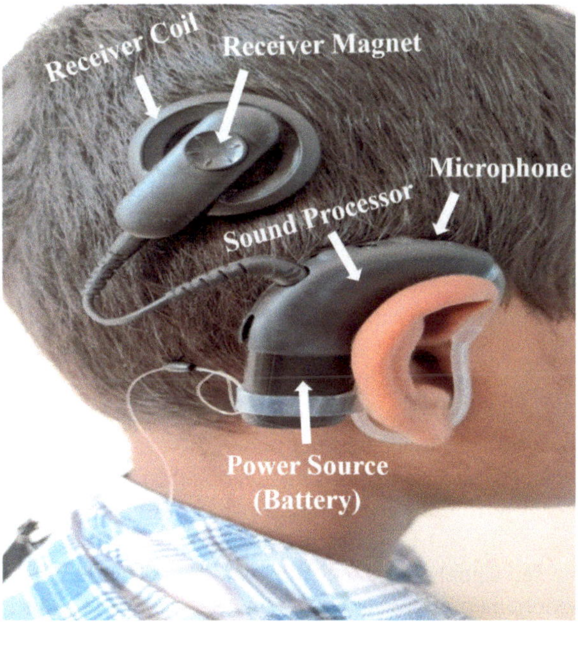

Fig. 10.6 External parts of a cochlear implant

Fig. 10.7 Internal parts of a cochlear implant

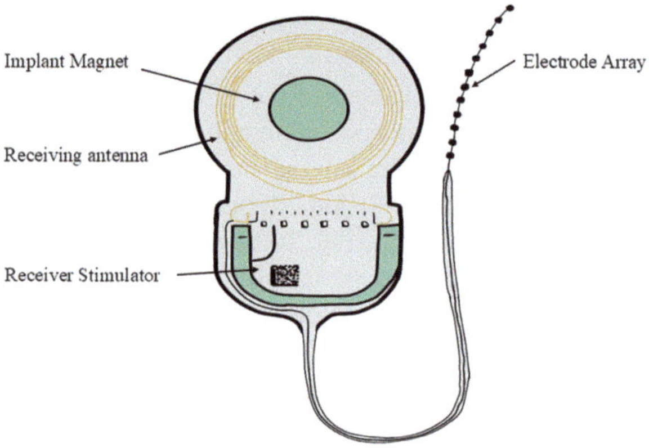

deliver the electric current from the receiver-stimulator to the electrode array. The electrode array consists of multiple electrode contacts (12–22 electrodes). The length of electrode array varies across different cochlear implant manufacturers. Few electrode arrays are designed to be inserted close to neural elements innervating the cochlea.

Basic Operation of the Cochlear Implant

The microphone of the external sound processor captures the incoming audio signals and converts into electrical signals. The electrical signal is delivered to the preamplifier where the amplitude of the signals is increased to improve the signal-to-noise ratio. After that signal is analyzed by digital signal processor to determine the composition of audio input in the frequency, time, and intensity domains. The signal is divided into different analysis bands or channels to allow for frequency-specific processing. The division of broadband input signal into spectral analysis bands is accomplished by digital filtering. In this stage, the sound processor attempts to classify the signal as speech and noise. The signal processing takes place with the goal of optimising signal delivery to the recipient. An audiologist programs the sound processor with the goal of determining the magnitude of electrical current required in each channel to facilitate audibility as well as to produce a sensation that is loud, but not uncomfortable. This process is popularly called "*mapping*". It helps in restoring audibility and normalizing loudness. Once the signal is spectrally analyzed and assigned to different analysis bands, the output of these different bands pass through low pass filter in order to capture the amplitude envelope of the input signal. Based on the information obtained through mapping process, sound processor determines the magnitude of the stimulation that should be delivered to elicit audibility and loudness percept. Later, digital signal processor converts the processed signals to a coded electrical signal that is delivered to the external coil. The external coil delivers the signal across the skin to the internal coil of the cochlear implant via radio frequency (RF) transmission with a carrier frequency ranging from 2.5 to 50 MHz. The sound processor determines how the implant should deliver electrical stimulation to the auditory nerve.

The internal components of the cochlear implant do not have any power source; the RF signal delivered from sound processor is used to operate cochlear implant. The digital signal processor of the cochlear implant analyzes the RF signals received from external coil. The stimulator of the cochlear implant continuously produces biphasic electrical pulses at a fixed moderate-to-fast rate. The amplitude of these pulses is modulated by the magnitude of the amplitude envelope of the signal in each analysis band i.e. amplitude of the electrical pulses is directly proportional to the magnitude of the amplitude envelope of the original signal. The amplitude modulated electrical pulses are delivered to electrode contacts corresponding to the given analysis band. Multi channel cochlear implants take advantage of the natural tonotopic organization that exists in the cochlea by delivering high frequency signal to electrodes located towards the basal end of the cochlea and low frequency signal to the electrodes in the more apical location. The electrical pulse delivered across each electrode is highly staggered in time so that an electrical pulse is never simultaneously delivered to two different electrode contacts.

The sojourn of the electrical hearing which began with the unpleasant experience of electrical hearing by Alessandro Volta changed direction towards the first pleasant experience when Andre Djourno and Charles Eyries showed the world the way to directly stimulate auditory nerve electrically, and it never looked back ever since. The journey has culminated in a remarkable development in the treatment of individuals with severe to profound hearing loss with improved speech processing strategies, electrode shape, structure and numbers, and reduction in the size of speech processors from immovable clinical processors to the bulky body worn processor to behind-the-ear and now, in the current time, with off-the ear speech processor. The research is still ongoing across the world to achieve better technological advancement for improving the quality of life of individuals with hearing impairment.

References

Berliner, K. I., Stovall, R. A., House, W. F., & Maddox, H. E., III. (1990). Investigator differences in the cochlear implantation of children. *Otolaryngology—Head and Neck Surgery, 102*(6), 683–689.

Ching, T. Y., Dillon, H., Marnane, V., Hou, S., Day, J., Seeto, M., et al. (2013). Outcome of early- and late-identified children at 3 years of age. *Ear and Hearing, 34*(5), 535–552.

Clark, G. M. (2003). *Cochlear implants*. Springer Verlag.

Clark, G. M., Tong, Y. C., Black, R., Forster, I. C., Patrick, J. F., & Dewhurst, D. J. (1977). A multiple electrode cochlear implant. *The Journal of Laryngology & Otology, 91*(11), 935–945.

Clark, G. M., Black, R., Forster, I. C., Patrick, J. F., & Tong, Y. C. (1978). Design criteria of a multiple-electrode cochlear implant hearing prosthesis. *The Journal of the Acoustical Society of America, 63*(2), 631–633.

Dettman, S. J., Dowell, R. C., Choo, D., Arnott, W., Abrahams, Y., Davis, A., et al. (2016). Long-term communication outcomes for children receiving cochlear implants younger than 12 months: A multicenter study. *Otology & Neurotology, 37*(2), e82–e95.

Djourno, A., & Eyries, C. (1957). Auditory prosthesis by means of a distant electrical stimulation of the sensory nerve with the use of an indwelt coiling. *La Presse Médicale, 65*(63), 1417.

Eisenberg, L. S. (2015). The contributions of William F. House to the field of implantable auditory devices. *Hearing Research, 322*, 52–56.

Eisenberg, L. S., & House, W. F. (1982). Initial experience with the cochlear implant in children. *The Annals of Otology, Rhinology & Laryngology. Supplement, 91*(2 Pt 3), 67–73.

Eshraghi, A. A., Gupta, C., Ozdamar, O., Balkany, T. J., Truy, E., & Nazarian, R. (2012). Biomedical engineering principles of modern cochlear implants and recent surgical innovations. *The Anatomical Record: Advances in Integrative Anatomy and Evolutionary Biology, 295*(11), 1957–1966.

Geers, A., Bernner, C., & Davidson, L. (2003). Factors associated with development of speech perception skills in children implanted by age five. *Ear and Hearing, 24*(Suppl), 24S–35S.

Geers, A. E. (2004). Speech, language, and reading skills after early cochlear implantation. *Archives of Otolaryngology–Head & Neck Surgery, 130*(5), 634–638.

Geers, A. E., Moog, J. S., Biedenstein, J., Brenner, C., & Hayes, H. (2009). Spoken language scores of children using cochlear implants compared to hearing age-mates at school entry. *Journal of Deaf Studies and Deaf Education, 14*(3), 371–385.

House, W. F. (1974). Goals of the cochlear implant. *Laryngoscope, 84*(11), 1883–1887.

House, W. F. (1976). Cochlear implants. *Annals of Otology, Rhinology & Laryngology, 85*(Suppl. 27), 1–93.

House, W. F. (2011). *The struggle of a medical innovator: Cochlear implants and other ear surgeries*. CreateSpace.

House, W. F., & Urban, J. (1973). Long term results of electrode implantation and electronic stimulation of the cochlea in man. *Annals of Otology, Rhinology & Laryngology, 82*(4), 504–517.

Merzenich, M. M. (2015). Early UCSF contributions to the development of multiple-channel cochlear implants. *Hearing Research, 322*, 39–46.

Mudry, A., & Mills, M. (2013). The early history of the cochlear implant: A retrospective. *JAMA Otolaryngology–Head & Neck Surgery, 139*(5), 446–453.

Rance, G., & Barker, E. J. (2008). Speech perception in children with auditory neuropathy/dyssynchrony managed with either hearing aids or cochlear implants. *Otology & Neurotology, 29*(2), 179–182.

Volta, A. (1800). On the electricity excited by the mere contact of conducting substances of different kinds. *Philosophical Transactions of the Royal Society, 90*, 403–431.

Wilson, B. S. (2000). Cochlear implant technology. In J. K. Niparko, K. I. Kirk, N. K. Mellon, A. M. Robbins, D. L. Tucci, & B. S. Wilson (Eds.), *Cochlear implants: Principles & practices* (pp. 109–119). Lippincott Williams & Wilkins.

Wilson, B. S., & Dorman, M. F. (2008). Cochlear implants: A remarkable past and a brilliant future. *Hearing Research, 242*(1–2), 3–21.

World Health Organization. (2021). *Highlighting priorities for ear and hearing care - World report on hearing*. World Health Organization. Available from: https://www.who.int/activities/highlighting-priorities-for-ear-and-hearing-care [cited 2021 Mar 9].

Chapter 11
Cochlear Implants: Audiological Perspectives

Prawin Kumar, Prabuddha Bhatarai, Kumari Apeksha, and Niraj Kumar Singh

Abstract Cochlear Implants enhance communication, but they do not fully replicate natural hearing, making ongoing audiological support essential for optimal outcomes. Cochlear implants have played a pivotal role in improving the quality of life of children with pre-lingual hearing loss and adults with post-lingual hearing loss to re-enter the hearing and social world. Similarly, children with severe to profound hearing loss can now be integrated into mainstream education due to hearing restoration by cochlear implants. Therefore, the selection of suitable candidates is most important for the success of advanced technology like cochlear implants in this era. This chapter discusses the assessment of audiological candidacy for cochlear implantation from the findings of an extensive series of evaluations for children and adults.

Keywords Audiometric thresholds · Speech recognition scores · Single-sided deafness · Asymmetrical hearing loss · Cochlear implants

Introduction

Cochlear implant (CI) is an advanced prosthetic device that restores hearing in individuals with severe to profound sensorineural hearing loss. It bypasses the damaged parts of the ear, directly stimulating the auditory nerve. From an audiological

P. Kumar (✉) · N. K. Singh
Department of Audiology, All India Institute of Speech and Hearing, University of Mysore, Mysore, India

P. Bhatarai
Department of Speech, Language and Hearing Sciences, The University of Texas at Dallas, Richardson, TX, USA

K. Apeksha
MarThoma College of Special Education, Kerala University of Health Sciences, Kasaragod, Kerala, India

P. Kumar et al. (eds.), *Advances in Implantation Otology*,
https://doi.org/10.1007/978-981-96-8671-1_11

perspective, a cochlear implant offers significant benefits, improving speech perception and sound localization. The audiological assessment for CI candidacy requires an extensive series of evaluations for children and adults with hearing loss. In addition, the success of CI users depends on factors such as the age of implantation, duration of deafness, and auditory training. While CI enhances communication, it does not fully replicate natural hearing, making ongoing audiological support essential for optimal outcomes. The process of cochlear implantation is a team work, with the team including an otolaryngologist, an audiologist, and a habilitationist, who join hands to not only restore hearing in adults and children with hearing loss, but also help them overcome the obstacles caused by the presence of hearing loss. Cochlear implants have facilitated children with pre-lingual and adults with post-lingual hearing loss in overcoming the effects of hearing loss and connect with the social world. The children with severe to profound hearing loss can now be integrated into mainstream education due to hearing restoration by CI and with the help of extensive speech-language therapy/auditory verbal therapy/listening training. Technological improvements, the acceptance of the device, and the performance of the recipients in day-to-day life has led to the popularity of cochlear implantation. However, not everyone can benefit from cochlear implantation. Those fulfilling certain candidacy criteria tend to derive the highest possible benefits from this modern-day technological wonder.

Candidacy for Cochlear Implants

The Food and Drug Administration (FDA), initially in 1985 approved multichannel cochlear implants only for adults, but the criteria for cochlear implantation have rapidly evolved ever since. The FDA authorized pediatric cochlear implantation in June 1990 for children 2 years or older. It was later amended in the year 2000, which brought the lower age limit to 12 months and with the latest amendment in 2020, the minimum age of implantation was brought down to 9 months, subject to the fulfillment of certain other prerequisites. However, several children have been implanted under the lowest permissible age limit of 9 months. This can be permitted under special circumstances such as those in whom the imaging findings are suggestive of the beginning of meningitis-induced cochlear fibrosis and ossification. In such cases, the child should receive a CI as soon as possible because a completely ossified cochlea might prohibit full insertion of the electrode array, probably resulting in poor performance (Rotteveel et al., 2005; Roland et al., 2008; Liu et al., 2015). Many centers routinely implant infants (6 to 9 months) if they feel confident in the behavioral and physiological testing results. The literature supports the efficacy and safety of considering CI surgery between 6 months to 9 months with no higher risk of implantation-related complications (Roland et al., 2009; Friedmann et al., 2020).

Candidacy criteria depend on several aspects, such as the patient's age, etiology, implant manufacturer, and even within a manufacturer, the implant type (e.g., Nucleus Hybrid- L24 and MED-EL EAS). The prevalence of overlapping indications with cochlear implants, hearing aids, osseous integrated auditory prosthesis, middle ear implants, and shorter electrode, atraumatic cochlear implants for hearing preservation further complicates eligibility evaluation. Even for the most skilled members of a cochlear implant team, selecting potential cochlear implant candidates may be a challenging procedure with all of these variables at play. Clinicians who do not work with cochlear implants regularly may not realize how many patients may benefit from this technology.

Several factors must be examined when selecting the right candidates for cochlear implantation. While many of the difficulties are connected to the audiological examination, such as audiometric and speech recognition tests, the candidacy is also dependent on medical, radiological, and psychological aspects. Candidacy criteria also differ according to the age of implantation, with pre-lingual versus post-lingual deafness being a significant contributor to the eventual decision on the candidacy. This section will elaborate the audiological candidacy for cochlear implantation in adults and children.

Cochlear Implant Candidate Selection: Adults

Deciding on the candidacy for cochlear implantation for adults is nowhere near as straight forward as it might seem. Several aspects of audiological evaluation need assessment before deciding on it, in addition to the medical, radiologic, and psychological issues.

Audiological Tests-Based Criteria for Candidacy Evaluation of Adults

Almost all cochlear implant assessments begin at the audiology clinic. By the time an adult patient is referred for a cochlear implant examination, they have most likely been seen by an audiologist for hearing aid fits for several years. As a result, when adult patients come in for a cochlear implant candidacy examination, they are usually aware that hearing aids are insufficient for effective communication and are ready to move forward. From a professional standpoint, this is often a quite different experience than that of a rehabilitative audiologist suggesting hearing aids when rejection and hesitancy to use hearing aids are common.

Despite the fact that most patients present to the cochlear implant evaluation with prior audiograms, it is recommended that comprehensive audiometric testing be completed again. The cochlear implant candidacy evaluation comprises of basic speech audiometry, such as ear-specific speech reception thresholds and word recognition with recorded stimuli, and audiometric thresholds through air-conduction for octave frequencies between 125 Hz and 8000 Hz and bone conduction thresholds for at least 500 Hz to 4000 Hz. However, due to the increasing benefits of minimally traumatic surgical techniques and low-frequency hearing preservation following cochlear implantation (Carlson et al., 2010; Roland et al., 2016; Wanna et al., 2018), obtaining thresholds at 125 Hz and 250 Hz is crucial. Although oto-acoustic emissions (OAEs) are essential aspect of diagnostic audiology, most adult implant assessment procedures do not incorporate them. This is because most adult patients who come in for a cochlear implant examination have been wearing hearing aids for a long time. In reality, all three cochlear implant manufacturers specify limited benefits from "appropriately fitted biaural hearing aids" as a condition for eligibility determination. Thus, even if an adult previously possessed OAEs at lower frequencies, long-term use of amplification has been linked to the subsequent loss of OAEs (Deltenre et al., 1999). OAEs are typically present when the pure tone threshold is within 20 dBHL whereas they will be almost certainly absent if the pure tone threshold exceeds 35 dBHL. The presence of OAE despite poor audiometric thresholds might be an indication of retro-cochlear pathology. OAE assessment is also helpful in identifying sloping hearing loss; for example, the presence of OAEs in low-frequency regions could be an indication for the CI team to consider a short electrode array to avoid the alteration of the active cochlear amplifier in the apical region of the cochlea. While the general candidacy criteria for an adult to undergo cochlear implantation has a unanimous agreement, the requirements for adult cochlear implantation can vary among the device manufacturers. For adult implant candidacy, Advanced Bionics and MED-EL, for example, demand bilateral severe-to-profound sensorineural hearing loss. On the other hand, Cochlear Ltd. specifies bilateral moderate-to-profound sensorineural hearing loss to incorporate those with sloping hearing loss, who otherwise may not benefit from amplification for effective communication. The detailed manufacturer-specific basic candidacy criteria for an adult to undergo cochlear implantation is given in Table 11.1.

Table 11.1 Excerpts of manufacturer-specific audiological criteria for cochlear implantation candidacy for adults

Parameter	Cochlear Ltd	Med-EL	Advanced-Bionics
Age	≥18 years	≥18 years	≥18 years
Hearing loss	Bilateral SNHL	Bilateral SNHL	Bilateral SNHL
Degree of hearing loss	Low frequencies: moderate-profound; Mid-high frequencies: profound	Severe to profound (PTA = 70 dB HL for 500 Hz, 1000 Hz, & 2000 Hz)	Severe-to-profound (PTA > 70 dB HL)
Onset of hearing loss	Pre-lingual/peri-lingual/post-lingual	–	Post-lingual
Hearing aid use	Appropriately fitted binaural hearing aids	Appropriately fitted binaural hearing aids	Appropriately fitted binaural hearing aids
Aided speech recognition	≤50% in the to be implanted ear (≤60% in the best-aided condition) on recorded tests of open-set sentence recognition	≤40% in best-aided listening condition on recorded tests of open-set sentence recognition (HINT sentences)	<50% score on a test of open-set sentence recognition

Note. *HINT* Hearing in Noise test, *PTA* pure tone average, *SNHL* sensorineural hearing loss

Speech Recognition Tests for Candidacy Evaluation of Adults

Monosyllabic words, phrases, and sentences in noise are among the speech recognition materials used for the evaluation of cochlear implantation eligibility. Speech recognition performance should be assessed with both monosyllabic words [consonant nucleus consonant (CNC) words] (Peterson & Lehiste, 1962) and the Hearing in Noise Test (HINT) sentences (Nilsson et al., 1994) presented in quiet and in a fixed level noise background, according to the 1996 minimum speech test battery (MSTB) committee (Nilsson et al., 1997). Because there is evidence that HINT sentences suffer from ceiling effects, even for certain preoperative patients who struggle with communication and could benefit from cochlear implantation, the updated MSTB committee advises the use of CNC words and Arizona Bioindustry Association (AzBio) sentences (Spahr et al., 2012) and phrases (Gifford et al., 2008). The MSTB also suggests using AzBio phrases in quiet and noisy environments and the Bamford-Kowal-Bench Speech-in-Noise (BKB-SIN) test (Killion et al., 2001). Despite the recommendation of using the same test, manufacturer-specific cut-offs vary. For example, Advanced Bionics defined its candidacy criteria of HINT sentence recognition scores of up to 50% in the best-aided condition; Cochlear Americas stated speech recognition accuracy of up to 50% and up to 60% in the best-aided condition in the ear to be implanted; and MED-EL states the criteria of HINT sentence recognition up to 40% in the best-aided condition. Nonetheless, until at such time when a uniformity is arrived upon, the clinicians are best advised to follow the manufacturer-specific guidelines.

Hearing Aid Verification for Candidacy Evaluation of Adults

Before deciding whether speech metrics should be used to establish eligibility, we must first ensure that the patient is using appropriately fitted hearing aids. This is particularly essential because all implant manufacturers cite limited benefits from properly fitting hearing aids as a condition for implant eligibility. Hearing aid verification might imply various things to different audiologists; nonetheless, there are well-established practice guidelines for hearing aid verification. The American Academy of Audiology released the "*Guidelines for the Audiologic Management of Adult Hearing Impairment*" in 2006 (Valente, 2006). As per these guidelines, a clinician must verify that the prescribed gain from a standard prescriptive formula is indeed producing the desired sound pressure levels in the ear canal of the patient. Therefore, using functional gain measurements alone to verify hearing aid settings is unsuitable for the candidate selection process. Although the aided sound field thresholds give information on the audibility of low-level stimuli, they do not provide information on the audibility of typical conversational-level speech, which is a criterion for effective communication. The MSTB recommends a presentation level of 60 dB SPL for speech stimuli used in implant eligibility determination; hence, the stimulus utilized for hearing aid verification, whether speech or a speech-like signal, should be 60 dB SPL.

Subjective Evaluation of Perceived Performance Before Cochlear Implantation of Adults

The objective evaluations of speech perception and subjective assessments of benefit may not always coincide (Holder et al., 2018; Wackym et al., 2007). One possible explanation is that the audiometric test booth conditions may not accurately reflect real-world listening situations. Subjective assessment instruments can also verify the effectiveness of a treatment option, such as cochlear implantation. The popular and commonly used subjective measures of evaluation can be found in Table 11.2.

The American Cochlear Implant Alliance Task Force recommended a "*revised 60/60 guideline*" for determining cochlear implant candidacy in adults due to the addition of asymmetrical hearing loss and single-sided deafness (Zeitler et al., 2024). It advised to refer patients for cochlear implantation if they have unaided

Table 11.2 Questionnaire-based subjective measures used for cochlear implant users

Tests	Characteristics
Speech, Spatial, and Qualities (SSQ) (Gatehouse & Noble, 2004)	It assesses one's hearing abilities and experiences in the areas of speech communication, spatial hearing, and speech and sound quality. It employs an 11-point visual analogue scale ('0' being highly negative and '10' highly positive). For each of the 49 scenarios, the respondent is asked to select the number that best describes his or her hearing experience on a numerical scale.
Abbreviated Profile of Hearing Aid Benefit (APHAB) (Cox & Alexander, 1995)	It assesses listening difficulty in four areas: ease of communication, background noise, reverberation, and evasiveness of sound. The difference in listening difficulties found before and after cochlear implantation provides an index of the benefit associated with the procedure.
Client-Oriented Scale of Improvement (COSI) (Dillon et al., 1997)	It is a clinical assessment instrument developed by National Acoustical Laboratories for evaluating individually decided outcomes following amplification. The patient can indicate listening circumstances that he or she would like to enhance with cochlear implants.
Nijmegen Cochlear Implant Questionnaire (NCIQ) (Hinderink et al., 2000)	It is an instrument to assess Quality-of-life with 60 items created for adult cochlear implant recipients. Basic sound perception (for example, environmental sounds), advanced sound perception (for example, modulation of one's own voice, speech intelligibility), speech perception, self-esteem, activity, and social interactions are all assessed. It was created for use during pre- and post-implant evaluations.
Cochlear Implant Function Index (CIFI) (Coelho et al., 2009)	It is a 25-item self-assessment measure designed and validated for use with adult cochlear implant recipients. It assesses a person's dependence on visual cues, telephone use, workplace communication, and hearing in noisy group and large-room contexts.

PTA ≥60 dB HL and unaided word recognition score = 60% in one or both ears. In addition, those patients falling outside of the revised 60/60 guideline or those falling outside of traditional CI candidacy criteria who do not receive adequate benefit from their current technology should also be referred for a formal CI evaluation. The examples of such conditions are unilateral SNHL, asymmetric SNHL, low-frequency thresholds in the normal to the mild range with profound hearing loss in the higher frequencies. Zowlan and colleagues performed retrospective analyses of adult CI candidates using the 60/60 guideline and reported a 96% sensitivity rate (candidate met both criteria) and 65% specificity rate (non-candidate did not meet the 60/60 criteria) (Zowlan et al., 2020). It is also important to consider a poor correlation between unaided speech recognition scores and audiometric thresholds when making a decision on the eventual CI candidacy (McRackan et al., 2018). Therefore, if patients demonstrate limited benefits using appropriately fitted hearing aids, it is recommended to refer such cases for CI evaluation regardless of the performance on any single test or group of audiological tests.

Cochlear Implant Candidate Selection: Children

As mentioned in the previous section, determining cochlear implant candidacy can be a complex process. There are many aspects requiring careful consideration in pediatric cochlear implant candidate selection, including medical, radiologic, and psychological issues.

Audiological Test-Based Candidacy Evaluation of Children

Like candidacy examinations for prospective implantation in adults, almost all pediatric cochlear implant assessments begin in the audiology clinic. Behavioral hearing tests and objective assessments of auditory function, such as otoacoustic emissions and auditory brainstem response, are usually done at the diagnostic audiology clinic before the cochlear implant evaluation. The pediatric cochlear implant evaluation process does not begin with diagnosing severe-to-profound hearing loss because children and their families come to the evaluation with a confirmed diagnosis and hearing aid experience. As a result, the family comes to the appointment with knowledge and at least partial acceptance of the diagnosis. This often makes it easier to discuss cochlear implants without the raw emotional component of a newly diagnosed hearing loss. Audiologists who specialize in all areas of pediatric audiology treatment, from the initial diagnosis to hearing aid fits, follow-up, auditory progress evaluation, and cochlear implant eligibility decision, are required to carry out candidacy evaluation for a child. Given the high demand for highly skilled pediatric cochlear implant audiologists, a single provider is rarely involved in all previous diagnostic and amplification-related appointments. However, such continuity of care would be extremely beneficial to a family dealing with several new experiences following a hearing loss diagnosis.

Despite the fact that most families bring past audiograms and reports of other objective assessments when arriving for the first candidacy examination, it is suggested that extensive audiometric testing be conducted. This is a better way to get more ear-specific pure-tone and speech awareness information, especially for frequencies that may have been missing from previous audiograms. It is also a good idea to get tympanograms and, at the very least, ipsilateral middle ear muscle reflexes done. Since multiple assessments of behavioral hearing status and hearing aid fitting are recommended before finalizing candidate selection, it is typical for a child not to be seen by the cochlear implant team for assessment until at least 6 months of age, which is the age at which a reliable behavioral assessment of hearing can be completed. Thus, the earliest implant evaluation/workup appointments involve visual reinforcement audiometry, and/or behavioral observation audiometry. Concomitant conditions that may delay sitting up, independent head and neck control, and greater global developmental and/or cognitive capacities make assessing young children more difficult. OAEs are a valuable tool for evaluating cochlear implant candidacy. Although OAEs are used as a first-pass screening method in most newborn hearing screening programs in well-baby nurseries (White et al., 2005; Widen et al., 2005), not all children will have had this performed. Almost every cochlear implant audiologist has a story about a patient who comes in for an evaluation and then gets diagnosed with auditory neuropathy spectrum disorder (ANSD) after the evaluation. Although ANSD does not exclude a patient from receiving a cochlear implant (Alzhrani et al., 2019; Breneman et al., 2012; Kontorinis et al., 2014; Peterson et al., 2003; Rance & Barker, 2008; Shallop et al., 2001), it is crucial to have an accurate diagnosis to explore all possible habilitative options.

Audiometry-based criteria for cochlear implantation differ across implant manufacturers. For pediatric candidacy, there is an additional element of age-specific audiometric criteria. For children aged 12–24 months, the current criteria from all leading cochlear implant manufacturers specify bilateral profound sensorineural hearing loss. This is not to imply that children with less severe hearing losses would not benefit from cochlear implantation. This was due to the difficulty associated with obtaining accurate behavioral thresholds in such young groups. This is also an argument for lowering the FDA-approved age for cochlear implantation from 12 months to slightly younger, perhaps in the 6-months to 9-months range (Cosetti & Roland, 2010). Research has demonstrated significant benefits for children implanted in the first year of life, even as compared to children implanted in the second year of life, on measures of word and language acquisition (Bergeson et al., 2010; Houston & Miyamoto, 2010; Moog & Geers, 2010; Niparko et al., 2010), speech perception (Tajudeen et al., 2010), speech intelligibility (Habib et al., 2010), and vocabulary development (Hayes et al., 2009; Houston & Miyamoto, 2010; Tomblin et al., 2005). In a study by Spitzer and Waltzman (2023), the authors reported that cochlear implants are beneficial at any age. In general, younger age CI users receive greater benefits when considering pre-lingual deafness.

Audiometric Thresholds for Cochlear Implant Candidacy in Children

For a newborn with severe-to-profound hearing loss, the auditory input, at least partly, will be missed throughout the first year of life. This is true even for newborns who have hearing aids that are correctly fitted because audibility may be insufficient to provide constant auditory access to spoken language. Between the ages of 7.5 and 10.5 months, the ability for word segmentation develops quickly (Jusczyk, 2002). Babies have the potential for long-term storage of new words by 8 months, which is a requirement for auditory-based language development (Houston & Jusczyk, 2003; Jusczyk & Hohne, 1997). As a result, a newborn with severe-to-profound sensorineural hearing loss, who has limited assisted audibility, misses out on the critical auditory-based language learning opportunities in the first year of life (Levine et al., 2016).

The audiometric requirements are different across the manufacturers. For Cochlear Ltd., the criteria for implantation in children over the age of two years are more liberal, including bilateral severe-to-profound sensorineural hearing loss, allowing for somewhat greater residual acoustic hearing. However, both Advanced Bionics and MED-EL continue to mention bilateral profound sensorineural hearing loss as criteria for above 2 years of age. The cochlear implant team has the professional clinical judgment to assess candidacy if a child has moderate-to-profound sensorineural hearing loss and is not making auditory improvement with adequately fitting hearing aids and assistance (Table 11.4). Many studies have shown that children with bilateral sensorineural hearing impairments beyond the range of designated candidacy gain significantly in speech recognition and language after cochlear implantation (Carlson et al., 2015; Leigh et al., 2016; Schaefer et al., 2019).

Speech-Perception Metrics for Candidacy in Children

The Pediatric Minimum Speech Test Battery [PMSTB] (Uhler et al., 2017) is an appropriate reference for preoperative testing. Following 5 years of literature analysis and critical debate among almost 60 pediatric clinicians (audiologists and speech/language pathologists), hearing scientists, and business representatives, the PMSTB was released in 2017. This can yield useful information about a child's speech perception for various types of speech stimuli.

Multiple Estimates of Speech Recognition for Candidacy in Children

Unlike adult implant candidates and older children who use hearing aids may be asked to make multiple visits over the course of several months. This is especially true for borderline candidates, where many visits will be necessary to establish if a child is progressing with properly fitting hearing aids and assistance. FDA-approved indications stipulate that a 6-month hearing aid trial should be completed before evaluating eligibility; hence, each professional in the implant team is responsible for creating own protocol for prescribing the number of audiological tests performed during those 6 months.

In situations of meningitis, when cochlear ossification might restrict electrode placement and results, FDA-approved standards now indicate that a shorter hearing aid trial is permissible and suitable. In the case of older children with progressive hearing loss, rapid onset hearing loss, or late identification, shorter hearing aid trial periods are typical procedures. The main issue with a compressed hearing aid trial period is that the least intrusive treatment option should be thoroughly investigated before implant candidacy is determined.

Speech Discrimination and Recognition Tests in Children Under 3 Years of Age

Although closed-set speech perception metrics are not mentioned in the current labeled indications for pediatric cochlear implantation, they can be a valuable tool for clinicians to monitor speech recognition performance and improvement prior to evaluating implant eligibility. Auditory skills development in younger children is often assessed using data from auditory questionnaires, parental reports, and speech/language evaluations. This is especially true for children with severe to profound sensorineural hearing loss, for whom we predict limited improvement in auditory abilities and auditory/oral language development.

This criterion is broken in the case of younger children who have acquired and/or have progressive hearing loss. For a younger child, there is a range of standardized tests of speech discrimination or recognition that are adequate. Audiologists usually start with closed-set tests, which have a restricted number of options and do not need a spoken answer. The Early Speech Perception Test (Moog & Geers, 1990) has a low verbal version as a sub-component for use in children as young as 2 years of age. Similar tests are available in several other languages such as early speech perception test in Malayalam (Jijo & Yathiraj, 2010), modified-early speech perception test in Kannada (Priya, 2017).

Visual Reinforcement Infant Speech Discrimination (VRISD)

VRISD is based on the visual reinforcement audiometry (VRA) principle of a conditioned head turn, making it suited for usage with infants aged 6–24 months. Unlike traditional VRA, which needs a child to perceive a sound, VRISD allows us to detect scenarios in which a child detects a sound change. VRISD uses operant conditioning to reinforce a head turn as a correct response (or a hit) through animated video or mechanical toy reinforcement. Multiple sound contrasts can be used in a single test session or multiple test sessions to assess infant speech discrimination. Vowel contrasts such as /a/ versus /i/ and /a/ versus /u/, which are discriminated via spectral cues, are the most prevalent speech stimuli used in VRISD protocols. When compared to contrasts based on voice onset time (e.g., /ta/ vs. /da/) or place of articulation (e.g., /ba/ vs. /da/), vowel contrasts are easier for younger infants and emerge earlier (Boothroyd, 1984; Eilers et al., 1977, 1981; Uhler et al., 2011; Van Wieringen & Wouters, 1999). VRISD is usually used after a child has achieved a 75% discrimination competency in verified and normed contrasts such as /ba/ versus /da/ and /a/ versus /i/ (Uhler et al., 2015). Though there are no current recommendations for using VRISD to determine pediatric implant candidacy, it can be a valuable tool in an audiologist's toolbox because it allows to see if an infant is making expected developmental gains in speech sound discrimination after acoustic amplification and intervention. VRISD has traditionally been used more in research and has yet to acquire widespread clinical use; however, since its inclusion in the PMSTB protocol (Uhler et al., 2017), this tool has drawn more attention and is making its way into more clinical protocols (Table 11.3).

Table 11.3 Speech perception tests used for cochlear implant users

Tests Selected	Open or Closed Set	Stimulus	Listening Condition	Norming Population	Pros	Cons
VRISD	Closed	Syllable	Quiet	Normal hearing	Independent of language abilities	Requires conditioned head turn; norms required for additional contrasts
ESP, Low Verbal or Standard	Closed	Word	Quiet	Hearing loss	Assesses an array of speech discrimination abilities	Toys can be distracting
PSI	Closed	Word, Sentence	Quiet and noise	Normal hearing and hearing loss	Can be done in presence of semantic distractor	Limited number of lists
MLNT/ LNT	Open	Word	Quiet	N/A	Familiar words for children with limited vocabulary, lists with varying lexical difficulty	Limited number of lists, norms needed
CNC	Open	Word	Quiet	N/A	Use of prompt "ready" included in adult MSTB	50-word list is most reliable, child may need breaks

(continued)

Table 11.3 (continued)

Tests Selected	Open or Closed Set	Stimulus	Listening Condition	Norming Population	Pros	Cons
BKB	Open	Sentence	Quiet	N/A	Use of prompt "ready", low context for younger children	Norms not available for children younger than 5 year
BKB-SIN	Open	Sentence	Noise	Normal hearing	Adaptive test, norms across life span	Norms not available for children younger than 5 year (Schafer, 2010)
Pediatric AzBio (BabyBio)	Open	Sentence	Quiet and noise	Normal hearing	Norms for children 5–12 year, equivalent lists	16 lists, female talker Only
Modified early speech perception test-Kannada	Closed	Word	Quiet	Normal Hearing	Normative for children (3 to 5 years)	3 to 5 years

Note: *ESP* Early Speech perception test, *LNT* Lexical Neighborhood test, *MLNT* Multi-lexical Neighborhood test, *AzBio sentence test* Arizona Bioindustry Association sentence test, *PSI test* Pediatric speech intelligibility test, *CNC word test* Consonant-nucleus-consonant word test, *VRISD* Visual Reinforcement infant speech discrimination, *BKB-SIN* Bamford-Kowal-Bench- Speech-in-Noise test

The American Cochlear Implant Alliance Task Force guidelines for determining cochlear implant candidacy in children recommended "*50/70+ guidelines*" for referral to pediatric cochlear implant candidacy (Warner-Czyz et al., 2022). It is advised that the CI specialist clinicians deal with CI candidacy in children to follow the criteria for referral. The criteria of referral for cochlear implantation suggests that any child having word recognition scores of less than 50% correct (Dettman et al., 2004; Bittencourt et al., 2012), unaided pure-tone thresholds of greater than 70 dB HL (Davidson, 2006; Leigh et al., 2011; Leal et al., 2016) or, poor functional performance, limited progress in language or auditory development, or poor quality of life be referred for cochlear implantation (Mondain et al., 2002; Vickers et al., 2016). Nonetheless, differences exist in the candidacy criteria for pediatric cochlear implantation among the implant manufacturers (Table 11.4).

Table 11.4 Excerpts of pediatric audiological candidacy criteria for cochlear implants recommended by the leading cochlear implant manufacturers

Parameter	Cochlear Ltd	Med-EL	Advanced-Bionics
Age	12 months to 17 years	12–24 months >2 years	≥12 months
Hearing loss	Bilateral SNHL	Bilateral SNHL	Bilateral SNHL
Degree of hearing loss	Profound (= 90 dB HL)	Profound (12–24 months); Severe to profound (>2 years)	Profound; thresholds =90 dB HL at 1000 Hz
Duration of hearing aid use	Appropriately fitted binaural hearing aids for =6 months; at least 3 months in 12–23 months age group; no minimum duration if signs of cochlear ossification on x-rays	Appropriately fitted binaural hearing aids for 3–6 months	Appropriately fitted binaural hearing aids for 3–6 months
No benefits from hearing aid	*Child's age < 4 years*: Could not reach developmentally-appropriate milestones on IT-MAIS or MAIS <20% score on a simple open-set word recognition test at 70 dB SPL *Child's age = 4 years*: Score < 12% on a difficult open-set word recognition test Score < 30% on an open-set sentence test performed at 70 dB SPL	*In younger children*: Insignificant progress in the development of simple auditory skills, as quantified on MAIS or ESP, despite intensive habilitation for 6 months with appropriately fitting hearing aids *In older children*: Scores =30% on open set MLNT or LNT	*In younger children*: Lack of progress in the development of simple auditory skills despite intensive habilitation with appropriately fitting hearing aids *In older children*: Scores <20% on MLNT or LNT

Note. *IT MAIS* Infant-toddler Meaningful Auditory Integration Scale, *MAIS* Meaningful Auditory Integration Scale, *ESP* Early Speech Perception, *SNHL* sensorineural hearing loss, *MLNT* Multi-syllabic Lexical Neighborhood Test, *LNT* Lexical Neighborhood Test

Evaluation of Auditory Skills and Progress in Infants and Children 3 Years of Age or Less

The audiologist is most likely to assess a child's auditory skills subjectively based on parental history and the administration of validated questionnaires that measure a child's auditory-based reaction to sounds in their surroundings. The PSMTB recommends using the Auditory Skills Checklist (Meinzen-Derr et al., 2007) and the LittlEARS auditory questionnaire (Coninx et al., 2009; Weichbold et al., 2005) to evaluate auditory skills in children at both pre-and post-implant appointments.

Hearing Aid Trial, Verification, and Evaluation of Speech and Language

Hearing aids must be verified using either probe-microphone measurements or test-box verification with patient-specific real ear to coupler difference (RECD) adjustments, according to the American Academy of Audiology's Pediatric Amplification Protocol (2003). In addition, because nonlinear hearing aid circuitry is commonly used to achieve audibility at various input levels, a prescriptive formula, such as DSL v5.0 (Cornelisse et al., 1995; Richard et al., 1985; Scollie et al., 2005), should be used to verify target audibility at speech-input levels corresponding to soft, medium, and loud, such as 50, 60, and 70 dB SPL.

When starting a hearing aid trial for a very young child who is a cochlear implant candidate based on the severity of the hearing loss, it is also essential to arrange a speech/language examination to establish baseline language abilities against which future progress may be compared. The SLP's exact metrics are determined by the child's chronological age and his or her "hearing" age. In order to get appropriate benefits from hearing aids, it is anticipated that the child will display a monthly growth curve in auditory abilities and speech and language development with amplification during the hearing aid trial period. After 6 months of wearing hearing aids, a child should have made at least 6 months of growth in auditory skills and speech-language development. If this is not the case for a child who uses amplification, has been undergoing appropriate therapeutic intervention with regularity, and has no developmental or cognitive delays, cochlear implantation should be explored.

During the candidacy evaluation process using hearing aid trial, it is suggested that a child gets at least two speech-language tests. Although norm-referenced measurements are unlikely to be accessible in such a short amount of time, several criterion-referenced measures can give important information regarding the child's progress with properly fitting hearing aids. Children must get appropriate intervention, including frequent visits from or to a member of the early intervention team, speech-language therapy, and active parental participation to augment therapy with effective modeling of spoken-language development. During the candidacy screening process, the cochlear implant team may gather information from the parents about the regularity with which the child has been using the hearing aid and attending the prescribed therapy program. It sets a high bar for what to expect after cochlear implant surgery in terms of extensive intervention.

An international survey about cochlear implant candidacy revealed differences in audiometric and speech perception measures, funding structure to support cochlear implantation, and access to implants within different countries (Vickers et al., 2016). The study included participants from 17 countries, and revealed that unilateral implants for children and adults were being supported through national funding in most of the countries (30% used medical insurance & 10% self-funding). For those countries using speech perception-based tests, 40% use word tests, 24% use sentence tests, and 36% use both. Among the countries using audiometric thresholds for candidacy, the majority use a criteria of pure tone thresholds exceeding 75–85 dB

HL at frequencies above 1 kHz as the candidacy criteria. The United Kingdom and Belgium were reported to have the most conservative audiometric criteria whereas countries like Australia, Germany, and Italy were the most lenient.

Care and Maintenance of the Device

The sound delivered via a cochlear implant can be abruptly turned off by anything as simple as a dead battery, despite meticulous consideration of eligibility criteria, surgeries performed by skilled surgeons, and highly advanced programming techniques. For a young child, routine school staff's attention to the care and maintenance of the cochlear implant device can be the difference between a world of sound and a world of quiet. This section will delve deep in to use and care of a cochlear implant.

Appropriate Handling and Storage of the Cochlear Implant

A basic rule on where an implant should be handled could make a world of difference between recurring damage and uninterrupted functioning of the implant. As much as possible, the cochlear implant should be handled when standing or sitting on a carpeted surface. Despite the fact that the speech processor is designed for children and is quite sturdy, it should not be dropped or banged needlessly. The cables connecting various implant components are more prone to damage than any other external component of the device. The device should be handled with utmost care, avoiding using any wires connected to external components to support the device's weight. Children should be warned to avoid twisting or spinning the cables unnecessarily. In fact, unless a dire need arises, the implant cables should be only handled by parents or care givers at home and the supporting school staff, including teachers, at the school. Most school activities can be done with the cochlear implant in place. When not in use for various reasons, the device should be stored in its dedicated case and kept out of the reach of children and away from windows and water sources. One must avoid exposing the device to excessive temperature swings of more than 115 °F or less than 32 °F. The device should be kept at room temperature while not in use.

Daily Maintenance

The cochlear implant should be checked for appropriate functioning at the start of each day and before therapy sessions. This evaluation involves a visual inspection of the external implant components to detect any signs of physical damage, and to confirm that the cables are correctly connected. The troubleshooting part goes over a more in-depth examination of the cochlear implant. Because a cochlear implant cannot be listened to the same way that hearing aids can, we must rely on the child to offer input on how the device sounds. The Ling's 6-Sound Test is one method for doing so (Ling 2002).

The Ling's 6-Sound test represents the spectrum of speech sounds heard in everyday conversation. These six sounds, presented daily, assist in testing the spectrum of auditory responsiveness of cochlear implant users and can be used to detect any change or reduction in auditory awareness. The sounds /a/, /i/, /u/, /s/, /?/, and /m/ should all be delivered solely in auditory modality, completely avoiding visual cues. This can be done by emitting noises from behind the child on the implanted ear's side or directly in front of the child using a speech screen (audio speaker mesh over an embroidery hoop) positioned in front of the speaker's face to conceal any visual cues. The child is requested to raise his or her hand when each sound is heard.

Older children and adults may be asked to make the sound they hear. If a decline in responsiveness is noted, the external components should be examined, provided the child was alert during the activity. If the teachers or the therapist identifies the decline in responsiveness during the Ling's 6-Sound test, the audiologist or parent should be notified if the device looks to be working adequately. A change in auditory responsiveness could also suggest that more programming is needed or that the map stored on the speech processor needs to be changed. Classroom observations of a cochlear implant user's performance can help the audiologist fine-tune the map for maximum benefit. In order to maximize the auditory potential of the cochlear implant user, the classroom teacher and other school staff must join hands with the cochlear implant audiologist.

Cochlear Implant's Battery

The cochlear implant's battery is essential to its optimal operation. For functioning of the device, special rechargeable batteries or battery packs are required; however, some cochlear implants can also function adequately on power from AA or 675 HP batteries (HP means high power and is critical for delivering appropriate battery power to operate behind-the-ear speech processors). It is recommended that a spare set of batteries be kept at school for cochlear implant systems that do not require a specialized rechargeable battery pack. This spare set of batteries can be used if the implant batteries run out during the school day. Parents should be advised to send at least one spare, fully charged battery in their child's bag every day for devices that need to use a specific rechargeable battery pack. A device-specific charger must be used to charge rechargeable batteries. Batteries that are discarded cannot be recharged. Attempting to recharge non-rechargeable disposable batteries can damage the battery charger. Additionally, failing to charge a rechargeable battery fully reduces the battery's life. A battery to get fully charged may take 2–10 hours, depending on the device.

The duration for which the charge of a set of batteries lasts should be known to the classroom teacher so that batteries can be checked and replaced as needed. Most speech processors have a light-emitting diode (LED) that illuminates when the batteries are adequately charged. The batteries or the battery pack should be replaced if the LED does not illuminate despite the power to the charger being turned on. The batteries must be inserted appropriately for proper operation, and the battery compartment must be entirely closed and kept in the correct position. A cotton swab dipped in sanitizer can be used to gently clean any dirt on the battery connections.

Moisture

Moisture can harm the microphone and the speech processor. Dirt and debris from the external components should be removed by wiping with a soft, dry cloth. The external components of the cochlear implant should never be submerged or cleaned with water or other cleaning agents. A hairdryer or other electrical appliance should not be used to dry the device after it has been exposed to moisture. To dry the device, it should be placed in a drying pouch after removing the batteries. A drying kit is a container filled with moisture-absorbing crystals (desiccant) that help aerate and protect the external device components from moisture-related damage.

Overall, cochlear implants require regular care and maintenance to ensure optimal function. Patients/caregivers should keep the external components, such as the processor and microphone, clean by wiping them with a dry cloth daily. They must avoid moisture exposure and use protective covers when needed. They need to check the battery regularly, replacing it when it's low to ensure proper function. The regular physical inspection should be done by the caregivers for any signs of damage or wear, and address any issues promptly. It is important to ensure that the implant is programmed correctly through follow-up appointments with the Audiologist. The device should be kept safely when not in use and further periodic maintenance checks will extend the life and effectiveness of the implant.

References

Alzhrani, F., Yousef, M., Almuhawas, F., & Almutawa, H. (2019). Auditory and speech performance in cochlear implanted ANSD children. *Acta Oto-Laryngologica, 139*(3), 279–283.

Bergeson, T. R., Houston, D. M., & Miyamoto, R. T. (2010). Effects of congenital hearing loss and cochlear implantation on audiovisual speech perception in infants and children. *Restorative Neurology and Neuroscience, 28*(2), 157–165.

Bittencourt, A. G., Torre, A. A., Bento, R. F., Tsuji, R. K., & Brito, R. D. (2012). Prelingual deafness: Benefits from cochlear implants versus conventional hearing aids. *International Archives of Otorhinolaryngology, 16*, 387–390.

Boothroyd, A. (1984). Auditory perception of speech contrasts by subjects with sensorineural hearing loss. *Journal of Speech and Hearing Research, 27*(1), 134–144.

Breneman, A. I., Gifford, R. H., & DeJong, M. D. (2012). Cochlear implantation in children with auditory neuropathy spectrum disorder: Long-term outcomes. *Journal of the American Academy of Audiology, 23*(1), 5–17.

Carlson, M. L., Breen, J. T., Gifford, R. H., Driscoll, C. L. W., Neff, B. A., Beatty, C. W., Peterson, A. M., & Olund, A. P. (2010). Cochlear implantation in the octogenarian and nonagenarian. *Otology and Neurotology, 31*(8), 1343–1349.

Carlson, M. L., Sladen, D. P., Haynes, D. S., Driscoll, C. L., DeJong, M. D., Erickson, H. C., Sunderhaus, L. W., Hedley-Williams, A., Rosenzweig, E. A., Davis, T. J., & Gifford, R. H. (2015). Evidence for the expansion of pediatric cochlear implant candidacy. *Otology and Neurotology, 36*(1), 43–50.

Coelho, D. H., Hammerschlag, P. E., Bat-Chava, Y., & Kohan, D. (2009). Psychometric validity of the Cochlear Implant Function Index (CIFI): A quality of life assessment tool for adult cochlear implant users. *Cochlear Implants International, 10*(2), 70–83.

Coninx, F., Weichbold, V., Tsiakpini, L., et al. (2009). Validation of the LittlEARS® auditory questionnaire in children with normal hearing. *International Journal of Pediatric Otorhinolaryngology, 73*(12), 1761–1768.

Cornelisse, L. E., Seewald, R. C., & Jamieson, D. G. (1995). The input/output formula: A theoretical approach to the fitting of personal amplification devices. *Journal of the Acoustical Society of America, 97*(3), 1854–1864.

Cosetti, M., & Roland, J. T. (2010). Cochlear implantation in the very young child: Issues unique to the Under-1 population. *Trends in Amplification, 14*(1), 46–57.

Cox, R. M., & Alexander, G. C. (1995). The abbreviated profile of hearing aid benefit. *Ear and Hearing, 16*(2), 176–186.

Davidson, L. S. (2006). Effects of stimulus level on the speech perception abilities of children using cochlear implants or digital hearing aids. *Ear and Hearing, 27*, 493–507.

Deltenre, P., Mansbach, A. L., Bozet, C., Christiaens, F., Barthelemy, P., Paulissen, D., & Renglet, T. (1999). Auditory neuropathy with preserved cochlear microphonics and secondary loss of otoacoustic emissions. *International Journal of Audiology, 38*(4), 187–195.

Dettman, S. J., D'Costa, W. A., Dowell, R. C., Winton, E. J., Hill, K. L., & Williams, S. S. (2004). Cochlear implants for children with significant residual hearing. *Archives of Otolaryngology and Head Neck Surgery, 130*, 612–618.

Dillon, H., James, A., & Ginis, J. (1997). Client Oriented Scale of Improvement (COSI) and its relationship to several other measures of benefit and satisfaction provided by hearing aids. *Journal of the American Academy of Audiology, 8*(1), 27–43.

Eilers, R. E., Wilson, W. R., & Moore, J. M. (1977). Developmental changes in speech discrimination in infants. *Journal of Speech and Hearing Research, 20*(4), 766–780.

Eilers, R. E., Morse, P. A., Gavin, W. J., & Oiler, D. K. (1981). Discrimination of voice onset time in infancy. *Journal of the Acoustical Society of America, 70*(4), 955–965.

Friedmann, D. R., Tona, K. M., Roland, J. T. Jr, Spitzer, E. R., Waltzman, S. B. (2020). Cochlear implantation in children under 12 months: Prevalence and implications of 'hidden' disabilities. *Cochlear Implants International, 21*, 307–312.

Gatehouse, S., & Noble, I. (2004). The speech, spatial and qualities of hearing scale (SSQ). *International Journal of Audiology, 43*(2), 85–99.

Gifford, R. H., Shallop, J. K., & Peterson, A. M. (2008). Speech recognition materials and ceiling effects: Considerations for cochlear implant programs. *Audiology and Neurotology, 13*(3), 193–205.

Habib, M. G., Waltzman, S. B., Tajudeen, B., & Svirsky, M. A. (2010). Speech production intelligibility of early implanted pediatric cochlear implant users. *International Journal of Pediatric Otorhinolaryngology, 74*(8), 855–859.

Hayes, H., Geers, A. E., Treiman, R., & Moog, J. S. (2009). Receptive vocabulary development in deaf children with cochlear implants: Achievement in an intensive auditory-oral educational setting. *Ear and Hearing, 30*(1), 128–135.

Hinderink, J. B., Krabbe, P. F. M., & Van Den Broek, P. (2000). Development and application of a health-related quality-of-life instrument for adults with cochlear implants: The Nijmegen Cochlear Implant Questionnaire. *Otolaryngology - Head and Neck Surgery, 123*(6), 756–765.

Holder, J. T., Reynolds, S. M., Sunderhaus, L. W., & Gifford, R. H. (2018). Current profile of adults presenting for preoperative cochlear implant evaluation. *Trends in Hearing, 22*. https://doi.org/10.1177/2331216518755288

Houston, D. M., & Jusczyk, P. W. (2003). Infants' long-term memory for the sound patterns of words and voices. *Journal of Experimental Psychology: Human Perception and Performance, 29*(6), 1143–1154.

Houston, D. M., & Miyamoto, R. T. (2010). Effects of early auditory experience on word learning and speech perception in deaf children with cochlear implants: Implications for sensitive periods of language development. *Otology and Neurotology, 31*(8), 1248–1253.

Jijo, P. M., & Yahtiraj, A. (2010). *Early speech perception test in Malyalam hearing impaired children* (pp. 105–119). [Dissertation based article published at All India Institute of Speech and Hearing].

Jusczyk, P. W. (2002). Some critical developments in acquiring native language sound organization during the first year. *Annals of Otology, Rhinology and Laryngology, 111*(5 II), 11–15.

Jusczyk, P. W., & Hohne, E. A. (1997). Infants' memory for spoken words. *Science, 277*(5334), 1984–1986.

Killion, M. C., Niquette, P. A., Revit, L. J., & Skinner, M. W. (2001). Quick SIN and BKB-SIN, two new speech-in-noise tests permitting SNR-50 estimates in 1 to 2 min. *The Journal of the Acoustical Society of America, 109*(5), 2502.

Kontorinis, G., Lloyd, S. K. W., Henderson, L., Jayewardene-Aston, D., Milward, K., Bruce, I. A., O'Driscoll, M., Green, K., & Freeman, S. R. M. (2014). Cochlear implantation in children with auditory neuropathy spectrum disorders. *Cochlear Implants International, 15*(Suppl), S51–S54.

Leal, C., Marriage, J., & Vickers, D. (2016). Evaluating recommended audiometric changes to candidacy using the speech intelligibility index. *Cochlear Implants International, 17*(Suppl 1), 8–12.

Leigh, J. R., Dettman, S. J., & Dowell, R. C. (2016). Evidence-based guidelines for recommending cochlear implantation for young children: Audiological criteria and optimizing age at implantation. *International Journal of Audiology, 55*, S9–S18.

Leigh, J., Dettman, S., Dowell, R., Sarant, J. (2011). Evidence-based approach for making cochlear implant recommendations for infants with residual hearing. *Ear and Hearing, 32*, 313–322.

Ling, D. (2002) *Speech and the Hearing Impaired Child* (2nd ed.) Washington, DC: A. G. Bell Association for the Deaf and Hard of Hearing.

Liu C. C., Sweeney M., Booth T. N., Lee K. H., Kutz J. W., Roland P., Isaacson B. (2015). The impact of postmeningitic labyrinthitis ossificans on speech performance after pediatric cochlear implantation. *Otology and Neurotology, 36*, 1633–1637.

Levine, D., Strother-Garcia, K., Golinkoff, R. M., & Hirsh-Pasek, K. (2016). Language development in the first year of life: What deaf children might be missing before cochlear implantation. *Otology and Neurotology, 37*(2), e56–e62.

McRackan, T. R., Fabie, J. E., Burton, J. A., Munawar, S., Holcomb, M. A., & Dubno, J. R. (2018). Earphone and aided word recognition differences in cochlear implant candidates. *Otology and Neurotology, 39*(7), e543–e549.

Meinzen-Derr, J., Wiley, S., Creighton, J., & Choo, D. (2007). Auditory skills checklist: Clinical tool for monitoring functional auditory skill development in young children with cochlear implants. *Annals of Otology, Rhinology and Laryngology, 116*(11), 812–818.

Mondain, M., Sillon, M., Vieu, A., Levi, A., Reuillard-Artieres, F., Deguine, O., Fraysse, B., Cochard, N., Truy, E., & Uziel, A. (2002). Cochlear implantation in prelingually deafened children with residual hearing. *International Journal of Pediatric Otorhinolaryngology, 63*, 91–97.

Moog, J., & Geers, A. E. (1990). *Early speech perception test for profoundly hearing-impaired children*. Central Institute for the Deaf.

Moog, J. S., & Geers, A. E. (2010). Early educational placement and later language outcomes for children with cochlear implants. *Otology and Neurotology, 31*(8), 1315–1319.

Nilsson, M., Soli, S. D., & Sullivan, J. A. (1994). Development of the hearing in noise test for the measurement of speech reception thresholds in quiet and in noise. *Journal of the Acoustical Society of America, 95*(2), 1085–1099.

Nilsson, M., McCaw, V., & Soli, S. (1997). *Minimum speech test battery for adult cochlear implant users. User's manual.* House Ear Institute.

Niparko, J. K., Tobey, E. A., Thal, D. J., Eisenberg, L. S., Wang, N. Y., Quittner, A. L., & Fink, N. E. (2010). Spoken language development in children following cochlear implantation. *JAMA - Journal of the American Medical Association, 303*(15), 1498–1506.

Peterson, G. E., & Lehiste, I. (1962). Revised CNC lists for auditory tests. *The Journal of Speech and Hearing Disorders, 27*, 62–70.

Peterson, A., Shallop, J., Driscoll, C., Breneman, A., Babb, J., Stoeckel, R., & Fabry, L. (2003). Outcomes of cochlear implantation in children with auditory neuropathy. *Journal of the American Academy of Audiology, 14*(4), 188–201.

Priya, K. (2017). *Modified early speech perception test in Kannada (MESP-K).* [Unpublished Master's Dissertation, University of Mysore, Mysore].

Rance, G., & Barker, E. J. (2008). Speech perception in children with auditory neuropathy/dyssynchrony managed with either hearing aids or cochlear implants. *Otology and Neurotology, 29*(2), 179–182.

Richard, S., Ross, M., & Mark, S. (1985). Selecting amplification characteristics for younghearing-impaired children. *Ear and Hearing, 6*(1), 48–53.

Roland, J. T. Jr, Coelho, D. H., Pantelides, H., Waltzman, S. B. (2008). Partial and double-array implantation of the ossified cochlea. *Otology and Neurotology, 29*, 1068–1075.

Roland, J. T. Jr, Cosetti, M., Wang, K. H., Immerman, S., Waltzman, S. B. (2009). Cochlear implantation in the very young child: Long-term safety and efficacy. *Laryngoscope, 119*, 2205–2210.

Roland, J. T., Gantz, B. J., Waltzman, S. B., & Parkinson, A. J. (2016). United States multicenter clinical trial of the cochlear nucleus hybrid implant system. *Laryngoscope, 126*(1), 175–181.

Rotteveel, L. J., Snik, A. F., Vermeulen, A. M., Mylanus, E. A. (2005). Three-year follow-up of children with postmeningitic deafness and partial cochlear implant insertion. *Clinical Otolaryngology, 30*, 242–248.

Schafer, E. C. (2010). Speech perception in noise measures for children: A critical review and case studies. *Journal of Educational Audiology, 16*, 4–15.

Schaefer, S. M., de Kruijf, M., Henderson, L., Metryka, A., O'Driscoll, M., & Bruce, I. A. (2019). Improved speech and language development after unilateral cochlear implantation in children with a potentially useable contralateral ear. *Cochlear Implants International, 20*(1), 39–46.

Scollie, S., Seewald, R., Cornelisse, L., Moodie, S., Bagatto, M., Laurnagaray, D., Beaulac, S., & Pumford, J. (2005). The desired sensation level multistage input/output algorithm. *Trends in Amplification, 9*(4), 159–197.

Shallop, J. K., Peterson, A., Facer, G. W., Fabry, L. B., & Driscoll, C. L. W. (2001). Cochlear implants in five cases of auditory neuropathy: Postoperative findings and progress. *Laryngoscope, 111*(4), 555–562.

Spahr, A. J., Dorman, M. F., Litvak, L. M., Van Wie, S., Gifford, R. H., Loizou, P. C., Loiselle, L. M., Oakes, T., & Cook, S. (2012). Development and validation of the azbio sentence lists. *Ear and Hearing, 33*(1), 112–117.

Spitzer, E. R., & Waltzman, S. B. (2023). Cochlear implants: The effects of age on outcomes. *Expert review on Medical devices., 20*, 1131–1141.

Tajudeen, B. A., Waltzman, S. B., Jethanamest, D., & Svirsky, M. A. (2010). Speech perception in congenitally deaf children receiving cochlear implants in the first year of life. *Otology and Neurotology, 31*(8), 1254–1260.

Tomblin, J. B., Barker, B. A., Spencer, L. J., Zhang, X., & Gantz, B. J. (2005). The effect of age at cochlear implant initial stimulation on expressive language growth in infants and toddlers. *Journal of Speech, Language, and Hearing Research, 48*(4), 853–867.

Uhler, K., Yoshinaga-Itano, C., Gabbard, S. A., Rothpletz, A. M., & Jenkins, H. (2011). Longitudinal infant speech perception in young cochlear implant users. *Journal of the American Academy of Audiology, 22*(3), 129–142. https://doi.org/10.3766/jaaa.22.3.2

Uhler, K. M., Baca, R., Dudas, E., & Fredrickson, T. (2015). Refining stimulus parameters in assessing infant speech perception using visual reinforcement infant speech discrimination: Sensation level. *Journal of the American Academy of Audiology, 26*(10), 807–814.

Uhler, K., Warner-Czyz, A., & Gifford, R. (2017). Pediatric minimum speech test battery. *Journal of the American Academy of Audiology, 28*, 232–247.

Valente, M. (2006). Guideline for audiologic management of the adult patient. *Internationale Konferenz Chicago 2006 (Phonak), 2002*, 333–339.

Van Wieringen, A., & Wouters, J. (1999). Natural vowel and consonant recognition by Laura cochlear implantees. *Ear and Hearing, 20*(2), 89–103.

Vickers, D., Raeve, L. D., & Graham, J. (2016). International survey of cochlear implant candidacy. *Cochlear Implants International, 17*(Suppl), 36–41.

Wackym, P. A., Runge-Samuelson, C. L., Firszt, J. B., Alkaf, F. M., & Burg, L. S. (2007). More challenging speech-perception tasks demonstrate binaural benefit in bilateral cochlear implant users. *Ear and Hearing, 28*(Suppl), S80–S85.

Wanna, G. B., O'Connell, B. P., Francis, D. O., Gifford, R. H., Hunter, J. B., Holder, J. T., Bennett, M. L., Rivas, A., Labadie, R. F., & Haynes, D. S. (2018). Predictive factors for short- and long-term hearing preservation in cochlear implantation with conventional-length electrodes. *Laryngoscope, 128*(2), 482–489.

Warner-Czyz, A. D., Roland, T., Jr., Thomas, D., Uhler, K., & Zombek, L. (2022). American cochlear implant alliance task force guidelines for determining cochlear implant candidacy in children. *Ear and Hearing, 43*, 268–282.

Weichbold, V., Tsiakpini, L., Coninx, F., & D'Haese, P. (2005). Development of a parent questionnaire for assessment of auditory behaviour of infants up to two years of age. *Laryngo- Rhino-Otologie, 84*(5), 328–334.

White, K. R., Vohr, B. R., Meyer, S., Widen, J. E., Johnson, J. L., Gravel, J. S., James, M., Kennalley, T., Maxon, A. B., Spivak, L., Sullivan-Mahoney, M., & Weirather, Y. (2005). A multisite study to examine the efficacy of the otoacoustic emission/automated auditory brainstem response newborn hearing screening protocol: Research design and results of the study. *American Journal of Audiology, 14*(Suppl), S200–S216.

Widen, J. E., Johnson, J. L., White, K. R., Gravel, J. S., Vohr, B. R., James, M., Kennalley, T., Maxon, A. B., Spivak, L., Sullivan-Mahoney, M., Weirather, Y., & Meyer, S. (2005). A multisite study to examine the efficacy of the otoacoustic emission/automated auditory brainstem response newborn hearing screening protocol: Results of visual reinforcement audiometry. *American Journal of Audiology, 14*(Suppl), S217–S228.

Zeitler, D. M., Prentiss, S. M., Sydlowski, S. A., & Dunn, C. C. (2024). American cochlear implant alliance task force: Recommendations for determining cochlear implant candidacy in adults. *The Laryngoscope, 134*(Suppl), S1–S14.

Zwolan, T. A., Schvartz-Leyzac, K. C., & Pleasant, T. (2020). Development of a 60/60 guideline for referring adults for a traditional cochlear implant candidacy evaluation. *Otology and Neurotology, 41*(7), 895–900.

Chapter 12
Surgical Perspective of Cochlear Implants: Preoperative Preparation

Gaurav Gupta, Kranti Bhavana, and Neha Shakrawal

Abstract The preparation before cochlear implant surgery focuses on thoroughly assessing the patient's hearing function to identify those who will benefit most from the procedure. This process also helps detect potential surgical complications and ensures the patient's readiness for postoperative care. Typically, an ENT surgeon is the first to assess individuals with congenital hearing loss. The evaluation includes a series of tests conducted by an audiologist, speech and language pathologist, child psychologist, and paediatrician, followed by counselling for the family and setting up a vaccination timeline. This chapter highlights the importance of preoperative preparation before cochlear implant surgery.

Keywords Immunization · HRCT · MRI · Audiological Tests · Speech Language assessment

Introduction

The preoperative preparation in cochlear implantation aims for a thorough evaluation of patient's functional hearing abilities and selecting the patients who will significantly improve after the intervention. It also aids in spotting potential surgical problems and postoperative compliance of the patient. An Otorhinolaryngologist is often the first to encounter the visits of congenital hearing loss. The evaluation

G. Gupta (✉)
Department of Oto-rhino-laryngology, Sardar Patel Medical College, Bikaner, Rajasthan, India

K. Bhavana
Department of Oto-rhino-laryngology, All India Institute of Medical Sciences, Patna, Bihar, India

N. Shakrawal
Department of Oto-rhino-laryngology, Dr. Sampurnanand Medical College, Jodhpur, Rajasthan, India

P. Kumar et al. (eds.), *Advances in Implantation Otology*,
https://doi.org/10.1007/978-981-96-8671-1_12

proceeds with an array of assessments by an audiologist, a speech and language pathologist, a child psychologist, and a pediatrician followed by family counselling and a schedule of vaccination. The flow chart in Fig. 12.1 outlines the broad concepts involved in the preoperative evaluation. A detailed description is given in the individual section.

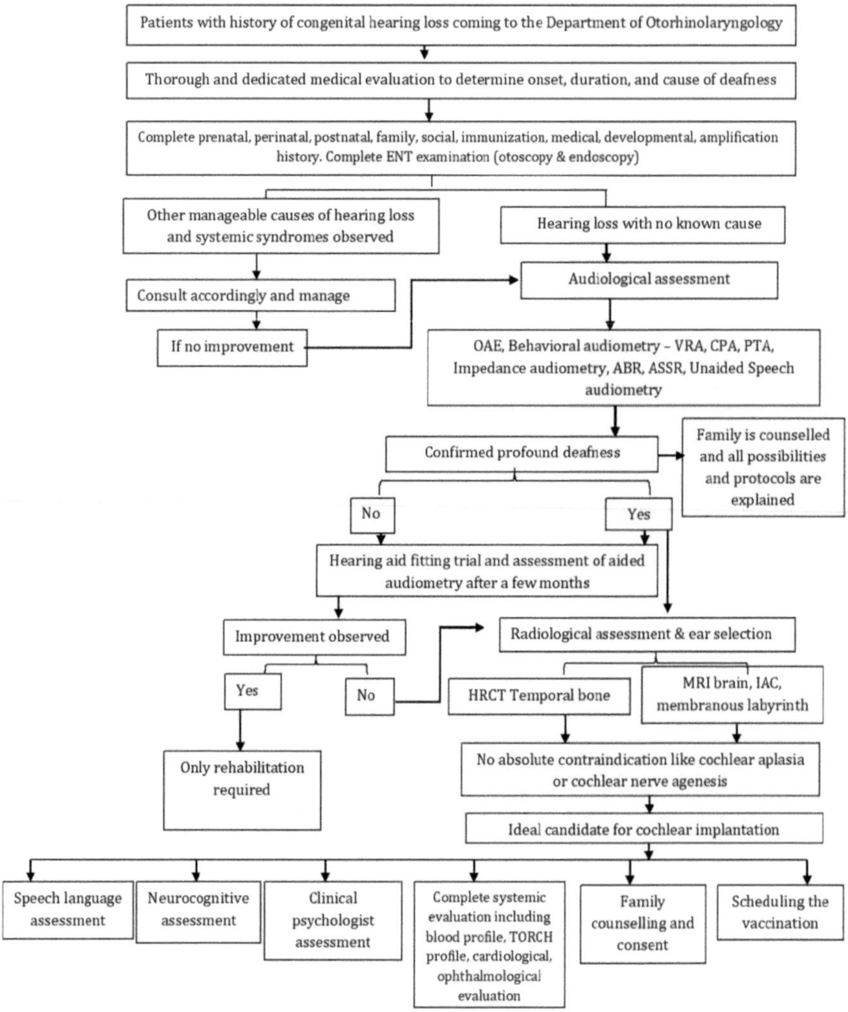

Fig. 12.1 Flowchart showing the components of preoperative preparation in cochlear implantation

Medical Evaluation and Local Examination

It includes evaluation of deafness which includes a complete history and otorhinolaryngological examination. A detailed history is taken to determine the onset, cause, duration, bilaterality, and progression of deafness. Significant history in relation to prenatal, perinatal, postnatal development, immunization status, and socioeconomic background is gathered along with amplification history. Delayed motor milestones, difficulty in walking or maintaining balance should be noted to rule out vestibular dysfunction.

The local examination includes inspection for previous surgical scars or the presence of active infection. Active infection of the external or middle ear (acute/chronic otitis media or cholesteatoma) is a contraindication to surgery as it increases the risk of meningitis and other intracranial infections (Wei et al., 2007a). Any tympanic membrane perforation or middle ear effusion should be managed beforehand. Open mastoid cavities should be treated first followed by staged cochlear implantation. Failure in the management of chronic infection often results in implant extrusion.

The systematic examination helps to detect problems that might interfere with patients' ability for successful results or attending surgical rehabilitation programs. Syndromic association of profound deafness must be ruled out. The various syndromes associated with deafness are Waardenburg, Usher, Klippel-Fiel, Pendred, Treacher Collins, Trisomy 13 and 18, Retinitis pigmentosa, Lange-Neilsen, Refsum, and Hunter's syndrome.

Audiological Assessment It is the primary assessment to evaluate patient's functional hearing abilities, identification of degree of deafness with amount of residual hearing and assessment of results after amplification trial. Its importance is discussed in brief here. The detailed overview is described in Chapter 11. The various constituents of complete audiological assessment are:

(a) Behavioural (Pure tone) audiometry
(b) Impedance evaluation
(c) Auditory brainstem responses (ABR)
(d) Auditory steady-state responses (ASSR)
(e) Oto-acoustic emissions (OAE)
(f) Unaided speech audiometry
(g) Hearing aid trial and aided audiometry
(h) Comparison of a candidate's pre implantation performance with that of current cochlear implant users.

Radiological Assessment and Ear Selection

The main purpose of diagnostic imaging is to identify cochlear patency and a functional cochlear nerve. They aid in choosing the side of implantation and acts as a roadmap for surgery. They are important tools in teaching and operative planning.

High Resolution Computed Tomographic (HRCT) Temporal Bone

Proper magnification and slice thickness provide essential information about the anatomy and variations of the inner ear. HRCT scan is superior in defining bony landmarks along with detecting inner ear morphology. Various structures examined are otic capsule, various turns of cochlea, vestibule, semi-circular canals, internal acoustic canal (IAC), cochlear duct, fallopian canal, cochlear nerve, facial recess, mastoid emissary vein, carotid canal, sigmoid sinus, mastoid air cells, height of jugular bulb and parietal bone thickness. Evaluation of scala tympani is of utmost importance to ensure proper electrode insertion (Fig. 12.2). Axial sections better demonstrate the basal turn, round window, horizontal part of facial nerve and tympanum, while coronal sections are superior in exposing basal and middle turns of cochlea, vertical part of facial nerve, and jugular bulb (Fig. 12.3). Associated inner ear malformations like Mondini's deformity, incomplete partition, dilated vestibule, enlarged vestibular aqueduct, common cavity, or cochlear hypoplasia are also assessed (Fig. 12.4). Anticipated CSF gusher intraoperatively will be acknowledged on HRCT scan. Other variations in the pneumatization around the cochlea and facial

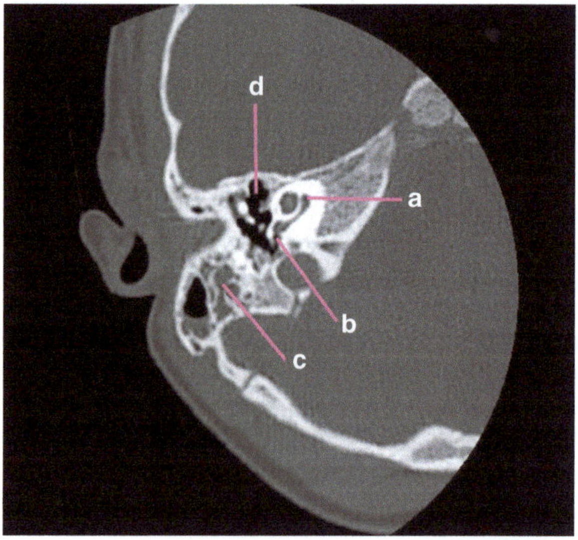

Fig. 12.2 An axial HRCT section of the temporal bone demonstrating (**a**) basal turn of the cochlea, (**b**) round window, (**c**) mastoid air cells, and (**d**) tympanum

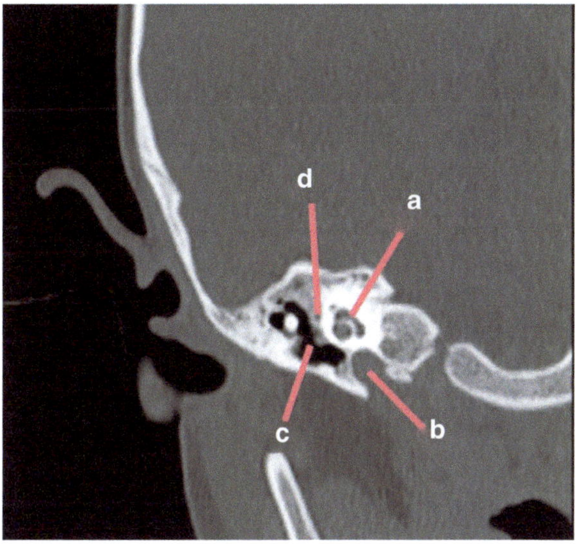

Fig 12.3 A coronal HRCT section of temporal bone demonstrating (**a**) basal turn of the cochlea, (**b**) jugular bulb, (**c**) tympanum, and (**d**) horizontal part of the facial nerve

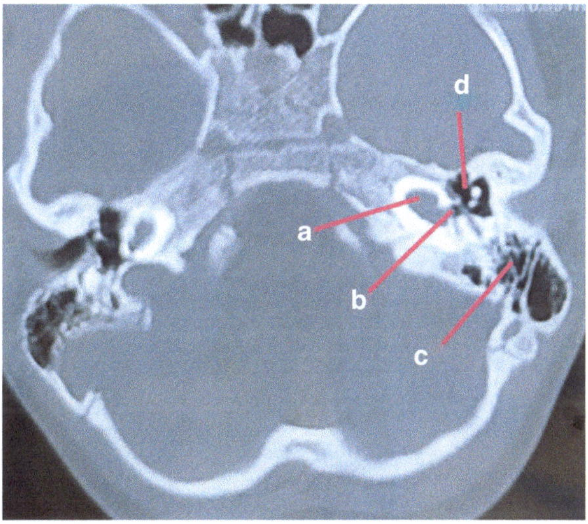

Fig. 12.4 An axial section HRCT of the temporal bone demonstrating (**a**) common cavity (**b**) round window, (**c**) mastoid air cells, and (**d**) tympanum

nerve are important preoperative indicators. An intracochlear calcification needs excessive drilling during cochleostomy which potentially damages the spiral ganglion afferents (Arts et al., 2002), and therefore need to be identified. A large infracochlear cell might be confused with a round window necessitating careful examination and inferencing. Variations of facial nerve dehiscence near facial recess necessitate caution towards posterior tympanotomy. Sennaroglu and Emel (2016) found that narrow (<2 mm) facial recess is a negative indicator of cochleostomy and results in difficult electrode insertion.

Otosclerosis results in opacification of otic capsule or round window along with an increased diameter of cochlear duct which can be appreciated on HRCT. Patients having cochlear ossification might not respond to usual electrical stimulation and need high power output from the signal processor (Eisenberg et al., 1984). Although MRI is better in delineating the new onset or partial ossification and fibrosis of inner ear structures, complete ossification is visualized in HRCT as well. The knowledge of ossification or fibrous occlusion of inner ear structures before the implantation plays an integral role in choosing surgical approaches and device selection. It is always wise to compare the anatomy of both sides to choose the best ear for implantation.

Magnetic Resonance Imaging (MRI) Brain, IAC, Membranous Labyrinth

It allows better soft tissue delineation and identifies the status of cochlear nerve, membranous labyrinth, and endolymphatic sac. A patent cochlear duct and a functional cochlear nerve is an essential requirement for cochlear implantation. The hypoplastic cochlea has a short length cochlea and ranges from the common cavity to incomplete partition at the apex of cochlea. The thickness and caliber of the cochlear nerve (specifically T2 sagittal section of IAC demonstrating the four nerves) can be assessed (Fig. 12.5). It is better in demonstrating post-meningitic intracochlear fibrosis, or superficial siderosis which narrows the diameter of internal acoustic meatus (Connor et al., 2009; Digge et al., 2016). Complete cochlear agenesis or abnormal dimensions of internal acoustic meatus indicating possible nerve

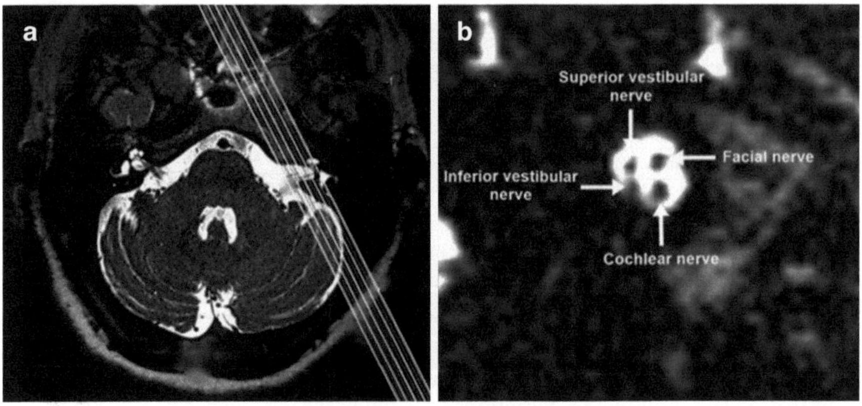

Fig. 12.5 (**a**) An axial T2 weighted MRI showing bilateral vestibulocochlear nerve bundles. (**b**) Parasagittal multiplanar reconstruction at the level of midpoint of IAC for the assessment of four nerves (cochlear, facial, superior and inferior and inferior vestibular nerves)

aplasia are contraindications for cochlear implantation. In meningitis, repeat scans in an immediate preoperative period are advised (Luxford & Cullen, 2010).

While HRCT has a risk of ionizing radiation exposure, there are no associated radiation risks in MRI. Moreover, it serves as a baseline for brain parenchyma before implant artifacts observed postoperatively. It has the advantage of detecting any retro cochlear or intracranial pathology (Hong et al., 2010).

Ear Selection

Ideally, bilateral cochlear implantation results in the best outcomes. In cases of unilateral implantation, characteristics in the temporal bone radiology help in deciding the best ear to be implanted. The presence of functional cochlear nerve, patent cochlea, facial nerve course, along with any ongoing dysplasia, ossification, or active infection, such as chronic otitis media, are weighed together to determine the best side for implantation. Use of contralateral hearing aid in unilateral implantation should be recommended. In such cases, the best ear to implant is the one that has no or minimal residual hearing, or the one which is not getting any benefit from the amplification. The electrode insertion destroys the residual hearing making the amplification useless. If all the factors are similar on both sides, the right ear is chosen as the center for speech recognition lies in the left hemisphere. In ears with bilateral prolonged anacusis, the one with residual hearing is implanted.

Speech and Language Assessment

Evaluation of a child's speech and communication performances helps in establishing a baseline level before implantation. Speech and language therapists ensure that the patient is using the hearing aids during the wake hours and is habitual with speech therapy. They assess the benefits after amplification and motivate the parents for enrolment in rehabilitation programs.

Neurocognitive/Psychosocial Assessment

A detailed evaluation of patients' ability to cope with the implantation and rehabilitation is done by a clinical psychologist. Good mental and physical health is paramount for successful results. A clinical psychologist assesses patients' verbal and non-verbal intelligence, memory skills, attention, and visual and motor integration. Any developmental delay will affect hearing and speech performances after cochlear implantation. The patient is referred to a pediatrician for clinical or genetic evaluation if needed. This section is discussed in detail in Chapter 11.

Family Counselling and Informed Consent

It begins with explaining and motivating the family members about the surgery, post-surgical rehabilitation, and keeping realistic expectations. The surgical procedure is explained with anticipated risks during and after the surgery. The expenses, cost, switch on, mapping, handling, and maintenance of implant are discussed with a demonstration of hearing by showing dummy implants and external devices. The prospective cochlear implant recipients or their care givers are counselled regarding no instant improvement in speech and auditory performances after implantation and the utility of post-operative rehabilitation for better results (Degive & Archinard, 1992). A detailed consent is obtained after explaining all the concerns to avoid any future medico-legal litigation. They should be having prior knowledge of certain difficulties which a surgeon might encounter intraoperatively, like incomplete electrode insertion, inadvertent facial nerve injury, or profuse bleeding. Parents are counselled to take care of their child to prevent any potential damage to the device from any kind of trauma or sports.

Vaccination Protocol

To prevent post-implant meningitis by Streptococcus pneumoniae and Hemophilus influenzae, vaccination is advised against these pathogens. The Centre for disease control and prevention (CDC) and the advisory committee on immunization practices (ACIP) have given vaccination guidelines for cochlear implant recipients. The guidelines are summarized in Table 12.1. PPSV 23 is not recommended for children <2 years as they may show a poor immune response to pure capsular antigen (Wei et al., 2007b).

Adequate evaluation of implant candidacy with accurate management to gain maximum benefit is the aim of preoperative assessment. Patient selection is best achieved by collaborative and cooperative teamwork. The patient and family members should become familiar with all team members to ease the procedure and for maximum success.

Table 12.1 Routine vaccination guidelines and variations in cochlear implant recipients

Vaccination Schedule		Administration of Doses									
		1 month	2 months	4 months	6 months	9 months	12 months	15 months	2–5 years		6–18 years
Routine	Pneumocccal conjugate (PCV 13)		1st dose	2nd dose	3rd dose		4th dose		If the series is incomplete or any dosing is missed, 1 dose of PCV 13 should be given		
	Haemophilus influenzae type b (Hib)		1st dose	2nd dose			3rd and 4th dose				Previously unvaccinated children- need no vaccination
							If only 1 dose is administered by now, no further dosing required				
							If unvaccinated at age15 months to 5 years, 1 dose should be administered				
In Cochlear Implant surgery	Pneumococcal polysaccharide (PPSV 23)								History of Incomplete series of PCV 13 vaccination	If 3 doses of PCV 13 taken, 1 dose of PCV 13 should be given	In case of no history of PCV 13 or PPSV 23 dosing, 1 dose of PCV 13 and 1 of PPSV 23 should be administered
										If less than 3 doses of PCV 13 taken, 2 doses of PCV 13 should be given	
									If no history of PPSV 23, 1 dose of PPSV 23 should be given		In case of a history of any PCV 13 but no PPSV 23, 1 dose of PPSV 23 must be given
											In case of history of PPSV 23 but no PCV 13, 1 dose of PCV 13 should be administered

There should be at least 8 weeks of interval between two vaccine doses

References

Arts, H. A., Garber, A., & Zwolan, T. A. (2002). Cochlear implants in young children. *Otolaryngologic Clinics of North America, 35*(4), 925–943.

Connor, S. E., Bell, D. J., O'gorman, R., & Fitzgerald-O'Connor, A. (2009). CT and MR imaging cochlear distance measurements may predict cochlear implant length required for 360 insertion. *AJNR: American Journal of Neuroradiology, 30*(7), 1425–1430.

Degive, C., & Archinard, M. (1992). Psychological adaptations and emotional observations of eight multichannel cochlear implant patients. *ORL: Journal for Otorhinolaryngology and Its Related Specialties, 54*, 317–319.

Digge, P., Solanki, R. N., Shah, D. C., Vishwakarma, R., & Kumar, S. (2016). Imaging modality of choice for pre-operative Cochlear imaging: HRCT vs. MRI Temporal Bone. *Journal of Clinical and Diagnostic Research: JCDR, 10*(10), TC01–TC04.

Eisenberg, L. S., Luxford, W. M., Becker, T. S., & House, W. F. (1984). Electrical stimulation of the auditory system in children deafened by meningitis. *Otolaryngology and Head and Neck Surgery, 92*, 700–705.

Hong, P., Jurkowski, Z. C., & Carvalho, D. S. (2010). Preoperative cerebral magnetic resonance imaging and white matter changes in pediatric cochlear implant recipients. *International Journal of Pediatric Otorhinolaryngology, 74*(6), 658–660.

Luxford, W., & Cullen, R. (2010). Surgery for cochlear implantation. In Arriaga (Ed.), *Otologic surgery* (3rd ed., pp. 373–381). Saunders.

Sennaroglu, L., & Emel, T. (2016). Cochlear implantation in a subject with a narrow facial recess: Importance of preoperative radiological findings. *Cochlear Implants International, 17*(3), 158–161.

Wei, B. P., Clark, G. M., O'Leary, S. J., Shepherd, R. K., & Robins-Browne, R. M. (2007a). Meningitis after cochlear implantation. *BMJ (Clinical research ed.), 335*(7629), 1058.

Wei, B. P., Robins-Browne, R. M., Shepherd, R. K., Azzopardi, K., Clark, G. M., & O'Leary, S. J. (2007b). Assessment of the protective effect of pneumococcal vaccination in preventing meningitis after cochlear implantation. *Archives of Otolaryngology—Head & Neck Surgery, 133*(10), 987–994.

Chapter 13
Cochlear Implants: Surgical Techniques

Mohnish Grover, Ashima Saxena, and Divya Jangid

Abstract Cochlear implantation surgery is a precision surgery that involves the common principles of gentle tissue handling, meticulous hemostasis, landmark identification with a thorough understanding of the complex temporal bone anatomy, preservation of critical structures including the facial nerve, and accurate placement of the electrodes in the cochlear lumen. Cochlear implantation surgery, characterized as an aseptic procedure with minimal infection risk, advocates a singular preoperative intravenous antibiotic dose for infection mitigation. Elevated risk factors, such as obesity and diabetes, underscore the importance of prophylaxis, commonly employing a cephalosporin.

Keywords Skin Flap · Cortical Mastoidectomy · Posterior Tympanotomy · Round Window Membrane · Cochleostomy

Introduction

Cochlear implantation surgery is a precision surgery that involves the common principles of gentle tissue handling, meticulous hemostasis, landmark identification with a thorough understanding of the complex temporal bone anatomy, preservation of critical structures including the facial nerve, and accurate placement of the electrodes in the cochlear lumen. Since the implant is a neuro-prosthetic device that should desirably last for a few decades, surgeons take strict precautions to maintain

M. Grover (✉) · D. Jangid
SMS Medical College and Hospital, Jaipur, Rajasthan, India

A. Saxena
Soni Hospital, Jaipur, Rajasthan, India

P. Kumar et al. (eds.), *Advances in Implantation Otology*,
https://doi.org/10.1007/978-981-96-8671-1_13

a sterile environment during the procedure to ensure the best possible outcome for the patient preparation (Alessa et al., 2016).

Cochlear implantation surgery, characterized as an aseptic procedure with minimal infection risk, advocates a singular preoperative intravenous antibiotic dose for infection mitigation. Elevated risk factors, such as obesity and diabetes, underscore the importance of prophylaxis, commonly employing a cephalosporin. Preoperative glucocorticoids, particularly intraoperative dexamethasone, are frequently administered to preserve residual hearing, offering ancillary advantages such as mitigating postoperative nausea and reducing intubation discomfort (Cho et al., 2016). Preoperative preparation includes shaving the periauricular area of the scalp.

Positioning, Infiltration and Draping for Surgery

Under general anesthesia, the patient is positioned supine, with the head turned 45 to 60 degrees away from the surgeon. Sterile preparation involves meticulous cleansing of the pinna, half of scalp, and cheek with povidone iodine scrub. Authors also advise putting this solution in the external auditory canal to detect any injury to the external auditory canal while doing posterior tympanotomy later. If such a thing happens the field in posterior tympanotomy will show brown color of povidone iodine even if there is a minute damage (Carfrae, 2009). Incision is marked along with the site of the proposed RS stimulator package as shown in the Fig. 13.1. An occlusive drape impregnated with povidone iodine is used to retract the pinna anteriorly and seal off the external auditory meatus (Fig. 13.1).

Prolonged neuromuscular blockade is avoided if facial nerve monitoring is done (Blair et al., 1994). The authors do not like using any head ring, however this can be a personal choice of the operating surgeon. If at all a head ring is being used, it

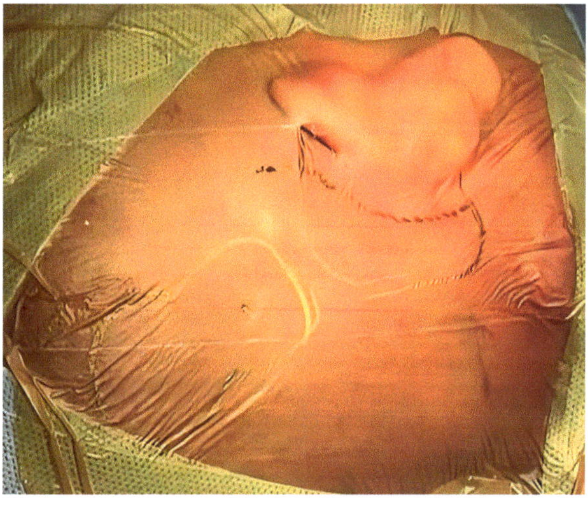

Fig. 13.1 Draping and marking done before starting surgery. Care must be taken that the proposed site for receiver stimulator package is such that it does not overlap the processor which will be placed behind the ear after switch-on of the device. Such overlap may lead to pressure necrosis of skin. (*Pic courtesy: Dr Sunil Narayan Dutt*)

should be a very thin one so that the neck is not flexed a lot, which would limit the comfort of surgeons hands.

Infiltration is done using a 26 gauge needle and 5 ml syringe loaded with commercially available 2% adrenaline:lignocaine (1:1,00,000) local anesthetic solution. Maximum dose is calculated according to the body weight of the patient and a simplified way to calculate is as follows.

The maximum safe dose of lignocaine with adrenaline is 7 mg/kg and concentration of lignocaine used is 2% (20 mg/ml) thus the maximum volume of lignocaine, which can be safely used is 0.35 ml/kg. In an average 60 kg adult, the maximum volume of Lignocaine with Adrenaline which can be used is 21 ml. Similarly, it can be calculated for pediatric cases and should not exceed the maximum safe dose. Care is taken to always inform the anesthetist before infiltrating and aspirating prior to injecting. Infiltration is done along the proposed incision site which lies approximately 0.5–1 cm posterior to the post auricular groove.

Incision and Skin Flap Design

Cochlear implant incisions have undergone evolutionary changes, yet the fundamental principles of incision design persist. Authors prefer a minimal access post auricular incision (Wilde's incision) akin to the one used for routine tympanoplasties is considered sufficient (Fig. 13.2).

The incision is made 0.5–1 cm behind the postauricular groove. This may however be extended superior a bit for surgeons comfort. The ensuing skin flap must be superficial to postauricular muscles in the avascular plane while preserving a robust blood supply. The flap needs to be retracted with help of stay sutures (Otologic surgery atlas/Stanford medicine/cochlear implants 2025) (Fig. 13.3).

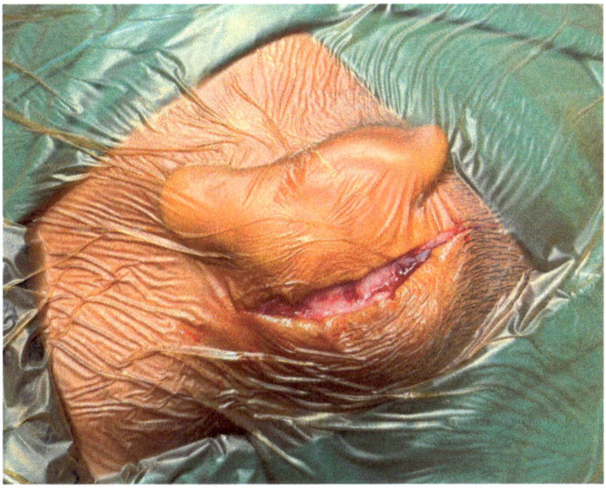

Fig. 13.2 Post-auricular incision used for cochlear implant surgery. Slight superior extension may be given as per surgeon's comfort

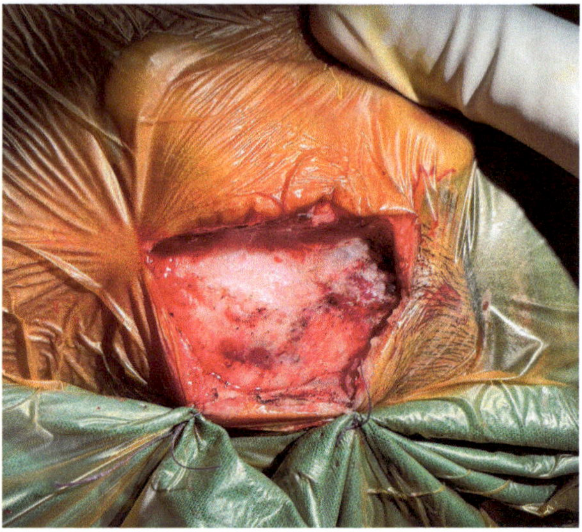

Fig. 13.3 Skin flap is raised superficial to the postauricular muscles and is secured with stay sutures

Some surgeons prefer using self-retaining mastoid retractors. Unobstructed access to the linea temporalis, mastoid tip, and spine of Henle is imperative. Care is taken not to extend the skin flap below the attachment of strap muscles to avoid larger branches of the occipital and posterior auricular vessels. It is advisable to minimize the use of electrocautery and respect the tissues (Qin et al., 2016).

Surgeons can prefer to use a scalpel, tissue dissecting scissors or monopolar cautery for skin flap elevation but care must be given that an adequate skin flap thickness is maintained. Efficient magnetic attraction and radio frequency transmission to the receiver stimulator package depends on skin flap thickness (6–8 mm). In thick-skin cases, if surgical thinning, is needed, it requires well-illuminated access to the undersurface of the most distal skin flap and to avoid dissection into follicles (Zaubitzer et al., 2022).

Musculoperiosteal Flap

This flap acts as a second layer of protection. Authors prefer using anteriorly based Palva's flap. The superior incision of Palva's flap starts 0.5–1 cm below the superior attachment of the pinna and goes posteriorly in a horizontal manner. The landmark of the inferior incision is 0.5 cm below the attachment of the pinna. The incision starts from there and then goes posteriorly. Authors prefer to curve it up as it goes posteriorly and meet the superior incision (Panda et al., 2020) (Fig. 13.4).

This curvature of inferior incision helps avoid the mastoid emissary vein which if injured can lead to unnecessary bleeding, which at times can be bothersome. Again minimal use of electrocautery is advisable to prevent retraction of this flap and preserve the vascular supply. Once incisions have been made, the flap is

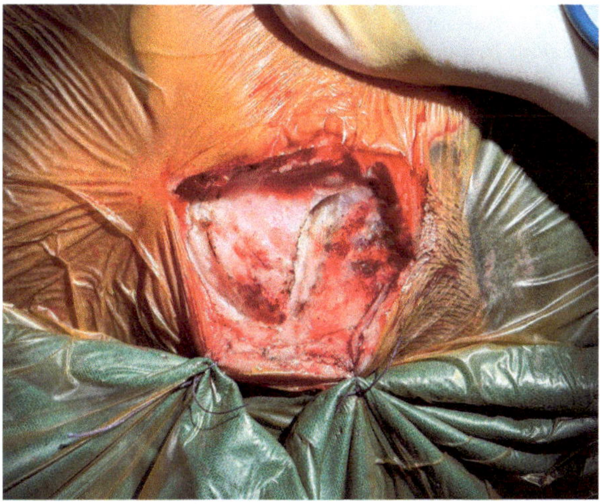

Fig. 13.4 Cuts for the anterior based musculo-periosteal flap

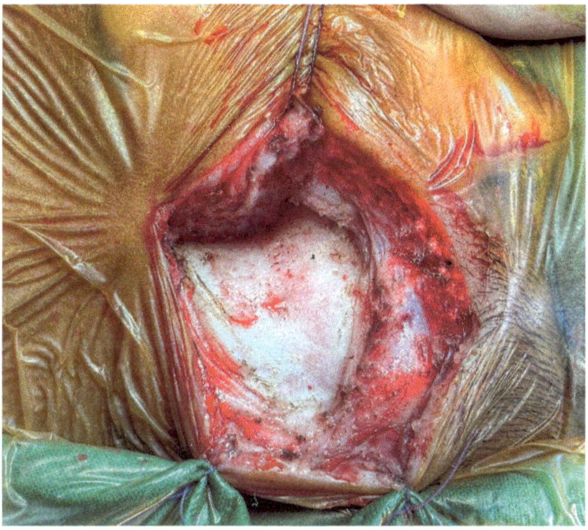

Fig. 13.5 Anteriorly based musculoperiosteal Palva flap raised and secured with a stay suture giving good exposure to the mastoid cortex

elevated anteriorly with help of periosteal elevator. The flap should be elevated to the extent that the flap over the lateral part of bony external auditory canal is also elevated. Visualising this is helpful while doing posterior tympanotomy so that the surgeon can predict the slope of the canal and prevent its injury. The flap is then secured with help of stay sutures or mastoid retractor (Fig. 13.5). The latter is preferred since it allows more manoeuvrability and working space (Otologic surgery atlas/Stanford medicine/cochlear implants, n.d.).

Some surgeons prefer elevating the superiorly based musculoperiosteal flap as shown in Fig. 13.6. However, care must be taken that the anterior incision of this flap does not lie directly deep into the skin incision to provide good strength to the soft tissues (Fig. 13.7).

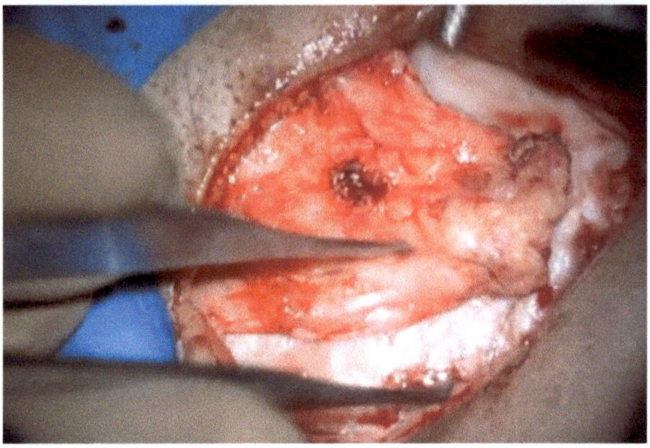

Fig. 13.6 Cuts for the superiorly based musculoperiosteal flap

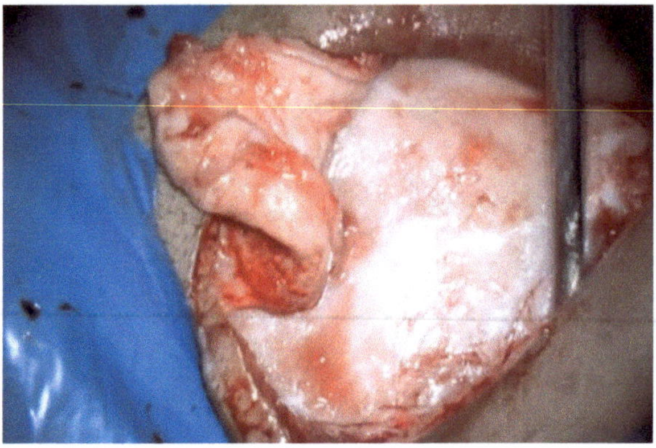

Fig. 13.7 Superiorly based musculoperiosteal flap raised exposing mastoid cortex

Whichever flap is preferred, it should be meticulously crafted to achieve maximum dimensions for ease of closure later on while giving good coverage to the implant and it is preferable that the closure suture line does not directly overlie the implant package.

Raising Periosteal Pocket

After elevating the musculoperiosteal flap, the periosteal pocket is elevated posteriorly with the help of a periosteal elevator. Care must be taken that it is just appropriate as per the implant being used. The tightness of this pocket prevents undue displacement of the implant later on (Jethanamest et al., 2014). At this point, some soft tissues may be harvested to be used later on for sealing the round window/ cochleostomy (Clark et al., 2009).

Cortical Mastoidectomy

A cortical mastoidectomy is performed, exposing the fossa incudis along with the short process of the incus. It is different from a standard mastoidectomy in that the edges of the cavity are kept in an overhanging manner to accommodate the lead securely, eliminating the need for additional compression. The limits of mastoidectomy are tegmen mastoideum superiorly, tip area inferiorly, sigmoid sinus posteriorly and thinning of the posterior bony wall of the external auditory canal (EAC) anteriorly. Again, as compared to a standard simple mastoidectomy the surgeon may not exenterate all the air cells and drilling anteriorly is given more emphasis to thin out the posterior EAC (Fig. 13.8).

Thinning the posterior canal wall is a crucial precursor step to perform a good posterior tympanotomy. To prevent overzealous thinning and to identify damage to the tympanomeatal flap or annulus, the external auditory canal is filled with povidone iodine at the start of the procedure. In case the surgeon accidentally goes through the annulus or tympanomeatal flap, leakage of povidone iodine can be seen which is popularly referred to as 'betadine sign'. Timely identification limits the extent of injury and allows the surgeon to repair the defect at the end of the surgery using fascia, cartilage or bone pate.

Posterior Tympanotomy

After a good cortical mastoidectomy, a posterior tympanotomy is created by opening the facial recess, which is bounded superiorly by the fossa incudis, laterally by the chorda tympani and medially by the facial nerve (Fig. 13.9).

Care must be taken to drill in strokes parallel to the facial nerve with copious irrigation. Many surgeons prefer using a coarse diamond burr and carry out this step with careful attention paid to preserving a layer of bone that overlays the vertical facial nerve using the axis of short process of incus as a landmark (Jain et al., 2019). The bony EAC wall is maximally thinned without penetration. Preservation of the

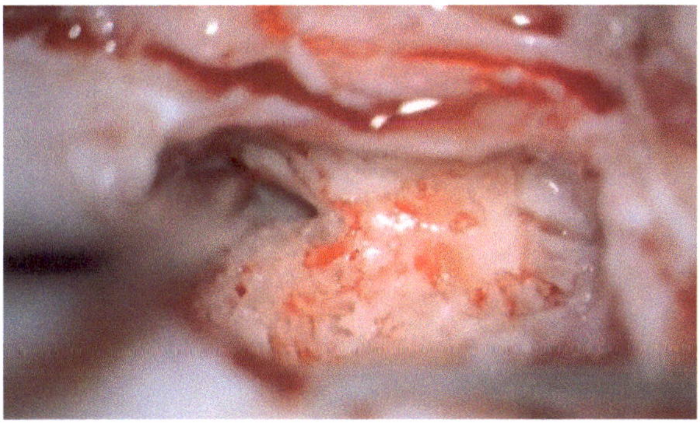

Fig. 13.8 Surgical field right ear showing a well-done cortical mastoidectomy for cochlear implant with adequately thinned posterior canal wall, lateral semicircular canal, aditus and incus

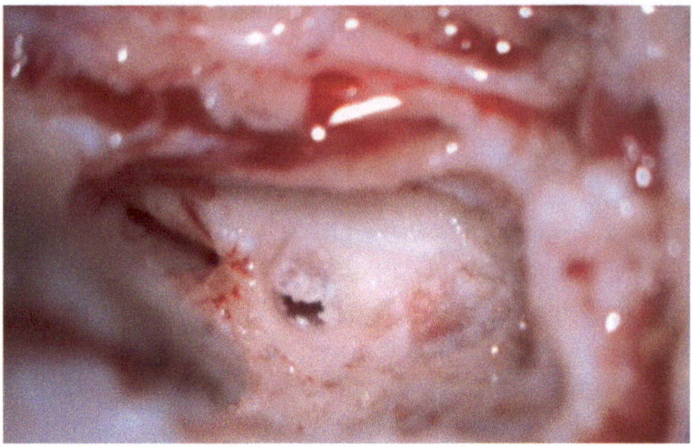

Fig. 13.9 Surgical field right ear showing short process of incus, thinned out posterior canal wall, chorda tympani nerve and initial part of posterior tympanotomy. (Herald cell)

chorda tympani is typically important. In many cases, a 'herald' air cell will be encountered in the region of the facial recess which communicates with the middle ear. Widening it will allow the surgeon to enter the middle ear safely. Presence of any bleeding soft tissue in this area should be approached with care. The use of gelatin sponge soaked with adrenaline is advocated. It is prudent to wait after the application of adrenaline soaked gelatin sponge to achieve good control of bleeding before proceeding and confirming the nature of the soft tissue under high magnification. This is done to avoid causing injury to the facial nerve. When available, a facial nerve monitor can be a great adjunct for surgeons in confidently identifying the course of the facial nerve. The opening of the facial recess can be confirmed using a saline flush which is given through the antrum via aditus and sucked out through the posterior tympanotomy opening created.

Upon entering the middle ear via posterior tympanotomy approach, the surgeon should widen it enough so that adequate light can pass through. It should also be adequate enough to allow passing of instruments later on. The structures that can be identified through an adequate sized posterior tympanotomy include the pyramid, the stapedius tendon, the incudostapedial joint, the jacobson's nerve, the bulge of the promontory and the round window niche (Fig. 13.10). In certain cases, bone removal on the anterior medial surface of the fallopian canal, just below the pyramidal process, may be necessary to ensure adequate access to the round window (RW). Authors prefer to pack the facial recess with dexamethasone soaked gelfoam prior to opening the inner ear and create the well for the RS package in the meantime. This allows for any edema in the middle ear to settle down and also minimises the duration for which the inner ear is open and exposed.

Drilling the Well for Receiver Stimulator Package

Securing the receiver-stimulator (RS) package in cochlear implantation is an important step of surgery, while the technique used is still dependent on the type of implant and surgeon preference. There are many RS fixation techniques described

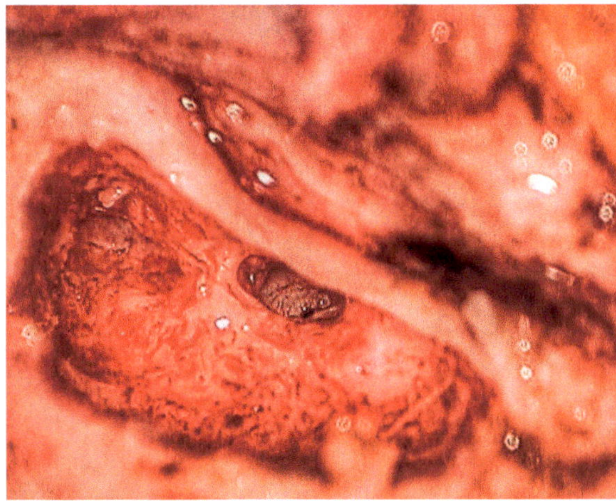

Fig. 13.10 Posterior tympanotomy showing IS Joint, bulge of the promontory and round window niche

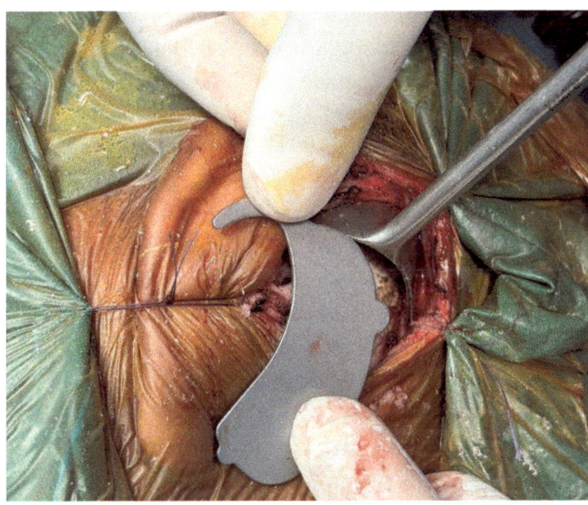

Fig. 13.11 Template to mark the site of the processor and use of Dr. Kirtane's retractor to drill the site of well for the RS package

in the literature. These techniques fall mainly into one of two categories: bony recess techniques (opted by most surgeons) and tight periosteal pocket techniques (opted by a minority but increasing as the implants are becoming thinner and smaller in size) (Markodimitraki et al., 2021). Expert drilling carves out a bony recess behind the mastoid cavity, utilizing specific templates tailored for each device to delineate boundaries and maintaining a 2–2.5-cm-wide ridge between the recess and mastoid cavity. Use of soft tissue retractors make this step easier and more comfortable for the surgeon. The authors prefer using a retractor developed by (Kirtane et al., 2018) (Fig. 13.11).

The depth of the recess accommodates the entire thickness of the employed RS, emphasizing the minimization of dural exposure. Diamond and coarse diamond burrs, ranging from 3.5 to 2.3 or less in size, are utilized to polish the bed so that the

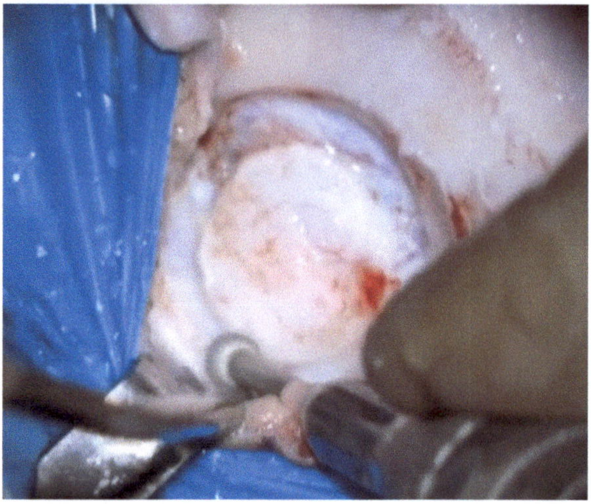

Fig. 13.12 Well being drilled to accommodate the RS package

implant does not rock on it when placed there later. If the bony thickness is too less, in order to achieve adequate depth, authors prefer creating a bony island in the center and exposing the dura all around which can be depressed to accommodate the RS package (Clark et al., 1991). The anterior edge of the well should be drilled such that it has a right angle to the base of the well. This prevents anterior dislocation of the implant. The size of the well should be as per the size of the implant being used. Implant model specific templates should be used for gauging this size. A tunnel connecting the well to the mastoid cavity is drilled. Care should be taken that the two ends of the tunnel should be crafted differently. The part near the well should be wider to accommodate the fantail of the implant. The part of the tunnel near the mastoid cavity should be drilled such that a ridge or notch is created which would support the electrode array from bouncing out of the mastoid cavity. Additionally, a slope is introduced in the tunnel floor towards the anterior side to facilitate the smooth placement of the lead in the mastoid cavity. For the newer generation of implants which are thinner, drilling a bony recess is not mandatory and a tight subperiosteal pocket usually suffices. However, authors prefer making a well in all implants (Figs. 13.12 and 13.13).

Securing the Receiver-Stimulator

The pocket for the RS package is thoroughly irrigated with saline and hemostasis is verified. Securing the RS package should precede the opening of the cochleostomy to enable the immediate insertion of the electrode, thereby reducing the escape of perilymph and the entry of air, blood, or bone dust. Some surgeons prefer making tie down holes in the bone to pass anchoring sutures (Markodimitraki et al., 2021),

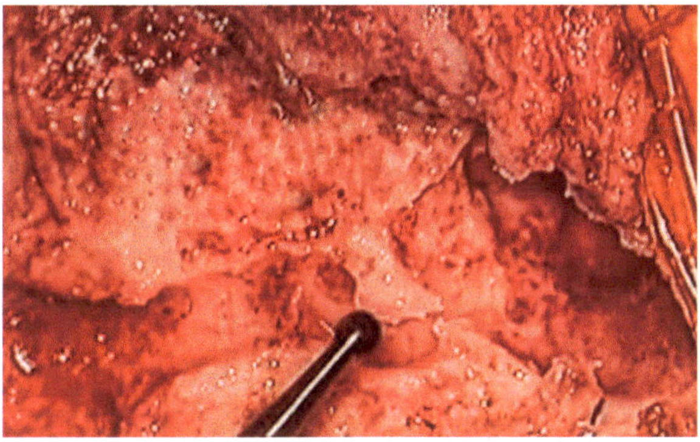

Fig. 13.13 Tunnel from the well upto the mastoid cavity with a notch for securing the electrodes

however authors believe that this is not needed if the periosteal pocket is kept tight and well is drilled optimally.

Before opening the implant, authors recommend covering the operative field with fresh linen and change of gloves for the operating team. The implant is unpacked by a floor nurse and its impedances checked by an audiologist to ensure that electrodes are intact and functioning. Implant is opened and kept carefully in the surgical field so that it snugly fits the well created for it. A periosteal stitch may be taken to anchor the implant firmly. The electrode array is gently kept away from the mastoid cavity with the help of a gauze piece.

Entry Inside the Cochlea

Cochlea can be entered in many ways. The most important principle is to have 'soft' entry inside the cochlea. Let's look at the ways to enter the cochlea:

Round Window

Entry through the round window membrane offers the advantage of minimizing drill trauma, although drilling on the overhang of the RW niche is usually necessary. The niche is drilled to expose the anteroinferior part of the round window membrane. Using a 1.5-mm diamond burr, bone is meticulously removed from the tegmen of the round window (RW) to establish visual and surgical access to the round window membrane (RWM). Dissection typically progresses from anteroinferior to posterosuperior, following the annulus of the RWM. This method prevents the entry of air, bone dust, and blood into the vestibule, leading to a reduced loss of perilymph. Once exposed enough, it is incised under a pool of dexamethasone with a sharp curved pick (Richard et al., 2012) (Fig. 13.14).

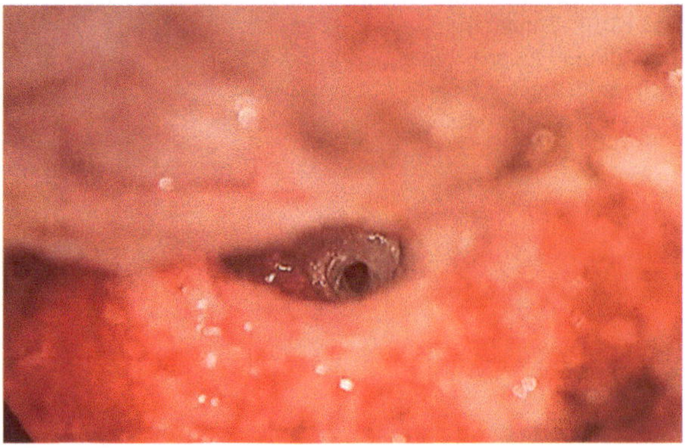

Fig. 13.14 Round window incised for entry into the cochlea

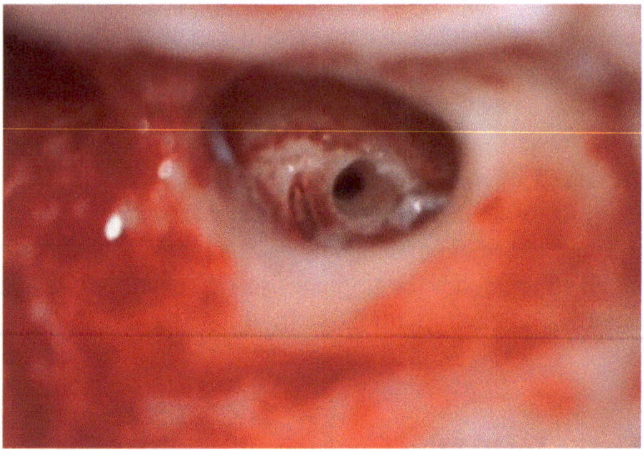

Fig. 13.15 Separate antero inferior cochleostomy

Cochleostomy

The traditional bony cochleostomy has the benefit of an insertion trajectory that more closely aligns with the axis of the scala tympani. It should be created antero-inferior to round window, more inferior, to prevent damaging osseous spiral lamina and entry into scala tympani. Once thinned to a blue line, the bone is delicately removed using a fine pick and membranous cochlea incised (Fig. 13.15).

Extended Round Window/Modified Round Window Entry

More recently, the extended RW cochleostomy has come into use and can be considered a compromise between the two approaches. In this technique, the round window is enlarged anteroinferiorly toward the location of a bony cochleostomy.

Due to variations in the anatomy of the RW niche and differences in electrode configurations, there isn't a universally superior cochleostomy type for all patients and electrodes. The concept of adaptive cochleostomy proposes that the choice of cochleostomy should be tailored to each individual case, rather than employing a single cochleostomy type across all situations (Balkany, 2012). The Author's first preference is round window entry but it is changed as per the need.

Insertion Vectors

Cochlear implant electrodes are ideally introduced along a trajectory that aligns with the lumen of the scala tympani. Surgeons need to carefully consider three insertion vectors: anterior (toward the nose), inferior (toward the feet), and medial (toward the opposite ear). The specific vectors involved may vary slightly depending on the type of cochleostomy.

In the case of a round window membrane (RWM) cochleostomy, the modiolus typically lies directly anterior to the cochleostomy site. It is crucial to emphasize the inferior vector to prevent any impact, particularly when employing a pre-curved electrode. For practical guidance during RWM insertion, the surgeon directs the electrode toward the presumed location of the bony cochleostomy, situated anterior and inferior to the RWM. Adjusting the medial vector involves slightly elevating the proximal end of the electrode from the fallopian canal, orienting the tip toward the opposite ear.

The anterior vector, during RWM insertion, naturally progresses from the mastoid toward the nose and usually does not require special attention. In the case of an extended round window (RW) cochleostomy, slightly anteroinferior to the RWM cochleostomy, a somewhat reduced inferior vector is needed. For the bony cochleostomy, located even more anteroinferiorly, the inferior vector is further minimized. Careful consideration of these vectors ensures precise and effective electrode placement (Breinbauer et al., 2015).

Electrode Insertion

A small amount of dexamethasone is instilled inside cochlea before insertion begins. This acts as a lubricant and facilitates smoother insertion of the electrode array into the cochlea. It also aids in the removal of bone dust and other debris by allowing them to "float out" of the sealing of the round window before electrode insertion. Furthermore, it also decreases the cochlear trauma when electrodes are being inserted. Studies also mention that it also decreases long term intracochlear fibrosis (Chambers et al., 2019). Using insertion forceps, carefully position the electrode tip within the cochleostomy. It is crucial to guide the electrode away from the modiolus and basilar membrane, aligning it with the principal axis of the scala tympani.

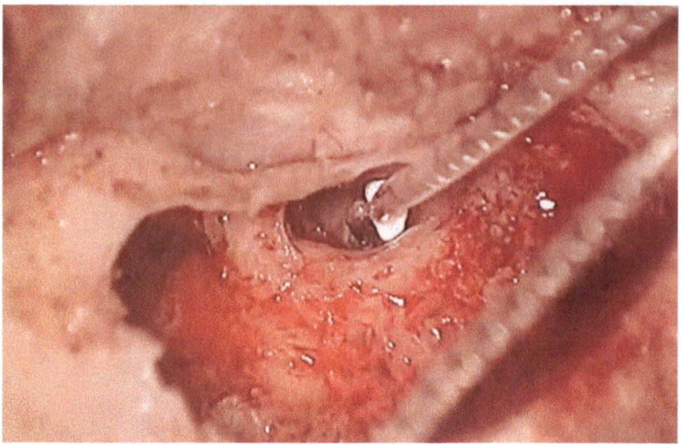

Fig. 13.16 Electrode array inserted into the round window upto the flange

Demonstrations have highlighted that the speed of electrode insertion is a crucial factor in hearing preservation surgery. Slower insertion rates, specifically lasting 30 seconds or more, have shown an association with superior hearing preservation outcomes and improved vestibular function (Kontorinis et al., 2011) (Fig. 13.16).

Insertion Speed

A slow and consistent insertion pace for cochlear implant electrodes, ideally lasting at least 30 seconds, is crucial for minimizing complications and optimizing outcomes. Authors prefer insertion over 60–90 seconds. It is considered that higher speed of insertion causes higher intracochlear pressures leading to damage to inner ear structures and higher chances of loss of any residual hearing (Kontorinis et al., 2011).

Intraoperative Monitoring in Cochlear Implantation

Two specific technologies are in common use for intraoperative real time monitoring.

Active Insertion Monitoring (AIM) (Mushtaq et al., 2022)

Intraoperative Electrocochleography (ECoG) during cochlear implant surgery involves monitoring electrical activity from the cochlea and auditory nerve in response to sounds or electrical stimuli. An acoustic tube is placed in the external auditory canal at the beginning of the surgery and taped properly (Fig. 13.17). This tube sends frequency specific acoustic stimuli which stimulate the remaining inner

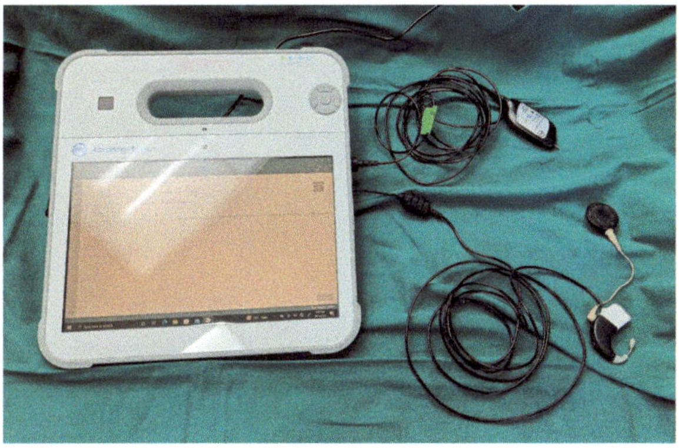

Fig. 13.17 Active monitoring system (AIM) by Advanced Bionics for intra-operative measurements

hair cells in the cochlea, enough to produce cochlear microphonics. These are recorded by the apical electrode as it progresses inside the cochlea and a real time feedback at 0.13 seconds interval is provided to the surgeon. The cochlear microphonics are recorded on a tablet attached to the acoustic tube and processor. A smooth slowly rising graph is seen as the electrode array is inserted inside the cochlea. As we go deeper the width of the lateral part of scala tympani starts getting lesser and any further insertion may damage the residual inner hair cells. At this juncture, the graph of cochlear microphonics starts declining and has a downslope. The surgeon is supposed to stop inserting any further. In the author's experience this usually comes when the insertion is around 22 mm depth, however the jury is still out to find out the ideal depth of insertion.

It's important to choose the patients who have residual hearing such that unaided hearing thresholds should be <80 dB in 250/500/750/1000 Hz. This tool is presently available with Advance Bionics Ltd. and goes by the name of Active Insertion Monitoring (AIM) system.

Smartnav (Page et al., 2018)

Smartnav (System for Management of Atraumatic Robotic Tool) is an advanced tool available with Cochlear Ltd. which provides wireless, real-time, actionable intraoperative insights to deliver added assurance in surgical outcomes for professionals and their patients.

Smartnav provides the following:

1. Angular insertion depth (lateral wall electrodes)
2. Depth of insertion
3. Real time speed and consistency of insertion
4. Final placement of electrode array to rule out any tip fold overs
5. Faster checking of impedances and ECAP thresholds

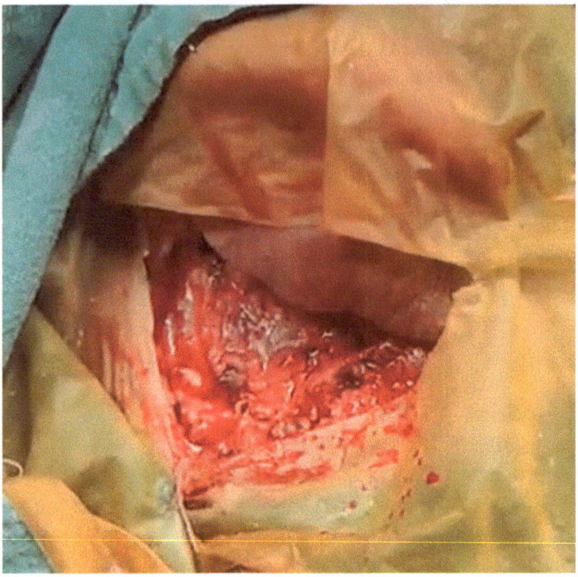

Fig. 13.18 Showing closure of the layers prior to skin closure

Authors find it useful and in future it may not be needed to do any intraoperative imaging if Smartnav provides adequate information.

Closure

Following the successful insertion of the electrode array, the cochleostomy should be securely sealed with a small piece of soft tissue (Cosett et al., 2010). Subsequently, the electrode cable is meticulously coiled into the mastoid cavity, underneath the overhanging edges of cortical mastoidectomy to resist extrusion (Fig. 13.16). Separate ground electrode, if present, should be placed under the temporal muscle on the bone. The incision is closed layer by layer (Fig. 13.18).

Hemostasis should be ensured before cleansing and if any oozing is there which needs to be cauterised then only bipolar cautery should be used. Finally, a delicate mastoid pressure dressing is applied.

References

Alessa, M., Shaikh, A., Aljedaani, Y., & Hassen, H. (2016). Complications of cochlear implantations. *Saudi Journal of Otorhinolaryngology Head and Neck Surgery, 18*(1). https://doi.org/10.4103/1319-8491.275260

Balkany, T. J. (2012). *Adaptive cochleostomy*. CI2012, Twelfth International Congress on Cochlear Implants and Other Implantable Auditory Technologies.

Blair, E. A., Teeple, E., Jr., Sutherland, R. M., Shih, T., & Chen, D. (1994). Effect of neuromuscular blockade on facial nerve monitoring. *The American Journal of Otology, 15*(2), 161–167.

Breinbauer, H. A., & Praetorius, M. (2015). Variability of an ideal insertion vector for cochlear implantation. *Otology and Neurotology, 36*(4), 610–617.

Carfrae, M. J., & Foyt, D. (2009). Intact meatal skin, canal wall down approach for difficult cochlear implantation. *The Journal of Laryngology and Otology, 123*(8), 903–906.

Chambers, S., Newbold, C., Stathopoulos, D., Needham, K., Miller, C., Risi, F., Enke, Y. L., Timbol, G., & Cowan, R. (2019). Protecting against electrode insertion trauma using dexamethasone. *Cochlear Implants International, 20*(1), 1–11.

Cho, H. S., Lee, K. Y., Choi, H., Jang, J. H., & Lee, S. H. (2016). Dexamethasone is one of the factors minimizing the inner ear damage from electrode insertion in cochlear implantation. *Audiology & Neuro-Otology, 21*(3), 178–186.

Clark, G., & Shepherd, R. (2009). Cochlear implant round window sealing procedures in the cat: An investigation of autograft and heterograft materials. *Acta Oto-laryngologica, 98.*

Clark, G. M., Cohen, N. L., & Shepherd, R. K. (1991). Surgical and safety considerations of multichannel cochlear implants in children. *Ear and Hearing, 12*(4 Suppl), 15S–24S.

Cosetti, M., et al. (2010). Cochlear implant electrode insertion. *Operative Techniques in Otolaryngology-Head and Neck Surgery, 21*(4), 223–232.

Jain, S., Deshmukh, P. T., Lakhotia, P., Kalambe, S., Chandravanshi, D., & Khatri, M. (2019). Anatomical study of the facial recess with implications in round window visibility for cochlear implantation: Personal observations and review of the literature. *International Archives of Otorhinolaryngology, 23*(3), e281–e291.

Jethanamest, D., Channer, G. A., Moss, W. J., Lustig, L. R., & Telischi, F. F. (2014). Cochlear implant fixation using a subperiosteal tight pocket without either suture or bone-recess technique. *The Laryngoscope, 124*(7), 1674–1677.

Kirtane, M., & Chavan, K. (2018). Cochlear implant surgical technique: Our experience. *Annals of Otology and Neurotology, 01*, 007–010.

Kontorinis, G., Lenarz, T., Stöver, T., & Paasche, G. (2011). Impact of the insertion speed of cochlear implant electrodes on the insertion forces. *Otology and Neurotology, 32*(4), 565–570.

Markodimitraki, L. M., Strijbos, R. M., Stegeman, I., & Thomeer, H. G. X. M. (2021). Cochlear implant fixation techniques: A systematic review of the literature. *Otology and Neurotology, 42*(7), 959–966.

Mushtaq, F., Soulby, A., Boyle, P., Nunn, T., & Hartley, D. E. H. (2022). Self-assessment of cochlear health by cochlear implant recipients. *Frontiers in Neurology, 13*, 1042408.

Page, J. C., Cox, M. D., Hollowoa, B., Bonilla-Velez, J., Trinidade, A., & Dornhoffer, J. L. (2018). Trends in intraoperative testing during cochlear implantation. *Otology and Neurotology, 39*(3), 294–298.

Panda, N. K., Nayak, G. R., Verma, R., Bakshi, J., & Virk, R. S. (2020). Cochlear implant surgery: Analysis of changes in surgical strategies for better outcomes. *Annals of Indian Academy of Otorhinolaryngology Head and Neck Surgery, 4*, 24. https://doi.org/10.4103/aiao.aiao_10_20

Qin, F., Li, W., Qiu, J., Zhang, L., & Zhong, M. (2016). After cochlear implantation: Complications related to flap around implants. *Journal of Otology, 11*(4), 198–201.

Richard, C., Fayad, J. N., Doherty, J., & Linthicum, F. H., Jr. (2012). Round window versus cochleostomy technique in cochlear implantation: Histologic findings. *Otology and Neurotology, 33*(7), 1181–1187.

Stanford Otologic Surgery Atlas. (n.d.) Postauricular Incision [Internet]. Stanford University; [cited 2025 Aug 24]. Available from: https://otosurgeryatlas.stanford.edu/otologic-surgery-atlas/fundamentals-of-ear-surgery/postauricular-incision/

Zaubitzer, L., Schaefer, E., Wallhaeuser-Franke, E., Burkart, J., Herrmann, K., Walter, B., Schell, A., Scherl, C., Servais, J., & Haeussler, D. (2022). Methods for measuring pre-, intra-, and postoperative skin thickness for cochlear implants. *Journal of Otology, 17*(2), 72–77.

Chapter 14
Cochlear Implants: Surgical Risks and Complications

Milind V. Kirtane, Sangeeta Varty, and Arpit Sharma

Abstract Cochlear Implantation (CI) is recognized as the most effective surgical treatment for those with hearing loss. As candidacy criteria have expanded over time, the number of CI surgeries has increased. With advancements in implant technology and surgical techniques, CI surgery has become a safe and routine procedure for skilled surgeons, though it can occasionally lead to complications. This chapter describes the risks and complications associated with a CI surgery.

Keywords Hematoma · Facial nerve paralysis · Hard failure · Soft failure · Meningitis

Introduction

Cochlear implantation (CI) has been established as the most effective surgical treatment for individuals with bilateral severe-to-profound hearing loss who are unable to derive benefit from Hearing Aids (HAs). Over the years, the number of cochlear implant surgeries has increased due to evolving candidacy criteria. With advances in implant technology and improved surgical techniques, cochlear implant surgery has become a safe and standard procedure in the hands of experienced Implant surgeons but can occasionally lead to complications (Antonelli et al., 2004). The likelihood of complications decreases as surgeons gain experience, and novice surgeons are encouraged to perform their first surgeries under the guidance of a mentor. Complex or challenging cases are best managed by more experienced surgeons. This chapter covers both major and minor complications in detail and discusses potential solutions for each.

The complications due to surgery can be classified in several ways such as (1) Major and Minor complications; (2) Early (within the first 2 weeks of implantation)

M. V. Kirtane · S. Varty · A. Sharma (✉)
Department of ENT, P. D. Hinduja Hospital and Medical Research Centre, Mumbai, Maharashtra, India

P. Kumar et al. (eds.), *Advances in Implantation Otology*,
https://doi.org/10.1007/978-981-96-8671-1_14

Table 14.1 Major and minor complications during cochlear implant surgery

Major Complications	Minor Complications
CSF leakage Hematoma or abscess Mastoiditis or middle ear infections with granulation tissue Cholesteatoma Skin necrosis and/or exposed implant Extrusion of the electrode or receiver-stimulator Meningitis Facial nerve paresis or paralysis Severe facial nerve stimulation Tinnitus or vertigo Dislocation or incorrect position of the electrode Device failure (Hard & Soft)	Injury to Chorda tympani (reversible or irreversible) Transient facial paresis Minor wound infection Otitis media Tympanic membrane perforation

and Late (more than 2 weeks after implantation) complications and (3) Device-related or Surgery-related complications (Cohen & Hoffman, 1991; Bhatia et al., 2004; Ikeya et al., 2013. The device-related complications are mostly concerned with failures of the device, malfunctions of various components, or external trauma. These complications may require the replacement of the device and therefore revision surgery. Whereas surgical complications are directly related to the surgical procedure and can be prevented. The complications can be divided into intraoperative complications, which include major bleeding, cerebrospinal fluid leakage, and injury to facial and chorda tympani nerves, and postoperative complications, which include wound infections, flap necrosis, hematomas, abscesses, otitis media tympanic membrane perforations, cholesteatoma, meningitis, facial paralysis, electrode displacement, device migration, processor failures, tinnitus, and vertigo (Bhatia et al., 2004; Ikeya et al., 2013). The major complications are device removal, additional surgery, facial nerve damage, or other significant problems causing persistent pain or impairment. (Table 14.1). Minor complications can be treated by medical or minor surgical intervention (Cohen & Hoffman, 1991; Ikeya et al., 2013).

Surgical complications can be avoided by following best practices which include careful preoperative evaluation and planning, meticulous surgery, and postoperative care. Further, radiological evaluation in the form of High-Resolution Computed Tomography (HRCT) and Magnetic Resonance Imaging (MRI) of the temporal bone are critical in understanding the temporal bone anatomy, candidacy, and surgical planning. This helps to avoid surgical pitfalls and is useful in the selection of a better ear for implantation.

Intraoperative Complications and Ways to Avoid and Manage Difficult Situations

1. **Facial nerve monitor**: In cochlear implant surgery, it is imperative to follow strict aseptic precautions. A facial nerve monitor should be used, especially in abnormal facial nerve courses or in congenital inner ear anomalies. A perioperative antibiotic is given prior to incision.
2. **Incision:** A vertical post-aural incision is taken from the mastoid tip, a few millimeters behind the post-aural groove, with a slight posterior curve superiorly. A small incision prevents flap-related complications. A large incision can lead to wound dehiscence and infections. To avoid injury to the facial nerve, the post-aural incision in children up to the age of 2 years should be positioned more posteriorly in the mastoid tip area.
3. **Musculo-periosteal layer**: The undermining of the flaps is done carefully in an avascular plane. A triangular postero-superior based musculo-periosteal flap is developed to expose the mastoid bone, exposing the areas for both the mastoidectomy and the well to house the receiver-stimulator. A pocket to accommodate the implant is made in a subperiosteal plane. Bleeding can occur during the elevation of the periosteal flap. Therefore, care must be taken not to create too large a pocket, as this can lead to hematoma formation and subsequent risk of infection. The damage to the mastoid emissary vein can cause significant blood loss and can result in cardio-vascular decompensation in the pediatric age group. Drilling using a diamond burr or use of bone wax will stop the bleeding from the mastoid emissary vein.
4. **Cortical Mastoidectomy**: A cortical mastoidectomy is carried out, ensuring that the edges of the mastoid cavity are not saucerized. The remaining bony overhang aids in securing the electrode leads within the cavity. To facilitate this, the posterior wall of the external auditory canal is appropriately thinned. Additionally, visualizing the short process of the incus, the lateral semicircular canal, and occasionally the digastric ridge can assist in locating the vertical segment of the facial nerve.
5. **The Well**: A template is utilized to drill the well to the correct size. For pediatric patients, the well should be drilled down to the dura to minimize the device profile. The well should be positioned sufficiently posterior to the postauricular incision. If the receiver or stimulator is placed directly beneath the ear-level processor, pressure between the components can lead to device exposure (Fig. 14.1). To prevent trauma to the dura, diamond burrs are employed. In case of accidental dural penetration, the defect should be sealed using fascia or fat and tissue glue. Once the well is formed, tie-down holes are drilled in the surrounding bone, or a periosteal stitch is placed to anchor the device to prevent its migration. With newer, thinner, and flatter implants, a shallow ramp is preferred over a deep well.
6. **The Facial Recess (Posterior Tympanotomy):** The facial recess approach is the standard procedure followed in cochlear implant surgery. The posterior

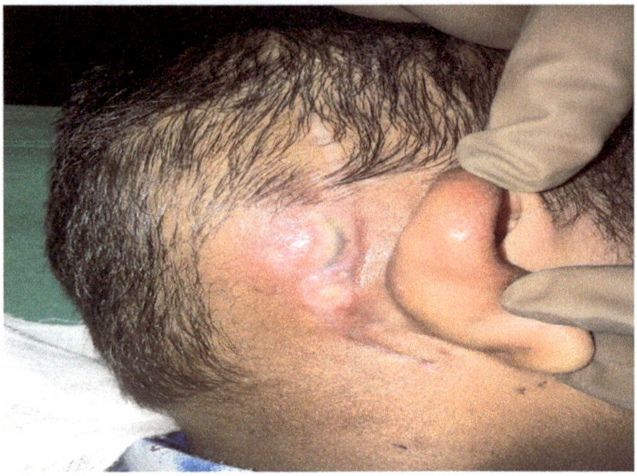

Fig. 14.1 Post-operative implant bulging due to improper placement close to incision

tympanotomy should be carefully planned. The facial and chorda tympani nerves should be routinely identified to prevent injuries to these nerves. If the external auditory canal wall is unintentionally breached during thinning, it should be repaired with bone pate and fascia or cartilage before the surgery concludes. This step helps prevent the formation of a retraction pocket at a later stage.

7. **Round window approach/Cochleostomy**: The anatomy of the Round Window Niche (RWN) can vary in some cases. It is typically located 2–3 mm inferior and slightly posterior to the oval window. Identifying the round window membrane is crucial for precise electrode array placement into the scala tympani. If possible, the electrode may be inserted through a small incision in the round window membrane. Alternatively, a cochleostomy is performed by drilling through the promontory, just anterior and inferior to the round window membrane, using a 1 mm diamond burr. Care must be taken to prevent bone dust or blood from entering the cochlea, and suction should be avoided on the opened cochlea to prevent loss of perilymph. The use of topical intratympanic steroids could be beneficial for hearing preservation.
8. **Fixation of Receiver and Stimulator and Insertion of electrode array**: The receiver-stimulator is fixed in the drilled well and then the electrode array is inserted in the Round Window/cochleostomy. The tip of the electrode array should be directed slightly anteriorly/inferiorly. The electrode array should be advanced very slowly and smoothly, and the insertion should stop at the point of first resistance. Care should be taken not to over-insert the electrode array. The cochleostomy opening must be sealed with connective tissue. This helps electrode stabilization, prevents electrode extrusion, and guards against ascending infections.
9. **Closure:** The wound should be closed in three layers. The previously created triangular flap should be sutured back to the periosteum. The receiver-stimulator and the electrode array must be covered with the flap.

10. **Postoperative Radiograph/Telemetry**: Intra-operative radiography is used to confirm the correct placement of the electrode into the cochlea and detect possible electrode misplacement or tip fold over. In addition, impedance testing and neural response measurements are done to confirm the proper functioning of the device and correct placement.

Complications

Infection after cochlear implant surgery is the most commonly reported complication. The incidence of infection ranges from 1.7% to 8.2% (Bhatia et al., 2004; Hopfenspirger et al. (2007). The complications related to surgical wounds include minor infections like tenderness over the receiver-stimulator, progressing to edema, erythema, cellulitis, and eventually an underlying abscess. There may be flap necrosis, gaping of the surgical incision, and extrusion of the receiver-stimulator and electrode array (Figs. 14.2 and 14.3). The initial treatment should be conservative with intravenous (IV) antibiotics.

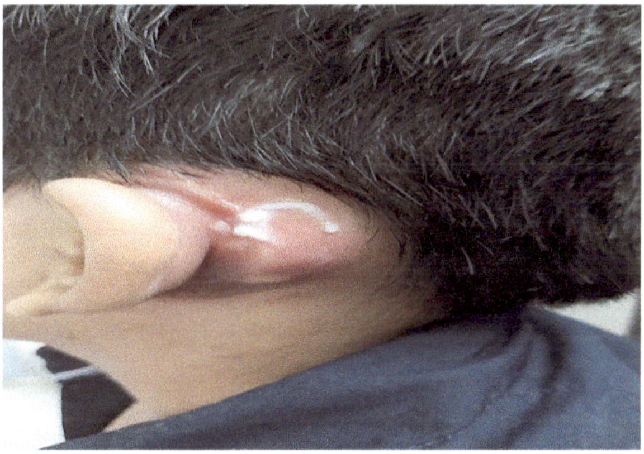

Fig. 14.2 Mastoiditis following cochlear implant surgery

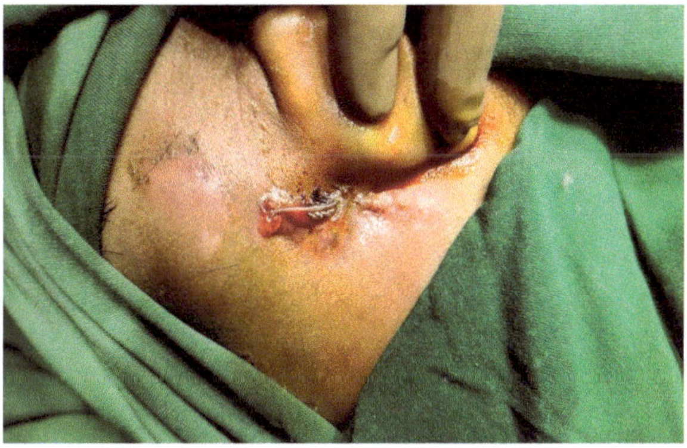

Fig. 14.3 Extruded electrode array through the incision

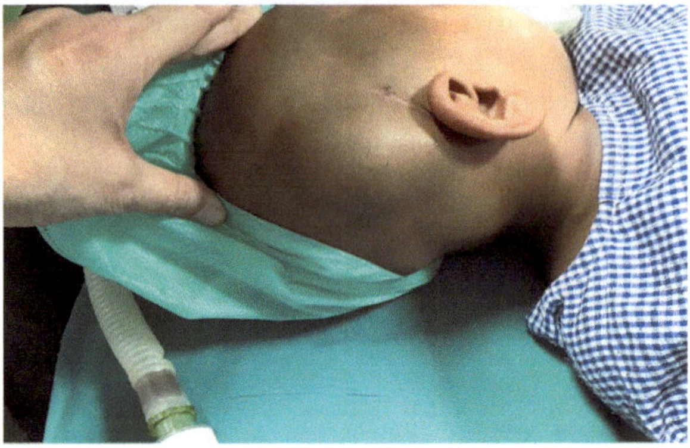

Fig. 14.4 Hematoma following cochlear implant surgery

In cases of recurrent or persistent infection, wound debridement, culture sensitivity, and appropriate antibiotics are advocated The hematoma formation over the implant site is observed or managed by pressure dressing or minor surgical drainage as required. To avoid hematoma formation, a tight pocket is created while elevating the periosteum (Fig. 14.4). The bacterial biofilms formation is a real challenge (Antonelli et al., 2004). If the infection persists, despite attempting the above measures, explantation may become necessary to eradicate the infection. When infection necessitates explantation and a second-stage re-implantation, the receiver-stimulator is removed, while the intra-cochlear electrode array remains in place. The electrode is cut at the facial recess to maintain the cochleostomy opening, preventing fibrosis or ossification. This approach helps optimize the likelihood of a successful re-implantation with complete electrode insertion once the infection has cleared.

Receiver-Stimulator or Electrode Extrusion

The receiver-stimulator can extrude through the skin even years after surgery. There are various factors which can result in the extrusion. The type of skin incision, fixation and position of the receiver-stimulator, the strength of the magnet, partial insertion, cochlear ossification, and general medical condition are important factors for extrusion. The migration of the electrode array usually presents with reduced speech perception. The use of peri-modiolar electrodes may prevent electrode extrusion. Additionally, tightly packing the cochleostomy site may help in keeping the electrode array in place. The intraoperative imaging can confirm the position and immediate recognition of this problem. The magnet strength of the transmitter coil can be adjusted to prevent local skin necrosis and device extrusion (Fig. 14.5).

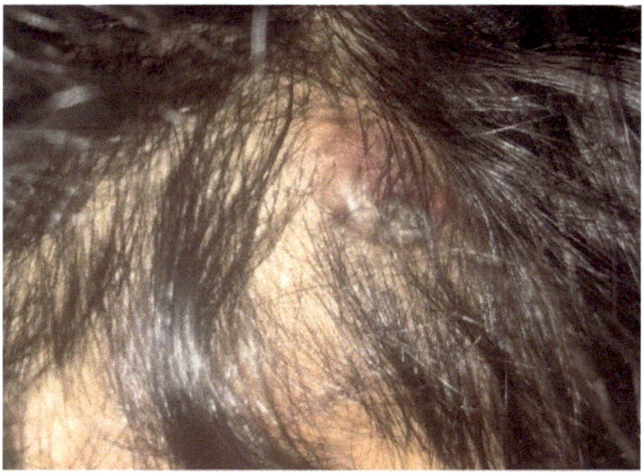

Fig. 14.5 Erythema post-Cochlear implantation due to high magnet strength

Meningitis

Meningitis, a life-threatening infection, is rarely seen now-a-days due to vaccination and good antibiotic coverage. It presents usually within the first year of implantation. It has been suggested that the incidence of meningitis in profoundly deaf patients is higher than in the general population. The patients with a history of otitis media and inner ear malformations are at higher risk of having meningitis.

The primary pathogens that cause meningitis in cochlear implant recipients are *Streptococcus pneumoniae* and *Haemophilus influenzae*. As this infection is preventable and can lead to serious outcomes, it is crucial to ensure proper vaccination for all implant recipients to lower the risk of meningitis. The most commonly recommended vaccines include the heptavalent pneumococcal conjugate vaccine (PCV7; Prevnar), the 23-valent pneumococcal polysaccharide vaccine (PPV23; Pneumovax 23), and the Hib (H. influenza type b conjugate) vaccine. Vaccination should be completed at least 1 month prior to the surgery.

Otitis Media and Cholesteatoma

Early diagnosis and prompt treatment of middle ear infection (otitis media) in cochlear implant recipients are crucial. The insertion of tympanostomy tubes before cochlear implant surgery in case of recurrent serous otitis media is advocated if conservative treatment does not resolve the middle ear effusion (Bhatia et al., 2004).

Cholesteatoma is reported as a late complication. Iatrogenic external auditory canal breach, undiagnosed tympanic membrane perforation, or pre-existing chronic ear disease can be predisposing factors for cholesteatoma formation. Iatrogenic injury to the external auditory canal and damage to the annulus can occur during drilling of posterior tympanotomy. These defects should be repaired using bone dust, fascia or perichondrium, and cartilage (Lin, 2009).

Facial Nerve Injury

Facial nerve injuries have become less frequent, but damage to the facial nerve can occur during cochlear implant surgery. In cochlear implantation, the vertical portion of the facial nerve and chorda tympani nerve serve as the boundaries of the posterior tympanotomy. To visualize the round window, a wide posterior tympanotomy must be created. The proximity of the two nerves to the recess may result in transient or permanent injury to the nerves. The incidence is more in the hands of inexperienced surgeons. Transient facial palsy can occur due to the heat generated by the shaft of the drill touching the facial nerve canal (House & Luxford, 1993; Alzhrani et al., 2016). Copious irrigation is used when drilling around the facial nerve. In approximately 15% of patients with inner ear anomalies, the facial nerve has an aberrant course. The variations in facial nerve anatomy can result in inadvertent injury to the facial nerve. A preoperative CT scan of the temporal bone will alert the surgeon on the abnormal course of the facial nerve and minimize inadvertent injury. Facial nerve monitoring in such a situation should be used, but it does not replace accurate knowledge of anatomy and proper training in performing a posterior tympanotomy. Other factors that can lead to facial paresis following cochlear implantation include reactivation of the herpes virus, acute nerve damage, and postoperative wound infections. Reactivation of the herpes simplex virus is a well-known cause of facial palsy after otologic procedures, particularly when the facial nerve is directly manipulated. Some research indicate that injury to the chorda tympani nerve may trigger viral reactivation. Acute nerve damage can occur from vasospasm caused by ischemia or venous obstruction, leading to nerve swelling.

In cases of minor facial nerve injury, a high dose of prednisone can help reduce swelling and prevent further damage. Facial nerve recovery typically takes several weeks, and physiotherapy is recommended. For more severe injuries or complete nerve disruption, surgical intervention, such as direct anastomosis or grafting, may be necessary. Best outcomes are achieved when a facial nerve graft is performed within the first few months after injury, while results are less favorable if performed after 6–12 months. In cases of delayed facial palsy, medical treatment with high-dose corticosteroids, possibly combined with antiviral therapy, is recommended (Fayad et al., 2003; Alzhrani et al., 2016).

Facial Nerve Stimulation

Facial nerve stimulation is a complication that can occur after cochlear implantation, with reported incidences ranging from 1% to 15% (Niparko et al., 1991; Alahmadi et al., 2023). This issue may be due to current leakage caused by changes in the electrical properties of the bone or the close proximity of the facial nerve to the cochlea's outer wall, combined with the high electrical current needed to stimulate the auditory nerve. Peri-modiolar electrodes, which are positioned closer to the modiolus, may reduce the likelihood of this problem as they direct less current toward the cochlea's outer wall (Battmer et al., 2006). The electrodes in the superior part of the cochlea are responsible for stimulating the facial nerve. The off-ending electrodes can be switched off to alleviate the problem. In some very severe cases, it can be challenging to program the implant, and re-implantation may be required (Alahmadi et al., 2023).

Chorda Tympani Injury

Due to its position, the chorda tympani nerve is vulnerable to damage during the drilling of the facial recess, which can lead to dysgeusia, or altered taste sensation. Patients often describe these taste changes as bitter, metallic, or salty. As bilateral cochlear implantation becomes more common, it is important to preserve the integrity of the chorda tympani nerve during the drilling process to avoid these sensory disturbances. One of the studies done by Kons and colleagues reported 17 out of 144 patients (incidence of 11.8%) had short-term taste change, whereas 26 out of 265 patients (incidence of 9.8%) reported long-term taste change (Kons et al., 2023). They reported that the taste change due to chorda tympani injury may be the most common adverse consequence of CI surgery.

Electrode Placement

Malpositioning or kinking of the electrode array can occur if the last few electrodes are forcefully inserted. Sometimes the electrodes may be found to be malpositioned outside the cochlea. There have been instances when the electrode array is found in the hypotympanum, in the superior semi-circular canal, internal auditory meatus, or even in the canal of the internal carotid artery. This is more likely to occur with cochlear malformation. Therefore, intra-operative radiography should be used in all cases, but more so in difficult cases or when malpositioning is suspected so that displaced electrodes can be readjusted immediately (Figs. 14.6, 14.7, 14.8 and 14.9).

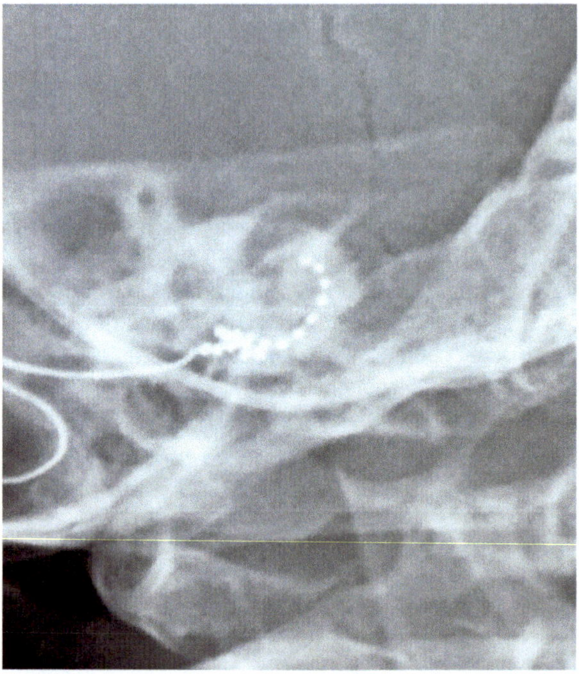

Fig. 14.6 An X-ray showing kinking of the electrode array after Cochlear Implantation

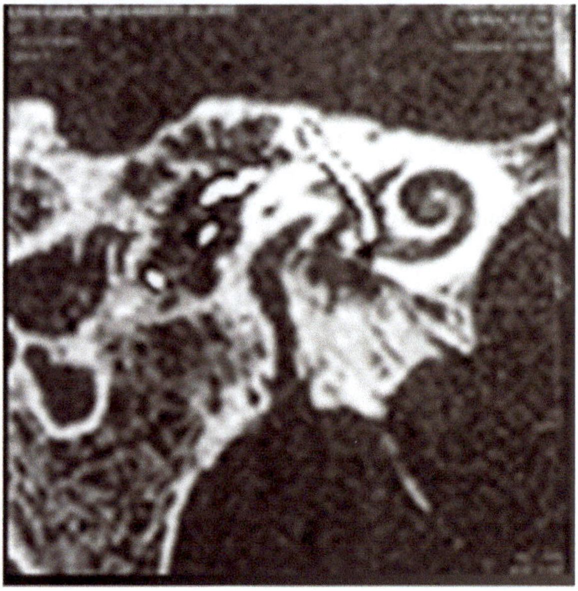

Fig. 14.7 CI electrode seen in Superior Semicircular Canal (SSCC) on CT scan

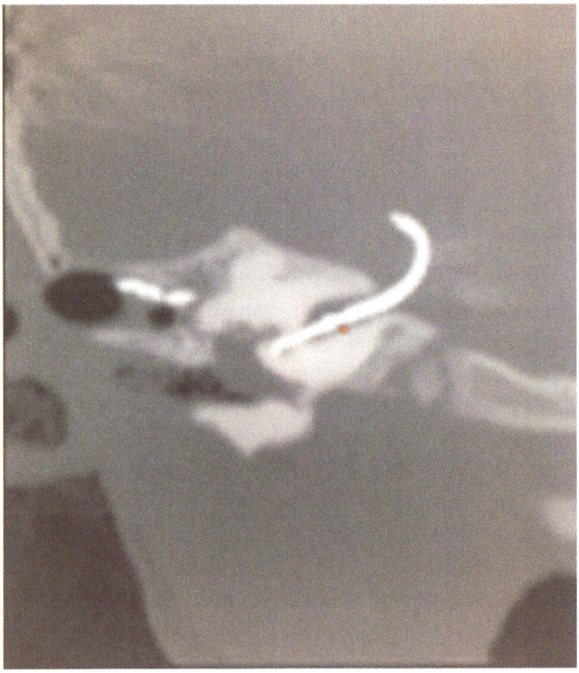

Fig. 14.8 Cochlear Implant electrode seen in Internal Auditory Canal (IAC)

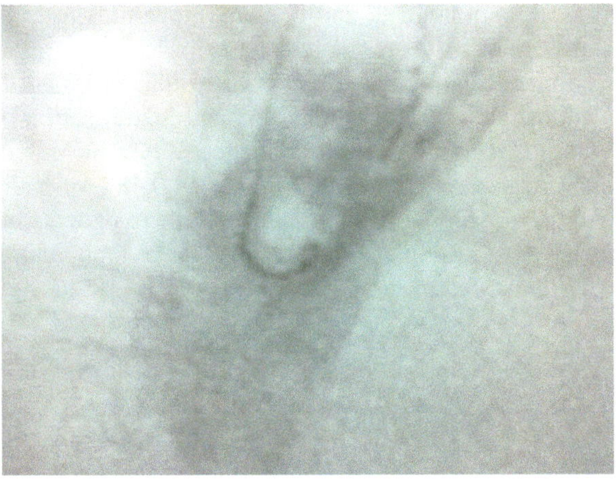

Fig. 14.9 An X-ray image showing the electrode array tip rollover after Cochlear Implantation

CSF Leakage from Cochleostomy

A CSF gusher should be anticipated in cases with an Incomplete partition type 1, common cavity, and an enlarged cochlear aperture as in Incomplete partition type 3. A gusher can be controlled by waiting for the flow to subside, which should take 10–15 minutes, and firmly packing the cochleostomy with soft tissue such as fascia, periosteum, or fat. It is prudent to consider doing a subtotal petrosectomy with blind sac closure in CSF gusher cases to prevent the possibility of future CSF leaks and meningitis. In patients with a Mondini deformity or an enlarged vestibular aqueduct, CSF may ooze from the cochleostomy or the round window. This can be easily sealed with connective tissue.

Device Failure

A confirmed device failure (hard failure) is characterized by the complete loss of auditory input or an electronic malfunction between the internal and external parts. CI patients report an abrupt loss of sound perception due to the lack of auditory input from the device. The evaluation confirms that no connection can be made with the device by external means, and revision of cochlear implant surgery is advised with the replacement of the device (Marlowe et al., 2010; Patnaik et al., 2016.

A potential device malfunction (soft failure) refers to a clinical issue with the cochlear implant where it continues to deliver some sound, but the patient experiences a decline in performance. This may involve irregular CI function, issues with programming, unusual sounds, heightened volume, or non-auditory effects such as discomfort, dizziness, or headaches (Nicholas & Geers, 2008). In such cases, revision cochlear implant surgery may be considered (Rivas et al., 2012). The diagnosis of suspected device malfunction must be investigated thoroughly by clinical, audiological, and imaging modalities to exclude medical problems and hardware or software-related causes of low performance. On completion of revision cochlear implant surgery, all explanted failed devices must be sent to the manufacturer for device analysis and identification of the source of the failure. The most common causes of device failure include case fracture or loss of hermetic seal. One of the studies reported 0.48% of patients (3 out of 627 CI cases) with device failure due to trauma. All three patients had the implant removed and underwent re-implantation at the same time and showed a good prognosis post-implantation.

Tinnitus and Vertigo

The risk of vertigo and tinnitus is significantly higher in the adult population than paediatric population (Rivas et al., 2008; Marlowe et al., 2010). Children rarely complain of post-operative giddiness which is usually transient. If vertigo is persistent or severe, a perilymph fistula should be suspected. With bilateral implantation, there is a potential risk of causing bilateral vestibular hypofunction. In patients with a pre-operative balance problem, vestibular assessment may help to select which ear to implant if unilateral implantation is proposed (i.e. opting for implanting the ear with poorer vestibular function). Cochlear implantation can have positive and negative effects on tinnitus, with 50–90% of CI patients reporting improvement in

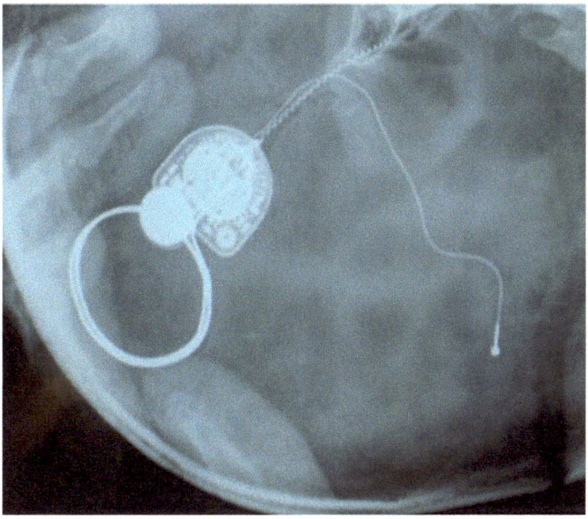

Fig. 14.10 An X-ray showing displaced magnet in a Cochlear Implant recipient

tinnitus after implantation and up to 28% having new or worsening tinnitus after implantation.

Magnet Displacement

Due to trauma at the implant site, it is possible for the magnet to become displaced from its silicone pocket. In such cases, the external component may not connect to the internal device, or the displaced magnet may be palpable through the skin in an abnormal position. An X-ray confirms the diagnosis. A minor surgical procedure is required to remove the displaced magnet and replace it with a new magnet (Fig. 14.10). One of the studies reported that 1.3% of patients had magnet migration. The most frequently reported cause for the magnet migration was MRI-induced movement (55.1%) followed by head trauma (32.1%). The most frequent possible management procedure reported was revision or exploratory surgery with surgical repositioning or replacement (Alahmadi et al., 2021).

Grisel Syndrome: Atlanto-Axial Rotation Subluxation

Grisel's syndrome is a non-traumatic atlantoaxial subluxation that is usually described after tonsil/adenoid surgery or drainage of neck abscess. The authors encountered this problem in one of the implantees in their series. A review of the literature showed only 1 case report after cochlear implant surgery (Nakashima et al., 2016). During otologic surgery, the neck of the patient might have been hyper-flexed and excessively rotated. The patient typically presented with painful torticollis which develops after operation/infection. The radiography of the cervical spine showed that the space between the atlas and the odontoid of the axis was more than 5 mm. The CT Scan of the cervical spine showed subluxation and rotation of the C1 and C2 vertebrae. The medical management consists of bed rest, antimicrobial therapy, anti-inflammatory agents with muscle relaxants, cervical traction, and a neck collar (Nakashima et al., 2016).

The rate of complications will become less as surgeons gain experience. The novice surgeon is advised to do his initial surgeries under the watchful eye of a mentor. Also, revision cases or cases where difficulties are anticipated are best dealt with by more experienced surgeons. For the novice surgeon, it is best to start off by observing cochlear implant surgeries, attending workshops to do hands-on cadaver dissections under supervision. While this does not guarantee a complication free coch;ear implantation, it is definitely a step in minimizing the instances of complications.

References

Alahmadi, A., Alenzi, S., Alsheikh, M., Alghamdi, S., Morra, M. E., & Badr, K. M. (2021). Magnet and receiver-stimulator displacement after cochlear implantation: Clinical characters and management approaches. *Saudi Medical Journal, 42*(8), 813–824.

Alahmadi, A., Abdelsamad, Y., Yousef, M., Alhabib, S. F., Alshalan, A., Hamed, N., & Alzhrani, F. (2023). Risk factors and management strategies of inadvertent facial nerve stimulation in cochlear implant recipients: A systematic review. *Laryngoscope Investigative Otolaryngology, 8*(5), 1345–1356.

Alzhrani, F., Lenarz, T., & Teschner, M. (2016). Facial palsy following cochlear implantation. *European Archives of Oto-Rhino-Laryngology and Head and Neck Surgery, 273*(12), 4199–4207.

Antonelli, P. J., Lee, J. C., & Burne, R. A. (2004). Bacterial biofilms may contribute to persistent cochlear implant infection. *Otology and Neurotology, 25*(6), 953–957.

Battmer, R., Pesch, J., Stöver, T., Lesinski-Schiedat, A., Lenarz, M., & Lenarz, T. (2006). Elimination of facial nerve stimulation by reimplantation in cochlear implant subjects. *Otology and Neurotology, 27*(7), 918–922.

Bhatia, K., Gibbin, K. P., Nikolopoulos, T. P., & O'Donoghue, G. M. (2004). Surgical complications and their management in a series of 300 consecutive paediatric cochlear implantations. *Otology and Neurotology, 25*(5), 730–739.

Cohen, N. L., & Hoffman, R. A. (1991). Complications of cochlear implant surgery in adults and children. *The Annals of Otology, Rhinology, and Laryngology, 100*(9 Pt 1), 708–711.

Fayad, J. N., Wanna, G. B., Micheletto, J. N., & Parisier, S. C. (2003). Facial nerve paralysis following cochlear implant surgery. *The Laryngoscope, 113*(8), 1344–1346.

Hopfenspirger, M. T., Levine, S. C., & Rimell, F. L. (2007). Infectious complications in pediatric cochlear implants. *The Laryngoscope, 117*(10), 1825–1829.

House, J. R., & Luxford, W. M. (1993). Facial nerve injury in cochlear implantation. *Journal of American Academy of Otolaryngology-Head and Neck Surgery, 109*(6), 1078–1082.

Ikeya, J., Kawano, A., Nishiyama, N., Kawaguchi, S., Hagiwara, A., & Suzuki, M. (2013). Long-term complications after cochlear implantation. *Auris, Nasus, Larynx, 40*(6), 525–529.

Kons, Z. A., Lee, L., & Coelho, D. H. (2023). Subjective and objective taste change after cochlear implantation systematic review and meta-analysis. *Otology and Neurotology, 44*(8), 749–757.

Lin, Y. S. (2009). Management of otitis media-related diseases in children with a cochlear implant. *Acta Oto-Laryngologica, 129*(3), 254–260.

Marlowe, A. L., Chinnici, J. E., Rivas, A., Niparko, J. K., & Francis, H. W. (2010). Revision cochlear implant surgery in children: The Johns Hopkins experience. *Otology and Neurotology, 31*(1), 74–82.

Nakashima, T., Matsuda, K., Okuda, T., Tono, T., Takaki, M., Hayashi, T., & Hanamure, Y. (2016). Case report of atlantoaxial rotatory fixation after cochlear implantation. *Case Reports in Otolaryngology, 2016*, 6486271.

Nicholas, J. G., & Geers, A. E. (2008). Expected test scores for preschoolers with a cochlear implant who use spoken language. *American Journal of Speech-Language Pathology, 17*(2), 121–138.

Niparko, J. K., Oviatt, D. L., Coker, N. J., Sutton, L., Waltzman, S. B., & Cohen, N. L. (1991). Facial nerve stimulation with cochlear implantation. VA Cooperative Study Group on Cochlear Implantation. *Journal of American Academy of Otolaryngology-Head and Neck Surgery, 104*(6), 826–830.

Patnaik, U., Sikka, K., Agarwal, S., Kumar, R., Thakar, A., & Sharma, S. C. (2016). Cochlear re-implantation: Lessons learnt and the way ahead. *Acta Oto-Laryngologica, 136*(6), 564–567.

Rivas, A., Marlowe, A. L., Chinnici, J. E., Niparko, J. K., & Francis, H. W. (2008). Revision cochlear implantation surgery in adults: Indications and results. *Otology and Neurotology, 29*(5), 639–648.

Chapter 15
Cochlear Implants: Signal Coding Strategies

Monita Chatterjee, Viral D. Tejani, and Kara C. Schvartz-Leyzac

Abstract In this chapter, we provide a general overview of how cochlear implants work, design considerations for cochlear implant signal processing, primary constraints and limitations, as well as contemporary efforts aimed at mitigating these limitations. We discuss spectral and temporal coding of sound by CI speech processors, as well as factors such as current spread and auditory-nerve health that limit the transmission of spectral and temporal features of sound. Finally, we discuss hearing preservation and signal processing for bilateral CIs, two areas that are receiving increasing attention in the field.

Keywords Cochlear implant · Compressed analog stimulation · Continuous interleaved sampling · Temporal cues · Place cues · Channel interaction

M. Chatterjee (✉)
Center for Hearing Research, Boys Town National Research Hospital, Omaha, NE, USA

The Roxelyn and Richard Pepper Department of Communication Sciences & Disorders, Northwestern University, Evanston, IL, USA
e-mail: Monita.Chatterjee@boystown.org; monita.chatterjee@northwestern.edu

V. D. Tejani
Department of Otolaryngology-Head and Neck Surgery, University of Iowa Hospitals and Clinics, Iowa City, IA, USA

Department of Communication Sciences and Disorders, University of Iowa, Iowa City, IA, USA

Department of Otolaryngology-Head and Neck Surgery, University Hospitals Cleveland Medical Center/Case Western Reserve University, Cleveland, OH, USA

K. C. Schvartz-Leyzac
Department of Otolaryngology-Head and Neck Surgery, Medical University of South Carolina, Charleston, SC, USA

P. Kumar et al. (eds.), *Advances in Implantation Otology*,
https://doi.org/10.1007/978-981-96-8671-1_15

Introduction

The cochlear implant (CI) is a neural prosthesis designed to restore hearing to those with significant hearing loss who may not benefit from traditional amplification. It is the first truly successful prosthesis of its kind and is now a routine option available to many patients around the world, from infants newly diagnosed with hearing loss to older individuals struggling with progressive hearing loss for decades. The success of the device represents a coming together of innovations in a number of otherwise distinct fields of research and development—engineering, medicine, neuroscience, materials sciences, psychology, audiology, and speech-language pathology. In this chapter, we provide a broad overview of cochlear implant technology from a signal processing perspective.

Evolution of Present-Day Cochlear Implant Processing Strategies

Early attempts at single-channel cochlear implants (CIs) used a version of what is now referred to as "compressed analog" (CA) stimulation— the electrical waveform transduced from the acoustic waveform was compressed and transmitted directly to the patient through wires connecting the speech processor to the implanted electrode (for example, the 3 M/House device) (Fretz & Fravel, 1985). These devices provided patients with sound awareness and noticeable improvements in closed-set speech recognition (Eddington, 1980; Gantz et al., 1988; Danhauer et al., 1990). A number of efforts by different groups led to the development of the first multichannel cochlear implants (for example, the Ineraid device and the Nucleus device), providing an opportunity for place-based coding of analog or pulsatile electrical stimuli. Multichannel devices allowed for improvements in speech understanding compared to single-channel devices (Eddington, 1980; Gantz et al., 1988). One limitation and concern of the CA approach implemented in multichannel devices was that multiple channels were stimulated simultaneously, leading to substantial overlap of electrical current and interaction between channels, which caused poorer spatial resolution and reduced speech understanding. The innovation of continuous interleaved sampling (CIS) (Wilson et al., 1991) provided both temporal and place-based spectral cues but also reduced simultaneous channel interaction, which substantially improved speech recognition by cochlear implant patients. An example of an early multichannel device, Cochlear Corporation's Nucleus 22 system, was designed to transmit pulsatile stimulation via radio-frequency transmission. The radio frequency transmitter coded the information about the pulse in successive durations of the 2.5 MHz radio frequency waveform to the implanted system, which included a receiving coil, decoding system, and the 22-electrode array within the cochlea (Shannon et al., 1990). Regardless of CI manufacturer, today's processors still use radio frequency transmission (generally at higher frequencies to accommodate faster pulse rates) to facilitate communication between the external processor and the implanted system, and interleaved pulsatile stimulation remains the method of choice. In the sections below, we will discuss the primary constraints in signal encoding for unilateral cochlear implants and some of the more widely used present-day processing strategies in the context of the perceptual capabilities of patients with CIs.

How a Basic Cochlear Implant Processor Works

Figure 15.1a outlines the general stages of signal processing in a cochlear implant system. Two types of speech processing strategies are currently employed by manufacturers. The first is the "continuous interleaved stimulation" (CIS) family of strategies, and the second is the "peak picking" family of strategies.

In the CIS type strategy (shown in Fig. 15.1b), the temporal envelope output of all active channels is transmitted to the corresponding electrodes. In all CIs, a miniature microphone picks up sound waves and transduces them to electrical signals. The electrical signals are transmitted to a processor which transforms the signals through several stages, including bandpass filtering into different frequency bands, selecting which bands are of interest (depending on the strategy or the noise reduction algorithm), and extracting temporal envelope information from those bands. A necessary element of all CI signal processing strategies is amplitude compression of

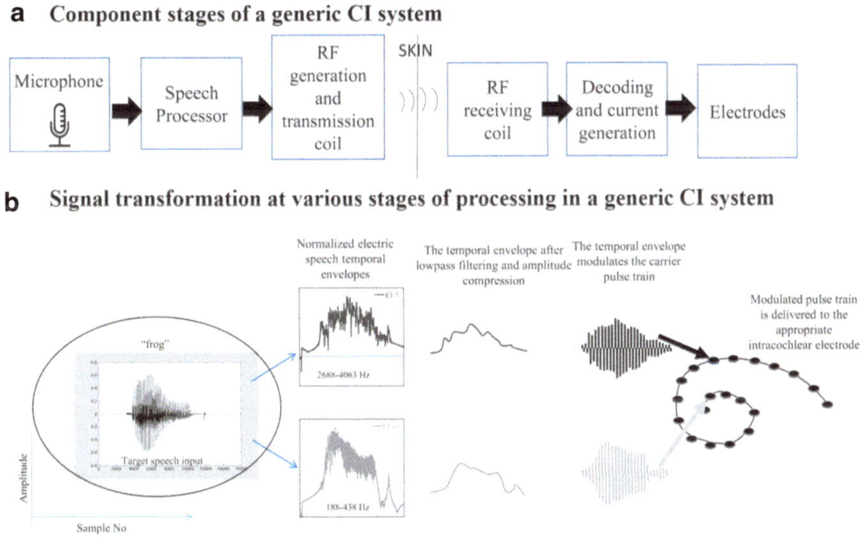

Fig. 15.1 Schematic representationof the signal processing stages of a generic cochlear implant device: (a) component stages of a generic CI system; (b) signal transformation at various stages of processing in a generic CI system

the temporal envelope from the acoustic to the electric domain. Compression is critical because of the vastly different dynamic range in acoustic versus electric hearing (discussed in detail later in this chapter). The compression distorts the temporal and spectral envelopes, reducing the contrast in both domains, but it is necessary because CI patients cannot tolerate sounds evoked by current pulses that are louder than 10–20 dB above the threshold. The compressed temporal envelope waveform is then used to modulate the amplitudes of current pulses that stimulate specific electrodes in the electrode array within the cochlea. The microphone and speech processor are housed in an earpiece that typically sits on or behind the external ear. Stimulation parameters from the speech processor for individual current pulses—for example, the electrodes to be stimulated, the timing of stimulation, and the amplitude of the stimulating current pulses—are transmitted via coded bursts of radio frequency waves across the skin to the internal part of the device (Fig. 15.1a). The internal components include a radio frequency receiver, electronics to decode the radio frequency signal, constant current generators to generate the desired current independent of the impedance in the path (up to the compliance limit), and the implanted electrodes. A frequency-to-electrode map (for example, Greenwood, 1990) determines which electrodes should be stimulated with input from the different frequency bands. Thus, in the two channels shown in the schematic representation (Fig. 15.1b), the temporal envelope from the low-frequency signal excites an apical electrode, while the temporal envelope from the higher-frequency signal excites a more basal electrode.

In the peak-picking type strategy, such as Advanced Combination Encoder (ACE), a predefined number of maxima are selected from the spectrum in each time frame, and information from these spectral peaks is transmitted to the corresponding electrodes.

Outcomes are similar across manufacturers, processing strategies, and devices. Effects of these different strategies vary with the listening condition and background noise, however. For instance, if the background noise is loud enough, the peak-picking strategy would pick more peaks from the noise than from the target speech, and the output information would be more representative of the background noise than the target speech. On the other hand, if the background were of a much lower frequency than the target (for example, wind noise), the output might miss the target information altogether, as all selected peaks might be associated with the background. In the CIS case, the transmitted envelope on all channels would be corrupted by the temporal envelope of the noise. The CIS strategy would transmit noisy temporal envelopes to the apical electrodes, and target-speech temporal envelopes to the high-frequency electrodes. This might make the speech just as challenging to identify as the output from the ACE strategy. Thus, background noise can interfere with speech perception differently in different processing strategies. However, the input dynamic range (IDR) also varies between CIS and peak-peaking strategies in order to accommodate these differences. The IDR is the range of acoustic stimulation (in dB SPL) that is mapped to electrical current units for CI stimulation. CIS type strategies typically use a fixed IDR which is broader in range (>60 dB), whereas peak-peaking strategies will generally use a narrower IDR window that automatically roves according to the level of background noise present. The IDR can be manipulated by the programming clinician.

Considerations and Constraints in Designing a Speech Processing Strategy for Cochlear Implants

Place Coding Constraints

Three constraints limit our ability to apply the place code (von Bekesy, 1956) when deciding which electrode receives information from which frequency region. The first is simply mechanical: it is not easy to insert a linear wire into a spiraling cavity. Electrode arrays are inserted "blind" by the surgeon, and due to the curvature and narrowing of the scala tympani when moving from base to apex, insertion depths generally stop short of the apical end of the cochlea. This means that the apical-most electrode may not stimulate neurons innervating the apical-most regions of the cochlea. The second constraint is that of current spread: the ideal design would limit the region of excitation to a "critical-band" around the electrode of interest. However, the conducting medium and tissue within the cochlea allow current to spread broadly, so neurons remote from the stimulated electrode receive unwanted information ("channel interaction") (Chatterjee & Shannon, 1998; Tang et al., 2011). The current spread is likely also greater for electrodes located further away from the modiolus. The third constraint is that the patient's neural survival pattern is unknown. Thus, a current pulse could be stimulating an electrode that does not have excitable tissue near it, and the current from that electrode might only excite remote surviving neurons. Such issues would impose a strong distortion on the neural spectrogram representation to higher centers of the brain. Electrode designs have been developed in attempts to address the problems of frequency-place mismatch and channel interaction, but these issues are more difficult to fully overcome.

Electrode Design to Address Place-Coding Problems

Apical electrodes are responsible for encoding low-frequency information; however, the limited insertion depth of CIs results in these same apical electrodes stimulating regions of the cochlea and auditory neurons that are primed to code higher-frequency information than what is actually delivered. That is, low-frequency information is delivered to higher-frequency regions of the cochlea, resulting in a mismatch between the place of cochlear stimulation and the pitch conveyed by the electrode, regardless of the CI manufacturer (Landsberger et al., 2015; Canfarotta et al., 2020, 2021). Though the impact of place-pitch mismatches on speech recognition outcomes is not entirely known, recent studies have suggested that longer electrodes / deeper insertions allowed by lateral wall electrode arrays result in a wider range of pitch percept and possibly better speech recognition outcomes (Landsberger et al., 2014; Buchman et al., 2014; Chakravorti et al., 2019, Canfarotta et al., 2021). Generally, results show better speech outcomes when the frequency-to-place mismatch is limited (Canfarotta et al., 2020, 2021; O'Connell et al., 2017).

While lateral wall electrodes allow for deeper insertions, their placement along the lateral wall means that the distance between the electrode and the modiolus is larger compared to pre-curved electrode arrays which are closer to the modiolus. The increased electrode-to-nerve distance means that current levels to achieve a comfortable loudness percept are higher (Davis et al., 2016; Chakravorti et al., 2019). The higher current levels in theory lead to greater channel interaction for lateral wall electrodes; this has been hypothesized to limit speech recognition outcomes in lateral wall CI recipients when compared to a matched cohort of pre-curved CI recipients in some studies (Holder et al., 2019). However, other studies have shown that speech recognition outcomes for patients implanted with lateral wall arrays are slightly better than those implanted with pre-curved arrays (O'Connell et al., 2016). A recent study that considered both electrode and patient demographic factors revealed that for pre-curved arrays, the outcomes were most influenced by modiolar proximity and complete insertion in the scala tympani. For lateral arrays, the insertion depth was the primary factor contributing to speech recognition outcomes (Chakravorti et al., 2019).

In an effort to overcome frequency-to-place mismatch, novel methods have been recently developed by incorporating pre- or post-operative computerized tomography (CT) data. Advanced pre-operative CT methods and analyses (Noble et al., 2014; Fan et al., 2023; Teymouri et al., 2011; Micuda et al., 2024; Helpard et al., 2021) allow for precise measurements of cochlear duct length thereby allowing more precise selection of electrode length that best aligns with cochlear measures. This ensures that longer electrode arrays can be adequately contained completely within the cochlea, lessening the chance of extra-cochlear electrodes. Moreover, post-operative CT data can be used to assess the frequency-to-place map for each individual and then adjust CI programming appropriately. Specifically, using estimated human cochlear frequency maps (Stakhovskaya et al., 2007), CT scans can be used to determine the approximate frequency place for each electrode. Then, the assigned frequency bandwidths for each electrode can be adjusted by the clinician (audiologist) to best align with the tonotopic placement of the array. If, for example, the insertion angle of the electrode allows for the most apical electrode to reach an estimated cochlear place frequency of 300 Hz, then the assigned bandwidth can be set to 300 Hz in the clinical programming software. It should be noted that the electrode lengths (and therefore corresponding frequency place) vary across manufacturers and electrode design. Therefore, the frequency-to-place mismatch will vary across recipients.

Only one CI manufacturer (Med-EL) offers automated clinical software (Otoplan) to analyze CTs and adjust CI programming accordingly. Emerging research among Med-EL recipients notes significant improvements when comparing speech recognition performance between default frequency-to-place maps and those created using frequency-to-place matching via Otoplan (Dillon et al., 2023; Muller-Graff et al., 2024). While this work is promising, further research is needed to better determine applicability to other CI manufacturers. There are other CT technologies analogous to Otoplan but are not yet as automated; such CT methods allow for sufficiently precise cochlear measures (Noble et al., 2014; Fan et al., 2023; Teymouri et al., 2011) which are required for frequency–to-place realignment. They can also be applied to all CI recipients regardless of manufacturer or model. However, novel frequency-to-place alignment approaches have not been adequately investigated among CI users other than those with Med-EL devices. Due to the variance in electrode length, electrode number, insertion angle, and assigned frequencies across manufacturers, the efficacy of reassigning frequency-to-place for manufacturers other than Med-EL is unknown.

Channel Interaction

Current spread along the cochlea leading to overlapping current between adjacent and distant electrodes is a significant limitation of CIs, leading to channel interaction and loss of spatial resolution at the peripheral level. This consequently impacts higher-order spectral resolution and speech perception (Hughes & Stille, 2008; Won et al., 2014; Scheperle & Abbas, 2015). A key innovation in CI technology was the introduction of interleaved sampling, in which the current pulses directed to multiple channels in a CI electrode array are interleaved in time, such that no two channels are stimulated simultaneously (Wilson et al., 1991). However, even with this improvement, channel interaction persists in CIs because of current spreading from successive pulses to remote neurons. Thus, neurons in regions in between two physical electrodes may be excited by current pulses from both. Newer current focusing and current steering processing strategies have attempted to address these issues by providing greater spectral resolution.

Modern-day CIs are typically programmed in the monopolar mode, in which the intracochlear electrode is stimulated relative to the extracochlear ground electrode. Contrast this with bipolar stimulation, in which an adjacent intracochlear electrode is used as the ground. A major advantage of monopolar stimulation as used presently over bipolar stimulation (as used in first-generation CIs) is that lower current levels are needed to achieve the same loudness percept, leading to longer battery life, without sacrificing speech understanding (Zwolan et al., 1996). However, monopolar stimulation consequently causes the current to traverse through the cochlea to the extracochlear ground electrode, and this broad current spread was thought to negatively affect speech perception. Bipolar and tripolar stimulation restrict the electric field spread since one or two intracochlear electrodes, respectively, are used as the return electrode (Kral et al., 1998). Despite this, early studies showed that speech recognition outcomes were either comparable when using monopolar and bipolar current configurations, or in some cases slightly better with a broader stimulation configuration (Pfingst et al., 1997, 2001; Zwolan et al., 1996).

However, these studies might not necessarily translate to modern CI technology or implant recipients. Generally, psychophysical studies have shown that using a focused rather than monopolar stimulation pattern narrows the electrical current excitation pattern (Chatterjee et al., 2006; Zhu et al., 2012; Saoji et al., 2013; Padilla & Lansberger, 2016). However, the current level required to excite equal loudness perception is typically higher for tripolar compared to monopolar stimulation, and therefore spread of excitation for tripolar stimulation might also be equally broad at sufficiently loud stimulation levels in some listeners (Landsberger et al., 2012). Related to this point, appropriate current levels for stimulation sometimes exceed the voltage compliance limitations of the system, preventing accurate transmission of the current. Lastly, data suggest that focused tripolar stimulation can result in 'side lobes' from the return electrodes, which is more likely to occur at higher stimulation levels and for electrodes closer to the modiolus (Bonham & Litvak, 2008). When present, side lobes might stimulate the auditory nerve at a site distant to the intended electrode, thereby affecting spectral resolution. Studies have produced mixed results when examining the potential benefit of a tripolar versus monopolar stimulation strategy for speech recognition outcomes (Berenstein et al., 2008; Srinivasan et al., 2013; Smith et al., 2013). However, a study using adaptive tripolar stimulation, which adjusts the current focus based on the stimulation level for each electrode, showed promising results for improving speech recognition (Arenberg et al., 2018).

Others have proposed the use of current steering technology to improve spectral resolution for CI users (Firszt et al., 2007; Koch et al., 2007). Current steering involves dividing the total charge, normally delivered to one electrode, between two adjacent electrodes in order to evoke an intermediate pitch percept. The ratio of current between the two electrodes () can be systematically adjusted to theoretically create more than one intermediate pitch, which is sometimes referred to as "virtual" electrodes or pitches. While studies have demonstrated the efficacy of this approach for simple pitch perception (Firszt et al., 2007), implementation of current steering in an effort to improve speech recognition has yielded mixed results (Buechner et al., 2008; Chang et al., 2009; Melo et al., 2012).

Focused, tripolar current has also been used in an effort to control for facial nerve stimulation in CI patients (Bahmer & Baumann, 2016; Bahmer et al., 2017; Braun et al., 2019). Depending on cochlear anatomy, electrode insertion and electrode type, facial nerve stimulation can sometimes accompany auditory sensation during cochlear implant stimulation. However, recent studies have shown that this undesirable side effect can also be better controlled when a tripolar stimulation method is used. Bahmer and Baumann (2016) used EMG measurements in four CI patients to reveal that, when compared to biphasic stimulation, triphasic pulses require higher stimulation levels to elicit an equal amount of facial nerve stimulation, as shown in EMG amplitudes. Further work showed that cathodic-first tripolar stimuli were more effective compared to anodic-first tripolar stimuli in limiting facial nerve stimulation (Bahmer et al., 2017). As a result, Med-EL now offers the option for tripolar stimulation in their most recent programming software.

Time Coding Constraints

For all cochlear implant strategies, the temporal fine structure of the incoming signal is replaced with a fixed-rate pulse train that does not reflect the acoustic properties of the speech signal. The pulse rate varies depending upon the manufacturer and individual, but modern-day processing strategies use pulse rates in the range of 900–3000 Hz on each channel. However, the effects of pulse rate on perception with a CI are unclear and vary across patients. Psychophysical studies reveal that while some CI patients are able to detect pulse rate differences at higher rates, many are not sensitive to changes in pulse rate ("temporal fine structure") at rates higher than 300 Hz (e.g., Zeng, 2002). Some studies have shown that speech recognition performance with CIs improves when increasing the pulse rate on each electrode from a lower rate (i.e., 250 Hz) to a higher rate. Additional studies show preferential speech recognition performance using pulse rates varies across CI users but those preferences are not necessarily well understood or predictable (Plant et al., 2007; Brochier et al., 2017; Friesen et al., 2005; Shader et al., 2020).

Temporal fine structure within the range of 50–600 Hz is important for the perception of musical pitch and voice pitch, as well as for speech perception in noise (Rosen, 1992; Oxenham, 2008). CI patients do not perceive sinusoidal or pulse train stimuli within these rates as musical, and their pitch discrimination within this range is significantly impaired relative to their hearing peers (Shannon, 1983; Zeng, 2002). In most processing strategies, speech processors transmit temporal envelope information at a fixed carrier pulse rate. Thus, temporal fine structure is largely ignored. Some strategies offered by Med-EL include limited transmission of temporal fine structure, but as indicated previously, the evidence regarding tangible improvements in speech perception in noise or in melody recognition is mixed.

Intensity Coding Constraints

Unlike those with typical hearing who enjoy a wide dynamic range in excess of 120 dB, electrical stimulation provides a narrow range of 6–20 dB, with expansive loudness functions (i.e., loudness growing slowly near threshold and with an accelerating pace at higher levels) (Kiang & Moxon, 1972; Shannon, 1985; Chatterjee, 1999; Wilson & Dorman, 2008). This limits the ability of cochlear implant processors to transmit information about large swings in amplitude within and across channels. This constraint limits the transmission of both temporal and spectral envelopes, as well as dynamic aspects of spectral envelopes. Loudness growth in CIs can vary depending on pulse parameters used to change the charge per pulse. Loudness increases differently with increasing pulse amplitude than with increasing pulse phase duration (Chatterjee et al., 2000), and the difference depends on the degree of focusing of the electric field. Coding intensity changes with pulse phase duration limits the ability to transmit pulses at a very high carrier rate, but there is no evidence to show a significant difference in speech perception when intensity is coded in either way.

Examples of Contemporary Processing Strategies and Electrode Designs

Advanced Bionics

Historically, Advanced Bionics has used a CIS-like strategy with more contemporary strategies incorporating current steering. The default programming strategy is Optima-S, which is a sequential stimulation, CIS-like strategy that also offers current steering technology. The Optima-S strategy is theoretically similar to its predecessor, Fidelity120, with the primary improvement of battery life/reduced power requirements for the former than the latter. Currently, Advanced Bionics offers two electrode arrays- one that is narrow in diameter and typically resides more lateral from the modiolus, and another placed slightly more medial. Both electrode arrays have 16 physical electrode contacts and use monopolar configurations as the only option. Both the pulse rate and pulse width are variable in Optima-S strategies, depending on the current levels required for adequate stimulation. For example, lower current/power requirements will often result in shorter pulse width duration and higher pulse rates. As current levels required for minimum stimulation levels increase, the pulse width duration will increase and the pulse rate will decrease automatically. If desired, the pulse width can be fixed by the clinician, which will subsequently affect the pulse rate. The pulse rate is fixed and equal on each of the 16 electrodes and can be as high as about 3700 pps.

Cochlear

Cochlear's default processing strategy (Advanced Combination Encoder or 'ACE') is a peak-picking strategy. The default number of peaks used for the strategy is eight ('maxima') but can be manipulated by the programming clinician if needed. In a few cases, the maxima might be constrained to a lower value if the number of electrodes used for stimulation is limited and/or if the pulse rate is increased. The default pulse rate for the ACE strategy is 900 pps and the pulse width duration is typically 25 or 37μs/phase. Both of these variables can be set independently by the programming clinician. While the highest pulse rate available for programming is 3500 pps, higher pulse rates are not often used for programming and can significantly limit the maxima value, which can have negative implications for speech understanding (Plant et al., 2002; Vandali et al., 2000). The ACE strategy uses a monopolar configuration. However, if required, more historical peak-picking programming strategies can be used (for example, SPEAK) with alternative electrode configurations (for example, bipolar, common ground, and pseudomonopolar). While not often required, these alternative strategies can offer some improvement in complex programming cases. Cochlear currently offers five electrode designs, all of which have 22 physical electrode contacts but vary in diameter, length, and intent to reside laterally or closer to the modiolus within the scala tympani.

Med-EL

For several years, Med-EL used a CIS-like approach until the recent development of a newer strategy called "Fine Structure Processing" or FSP. This strategy uses a fixed higher pulse rate signal on the medial and basal electrodes (around 1000–2000 pps) while using a lower and variable pulse rate on the most apical electrodes. The lower variable pulse rate is designed to mimic the low-frequency fine structure information in the original incoming signal. Results when using the FSP strategy are somewhat mixed, and there is not a clear indication that this type of processing yields significantly improved speech understanding or music perception compared to a CIS strategy (for example, Riss et al., 2011; Roy et al., 2015). Pulse width is usually fixed, although it can be manipulated by the programming clinician. For non-FSP channels, the pulse rate can also be changed somewhat (although there is not much flexibility) and the rate is largely pre-determined based on other programming parameters and power requirements individual to each recipient. Med-EL offers bipolar or tripolar electrode configurations, with the latter typically only used to reduce facial nerve stimulation. All electrode arrays have 12 physical electrode contacts and vary primarily in length. Otherwise, they are designed to be slim and flexible and reside in the middle or lateral portion of the scala tympani.

Oticon Medical (Recently Acquired by Cochlear Corporation)

Available since 2015, Oticon's Neuro System uses a peak-picking strategy, with a pre-determined number of maxima. The stimulation mode is unique compared to other devices, and uses a stimulation mode that combines common-ground and a monopolar pathway. Further, it uses pseudomonophasic electrical pulses with an anodic-leading phase and a capacitive discharge for charge balancing. Also unique to this system, loudness is not modulated by current amplitude (which is fixed) but rather by pulse width duration. Two electrode arrays are offered, both of which have 20 physical electrode contacts, and vary slightly in length as well as diameter and flexibility (Franco-Vidal et al., 2020). In 2022, Oticon Medical withdrew from manufacturing cochlear implants and was acquired by Cochlear Corporation.

Nurotron

The Nurotron CI system, the only CI system designed and manufactured in a developing country (China), offers both CIS and peak-peaking strategies, with the latter typically using about 6–8 maxima. In addition, it offers a third strategy which combines peak-picking and virtual channels. The default electrode configuration is monopolar, and the system uses cathodic-leading biphasic pulses for stimulation. Loudness is increased by adjusting the current level, and the pulse width fixed. The electrode array has 24 physical electrode contacts (Zeng et al., 2015).

Impact of Cochlear Implant Array Design on Outcomes

Alongside advances in digital signal processing to reduce current spread and improve encoding of spectral and temporal cues, the choice of electrode array design and their impact on patient performance has been researched in recent years. Regardless of cochlear implant manufacturer, two major electrode array designs exist presently—perimodiolar and lateral wall. Figure 15.2 shows a schematic representation of these two electrode arrays in the cochlea. Perimodiolar electrodes (such as the Nucleus CI532 Slim Modiolar depicted in Fig. 15.2, right panel) are precurved and sit close to the neural structures, while lateral wall electrodes (such at the CI522 Slim Straight depicted in Fig. 15.2, left panel) are straight arrays that are seated along the lateral wall of the cochlea. The electrode array type used for patients relies on the clinical judgment of audiologists and surgeons, as they consider surgeon experience/technique, cochlear anatomy, pre-operative residual hearing, and current clinical / research data.

Retrospective chart reviewers comparing speech perception outcomes between perimodiolar and lateral wall arrays have favored perimodiolar arrays (Holder et al.,

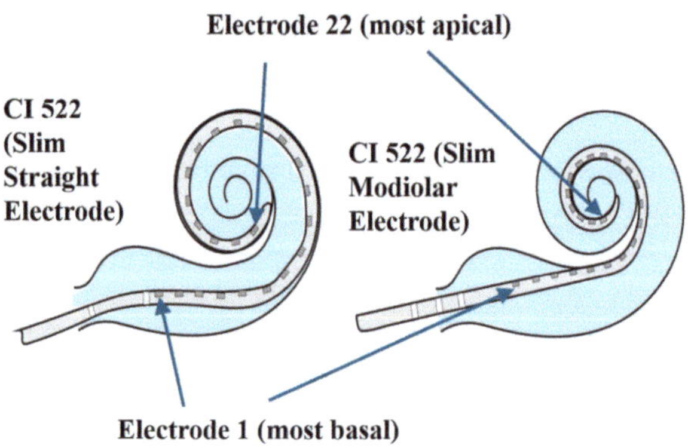

Fig. 15.2 Schematic representation of lateral wall (left panel) and perimodiolar (right panel) electrodes. (Adapted from McPhail et al., 2022, Fig. 1B)

2019), lateral wall arrays (O'Connell et al., 2016), or shown equivocal results (Fabie et al., 2018; MacPhail et al., 2022). Variability in test materials used across different clinics contributes to the lack of clear findings on the superiority of one electrode array design over the other. Differences have been shown in consonant-nucleus-consonant (CNC) word recognition (Holder et al., 2019), but no differences shown for AzBio sentence recognition in noise (Fabie et al., 2018; Holder et al., 2019), and conflicting results regarding AzBio sentence recognition in quiet (O'Connell et al., 2016; Fabie et al., 2018; Holder et al., 2019; MacPhail et al., 2022). The retrospective nature of these studies are a limitation likely also contributing to the lack of a consensus. More sensitive test materials are also necessary to evaluate any performance differences between perimodiolar and lateral wall electrode arrays (MacPhail et al., 2022). As will be discussed, the different electrode array design types may offer differing advantages.

Current Challenges

Number of Effective Channels

Maximizing performance with a CI is a goal of clinicians, researchers, and patients. Depending on the manufacturer, a given CI internal electrode array can feature up to 24 electrodes. Despite several advances / proposed signal processing (for example, CIS programming, tripolar stimulation, site-selection studies), channel interaction and smearing inevitably occur across the electrode array and potentially affect speech perception (Landsberger et al., 2012; Scheperle & Abbas, 2015; Arenberg et al., 2018). Thus, the number of effective channels (i.e., the number of independent channels of information conveying unique speech information) is often less than the number of electrodes implanted. In addition, the impoverished spectral information delivered by the CI forces listeners to rely on temporal information for speech understanding (Fu et al., 2004; Xu et al., 2005; Xu & Zheng, 2007; Xu & Pfingst, 2008). Normal hearing listeners listening to vocoded speech require few spectral bands for adequate speech recognition in quiet (Shannon et al., 1995; Xu & Zheng, 2007), but more bands are needed for speech recognition in noise (Qin & Oxenham, 2003; Xu & Zheng, 2007; Friesen et al., 2001), indicating that limited temporal resolution is not very detrimental to speech understanding in quiet, but can adversely affect speech understanding in noise. Parallel studies with early CI users showed similar limitations—speech recognition in quiet tended to plateau at about 8 channels. Unlike hearing peers, CI users could not benefit from increasing the number of active channels beyond 8 in noise backgrounds (Fishman et al., 1997; Friesen et al., 2001), suggesting a fundamental limitation that could not be alleviated by increasing the number of electrodes. These studies were performed in CI users using older technology and implanted under more stringent criteria. Over the years, surgical techniques have improved, electrode arrays have been redesigned, and CI candidacy criteria have evolved to include patients with better preoperative hearing / auditory status. More recent studies have revisited the issue of the limited number of channels with the idea that these factors may contribute to the auditory system making more effective use of the current state of the art in cochlear implant stimulation. Current generation CI users can certainly benefit from using up to 8 channels, but unlike older studies, the provision of additional channels up to 16 and even 22 can improve speech understanding in quiet and noise in newly implanted CI users. This is particularly the case for CI users with good spectral-temporal resolution (Croghan et al., 2017; Berg et al., 2019; Schvartz-Leyzac et al., 2017). Similarly, newly implanted CI users demonstrate better performance on spectral ripple density discrimination compared to older generation CI users, even when the experiments were conducted in the same lab using identical stimuli (compare Jeon et al., 2015 with Henry et al., 2005). While preoperative audiograms were not significantly different between the older and newly implanted CI users of the two studies, the newly implanted group had better preoperative speech perception. This could reflect relaxed CI candidacy criteria seen in the last decade, and also possibly a better neural substrate for electrical stimulation.

Complex Harmonic/Musical/Voice Pitch Coding

Sounds such as voices and musical instruments generate a harmonic complex [i.e., a component at the "fundamental frequency" (F0) accompanied by a number of overtones, or components at integer multiples of the F0 sinusoid]. The healthy auditory system decomposes this complex into its component parts within the low to mid-frequency region of the cochlea (resolved harmonics) and is sensitive to the spectro-temporal properties of the harmonic components. The perceived pitch of such harmonic complexes is musical and corresponds to the pitch evoked by the F0. The ability to perceive this musical pitch appears to rely on the high-fidelity representation of the spectro-temporal fine structure of F0 and its overtones (e.g., Oxenham, 2008, 2012). As CIs do not provide F0 information in either the spectral or temporal fine structure domains, CI users show deficits in several areas requiring sensitivity to harmonic pitch—for example, music perception, lexical tone recognition, indexical information in speech, question/statement identification, and identification of emotional prosody (Galvin et al., 2007; Fu & Zeng, 2000; Wang et al., 2011; Peng et al., 2012; Luo et al., 2007; Chatterjee et al., 2015; Barrett et al., 2020; Peng et al., 2017). In prelingually deaf children with CIs, these limitations also translate to deficits in their production of prosodic cues and lexical tones (e.g., Zhou et al., 2013; Peng et al., 2004; Xu et al., 2011; Deroche et al., 2019; Chatterjee et al., 2019; van de Velde et al., 2019). As a by-product of CI processing, F0 information may be available in the form of temporal envelope periodicity cues, and a weak form of pitch can be perceived from these periodicities in the envelope. However, this perceived pitch is not salient, and cannot support the perception of musicality in sounds (Burns & Viemeister, 1981). CI patients, however, exhibit sensitivity to such temporal envelope periodicity (Chatterjee & Oberzut, 2011). Their sensitivity to this cue has been shown to be correlated with their ability to discriminate complex harmonic pitch (Deroche et al., 2014) and to identify prosodic cues in speech, such as lexical tones and question/statement contrasts (Chatterjee & Peng, 2008; Luo et al., 2008). Attempts to improve the coding of F0 cues in CIs by deepening the temporal envelope modulations and synchronizing them across channels have met with some positive results, particularly in tone-language speakers (Vandali & van Hoesel, 2012; Vandali et al., 2019). However, the inability to provide salient F0 cues continues to present a significant challenge in the field of CIs.

Variable Neural Health

Post-mortem temporal bone studies in humans reveal that the surviving neural population in patients with hearing loss is not uniform from base to apex, but rather the spiral ganglion (SG) cell bodies are often present and healthier at some locations and can be absent or of poorer health at others (Nadol, 1997; Nadol & Eddington, 2006; Khan et al., 2005a, Khan et al., 2005b; Nadol et al., 1989; Linthicum & Fayad, 2009; Rask-Andersen et al., 2010). These studies also show variable survival of hair cells and supporting cells, both within and across ears. Early temporal bone studies showed that speech recognition in CI users was relatively independent of surviving SG counts and/or density (Khan et al., 2005a, b), but more recent studies do support a relationship between these two variables (Kamakura & Nadol, 2016; Seyyedi et al., 2014). A meta-analysis of studies examining SG counts and CI outcomes suggests little correlation between these two variables; it may be that a small number of SG neurons is necessary for speech perception or that multiple factors beyond SG counts largely contribute to CI outcomes (Cheng & Svirsky, 2021).

Animal studies reveal that the survival of SG cells affects electrical stimulation of the cochlea and that current stimulation parameters interact with SG survival during CI stimulation (Pfingst et al., 2011, 2015, 2017; Ramekers et al., 2014, 2015). The same animal studies reveal that specific electrophysiologic and psychophysical measures reflect the underlying condition of the SG cell bodies, and these same measures can be used in humans to infer information about the condition of the cochlea in implanted patients (Schvartz-Leyzac et al., 2019, 2020a, 2020b; Zhou et al., 2015, 2018; Zhou & Pfingst, 2016; Schvartz-Leyzac & Pfingst, 2016; Schvartz-Leyzac et al., 2020a, b). In agreement with histological studies of cadaver temporal bones, electrophysiologic and psychophysical measures in humans are not uniform from base to apex, but rather differ across electrodes within an ear and also across ears in CI users (Schvartz-Leyzac & Pfingst, 2016; Schvartz-Leyzac et al., 2020a, b; Zhou & Pfingst, 2014; Brill et al., 2009; Pfingst et al., 2004). Although findings are mixed, the evidence suggests that the same electrophysiological and psychophysical measures are related to speech recognition outcomes in CI users, indicating that the condition of the cochlea is important for speech understanding with a CI. Generally, in keeping with most recent post-mortem temporal bone studies, results suggest that a higher density of survival in SG cells is correlated with better post-operative speech recognition scores (Schvartz-Leyzac & Pfingst 2018; Schvartz-Leyzac et al., 2021 ; Zhou & Pfingst, 2014; Kim et al., 2010).

Standard clinical practice typically involves using all available electrodes for stimulation, and electrodes are usually only deactivated if adverse effects are noted such as facial nerve stimulation, dizziness, or an uncomfortable pitch perception. However, a recent study showed that, by selecting electrodes estimated to stimulate higher rather than lower SG cell populations, speech recognition could be improved (Schvartz-Leyzac et al., 2021). This so-called 'site-selection' approach has been used in other studies using various electrophysiologic, psychophysical, or radiologic measures to select specific electrodes for activation in CI processing with the goal of improving CI performance (Goehring et al., 2019; Noble et al., 2014; Zhou, 2019; Garadat et al., 2013). Taken together, these results show some promise that using a select number of electrodes might be more beneficial for some listeners compared to using the full complement of electrodes. This could be due to enhanced coding of spectral or temporal information, depending on the site selection method chosen. While not yet implemented into standard clinical programming, such approaches could be used in future processing or programming strategies.

Hearing Preservation

Changes in electrode array design and surgical techniques have allowed for the preservation of residual acoustic hearing in the implanted ear post-operatively. This allows CI users to utilize combined electric-acoustic stimulation (EAS) in the implanted ear, where low-frequency acoustic amplification is provided by an integrated hearing aid component and high-frequency stimulation is provided by the electrode array.

Research in hearing preservation was inspired by a growing population of patients with normal hearing / mild-moderate low-frequency hearing loss and severe to profound high-frequency hearing loss who could not benefit from traditional hearing aid amplification (Ching et al., 1998; Hogan & Turner, 1998; see Turner, 2006 for review). These patients did not qualify for cochlear implantation at the time as they had a substantial amount of residual hearing. There was initial evidence that acoustic hearing could be preserved post-implantation (von Illberg et al., 1999), leading to the conceptualization of the Nucleus Hybrid S8 short electrode array, featuring 6 electrodes spaced over a 6 mm or a 10 mm array that was inserted shallowly (Gantz & Turner, 2003). It is now possible to preserve hearing even with conventional length lateral wall electrodes (van Abel et al., 2015; Pillsbury et al., 2018; Lenarz et al., 2020) as well as pre-curved electrodes (Hunter et al., 2016; Nassiri et al., 2020).

Superior outcomes with EAS relative to electric-only stimulation have also been demonstrated for speech understanding in noise, localization, music perception, and perception of spectral/temporal cues (Gantz & Turner, 2003; Turner et al., 2004; Gfeller et al., 2006; Gifford et al., 2008, 2010; Brockmeier et al., 2010; Dunn et al., 2010, 2020; Helbig et al., 2011; Lenarz et al., 2013; Gantz et al., 2016, 2018; Roland et al., 2016, 2018; Pillsbury et al., 2018; Tejani & Brown, 2020). An underlying reason for the demonstrated benefits in these studies is that spectral and temporal cues are more accessible via acoustic hearing than electric hearing, and such cues are needed for more complex listening tasks.

From a signal processing perspective, the strategies used in electrical stimulation in EAS are similar to those of standard CIs, while the strategies of the hearing aid component are similar to those of conventional hearing aids. The key difference is the bandwidth of acoustic and electrical stimulation. The hearing aid component and the CI do not necessarily provide wideband stimulation. For example, a patient with good hearing preservation up to 500 Hz may only get acoustic amplification up to that frequency, while frequencies higher than 500 Hz may be encoded electrically. The bandwidth of acoustic and electric stimulation available varies depending on the patient's residual hearing; those with poorer residual hearing get more electrical stimulation while those with better residual hearing get more acoustic stimulation. However, determining the amount of bandwidth of acoustic and electric stimulation needed to optimize the benefit with EAS is not necessarily straightforward, as discussed in many recent studies (Fraysse et al., 2006; Vermeire et al., 2008; Karsten et al., 2013; Gifford et al., 2017). Additionally, the risk of hearing loss post-surgery necessitates reassignment of bandwidth.

One risk of hearing preservation implantation is the loss of residual acoustic hearing post-operatively. Regardless of electrode manufacturer and length, a partial loss up to 30 dB immediately and/or several months post-surgery is expected in 30–40% of patients. This loss does not necessarily preclude the use of acoustic amplification (Lenarz et al., 2013; van Abel et al., 2015; Scheperle et al., 2017; Pillsbury et al., 2018; Roland et al., 2018), as low-frequency audiometric thresholds (125, 250, and 500 Hz) of 50–70 dB HL can be maintained even 5 years after implantation (Gantz et al., 2018; Roland et al., 2018). In cases where patients do lose residual hearing, it is necessary to readjust the bandwidth of acoustic and electric stimulation, such that a greater bandwidth of electrical stimulation is provided. One downside is that earlier hearing preservation arrays were shorter in length (Gantz & Turner, 2003; Dunn et al., 2020), which means that compressing a wider frequency range into a short electrode further disrupts tonotopic matching (Landsberger et al., 2015) and may compromise speech understanding (Başkent & Shannon, 2004, 2005). This may not be as problematic nowadays as longer electrode arrays can be used for hearing preservation. Additionally, there is anecdotal evidence that patients have difficulty adjusting to a new frequency allocation, especially after having been acclimated to a previous allocation for a long period of time.

Signal Processing for Bilateral Cochlear Implants

Spatial hearing requires sound information in both ears. Binaural auditory processing enables us to localize the source of sound and is a powerful way to perceptually separate one sound source from another, thus improving our ability to hear speech in noise. In cochlear implant patients, binaural information may be theoretically provided with bilateral cochlear implantation. When both cochleae are implanted in the same surgery, the process is called "simultaneous bilateral implantation" and when some time elapses between surgeries on the two sides, the process is called "sequential bilateral implantation". Patients show a diversity of outcomes with bilateral implantation-- some are able to fuse the two signals from the two sides well and report improved ability to navigate their environments with the increased information, while others have more difficulty integrating the two inputs, sometimes experiencing interference between the two ears. Overall, bilateral cochlear implantation has a generally positive outcome in patients and has been suggested as a cost-effective solution (for example, Health Quality Ontario, 2018).

Signal processing for bilateral cochlear implants would ideally provide three characteristics: (1) synchronized electrical stimulation to the two ears so that interaural time and level difference cues can be available to the auditory system to compute the spatial location of the sound source; (2) synchronized information would be tonotopically matched in the two ears; (3) electrical stimulation pattern for interaural timing cues would be one that cochlear implant patients are sensitive to. Present-day bilateral implantation falls short of these ideals on multiple counts. First, only recently devices that are synchronized between the two sides have begun to be commercially conceptualized. Second, tonotopic matching between the two ears remains a challenging requirement, as the precise location of each electrode contact depends on the individual surgery, with the end result being a significant tonotopic mismatch between the devices in the two ears. Third, careful research has shown that cochlear implant patients are not as sensitive to interaural timing cues as needed for good sound localization outcomes, even in the best-case scenario (e.g., Long et al., 2003). The various factors discussed above for each device—neural health and survival, channel interaction, etc.—influence hearing with the device in each ear differently. For instance, the neural health in the two ears may be different depending on the duration of deafness prior to implantation and the pattern of hearing loss in each ear. In fact, results from human temporal bones (Seyyedi et al., 2014) and when using objective neural health measures in humans (Schvartz-Leyzac & Pfingst, 2018) suggest different neural patterns across ears for some CI recipients. This would influence binaural signal processing between the two ears. Even if tonotopically matched, synchronized signals were presented to the two implanted electrodes as in the idealized case, the difference in neural responsivity on the two sides would degrade the binaural processing of these inputs.

Signal processing strategies have typically been designed for unilateral cochlear implants. To date, a binaural signal processing strategy has not been available from manufacturers. Specific aspects of present-day signal processing strategies may distort binaural cues for bilateral cochlear implant patients in ways that are unique to the processing strategy (for example, Gray et al., 2021). In general, cochlear implant patients show better sensitivity to interaural level difference cues and interaural temporal envelope cues than to interaural timing cues, even with processing strategies that attempt to convey timing cues with greater precision (Ausili et al., 2020).

Current attempts at improving bilateral hearing with cochlear implants include addressing each of these issues individually, which is likely to result in improvements cumulatively over time. As an example, Potts et al. (2019) showed improvements in patients' access to interaural level difference cues and their speech perception in noise by reducing the distortion due to automatic gain control while providing synchronized input to the two sides.

References

Arenberg, J. G., Parkinson, W. S., Litvak, L., Chen, C., Kreft, H. A., & Oxenham, A. J. (2018). A dynamically focusing cochlear implant strategy can improve vowel identification in noise. *Ear and Hearing, 39*(6), 1136–1145.

Ausili, S. A., Agterberg, M. J. H., Engel, A., Voelter, C., Thomas, J. P., Stefan Brill, A. F. M., Snik, S. D., John Van Opstal, A., & Mylanus, E. A. M. (2020). Spatial hearing by bilateral cochlear implant users with temporal fine-structure processing. *Frontiers in Neurology, 11*, 915.

Bahmer, A., & Baumann, U. (2016). The underlying mechanism of preventing facial nerve stimulation by triphasic pulse stimulation in cochlear implant users assessed with objective measure. *Otology & Neurotology, 37*(9), 1231–1237.

Bahmer, A., Adel, Y., & Baumann, U. (2017). Preventing facial nerve stimulation by triphasic pulse stimulation in cochlear implant users: Intraoperative recordings. *Otology & Neurotology, 38*(10), e438–e444.

Barrett, K. C., Chatterjee, M., Caldwell, M. T., Deroche, M. L., Jiradejvong, P., Kulkarni, A. M., & Limb, C. J. (2020). Perception of child-directed versus adult-directed emotional speech in pediatric cochlear implant users. *Ear and Hearing, 41*(5), 1372–1382.

Başkent, D., & Shannon, R. V. (2004). Frequency-place compression and expansion in cochlear implant listeners. *The Journal of the Acoustical Society of America, 116*(5), 3130–3140.

Başkent, D., & Shannon, R. V. (2005). Interactions between cochlear implant electrode insertion depth and frequency-place mapping. *The Journal of the Acoustical Society of America, 117*(3 Pt 1), 1405–1416.

Berenstein, C. K., Mens, L. H., Mulder, J. J., & Vanpoucke, F. J. (2008). Current steering and current focusing in cochlear implants: Comparison of monopolar, tripolar, and virtual channel electrode configurations. *Ear and Hearing, 29*(2), 250–260.

Berg, K. A., Noble, J. H., Dawant, B. M., Dwyer, R. T., Labadie, R. F., & Gifford, R. H. (2019). Speech recognition as a function of the number of channels in perimodiolar electrode recipients. *The Journal of the Acoustical Society of America, 145*(3), 1556–1564.

Bonham, B. H., & Litvak, L. M. (2008). Current focusing and steering: Modeling, physiology, and psychophysics. *Hearing Research, 242*(1–2), 141–153.

Braun, K., Walker, K., Sürth, W., Löwenheim, H., & Tropitzsch, A. (2019). Triphasic pulses in cochlear implant patients with facial nerve stimulation. *Otology & Neurotology, 40*(10), 1268–1277.

Brill, S., Müller, J., Hagen, R., Möltner, A., Brockmeier, S. J., Stark, T., et al. (2009). Site of cochlear stimulation and its effect on electrically evoked compound action potentials using the MED-EL standard electrode array. *Biomedical Engineering Online, 8*, 1–10.

Brochier, T., McDermott, H. J., & McKay, C. M. (2017). The effect of presentation level and stimulation rate on speech perception and modulation detection for cochlear implant users. *The Journal of the Acoustical Society of America, 141*(6), 4097–4105.

Brockmeier, S. J., Peterreins, M., Lorens, A., Vermeire, K., Helbig, S., Anderson, I., et al. (2010). Music perception in electric acoustic stimulation users as assessed by the Mu. SIC test. In *Cochlear implants and hearing preservation* (Vol. 67, pp. 70–80). Karger Publishers.

Buchman, C. A., Dillon, M. T., King, E. R., Adunka, M. C., Adunka, O. F., & Pillsbury, H. C. (2014). Influence of cochlear implant insertion depth on performance: A prospective randomized trial. *Otology & Neurotology, 35*(10), 1773–1779.

Buechner, A., Brendel, M., Krüeger, B., Frohne-Büchner, C., Nogueira, W., Edler, B., & Lenarz, T. (2008). Current steering and results from novel speech coding strategies. *Otology & Neurotology, 29*(2), 203–207.

Burns, E. M., & Viemeister, N. F. (1981). Played-again SAM: Further observations on the pitch of amplitude-modulated noise. *The Journal of the Acoustical Society of America, 70*(6), 1655–1660.

Canfarotta, M. W., Dillon, M. T., Buss, E., Pillsbury, H. C., Brown, K. D., & O'Connell, B. P. (2020). Frequency-to-place mismatch: Characterizing variability and the influence on speech perception outcomes in cochlear implant recipients. *Ear and Hearing, 41*(5), 1349–1361.

Canfarotta, M. W., O'Connell, B. P., Giardina, C. K., Buss, E., Brown, K. D., Dillon, M. T., Rooth, M. A., Pillsbury, H. C., Buchman, C. A., Adunka, O. F., & Fitzpatrick, D. C. (2021). Relationship between electrocochleography, angular insertion depth, and cochlear implant speech perception outcomes. *Ear and Hearing, 42*(4), 941–948.

Chakravorti, S., Noble, J. H., Gifford, R. H., Dawant, B. M., O'Connell, B. P., Wang, J., & Labadie, R. F. (2019). Further evidence of the relationship between cochlear implant electrode positioning and hearing outcomes. *Otology & Neurotology, 40*(5), 617–624.

Chang, Y. T., Yang, H. M., Lin, Y. H., Liu, S. H., & Wu, J. L. (2009). Tone discrimination and speech perception benefit in Mandarin-speaking children fit with HiRes fidelity 120 sound processing. *Otology & Neurotology, 30*(6), 750–757.

Chatterjee, M. (1999). Effects of stimulation mode on threshold and loudness growth in multielectrode cochlear implants. *The Journal of the Acoustical Society of America, 105*(2), 850–860.

Chatterjee, M., & Oberzut, C. (2011). Detection and rate discrimination of amplitude modulation in electrical hearing. *The Journal of the Acoustical Society of America, 130*(3), 1567–1580.

Chatterjee, M., & Peng, S. C. (2008). Processing F0 with cochlear implants: Modulation frequency discrimination and speech intonation recognition. *Hearing Research, 235*(1–2), 143–156.

Chatterjee, M., & Shannon, R. V. (1998). Forward masked excitation patterns in multielectrode electrical stimulation. *The Journal of the Acoustical Society of America, 103*(5), 2565–2572.

Chatterjee, M., Fu, Q. J., & Shannon, R. V. (2000). Effects of phase duration and electrode separation on loudness growth in cochlear implant listeners. *The Journal of the Acoustical Society of America, 107*(3), 1637–1644.

Chatterjee, M., Galvin, J. J., Fu, Q. J., & Shannon, R. V. (2006). Effects of stimulation mode, level and location on forward-masked excitation patterns in cochlear implant patients. *Journal of the Association for Research in Otolaryngology, 7*, 15–25.

Chatterjee, M., Zion, D. J., Deroche, M. L., Burianek, B. A., Limb, C. J., Goren, A. P., et al. (2015). Voice emotion recognition by cochlear-implanted children and their normally-hearing peers. *Hearing Research, 322*, 151–162.

Chatterjee, M., Kulkarni, A. M., Siddiqui, R. M., Christensen, J. A., Hozan, M., Sis, J. L., & Damm, S. A. (2019). Acoustics of emotional prosody produced by prelingually deaf children with cochlear implants. *Frontiers in Psychology, 10*, 2190.

Cheng, Y. S., & Svirsky, M. A. (2021). Meta-analysis—Correlation between spiral ganglion cell counts and speech perception with a Cochlear implant. *Audiology Research, 11*(2), 220–226.

Croghan, N. B., Duran, S. I., & Smith, Z. M. (2017). Re-examining the relationship between number of cochlear implant channels and maximal speech intelligibility. *The Journal of the Acoustical Society of America, 142*(6), EL537-EL543.

Danhauer, J. L., Ghadialy, F. B., Eskwitt, D. L., & Mendel, L. L. (1990). Performance of 3M/house cochlear implant users on tests of speech perception. *Journal of the American Academy of Audiology, 1*(4), 236–239.

Davis, T. J., Zhang, D., Gifford, R. H., Dawant, B. M., Labadie, R. F., & Noble, J. H. (2016). Relationship between electrode-to-modiolus distance and current levels for adults with cochlear implants. *Otology & Neurotology, 37*(1), 31–37.

Deroche, M. L., Lu, H. P., Limb, C. J., Lin, Y. S., & Chatterjee, M. (2014). Deficits in the pitch sensitivity of cochlear-implanted children speaking English or Mandarin. *Frontiers in Neuroscience, 8*, 282.

Deroche, M. L., Lu, H. P., Lin, Y. S., Chatterjee, M., & Peng, S. C. (2019). Processing of acoustic information in lexical tone production and perception by pediatric cochlear implant recipients. *Frontiers in Neuroscience, 13*, 639.

Dillon, M. T., Buss, E., Johnson, A. D., Canfarotta, M. W., & O'Connell, B. P. (2023). Comparison of two place-based mapping procedures on masked sentence recognition as a function of electrode array angular insertion depth and presence of acoustic low-frequency information: A simulation study. *Audiology and Neurotology, 28*(6), 478–487.

Dunn, C. C., Perreau, A., Gantz, B., & Tyler, R. S. (2010). Benefits of localization and speech perception with multiple noise sources in listeners with a short-electrode cochlear implant. *Journal of the American Academy of Audiology, 21*(01), 044–051.

Dunn, C. C., Oleson, J., Parkinson, A., Hansen, M. R., & Gantz, B. J. (2020). Nucleus hybrid S12: multicenter clinical trial results. *The Laryngoscope, 130*(10), E548–E558.

Eddington, D. K. (1980). Speech discrimination in deaf subjects with cochlear implants. *The Journal of the Acoustical Society of America, 68*(3), 885–891.

Fabie, J. E., Keller, R. G., Hatch, J. L., Holcomb, M. A., Camposeo, E. L., Lambert, P. R., et al. (2018). Evaluation of outcome variability associated with lateral wall, mid-scalar, and perimodiolar electrode arrays when controlling for preoperative patient characteristics. *Otology & Neurotology, 39*(9), 1122–1128.

Fan, Y., Wang, J., Zhao, Y., Li, R., Liu, H., Labadie, R. F., et al. (2023, October). A unified deep-learning-based framework for cochlear implant electrode Array localization. In *International conference on medical image computing and computer-assisted intervention* (pp. 376–385). Springer Nature Switzerland.

Firszt, J. B., Koch, D. B., Downing, M., & Litvak, L. (2007). Current steering creates additional pitch percepts in adult cochlear implant recipients. *Otology & Neurotology, 28*(5), 629–636.

Fishman, K. E., Shannon, R. V., & Slattery, W. H. (1997). Speech recognition as a function of the number of electrodes used in the SPEAK cochlear implant speech processor. *Journal of Speech, Language, and Hearing Research, 40*(5), 1201–1215.

Franco-Vidal, V., Parietti-Winkler, C., Guevara, N., Truy, E., Loundon, N., Bailleux, S., et al. (2020). The Oticon Medical Neuro Zti cochlear implant and the Neuro 2 sound processor: Multicentric evaluation of outcomes in adults and children. *International Journal of Audiology, 59*(2), 153–160.

Fraysse, B., Macías, Á. R., Sterkers, O., Burdo, S., Ramsden, R., Deguine, O., et al. (2006). Residual hearing conservation and electroacoustic stimulation with the nucleus 24 contour advance cochlear implant. *Otology & Neurotology, 27*(5), 624–633.

Fretz, R. J., & Fravel, R. P. (1985). Design and function: A physical and electrical description of the 3M House cochlear implant system. *Ear and Hearing, 6*(3), 14S–19S.

Friesen, L. M., Shannon, R. V., Baskent, D., & Wang, X. (2001). Speech recognition in noise as a function of the number of spectral channels: Comparison of acoustic hearing and cochlear implants. *The Journal of the Acoustical Society of America, 110*(2), 1150–1163.

Friesen, L. M., Shannon, R. V., & Cruz, R. J. (2005). Effects of stimulation rate on speech recognition with cochlear implants. *Audiology and Neurotology, 10*(3), 169–184.

Fu, Q. J., & Zeng, F. G. (2000). Identification of temporal envelope cues in Chinese tone recognition. *Asia Pacific Journal of Speech, Language and Hearing, 5*(1), 45–57.

Fu, Q. J., Chinchilla, S., & Galvin, J. J. (2004). The role of spectral and temporal cues in voice gender discrimination by normal-hearing listeners and cochlear implant users. *Journal of the Association for Research in Otolaryngology, 5*, 253–260.

Galvin, J. J., III, Fu, Q. J., & Nogaki, G. (2007). Melodic contour identification by cochlear implant listeners. *Ear and Hearing, 28*(3), 302–319.

Gantz, B. J., & Turner, C. W. (2003). Combining acoustic and electrical hearing. *The Laryngoscope, 113*(10), 1726–1730.

Gantz, B. J., Tyler, R. S., Knutson, J. F., Woodworth, G., Abbas, P., McCabe, B. F., Hinrichs, J., Tye-Murray, N., Lansing, C., & Kuk, F. (1988). Evaluation of five different cochlear implant designs: Audiologic assessment and predictors of performance. *The Laryngoscope, 98*(10), 1100–1106.

Gantz, B. J., Dunn, C., Oleson, J., Hansen, M., Parkinson, A., & Turner, C. (2016). Multicenter clinical trial of the Nucleus Hybrid S8 cochlear implant: Final outcomes. *The Laryngoscope, 126*(4), 962–973.

Gantz, B. J., Dunn, C. C., Oleson, J., & Hansen, M. R. (2018). Acoustic plus electric speech processing: Long-term results. *The Laryngoscope, 128*(2), 473–481.

Garadat, S. N., Zwolan, T. A., & Pfingst, B. E. (2013). Using temporal modulation sensitivity to select stimulation sites for processor MAPs in cochlear implant listeners. *Audiology and Neurotology, 18*(4), 247–260.

Gfeller, K. E., Olszewski, C., Turner, C., Gantz, B., & Oleson, J. (2006). Music perception with cochlear implants and residual hearing. *Audiology and Neurotology, 11*(Suppl. 1), 12–15.

Gifford, R. H., Dorman, M. F., Spahr, A. J., Bacon, S. P., Skarzynski, H., & Lorens, A. (2008). Hearing preservation surgery: Psychophysical estimates of cochlear damage in recipients of a short electrode array. *The Journal of the Acoustical Society of America, 124*(4), 2164–2173.

Gifford, R. H., Dorman, M. F., & Brown, C. A. (2010). Psychophysical properties of low-frequency hearing: Implications for perceiving speech and music via electric and acoustic stimulation. *Cochlear Implants and Hearing Preservation, 67*, 51–60.

Gifford, R. H., Davis, T. J., Sunderhaus, L. W., Menapace, C., Buck, B., Crosson, J., et al. (2017). Combined electric and acoustic stimulation with hearing preservation: Effect of cochlear implant low-frequency cutoff on speech understanding and perceived listening difficulty. *Ear and Hearing, 38*(5), 539–553.

Goehring, T., Archer-Boyd, A., Deeks, J. M., Arenberg, J. G., & Carlyon, R. P. (2019). A site-selection strategy based on polarity sensitivity for cochlear implants: Effects on spectro-temporal resolution and speech perception. *Journal of the Association for Research in Otolaryngology, 20*, 431–448.

Gray, W. O., Mayo, P. G., Goupell, M. J., & Brown, A. D. (2021). Transmission of binaural cues by bilateral cochlear implants: Examining the impacts of bilaterally independent spectral peak-picking, pulse timing, and compression. *Trends in Hearing, 25*, 23312165211030411.

Greenwood, D. D. (1990). A cochlear frequency-position function for several species—29 years later. *The Journal of the Acoustical Society of America, 87*(6), 2592–2605.

Health Quality Ontario. (2018). Bilateral cochlear implantation: A health technology assessment. *Ontario Health Technology Assessment Series, 18*(6), 1.

Helbig, S., Van de Heyning, P., Kiefer, J., Baumann, U., Kleine-Punte, A., Brockmeier, H., et al. (2011). Combined electric acoustic stimulation with the PULSARCI100 implant system using the FLEXEAS electrode array. *Acta Oto-Laryngologica, 131*(6), 585–595.

Helpard, L., Li, H., Rohani, S. A., Zhu, N., Rask-Andersen, H., Agrawal, S., & Ladak, H. M. (2021). An approach for individualized cochlear frequency mapping determined from 3D synchrotron radiation phase-contrast imaging. *IEEE Transactions on Biomedical Engineering, 68*(12), 3602–3611.

Henry, B. A., Turner, C. W., & Behrens, A. (2005). Spectral peak resolution and speech recognition in quiet: Normal hearing, hearing impaired, and cochlear implant listeners. *The Journal of the Acoustical Society of America, 118*(2), 1111–1121.

Hogan, C. A., & Turner, C. W. (1998). High-frequency audibility: Benefits for hearing-impaired listeners. *The Journal of the Acoustical Society of America, 104*(1), 432–441.

Holder, J. T., Yawn, R. J., Nassiri, A. M., Dwyer, R. T., Rivas, A., Labadie, R. F., & Gifford, R. H. (2019). Matched cohort comparison indicates superiority of precurved electrode arrays. *Otology & Neurotology, 40*(9), 1160–1166.

Hughes, M. L., & Stille, L. J. (2008). Psychophysical versus physiological spatial forward masking and the relation to speech perception in cochlear implants. *Ear and Hearing, 29*(3), 435–452.

Hunter, J. B., Gifford, R. H., Wanna, G. B., Labadie, R. F., Bennett, M. L., Haynes, D. S., & Rivas, A. (2016). Hearing preservation outcomes with a mid-scala electrode in cochlear implantation. *Otology & Neurotology, 37*(3), 235–240.

Jeon, E. K., Turner, C. W., Karsten, S. A., Henry, B. A., & Gantz, B. J. (2015). Cochlear implant users' spectral ripple resolution. *The Journal of the Acoustical Society of America, 138*(4), 2350–2358.

Kamakura, T., & Nadol, J. B., Jr. (2016). Correlation between word recognition score and intracochlear new bone and fibrous tissue after cochlear implantation in the human. *Hearing Research, 339*, 132–141.

Kara C., Schvartz-Leyzac Teresa A., Zwolan Bryan E., Pfingst (2021) Using the electrically-evoked compound action potential (ECAP) interphase gap effect to select electrode stimulation sites in cochlear implant users Hearing Research 406108257-10.1016/j.heares.2021.108257

Karsten, S. A., Turner, C. W., Brown, C. J., Jeon, E. K., Abbas, P. J., & Gantz, B. J. (2013). Optimizing the combination of acoustic and electric hearing in the implanted ear. *Ear and Hearing, 34*(2), 142–150.

Khan, A. M., Handzel, O., Burgess, B. J., Damian, D., Eddington, D. K., & Nadol, J. B., Jr. (2005a). Is word recognition correlated with the number of surviving spiral ganglion cells and electrode insertion depth in human subjects with cochlear implants? *The Laryngoscope, 115*(4), 672–677.

Khan, A. M., Whiten, D. M., Nadol, J. B., Jr., & Eddington, D. K. (2005b). Histopathology of human cochlear implants: Correlation of psychophysical and anatomical measures. *Hearing Research, 205*(1–2), 83–93.

Kiang, N. Y., & Moxon, E. C. (1972). Physiological considerations in artificial stimulation of the inner ear. *Annals of Otology, Rhinology & Laryngology, 81*(5), 714–730.

Kim, J. R., Abbas, P. J., Brown, C. J., Etler, C. P., O'Brien, S., & Kim, L. S. (2010). The relationship between electrically evoked compound action potential and speech perception: A study in cochlear implant users with short electrode array. *Otology & Neurotology, 31*(7), 1041–1048.

Koch, D. B., Downing, M., Osberger, M. J., & Litvak, L. (2007). Using current steering to increase spectral resolution in CII and HiRes 90K users. *Ear and Hearing, 28*(2), 38S–41S.

Kral, A., Hartmann, R., Mortazavi, D., & Klinke, R. (1998). Spatial resolution of cochlear implants: The electrical field and excitation of auditory afferents. *Hearing Research, 121*(1–2), 11–28.

Landsberger, D. M., Padilla, M., & Srinivasan, A. G. (2012). Reducing current spread using current focusing in cochlear implant users. *Hearing Research, 284*(1–2), 16–24.

Landsberger, D. M., Mertens, G., Punte, A. K., & Van De Heyning, P. (2014). Perceptual changes in place of stimulation with long cochlear implant electrode arrays. *The Journal of the Acoustical Society of America, 135*(2), EL75-EL81.

Landsberger, D. M., Svrakic, M., Roland, J. T., Jr., & Svirsky, M. (2015). The relationship between insertion angles, default frequency allocations, and spiral ganglion place pitch in cochlear implants. *Ear and Hearing, 36*(5), e207–e213.

Lenarz, T., James, C., Cuda, D., Fitzgerald O'Connor, A., Frachet, B., Frijns, J. H., et al. (2013). European multi-centre study of the Nucleus Hybrid L24 cochlear implant. *International Journal of Audiology, 52*(12), 838–848.

Lenarz, T., Buechner, A., Lesinski-Schiedat, A., Timm, M., & Salcher, R. (2020). Hearing preservation with a new atraumatic lateral wall electrode. *Otology & Neurotology, 41*(8), e993–e1003.

Linthicum, F. H., Jr., & Fayad, J. N. (2009). Spiral ganglion cell loss is unrelated to segmental cochlear sensory system degeneration in humans. *Otology & Neurotology, 30*(3), 418–422.

Long, C. J., Eddington, D. K., Colburn, H. S., & Rabinowitz, W. M. (2003). Binaural sensitivity as a function of interaural electrode position with a bilateral cochlear implant user. *The Journal of the Acoustical Society of America, 114*(3), 1565–1574.

Luo, X., Fu, Q. J., & Galvin, J. J., III. (2007). Cochlear implants special issue article: Vocal emotion recognition by normal-hearing listeners and cochlear implant users. *Trends in Amplification, 11*(4), 301–315.

Luo, X., Fu, Q. J., Wei, C. G., & Cao, K. L. (2008). Speech recognition and temporal amplitude modulation processing by Mandarin-speaking cochlear implant users. *Ear and Hearing, 29*(6), 957–970.

MacPhail, M. E., Connell, N. T., Totten, D. J., Gray, M. T., Pisoni, D., Yates, C. W., & Nelson, R. F. (2022). Speech recognition outcomes in adults with slim straight and slim modiolar cochlear implant electrode arrays. *Otolaryngology–Head and Neck Surgery, 166*(5), 943–950.

Melo, T. M. D., Bevilacqua, M. C., & Costa, O. A. (2012). Speech perception in cochlear implant users with the HiRes 120 strategy: A systematic review. *Brazilian Journal of Otorhinolaryngology, 78*, 129–133.

Micuda, A., Li, H., Rask-Andersen, H., Ladak, H. M., & Agrawal, S. K. (2024). Morphologic analysis of the scala tympani using synchrotron: Implications for cochlear implantation. *The Laryngoscope, 134*(6), 2889–2897.

Müller-Graff, F. T., Spahn, B., Herrmann, D. P., Kurz, A., Völker, J., Hagen, R., & Rak, K. (2024). Comprehensive literature review on the application of the otological surgical planning software OTOPLAN® for cochlear implantation. *HNO, 72*, 1–12.

Nadol, J. B., & Eddington, D. K. (2006). Histopathology of the inner ear relevant to cochlear implantation. *Cochlear and Brainstem Implants, 64*, 31–49.

Nadol, J. B., Jr. (1997). Patterns of neural degeneration in the human cochlea and auditory nerve: Implications for cochlear implantation. *Otolaryngology-Head and Neck Surgery, 117*(3), 220–228.

Nadol, J. B., Jr., Young, Y. S., & Glynn, R. J. (1989). Survival of spiral ganglion cells in profound sensorineural hearing loss: Implications for cochlear implantation. *Annals of Otology, Rhinology & Laryngology, 98*(6), 411–416.

Nassiri, A. M., Yawn, R. J., Holder, J. T., Dwyer, R. T., O'Malley, M. R., Bennett, M. L., et al. (2020). Hearing preservation outcomes using a precurved electrode array inserted with an external sheath. *Otology & Neurotology, 41*(1), 33–38.

Noble, J. H., Gifford, R. H., Hedley-Williams, A. J., Dawant, B. M., & Labadie, R. F. (2014). Clinical evaluation of an image-guided cochlear implant programming strategy. *Audiology and Neurotology, 19*(6), 400–411.

O'Connell, B. P., Hunter, J. B., Gifford, R. H., Rivas, A., Haynes, D. S., Noble, J. H., & Wanna, G. B. (2016). Electrode location and audiologic performance after cochlear implantation: A comparative study between nucleus CI422 and CI512 electrode arrays. *Otology & Neurotology, 37*(8), 1032–1035.

O'Connell, B. P., Hunter, J. B., Haynes, D. S., Holder, J. T., Dedmon, M. M., Noble, J. H., et al. (2017). Insertion depth impacts speech perception and hearing preservation for lateral wall electrodes. *The Laryngoscope, 127*(10), 2352–2357.

Oxenham, A. J. (2008). Pitch perception and auditory stream segregation: Implications for hearing loss and cochlear implants. *Trends in Amplification, 12*(4), 316–331.

Oxenham, A. J. (2012). Pitch perception. *Journal of Neuroscience, 32*(39), 13335–13338.

Padilla, M., & Landsberger, D. M. (2016). Reduction in spread of excitation from current focusing at multiple cochlear locations in cochlear implant users. *Hearing Research, 333*, 98–107.

Peng, S. C., Tomblin, J. B., Cheung, H., Lin, Y. S., & Wang, L. S. (2004). Perception and production of Mandarin tones in prelingually deaf children with cochlear implants. *Ear and Hearing, 25*(3), 251–264.

Peng, S. C., Chatterjee, M., & Lu, N. (2012). Acoustic cue integration in speech intonation recognition with cochlear implants. *Trends in Amplification, 16*(2), 67–82.

Peng, S. C., Lu, H. P., Lu, N., Lin, Y. S., Deroche, M. L., & Chatterjee, M. (2017). Processing of acoustic cues in lexical-tone identification by pediatric cochlear-implant recipients. *Journal of Speech, Language, and Hearing Research, 60*(5), 1223–1235.

Pfingst, B. E., Zwolan, T. A., & Holloway, L. A. (1997). Effects of stimulus configuration on psychophysical operating levels and on speech recognition with cochlear implants. *Hearing Research, 112*(1–2), 247–260.

Pfingst, B. E., Franck, K. H., Xu, L., Bauer, E. M., & Zwolan, T. A. (2001). Effects of electrode configuration and place of stimulation on speech perception with cochlear prostheses. *JARO: Journal of the Association for Research in Otolaryngology, 2*(2), 87–103.

Pfingst, B. E., Xu, L., & Thompson, C. S. (2004). Across-site threshold variation in cochlear implants: Relation to speech recognition. *Audiology and Neurotology, 9*(6), 341–352.

Pfingst, B. E., Colesa, D. J., Hembrador, S., Kang, S. Y., Middlebrooks, J. C., Raphael, Y., & Su, G. L. (2011). Detection of pulse trains in the electrically stimulated cochlea: Effects of cochlear health. *The Journal of the Acoustical Society of America, 130*(6), 3954–3968.

Pfingst, B. E., Zhou, N., Colesa, D. J., Watts, M. M., Strahl, S. B., Garadat, S. N., et al. (2015). Importance of cochlear health for implant function. *Hearing Research, 322*, 77–88.

Pfingst, B. E., Colesa, D. J., Swiderski, D. L., Hughes, A. P., Strahl, S. B., Sinan, M., & Raphael, Y. (2017). Neurotrophin gene therapy in deafened ears with cochlear implants: Long-term effects on nerve survival and functional measures. *Journal of the Association for Research in Otolaryngology, 18*, 731–750.

Pillsbury, H. C., III, Dillon, M. T., Buchman, C. A., Staecker, H., Prentiss, S. M., Ruckenstein, M. J., et al. (2018). Multicenter US clinical trial with an electric-acoustic stimulation (EAS) system in adults: Final outcomes. *Otology & Neurotology, 39*(3), 299–305.

Plant, K. L., Whitford, L. A., Psarros, C. E., & Vandali, A. E. (2002). Parameter selection and programming recommendations for the ACE and CIS speech-processing strategies in the Nucleus 24 cochlear implant system. *Cochlear Implants International, 3*(2), 104–125.

Plant, K., Holden, L., Skinner, M., Arcaroli, J., Whitford, L., Law, M. A., & Nel, E. (2007). Clinical evaluation of higher stimulation rates in the nucleus research platform 8 system. *Ear and Hearing, 28*(3), 381–393.

Potts, W. B., Ramanna, L., Perry, T., & Long, C. J. (2019). Improving localization and speech reception in noise for bilateral cochlear implant recipients. *Trends in hearing, 23*, 2331216519831492.

Qin, M. K., & Oxenham, A. J. (2003). Effects of simulated cochlear-implant processing on speech reception in fluctuating maskers. *The Journal of the Acoustical Society of America, 114*(1), 446–454.

Ramekers, D., Versnel, H., Strahl, S. B., Smeets, E. M., Klis, S. F., & Grolman, W. (2014). Auditory-nerve responses to varied inter-phase gap and phase duration of the electric pulse stimulus as predictors for neuronal degeneration. *Journal of the Association for Research in Otolaryngology, 15*, 187–202.

Ramekers, D., Versnel, H., Strahl, S. B., Klis, S. F., & Grolman, W. (2015). Recovery characteristics of the electrically stimulated auditory nerve in deafened Guinea pigs: Relation to neuronal status. *Hearing Research, 321*, 12–24.

Rask-Andersen, H., Liu, W., & Linthicum, F. (2010). Ganglion cell and 'dendrite'populations in electric acoustic stimulation ears. In *Cochlear implants and hearing preservation* (Vol. 67, pp. 14–27). Karger Publishers.

Riss, D., Hamzavi, J. S., Selberherr, A., Kaider, A., Blineder, M., Starlinger, V., et al. (2011). Envelope versus fine structure speech coding strategy: A crossover study. *Otology & Neurotology, 32*(7), 1094–1101.

Roland, J. T., Jr., Gantz, B. J., Waltzman, S. B., Parkinson, A. J., & Multicenter Clinical Trial Group. (2016). United States multicenter clinical trial of the cochlear nucleus hybrid implant system. *The Laryngoscope, 126*(1), 175–181.

Roland, J. T., Jr., Gantz, B. J., Waltzman, S. B., & Parkinson, A. J. (2018). Long-term outcomes of cochlear implantation in patients with high-frequency hearing loss. *The Laryngoscope, 128*(8), 1939–1945.

Rosen, S. (1992). Temporal information in speech: Acoustic, auditory and linguistic aspects. *Philosophical Transactions of the Royal Society of London. Series B: Biological Sciences, 336*(1278), 367–373.

Roy, A. T., Carver, C., Jiradejvong, P., & Limb, C. J. (2015). Musical sound quality in cochlear implant users: A comparison in bass frequency perception between fine structure process-

ing and high-definition continuous interleaved sampling strategies. *Ear and Hearing, 36*(5), 582–590.
Saoji, A. A., Landsberger, D. M., Padilla, M., & Litvak, L. M. (2013). Masking patterns for monopolar and phantom electrode stimulation in cochlear implants. *Hearing Research, 298*, 109–116.
Scheperle, R. A., & Abbas, P. J. (2015). Relationships among peripheral and central electrophysiological measures of spatial and spectral selectivity and speech perception in cochlear implant users. *Ear and Hearing, 36*(4), 441–453.
Scheperle, R. A., Tejani, V. D., Omtvedt, J. K., Brown, C. J., Abbas, P. J., Hansen, M. R., et al. (2017). Delayed changes in auditory status in cochlear implant users with preserved acoustic hearing. *Hearing Research, 350*, 45–57.
Schvartz-Leyzac, K. C., & Pfingst, B. E. (2016). Across-site patterns of electrically evoked compound action potential amplitude-growth functions in multichannel cochlear implant recipients and the effects of the interphase gap. *Hearing Research, 341*, 50–65.
Schvartz-Leyzac, K. C., & Pfingst, B. E. (2018). Assessing the relationship between the electrically evoked compound action potential and speech recognition abilities in bilateral cochlear implant recipients. *Ear and Hearing, 39*(2), 344–358.
Schvartz-Leyzac, K. C., Zwolan, T. A., & Pfingst, B. E. (2017). Effects of electrode deactivation on speech recognition in multichannel cochlear implant recipients. *Cochlear Implants International, 18*(6), 324–334.
Schvartz-Leyzac, K. C., Colesa, D. J., Buswinka, C. J., Swiderski, D. L., Raphael, Y., & Pfingst, B. E. (2019). Changes over time in the electrically evoked compound action potential (ECAP) interphase gap (IPG) effect following cochlear implantation in Guinea pigs. *Hearing Research, 383*, 107809.
Schvartz-Leyzac, K. C., Colesa, D. J., Buswinka, C. J., Rabah, A. M., Swiderski, D. L., Raphael, Y., & Pfingst, B. E. (2020a). How electrically evoked compound action potentials in chronically implanted Guinea pigs relate to auditory nerve health and electrode impedance. *The Journal of the Acoustical Society of America, 148*(6), 3900–3912.
Schvartz-Leyzac, K. C., Holden, T. A., Zwolan, T. A., Arts, H. A., Firszt, J. B., Buswinka, C. J., & Pfingst, B. E. (2020b). Effects of electrode location on estimates of neural health in humans with cochlear implants. *Journal of the Association for Research in Otolaryngology, 21*, 259–275.
Seyyedi, M., Viana, L. M., & Nadol, J. B., Jr. (2014). Within-subject comparison of word recognition and spiral ganglion cell count in bilateral cochlear implant recipients. *Otology & Neurotology, 35*(8), 1446–1450.
Shader, M. J., Nguyen, N., Cleary, M., Hertzano, R., Eisenman, D. J., Anderson, S., et al. (2020). Effect of stimulation rate on speech understanding in older cochlear-implant users. *Ear and Hearing, 41*(3), 640–651.
Shannon, R. V. (1983). Multichannel electrical stimulation of the auditory nerve in man. I. Basic psychophysics. *Hearing Research, 11*(2), 157–189.
Shannon, R. V. (1985). Threshold and loudness functions for pulsatile stimulation of cochlear implants. *Hearing Research, 18*(2), 135–143.
Shannon, R. V., Adams, D. D., Ferrel, R. L., Palumbo, R. L., & Grandgenett, M. (1990). A computer interface for psychophysical and speech research with the nucleus cochlear implant. *The Journal of the Acoustical Society of America, 87*(2), 905–907.
Shannon, R. V., Zeng, F. G., Kamath, V., Wygonski, J., & Ekelid, M. (1995). Speech recognition with primarily temporal cues. *Science, 270*(5234), 303–304.
Smith, Z. M., Parkinson, W. S., & Long, C. J. (2013, July). Multipolar current focusing increases spectral resolution in cochlear implants. In *2013 35th annual international conference of the IEEE engineering in medicine and biology society (EMBC)* (pp. 2796–2799). IEEE.
Srinivasan, A. G., Padilla, M., Shannon, R. V., & Landsberger, D. M. (2013). Improving speech perception in noise with current focusing in cochlear implant users. *Hearing Research, 299*, 29–36.
Stakhovskaya, O., Sridhar, D., Bonham, B. H., & Leake, P. A. (2007). Frequency map for the human cochlear spiral ganglion: Implications for cochlear implants. *Journal for the Association for Research in Otolaryngology, 8*, 220–233.

Tang, Q., Benítez, R., & Zeng, F. G. (2011). Spatial channel interactions in cochlear implants. *Journal of Neural Engineering, 8*(4), 046029.
Tejani, V. D., & Brown, C. J. (2020). Speech masking release in Hybrid cochlear implant users: Roles of spectral and temporal cues in electric-acoustic hearing. *The Journal of the Acoustical Society of America, 147*(5), 3667–3683.
Teresa Y. C., Ching Harvey, Dillon Denis, Byrne (1998) (1998) Speech recognition of hearing-impaired listeners: Predictions from audibility and the limited role of high-frequency amplification The Journal of the Acoustical Society of America 103(2) 1128-1140 10.1121/1.421224
Teymouri, J., Hullar, T. E., Holden, T. A., & Chole, R. A. (2011). Verification of computed tomographic estimates of cochlear implant array position: A micro-CT and histologic analysis. *Otology & Neurotology, 32*(6), 980–986.
Turner, C. W. (2006). Hearing loss and the limits of amplification. *Audiology and Neurotology, 11*(Suppl. 1), 2–5.
Turner, C. W., Gantz, B. J., Vidal, C., Behrens, A., & Henry, B. A. (2004). Speech recognition in noise for cochlear implant listeners: Benefits of residual acoustic hearing. *The Journal of the Acoustical Society of America, 115*(4), 1729–1735.
Van Abel, K. M., Dunn, C. C., Sladen, D. P., Oleson, J. J., Beatty, C. W., Neff, B. A., et al. (2015). Hearing preservation among patients undergoing cochlear implantation. *Otology & Neurotology, 36*(3), 416–421.
Van De Velde, D. J., Schiller, N. O., Levelt, C. C., Van Heuven, V. J., Beers, M., Briaire, J. J., & Frijns, J. H. (2019). Prosody perception and production by children with cochlear implants. *Journal of Child Language, 46*(1), 111–141.
Vandali, A. E., & van Hoesel, R. J. (2012). Enhancement of temporal cues to pitch in cochlear implants: Effects on pitch ranking. *The Journal of the Acoustical Society of America, 132*(1), 392–402.
Vandali, A. E., Whitford, L. A., Plant, K. L., & Clark, G. M. (2000). Speech perception as a function of electrical stimulation rate: Using the Nucleus 24 cochlear implant system. *Ear and Hearing, 21*(6), 608–624.
Vandali, A., Dawson, P., Au, A., Yu, Y., Brown, M., Goorevich, M., & Cowan, R. (2019). Evaluation of the optimized pitch and language strategy in cochlear implant recipients. *Ear and Hearing, 40*(3), 555–567.
Vermeire, K., Anderson, I., Flynn, M., & Van de Heyning, P. (2008). The influence of different speech processor and hearing aid settings on speech perception outcomes in electric acoustic stimulation patients. *Ear and Hearing, 29*(1), 76–86.
von Békésy, G. (1956). Current status of theories of hearing. *Science, 123*, 779–783.
von Ilberg, C., Kiefer, J., Tillein, J., Pfenningdorff, T., Hartmann, R., Stürzebecher, E., & Klinke, R. (1999). Electric-acoustic stimulation of the auditory system. New technology for severe hearing loss. *ORL; Journal for Oto-Rhino-Laryngology and Its Related Specialties, 61*(6), 334–340.
Wang, W., Zhou, N., & Xu, L. (2011). Musical pitch and lexical tone perception with cochlear implants. *International Journal of Audiology, 50*(4), 270–278.
Wilson, B. S., & Dorman, M. F. (2008). Cochlear implants: current designs and future possibilities. *Journal of Rehabilitation Research and Development, 45*(5), 695–730.
Wilson, B. S., Finley, C. C., Lawson, D. T., Wolford, R. D., Eddington, D. K., & Rabinowitz, W. M. (1991). Better speech recognition with cochlear implants. *Nature, 352*(6332), 236–238.
Won, J. H., Humphrey, E. L., Yeager, K. R., Martinez, A. A., Robinson, C. H., Mills, K. E., et al. (2014). Relationship among the physiologic channel interactions, spectral-ripple discrimination, and vowel identification in cochlear implant users. *The Journal of the Acoustical Society of America, 136*(5), 2714–2725.
Xu, L., & Pfingst, B. E. (2008). Spectral and temporal cues for speech recognition: Implications for auditory prostheses. *Hearing Research, 242*(1–2), 132–140.
Xu, L., & Zheng, Y. (2007). Spectral and temporal cues for phoneme recognition in noise. *The Journal of the Acoustical Society of America, 122*(3), 1758–1764.

Xu, L., Thompson, C. S., & Pfingst, B. E. (2005). Relative contributions of spectral and temporal cues for phoneme recognition. *The Journal of the Acoustical Society of America, 117*(5), 3255–3267.

Xu, L., Chen, X., Lu, H., Zhou, N., Wang, S., Liu, Q., et al. (2011). Tone perception and production in pediatric cochlear implants users. *Acta Oto-Laryngologica, 131*(4), 395–398.

Zeng, F. G. (2002). Temporal pitch in electric hearing. *Hearing Research, 174*(1–2), 101–106.

Zeng, F. G., Rebscher, S. J., Fu, Q. J., Chen, H., Sun, X., Yin, L., et al. (2015). Development and evaluation of the Nurotron 26-electrode cochlear implant system. *Hearing Research, 322*, 188–199.

Zhou, N. (2019). Longitudinal effect of deactivating stimulation sites based on low-rate thresholds on speech recognition in cochlear implant users. *International Journal of Audiology, 58*(9), 587–597.

Zhou, N., & Pfingst, B. E. (2014). Relationship between multipulse integration and speech recognition with cochlear implants. *The Journal of the Acoustical Society of America, 136*(3), 1257–1268.

Zhou, N., & Pfingst, B. E. (2016). Evaluating multipulse integration as a neural-health correlate in human cochlear-implant users: Relationship to spatial selectivity. *The Journal of the Acoustical Society of America, 140*(3), 1537–1547.

Zhou, N., Huang, J., Chen, X., & Xu, L. (2013). Relationship between tone perception and production in prelingually deafened children with cochlear implants. *Otology & Neurotology, 34*(3), 499–506.

Zhou, N., Kraft, C. T., Colesa, D. J., & Pfingst, B. E. (2015). Integration of pulse trains in humans and Guinea pigs with cochlear implants. *Journal of the Association for Research in Otolaryngology, 16*, 523–534.

Zhou, N., Dong, L., & Hang, M. (2018). Evaluating multipulse integration as a neural-health correlate in human cochlear implant users: Effects of stimulation mode. *Journal of the Association for Research in Otolaryngology, 19*, 99–111.

Zhu, Z., Tang, Q., Zeng, F. G., Guan, T., & Ye, D. (2012). Cochlear-implant spatial selectivity with monopolar, bipolar and tripolar stimulation. *Hearing Research, 283*(1–2), 45–58.

Zwolan, T. A., Kileny, P. R., Ashbaugh, C., & Telian, S. A. (1996). Patient performance with the Cochlear Corporation "20 + 2" implant: Bipolar versus monopolar activation. *The American Journal of Otology, 17*(5), 717–723.

Chapter 16
Cochlear Implants: Pre-processing Strategies

Saji Maruthurkkara

Abstract Pre-processing strategies have led to the most significant improvements in speech perception in noise for cochlear implant recipients. These strategies: (a) enhance signals using wireless technologies, (b) isolate desired signals with beamforming, or (c) remove noise using broadband or spectral processing like automatic gain control, SNR-NR, ClearVoice, or wind noise reduction. The hearing device industry has rapidly developed new, highly effective technologies by leveraging innovations from the consumer device sector. Clinicians now have a wide array of pre-processing strategies to choose from. Understanding these technologies and their limitations is crucial for providing optimal care for cochlear implant recipients.

Keywords Automatic gain control · SNR · Clear voice · Wind noise · Wireless technologies · Beamforming

Introduction

A Cochlear Implant (CI) system works in four stages to stimulate the auditory nerve: (1) pre-processing, (2) sound coding, (3) radio frequency transmission, and (4) stimulation. The first two stages process sounds, the third stage transmits the processed sounds, and the final stage stimulates the auditory nerve. Pre-processing and sound coding play the most crucial roles in enhancing speech perception for a CI recipient. This chapter will focus on pre-processing, and a subsequent chapter will delve into sound coding (For more details, see Chap. 15).

In the bustling world that we live in, individuals with hearing impairment face even greater challenges in noisy environments including CI users compared to those with normal hearing (WHO, 2021). The main goal of any hearing device is to enhance the signal-to-noise ratio (SNR). There are two main ways to do this: (1)

S. Maruthurkkara (✉)
Cochlear Limited, Macquarie University, Sydney, NSW, Australia
e-mail: SMaruthurkkara@cochlear.com

P. Kumar et al. (eds.), *Advances in Implantation Otology*,
https://doi.org/10.1007/978-981-96-8671-1_16

enhancing the desired signal or (2) reducing unwanted noise. The best approach is often a mix of both the strategies.

Enhancing the Desired Signal

Enhancing the Signal by Collecting Close to the Source

The microphones that pick up the signals are typically located at the ear level. When a CI recipient listens to a person speaking in an environment with diffuse noise or noise coming from a specific location, moving closer to the speaker can enhance the signal. This adjustment increases the loudness of the desired signal relative to the background noise. It is a typical behaviour for individuals to lean towards the speaker when there is ambient noise. However, leaning towards or physically approaching a speaker may not always be practical. In such situations, an alternative approach is to 'collect signals closer to source', such as using a remote microphone to capture the desired signal directly from the speaker. The remote microphone then transmits the signals to the sound processor. Over the years, technology for collecting signals closer to the source or capturing only desired signals has evolved. Let's look at the evolution of some of these technologies and how they have changed over the years.

Lapel Microphones

Initially, wired lapel microphones were employed to collect signals closer to the source. They used a microphone to pick up the speaker's signal and transmit it via a long cable directly to the CI, thereby capturing the desired signals directly from the speaker without picking up environmental noise. However, practical limitations, such as the need for a cable between the speaker and the listener, hindered the adoption of this method in everyday life. Wireless methods for transmitting the signal from the remote microphone to the sound processor were required to make it practical.

Telecoil

The first wireless technology to collect desired signals close to the source was the use of telecoils (Fig. 16.1). A telecoil in the hearing device picks up electromagnetic signals that leak from a telephone receiver or a purpose-built loop system. Telecoils

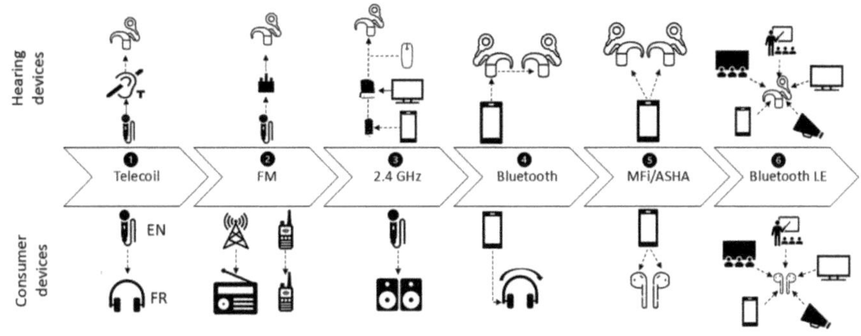

Fig. 16.1 Evolution of wireless technology to transmit audio signals in consumer devices and hearing devices. Dashed lines depict wireless transmission, and solid lines depict hardwired connections

have been a standard feature in hearing aids for decades, and several studies have shown improved speech perception in noise when telecoils have been used (Alfakir et al., 2015). However, the telecoil's frequency range typically spans from 200 Hz to 5000 Hz, and the lack of high-frequency signals can lead to deteriorated speech perception. Additionally, the telecoil's performance depends on its orientation within the hearing device or its position relative to the telephone receiver or loop, which is a hearing assistance system that uses a magnetic field to transmit sound directly to hearing devices. Signal quality diminishes as one moves away from the loop.

Furthermore, room loops are usually not portable, and the signal from one room's loop could spill over to an adjoining room. Interference from fluorescent lighting or electric power lines may distort the telecoil signal. Users must remember to switch on the telecoil to benefit from it, but sometimes they forget; thus, an auto-telecoil feature was introduced in the Nucleus® 6 sound processor (Cochlear Ltd), automatically activating the telecoil when a suitable electromagnetic signal is detected. While loop systems are available in public places like cinemas, airports, information counters, public transport, and taxis, their availability remains limited.

Loop systems were also used for normal-hearing individuals, providing immediate translation of presentations in different languages at international conferences (Katz, 2015). However, barring the limited use mentioned above, telecoil technology applications for normal-hearing people are quite constrained. Despite being a standard feature in hearing aids since the 1950s, telecoil technology hasn't seen significant advancements, likely due to its narrow scope of applications in the wider consumer device industry, as described by laws that govern economic principles.

Moore's Law (Moore, 1998) describes the exponential growth of computing power due to increasing transistor density on microchips. The law of supply and demand (Gale, 1955) states that as demand for a technology grows, its cost tends to decrease. These principles drive advancements, resulting in more efficient and accessible technology.

Two key factors drove the advancement of telephone technology: market forces and the shift to wireless communication. Initially, telephones were not widely popular due to limited accessibility. However, technological advancements ensued as market forces came into play and telephones transitioned into consumer devices. These improvements made telephones more affordable and significantly enhanced their performance. Additionally, the evolution of telephony from wired connections to wireless communication led to the advent of mobile phones, followed by smartphones and smartwatches. This proliferation of consumer devices further increased demand. Wireless technology emerged as a critical catalyst, propelling the industry forward.

Based on the number of devices sold, the hearing industry is a niche market compared to the vast consumer device market. Consequently, the hearing device industry alone does not have sufficient market force to drive technological growth. Fortunately, wireless audio transmission is a significant need in the consumer device industry, which has the necessary scale to create market forces that drive technological evolution. In other words, consumer-driven demand plays a pivotal role in realising the full potential of wireless audio technologies in hearing devices. Therefore, to understand the evolution of wireless audio technologies in the hearing device industry, it is essential first to understand their evolution in the consumer device space. Let's examine the evolution of wireless audio technology in both hearing and consumer devices. We will see that these technologies flourish in the hearing device space only when there is demand from the consumer device market.

Frequency Modulation (FM) Systems

The second generation of wireless audio, Frequency modulation (FM), came from the consumer device space (Fig. 16.1). FM is a popular method widely employed in walkie-talkies for telecommunication and radio broadcast systems for wirelessly transmitting audio signals with minimal distortion compared to other methods like amplitude modulation (AM). It involves transmitting data by altering the immediate frequency of a continuous wave. This technology was used in hearing devices with FM systems. It was widely used in schools where the teacher uses a remote microphone to transmit the signal wirelessly to one or more students in the classroom using an FM system connected to their hearing device. Research has demonstrated that using FM systems can significantly improve the speech perception in noise for CI recipients (Schafer et al., 2013). In the past, personal FM systems necessitated special adapters or cables to link the FM receiver with the sound processor. Unfortunately, this setup was cumbersome and error-prone due to the multiple connections involved. However, more recently, FM receivers have been purposefully designed for each sound processor, seamlessly integrating them. As a result, they are now user-friendly and less prone to errors. FM technology gained popularity primarily for radio listening in the consumer device realm. As a result, advancements were made in receiving FM signals. However, using microphones to capture sound from speakers and encode it into FM signals was less common in consumer devices. Consequently, this technology missed the technological innovations and economies of scale that benefited other consumer technologies.

2.4 GHz Wireless Transmission

The third generation of wireless audio transmission was a 2.4 gigahertz (GHz) signal, widely used in wireless microphones and Wi-Fi systems (Fig. 16.1). The 2.4 GHz signal operates at a higher frequency range (from 2.400 GHz to 2.483 GHz) compared to the FM system, which spans 72–76 MHz and 218–219 MHz. Due to its shorter wavelength, the 2.4 GHz signal can effectively penetrate molecular structures, making it more adept at passing through obstacles like walls and buildings. In contrast, FM signals are sensitive to reflection, rendering them less efficient when encountering walls.

Regulatory guidelines permit 2.4 GHz devices to transmit at higher power levels, enhancing their range and overall connectivity. Additionally, 2.4 GHz technology benefits from a broader range of transmission frequencies, providing more available channels. This reduces the likelihood of interference when multiple devices operate simultaneously. Despite congestion, 2.4 GHz devices can coexist harmoniously with Wi-Fi, Bluetooth, and other wireless technologies due to the abundance of available channels. These systems dynamically detect occupied frequencies and adjust their transmission to avoid interference. Globally accepted, the 2.4 GHz band simplifies international use. The 2.4 GHz systems have the potential to offer a higher SNR than FM systems due to their digital nature and techniques to reduce interference, leading to clearer audio transmission. In a commercially available public address system that utilises 2.4 GHz wireless audio technology, a wireless microphone captures the signal from the speaker, transmitting high-quality sound to a remote amplifier that reproduces the audio via loudspeakers. In the hearing device industry, this technology has been implemented across a wide range of wireless accessories, including the mini microphone, the TV streamer, and the phone clip. Studies that evaluated the benefits of a wireless, remote microphone accessory for CI recipients found that using the accessory significantly improved speech recognition in quiet and noise compared to using the CI sound processor alone (De Ceulaer et al., 2017; Wolfe et al., 2015). Other studies have found that using the Cochlear™ Wireless TV Streamer, which delivers audio signals directly to a CI sound processor from a television, significantly improved objectively measured speech recognition in quiet and noisy conditions compared to using the CI sound processor alone. Additionally, subjective reports indicated improved listening while watching TV, participating in conversations, and staying aware of surroundings (Duke et al., 2016; Neben, 2015). While 2.4 GHz wireless technology indeed offered significant improvements for audio streaming compared to earlier FM technology, its primary applications extended beyond audio streaming. It played a crucial role in data transfer, especially in Wi-Fi systems. Despite benefiting from economies of scale for data transmission, audio streaming capabilities did not receive the typical technological advantages associated with consumer device industry use due to their relatively limited application.

Bluetooth Classic

The fourth generation of wireless audio transmission was Bluetooth Classic (Fig. 16.1). Bluetooth Classic is an industry standard, wireless transmission technology that operates at 2.4 GHz. It offers more robust communication, improved security, and greater efficiency than its proprietary predecessors. While the earlier 2.4 GHz technology dynamically detects occupied frequencies and adjusts its transmission to avoid interference, Bluetooth Classic employs a superior frequency hopping spread spectrum (FHSS) technique. This method divides the available bandwidth into approximately 80 channels, and both devices follow a predetermined hopping sequence. This synchronisation ensures channel changes that prevent interference from other devices, such as Wi-Fi routers, microwaves, and cordless phones. Bluetooth Classic's FHSS approach enhances security, making it challenging for eavesdroppers to intercept data. Enhanced Data Rate (EDR), used in Bluetooth, enhances audio streaming quality by increasing the data rate. With faster transmission, EDR ensures smoother delivery of high-quality stereo audio. Essentially, it allows more data to flow between devices, reducing latency and enhancing the overall listening experience.

Bluetooth also introduced a more secure yet simple pairing method, where cryptographic keys are exchanged between devices. The pairing process involves device discovery, identification, authentication, and encryption. Older methods relied on PIN-based pairing, which was less secure. Bluetooth's affordability, low power consumption, compatibility, and ease of pairing contribute to its popularity across a wide range of consumer devices, including computers, mobile phones, and headphones.

Bluetooth Classic, however, transmitted audio for both the right and left ears together to the receiving device. The receiving device then separated the right and left audio signals to deliver stereo sound. This approach worked well for stereo systems, cars, and other setups where a hard wire connects the left and right speakers. However, when used in headphones, it requires a physical cable connecting the right and left earpieces. This technology was not widely implemented in hearing devices, where there are no physical connections between the right and left ears. In cases where it was used, the signal was sent to one hearing aid or sound processor, which then transmitted the signal to the other ear using a separate wireless connection. Unfortunately, this method increased the battery drain on the system.

Mfi and ASHA Proprietary Bluetooth Low-Energy

The next evolution—the fifth generation of wireless audio transmission, Bluetooth Low Energy—was popularised in the Made for iPhone (Mfi) feature in Apple AirPods (Fig. 16.1). Google later implemented this technology on Android devices using a protocol called Audio Streaming for Hearing Aids (ASHA). The technology enables faster data transfer rates, minimising the delay between sending audio data from a device and hearing it through headphones or speakers. This leads to smoother audio playback and better sound quality, especially when streaming high-quality music or videos. Additionally, this technology consumes less battery power because the connection remains dormant unless critical data is being shared. Furthermore, it features enhanced security protocols, making it more robust against potential vulnerabilities. Both Google and Apple technologies send separate signals to the left and right ears. As a result, new-generation earphones were developed without a cable connecting between the ears, making the earphones genuinely wireless. This innovation was also implemented in hearing aids, such as GN Resound hearing aids and the Nucleus 7 sound processor. The technology also allowed wireless audio streaming from iOS and Android devices to the sound processor and the contralateral hearing aid, enabling users to listen to music, watch videos, and make phone calls without intermediary devices. Before the advent of this technology, CI recipients had to rely on intermediary devices to connect their phones to the sound processor or use Bluetooth Classic. Phone calls can occur unexpectedly, and if the intermediary devices weren't set up correctly, the recipient would have to answer the call, explain to the caller that they were sorting out connection issues, and simultaneously troubleshoot the connection. This situation could lead to increased anxiety when a call came in and meant missing the first few moments of the conversation. However, with the current technology, there are no intermediate devices. Calls are directly routed to the sound processor, and recipients can answer them simply by tapping on their smartphone without fumbling with additional technology. A clinical study that evaluated direct audio streaming from a smartphone to the Nucleus 7 Sound Processor showed significant improvements in subjective benefits for hearing on the telephone while maintaining speech recognition in quiet and noise during standardised tests (Warren et al., 2019). This technology has opened up new avenues, including the ability to stream precisely calibrated audio signals. As a result, self-administered speech perception tests can now be conducted by directly streaming audio from a smartphone to the sound processor (Maruthurkkara et al., 2022).

Auracast Open Standard Audio Streaming

Since the introduction of truly wireless earbuds utilising proprietary Bluetooth Low Energy (BLE) technology in Apple and Android smartphones, wired headphones have largely been supplanted by wireless earbuds. This shift has engendered new habits among consumers. Many individuals now wear wireless earphones even when not actively listening to music or other audio. This behaviour has become commonplace due to the convenience and comfort offered by these devices. Whether for style, noise cancellation, or sheer habit, it is common to observe people with earbuds in their ears throughout the day. They may engage in everyday conversations while still wearing their earphones.

In the consumer device landscape, we are witnessing a proliferation of devices worn on the ear, poised for immediate audio consumption. This trend is driving the evolution of a new category of audio devices leveraging Auracast technology, the sixth generation of wireless audio transmission.

In June 2022, the Bluetooth special interest group established a new Bluetooth broadcast standard called Auracast, enabling users with BLE-compatible headphones to receive audio streams directly from sources such as TVs, cinemas, airports, and lecture theatres (Fig. 16.1). This innovative technology, designed for consumer devices, has already been implemented in several hearing aids, some over-the-counter hearing devices, and the Nucleus 8 sound processor. When a user is at an airport and wants to hear announcements specific to their gate, reception occurs seamlessly—there's no need to approach and handle a transmitting device for pairing physically. They open their phone, explore available broadcasts, and select their gate. It is akin to connecting to a Wi-Fi signal at an airport. Similarly, in a classroom setting, a person with an Auracast-enabled hearing device can receive the teacher's broadcast, while people with normal hearing can use Auracast-enabled headphones to receive the signal. The same principle applies to a cinema. Whether someone has a hearing impairment or normal hearing, everyone gains from the streamed audio. Compared with the proprietary Mfi and ASHA, Auracast employs stronger encryption protocols and better authentication mechanisms, enhancing privacy and security. By 2027, it is estimated that over three billion LE Audio-enabled devices will be on the market, incentivising approximately 2.5 million public venues to deploy Auracast broadcast transmitters globally by 2030 (ABI Research, 2022). The benefits of the proprietary Mfi and ASHA technology for listening on the telephone and streamed performance testing have already been proven (Maruthurkkara et al., 2022; Warren et al., 2019). However, these benefits are limited to streaming from personal smartphones or tablets. As Auracast technology becomes more widely available, CI recipients using compatible sound processors stand to benefit further as they can easily listen to streamed signals from various sources.

Enhancing the Signal by Collecting Only Desired Signals

Unfortunately, providing a remote microphone to a speaker may not always be practical, especially during brief interactions like those at a shop checkout or in group settings with multiple speakers. In such cases, an alternative approach is 'collecting only desired signals.' In the situations mentioned above, the listener instinctively looks at the speaker. By selecting signals only from the direction where the listener's head is oriented, the desired signal can be made clearer while still being captured by ear-level microphones.

Single Directional Microphones

A microphone has a diaphragm that moves in response to changes in air pressure caused by sound waves. This mechanical energy from the movement of the diaphragm is converted into an electrical signal using various methods, such as dynamic microphones (moving coil), ribbon microphones, or condenser microphones. Typically, microphones have a single port to capture sounds; this design captures sound waves from all directions, and such microphones are called omnidirectional microphones. Directional microphones have ports on both sides of the diaphragm. Sounds from the front and back are picked up well, but sounds from directions in the plane of the diaphragm produce no movement. The opposing forces cancel each other out, resulting in no sound being picked up from these directions. This design helps reduce the pickup of noise from certain directions. A polar plot is a circular graph that shows how a microphone responds to sounds coming from different directions. Figure 16.2 shows the polar plot with directional microphones. The distance from the centre represents the strength of the response: the farther from the centre, the stronger the response. The plot illustrates how the microphone's sensitivity changes as the sound source moves around it in a 360-degree circle. Polar plots are useful for visualising the directional characteristics of microphones. Directional microphones have a hypercardioid polar pattern (Fig. 16.2) where there is higher response from the front (0°) and the back (180°) and lower sensitivity to signals (noise) from the sides (90° & 270°).

The first commercial use of directional microphones in the 1940s was for cinema, TV, and radio. Directional mics were used in behind-the-ear style hearing aids from the 1960s. Studies comparing hearing aids with directional and omnidirectional microphones found that directional microphones perform better in noisy environments, with no significant disadvantages noted by hearing-impaired users (Mueller & Johnson, 1979; Nielsen & Ludvigsen, 1978). However, with the rise of in-the-ear and in-the-canal hearing aids in the 1980s, where the back of the microphone was inside the ear canal, the use of directional mics became impractical (Bentler, 2005).

Multiple Mic Beamforming

Directional microphones primarily reduce noise from the sides, resulting in a hypercardioid polar pattern. Often, the listener is more interested in capturing the signal from the front while minimising interfering noise from the sides and those from

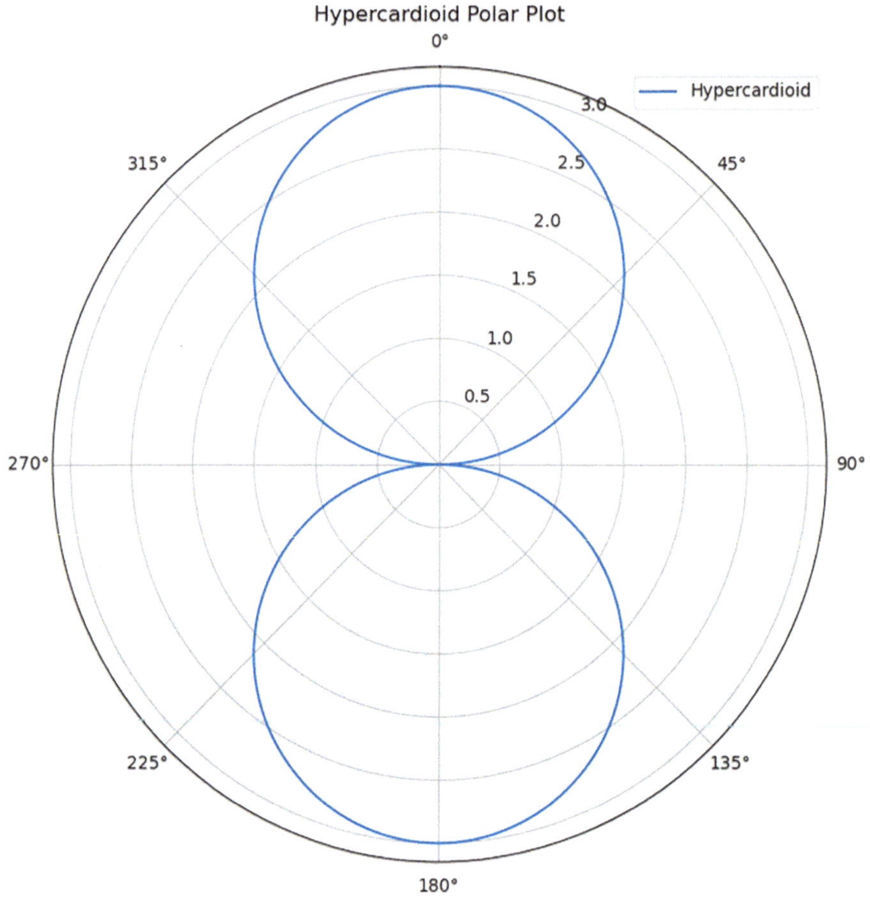

Fig. 16.2 Polar plot showing a single directional microphone's hypercardioid microphone response at all angles

behind. Beamforming is a technology that enhances front-facing signals while effectively reducing rear interference. To understand how this technology works, one must consider the principle of beamforming. Beamforming requires two microphones. When a signal originates from the front, there is a slight delay in the sound reaching the back microphone compared to the front microphone. This delay allows the system to determine that the sound is coming from the front. Conversely, when the sound comes from the side, there is no delay between the front and back microphones, enabling the system to identify the sound's lateral origin. When the sound arrives at an angle, there is a relative difference in the timing of the signal between the front and back microphones. By analysing this delay, the system can determine the sound's direction within a 360-degree range. The most advantageous aspect of this technology is the ability to dictate the system's response. By applying appropriate delays to sounds from specific angles, one can create a "null point," where no sound is picked up. Two types of beamforming technologies based on polar plots are fixed directionality and adaptive directionality beamforming.

Fixed Directionality Beamforming

In fixed directionality beamforming technologies, the system's response is designed to significantly attenuate the noise from the rear and the null points are set to static positions at the rear. Figure 16.3a shows the polar plot with the fixed directionality beamforming technology called 'Zoom' in Nucleus sound processors. Here, the speaker is positioned in front of the listener (0°), and there is maximum signal strength from this angle. The noise from the back (180°) is attenuated by 10 dB, and no sound is picked up at the null points. Early sound processors featured omnidirectional microphones that capture sounds from all directions, making them useful in quiet settings for picking up background sounds like microwave ping. Still, they can hinder speech perception in noisy environments by also collecting background noise. Fixed directionality beamforming technologies, such as Zoom, have been shown to enhance speech perception in noisy environments compared to omnidirectional microphones (Wolfe et al., 2012). Studies reveal that there are significant enhancements in speech perception scores in an S0NCI scenario, where speech is delivered from the front (0°) and noise is directed to the cochlear implant (CI) side. MED-EL's natural directionality setting shows a 3.4 dB improvement, Advanced Bionics' T-Mic, which functions similarly to the fixed directionality setting of Real Ear Sound, provides a 1.2 dB enhancement, and Cochlear's Zoom technology offers an improvement of 6.0 dB (Sivonen et al., 2020).

ForwardFocus is a new fixed directionality beamforming technology in Nucleus sound processors that increases microphone sensitivity to sounds in front while significantly reducing sensitivity to sounds from the rear (Fig. 16.3b). As a result, ForwardFocus significantly improves speech perception in noisy environments compared to other microphone directionality settings, especially when the noise comes from behind (Hey et al., 2019; Jones et al., 2023).

Adaptive Beamforming

In adaptive beamforming systems, the technology is designed to greatly reduce noise from the rear while dynamically adjusting null points based on the highest noise levels. Figure 16.3c, d, e & f displays the polar plots for the adaptive directionality beamforming technology called 'Beam' in Nucleus sound processors. In this configuration, the speaker is placed directly in front of the listener (0°), ensuring the strongest signal from this direction. The null points, where sound is not picked up, are adjusted to various directions (Fig. 16.3c–f) depending on the noise source's location. These adaptive beamforming technologies are particularly effective in

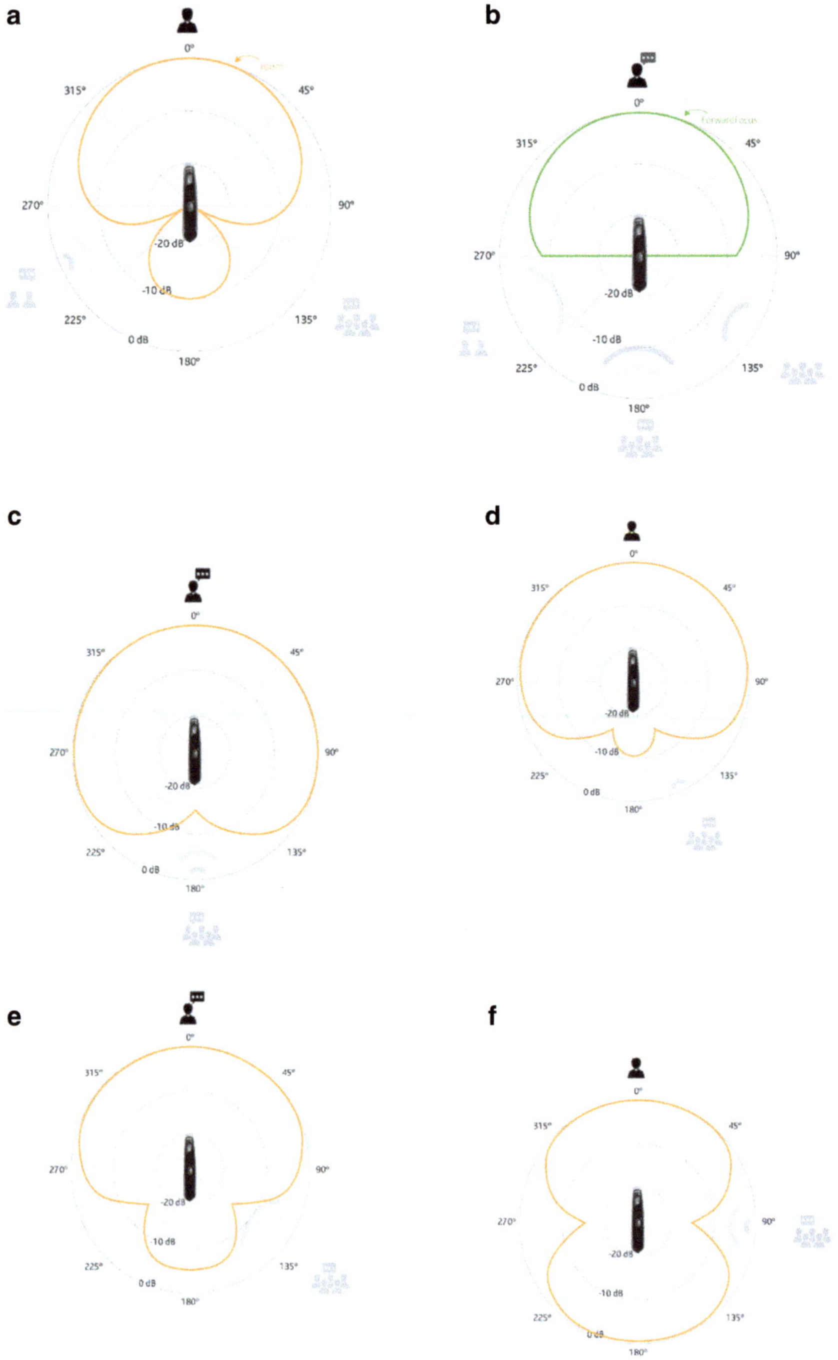

Fig. 16.3 Polar plots showing the microphone response at all angles for (**a**) Zoom and (**b**) forward focus with fixed directionality and (**c–f**) BEAM with adaptive directionality beamformer in Nucleus CI systems. The listener is depicted as a person in black, and the noise is depicted as a group of people in grey

challenging environments, such as restaurants or busy streets, where the direction of sound or noise can change significantly (Hersbach et al., 2012). Research indicates that there are notable improvements in speech perception scores in an S0NCI condition, where speech is presented at 0°, and noise is directed to the CI side. Specifically, MED-EL's adaptive directionality setting shows an improvement of 3.7 dB, Advanced Bionics' UltraZoom achieves an 11.0 dB improvement, and Cochlear's Beam® technology leads with a 12.7 dB improvement (Sivonen et al., 2020).

Scene Analysis

In the early days of sound processors, multiple program locations were available, allowing clinicians to save different noise reduction settings in each program. Users were instructed to switch programs as needed in various noisy environments. However, this required users to remember the purpose of each program. Clinicians often provided written instructions or small cards to help recipients recall which program to use. To address this, a remote assistant with a digital display was developed for the Nucleus 5 sound processor, clearly showing the label for each program. Despite this improvement, users still needed to manually change programs in challenging listening environments, which could be easily forgotten or sometimes embarrassing or cumbersome to do. Studies indicate that users of multiple memory hearing aids are likely to manually switch programs only if they can identify their current listening environment, understand the differences between settings, perceive a clear benefit from the new setting, are motivated to make the switch, and frequently encounter challenging listening situations that help them remember the appropriate settings and develop quick methods for changing programs (de Graaff et al., 2018). Therefore, even with multiple programs available, CI recipients might not manually switch programs in challenging listening environments. Implementing more automatic switching methods could be beneficial. Contemporary sound processors are equipped with automatic scene classifiers that identify the user's current environment. The SCAN program in Nucleus sound processors can detect six different environments: quiet, speech, noise, speech in noise, wind, or music. SCAN then automatically adjusts the directionality settings, such as standard, zoom, or Beam, or activates the wind noise reduction algorithm, eliminating the need for the user to change the settings manually. Similar automatic scene classifiers are available in Advanced Bionics and MED-EL sound processors, called AutoSound OS and Adaptive Sound Management. Clinical studies have shown that automatic scene analysis programs, which automatically select the appropriate microphone directionality settings like SCAN, significantly enhance speech understanding in various listening environments, resulting in successful user acceptance (Mauger et al., 2014).

Removing Unwanted Noise

The previous section, 'enhancing the desired signal,' discussed techniques for isolating the desired signal, either by capturing it close to the source or by collecting signals from the direction the listener is facing. However, since the main objective is to improve speech perception, the captured signal may still contain unwanted noise mixed with the desired speech. Therefore, additional methods are necessary to eliminate this noise. Two approaches to remove unwanted noise are broadband processing and spectral processing.

Removing the Noise Using Broadband Processing

Broadband processing entails eliminating all signals that fall outside the typical intensity range of speech. Another technique, spectral processing, focuses on isolating the desired speech signals within the specified intensity range and removing noise through spectral analysis, and will be explored further in the next subsection.

Input Dynamic Range (IDR)

People with normal hearing can generally detect sounds as quiet as 0 dB and tolerate sounds up to 100 dB. This span is known as the dynamic range (DR) and is about 100 dB for normal-hearing people. The DR is much narrower for electrical hearing, typically ranging from 3 to 20 dB (Moore, 2003). Within this range, individuals with normal hearing can distinguish between small steps in loudness, unlike those using CIs, who may have significantly fewer discernible loudness steps. In hearing aids, the entire range of input sounds from 0 to 100 dB is compressed into the output delivered through the receiver. However, in CI sound processors, compressing this range into the narrow DR available for electrical hearing would result in a poor auditory experience due to the lower hearing resolution. Therefore, the intensity range of the incoming signals must be adjusted to fit within the narrow DR available for CI stimulation.

Fortunately, the long-term average spectrum of conversational speech is approximately 30 dB (Byrne et al., 1994), meaning that very soft sounds do not significantly contribute to speech perception and can be disregarded. These low-level sounds are also likely to be masked by unwanted noise. Thus, instead of encoding the entire 0 to 100 dB range within the electrical DR, only a narrow DR of relevant signals is presented into the electrical DR. In Nucleus sound processors, the quietest sound chosen for stimulation is known as the threshold sound pressure level (T-SPL). Input signals at T-SPL are used for stimulation at T levels. The signal's loudness is increased following a loudness growth curve until it reaches a comfortable sound

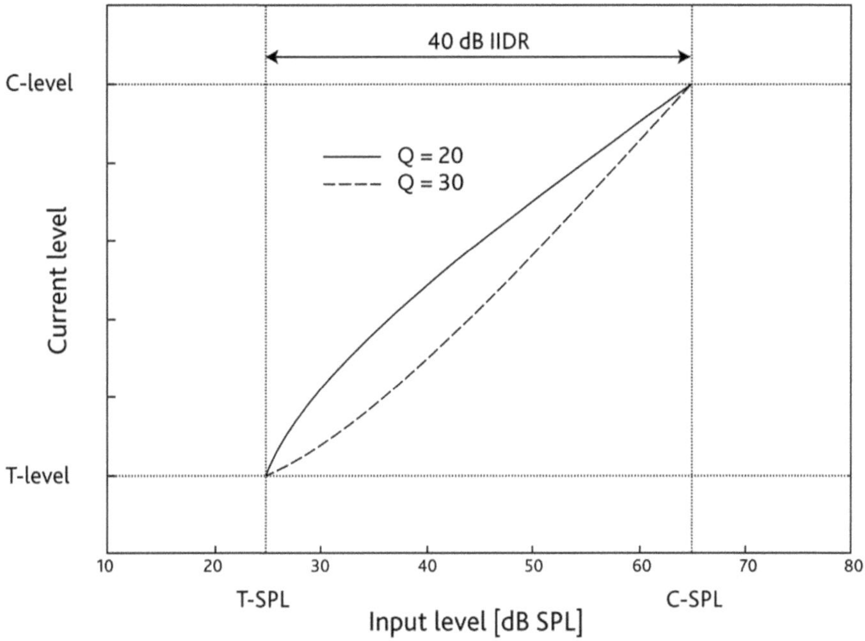

Fig. 16.4 Loudness growth

pressure level (C-SPL). Sounds at C-SPL are used for stimulation at the C level, while louder sounds beyond C-SPL undergo infinite compression and are also used for C-level stimulation.

In Nucleus sound processors, the default sensitivity setting places T-SPL and C-SPL at 25 dB and 65 dB, respectively. However, clinicians can adjust the instantaneous IDR (IIDR) to meet the CI recipient's needs during programming. For instance, if soft sounds are not audible even after adjusting T and C levels and using input processing options, the T-SPL can be lowered from 25 dB to 20 dB. Clinicians can also modify the loudness growth by changing the Q value. By default, Nucleus sound processors use a nearly linear loudness growth function (Q value of 20), as illustrated in Fig. 16.4. In other CI systems as well, a specific range of input sounds is also selected for stimulation. The IIDR is referred to as the "adaptive sound window" in MED-EL CI systems and the "input dynamic range" in Advanced Bionics CI systems.

Automatic Gain Control

In everyday life, many sounds occur at the same loudness level as conversational speech. However, we often encounter louder sounds from sources like blenders, hair dryers, and toilet flushes, or unexpectedly from an alarm clock, a baby crying, dishes clattering, or a door banging. Fast-acting automatic gain control (AGC) is used in hearing aids and all brands of CI sound processors to quickly reduce signal intensity when very loud sounds are detected. The system then gradually returns the intensity to previous levels once the loud sounds have passed. Sometimes, the environment remains consistently loud, such as at a rock concert, a busy restaurant, a school cafeteria, a bustling video arcade, or noisy industrial areas. In these situations, most brands of CI sound processors use a slow-acting AGC to make it easier to understand speech. This approach provides a smoother and more comfortable listening experience in such noisy environments. Since AGC applies to all sounds regardless of their spectral characteristics, it serves as another example of noise removal through broadband processing. Studies with hearing aids (Moore et al., 1991) and CI (Stöbich et al., 1999) have shown that the combination of slow and fast-acting AGCs helps improve speech perception for the listener.

Auto-Sensitivity (ASC)

As mentioned in the IDR section, a range of relevant sounds for speech perception, between T-SPL of 25 dB and C-SPL of 65 dB, is presented for stimulation within the electrical DR. This range of sounds (25–65 dB) may be relevant in a quiet environment; however, in a loud, noisy environment, low-level speech signals may be masked by the noise. People in such environments naturally raise their voices to be heard above the noise floor. In these situations, the default IDR sound window may not be suitable. The IDR can be adjusted using the microphone sensitivity setting (Fig. 16.5), while the instantaneous input dynamic range (IIDR)-the difference

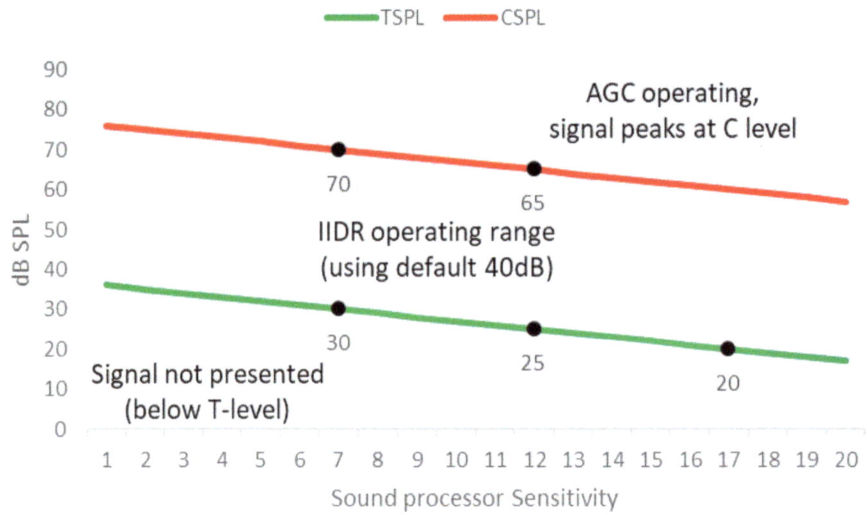

Fig. 16.5 Effect of microphone sensitivity on the IDR

between C-SPL and T-SPL-remains constant to ensure the recipient's audible range is consistent. When the microphone sensitivity is reduced from the default value of 12 to 7 in Nucleus sound processors, the IDR window shifts the T-SPL from 25 dB to 30 dB, meaning that all low-level noise up to 30 dB is ignored. The C-SPL changes from 65 dB to 70 dB, meaning that the sounds of people yelling over the noise will be captured and presented to the electrical DR. The CI recipient can adjust the microphone sensitivity using a remote control or a smartphone app. However, manually adjusting the sensitivity requires the user first to identify the type of environment they are in and then make the necessary adjustments, both of which can be pretty demanding. Autosensitivity (ASC) is a technology that automatically adjusts the microphone sensitivity based on the sound level in the environment. ASC is a slow-acting automatic volume control (AVC) algorithm that detects the level of stationary background noise in the environment and adjusts the sensitivity accordingly. When the noise floor exceeds 57 dB SPL, ASC lowers the microphone sensitivity to minimise the noise's impact. Clinicians can customise ASC for a CI recipient by adjusting the ASC breakpoint. They can decrease it from the default value of 57 dB SPL if the background noise is too loud or bothersome or increase it if ASC makes the desired signal too soft. A clinical study has shown that using ASC in Nucleus sound processors significantly enhances speech perception in noisy environments (Wolfe et al., 2009). Similar AVC algorithms are also used in MED-EL and Advanced Bionics sound processors.

Whisper™

As mentioned in the ASC section, reducing the microphone sensitivity manually or automatically in noisy environments can help mitigate the effects of low-level noise. However, in a quiet environment, one might need to increase the microphone sensitivity to better hear a speaker talking softly or from a distance. As shown in Fig. 16.5, when the microphone sensitivity is increased from the default value of 12 to 17, the T-SPL decreases from 25 dB to 20 dB, making soft speech at 20 dB audible. However, increasing sensitivity also amplifies other soft, unwanted noises, such as the sound of brushing against clothes. Adjusting the remote control or smartphone app can be challenging when already struggling to hear a speaker. The Whisper setting in Nucleus sound processors, which the recipient can manually select, provides quick access to softer speech sounds by boosting them by 10 dB. Clinical studies have shown significant improvement in speech understanding in quiet environments when using the Whisper setting (McDermott et al., 2002).

Removing the Noise Using Spectral Processing

As described in the previous section, broadband processing analyses the signal across all frequencies to isolate the typical intensity range of speech, discarding signals outside this range. However, unwanted noise may still be present within the speech range alongside the desired speech signal. Spectral processing can further reduce this noise by performing spectral analysis, emphasising frequencies associated with the desired signals and deemphasising those with higher noise levels. After the beamforming and broadband processing stages, the signal captured from the microphones is divided into multiple channels according to its frequency using a filterbank. Several methods have been employed for spectral processing in CI sound processors.

Adaptive Dynamic Range Optimisation (ADRO)

ADRO, or adaptive dynamic range optimisation used in Nucleus CI, is an adaptive algorithm designed to adjust the gain in each channel to ensure the signal remains audible and comfortable. It operates with predefined targets for audibility and comfort, determining the optimal range for sound levels. When the signal in any channel falls below the audibility target, ADRO increases the channel gain to make the sound audible. Conversely, if the signal exceeds the comfort target, ADRO decreases the channel gain to prevent discomfort. ADRO continuously monitors the incoming audio signal and dynamically adjusts the gain in real time to maintain the balance between audibility and comfort. By adjusting the gain based on the signal levels, ADRO helps manage background noise, making it easier to hear soft speech in quiet environments and speech in noisy conditions. Clinical studies (Dawson et al., 2004; James et al., 2002) have demonstrated that ADRO enhances the perception of soft speech in quiet environments as well as speech in noisy conditions.

Signal to Noise Ratio-Noise Reduction (SNR-NR)

While ADRO enhances audibility and reduces noise through spectral processing, it does so without distinguishing whether the signal in each channel is speech or noise. In contrast, SNR-NR, used in Nucleus CI, employs advanced algorithms to analyse incoming sounds, actively monitor the SNR in each channel, and identify noise-dominated frequency bands. It then reduces the gain in these noisy bands to minimise the impact of noise. SNR-NR has been shown to improve speech perception in environments with constant background noise, such as traffic or machinery noise (Mauger et al., 2012).

ClearVoice is an algorithm in Advanced Bionics CI that operates similarly to SNR-NR. It automatically analyses the listening environment and separates speech from background noise. By reducing the gain in frequency bands dominated by noise, ClearVoice makes speech clearer and easier to understand. Research indicates that ClearVoice greatly enhances speech understanding in noisy settings for cochlear implant users, who favour these settings and express high levels of satisfaction (Buechner et al., 2010; Kam et al., 2012). Ambient noise reduction is an algorithm in MED-EL cochlear implants that operates similarly to SNR-NR and has been shown to improve speech perception (Kurz et al., 2022).

Wind Noise Reduction (WNR)

CI users often experience wind noise during outdoor activities like walking, jogging, or cycling, especially on windy days or at higher speeds. Other everyday situations include driving with windows down, being in open spaces such as parks or beaches, engaging in sports like sailing or skiing, and walking through city streets with tall buildings that create wind tunnels. These conditions can make it challenging to hear essential sounds and speech. The microphones on sound processors are oriented forward to capture sounds from the front more effectively. However, when the user faces the wind, it can create turbulence around the microphones, leading to wind noise. Wind noise generally falls within the low-frequency range and tends to worsen when directional microphones are employed (Chung, 2012). Fortunately, multi-microphone technology can identify wind noise by detecting increased turbulence at one microphone compared to another. WNR algorithms implemented in Nucleus, MED-EL and Advanced Bionics sound processors are designed to enhance listening comfort in windy conditions. They work by switching to an omnidirectional microphone response and lowering the gain in low-frequency channels. WNR has been proven to improve speech perception for Nucleus and MED-EL CI users in windy environments (Goorevich et al., 2012; Hagen et al., 2020).

In noisy environments, hearing device users face more significant listening challenges than those with normal hearing. Pre-processing strategies play the most significant role in CI systems by enhancing the SNR. Over the years, methods to collect signals closer to the source have evolved from cumbersome wired lapel microphones to modern Auracast open standard audio streaming. These advancements, driven by the consumer device industry, have significantly improved SNR.

Strategies to capture only the desired signals have advanced from hardwired fixed directionality microphones to technologies that automatically adjust directionality patterns based on scene classifier analysis. Additionally, broadband spectral processing techniques further eliminate unwanted noise from the collected signals, enhancing speech perception in noisy environments.

Today's pre-processing strategies are highly effective in optimising speech perception for individuals with hearing impairments in various challenging listening situations. Future technological advancements will likely continue this trend of innovation in pre-processing technologies. However, clinicians have the authority to disable these settings based on their clinical judgment. Therefore, it is important for clinicians to make these powerful technologies accessible to CI recipients who need so that their hearing performance can be optimized.

References

ABI Research. (2022). *The Future of Bluetooth® Audio*. https://www.bluetooth.com/blog/le-audio-auracast-broadcast-audio-and-the-future-of-bluetooth-audio/

Alfakir, R., Holmes, A. E., Kricos, P. B., Gaeta, L., & Martin, S. (2015). Evaluation of speech perception via the use of hearing loops and telecoils. *Gerontology and Geriatric Medicine, 1*, 233372141559193.

Bentler, R. A. (2005). Effectiveness of directional microphones and noise reduction schemes in hearing aids: A systematic review of the evidence. *Journal of the American Academy of Audiology, 16*(7), 473–484.

Buechner, A., Brendel, M., Saalfeld, H., Litvak, L., Frohne-Buechner, C., & Lenarz, T. (2010). Results of a pilot study with a signal enhancement algorithm for HiRes 120 cochlear implant users. *Otology & Neurotology, 31*(9), 1386–1390.

Byrne, D., Dillon, H., Tran, K., Arlinger, S., Wilbraham, K., Cox, R., Hagerman, B., Hetu, R., Kei, J., Lui, C., Kiessling, J., Kotby, M. N., Nasser, N. H. A., El Kholy, W. A. H., Nakanishi, Y., Oyer, H., Powell, R., Stephens, D., Meredith, R., et al. (1994). An international comparison of long-term average speech spectra. *The Journal of the Acoustical Society of America, 96*(4), 2108–2120.

Chung, K. (2012). Wind noise in hearing aids: II. Effect of microphone directivity. *International Journal of Audiology, 51*(1), 29–42.

Dawson, P. W., Decker, J. A., & Psarros, C. E. (2004). Optimising dynamic range in children using the nucleus cochlear implant. *Ear and Hearing, 25*(3), 230–241.

De Ceulaer, G., Pascoal, D., Vanpoucke, F., & Govaerts, P. J. (2017). The use of cochlear's SCAN and wireless microphones to improve speech understanding in noise with the Nucleus6® CP900 processor. *International Journal of Audiology, 56*(11), 837–843.

de Graaff, F., Huysmans, E., Ket, J. C. F., Merkus, P., Goverts, S. T., Leemans, C. R., & Smits, C. (2018). Is there evidence for the added value and correct use of manual and automatically switching multimemory hearing devices? A scoping review. *International Journal of Audiology, 57*(3), 176–183.

Duke, M. M., Wolfe, J., & Schafer, E. (2016). Recognition of speech from the television with use of a wireless technology designed for cochlear implants. *Journal of the American Academy of Audiology, 27*(5), 388–394.

Gale, D. (1955). Law of supply and demand. *Mathematica Scandinavica, 3*, 155–169.

Goorevich, M., Zakis, J. A., Case, S., Harvey, T. I., Holmberg, P., Schall, F. S. J., Heasman, J., & Knight, M. (2012). Effect of a wind noise reduction algorithm on cochlear implant sound processing. In *12th international conference on cochlear implants and other implantable technologies*. Baltimore: John Hopkins Medical School.

Hagen, R., Radeloff, A., Stark, T., Anderson, I., Nopp, P., Aschbacher, E., Möltner, A., Khajehnouri, Y., & Rak, K. (2020). Microphone directionality and wind noise reduction enhance speech perception in users of the MED-EL SONNET audio processor. *Cochlear Implants International, 21*(1), 53–65.

Hersbach, A. A., Arora, K., Mauger, S. J., & Dawson, P. W. (2012). Combining directional microphone and single-channel noise reduction algorithms. *Ear and Hearing, 33*(4), e13–e23.

Hey, M., Hocke, T., Böhnke, B., & Mauger, S. J. (2019). ForwardFocus with cochlear implant recipients in spatially separated and fluctuating competing signals–introduction of a reference metric. *International Journal of Audiology, 58*(12), 869–878.

James, C. J., Blamey, P. J., Martin, L., Swanson, B., Just, Y., & Macfarlane, D. (2002). Adaptive dynamic range optimisation for cochlear implants: A preliminary study. *Ear and Hearing, 23*(1 SUPPL), 49S–58S.

Jones, M., Warren, C., Mashal, M., Greenham, P., & Wyss, J. (2023). Speech understanding in noise for cochlear implant recipients using a spatial noise reduction setting in an off the ear sound processor with directional microphones. *Cochlear Implants International, 24*(6), 311–324.

Kam, A. C. S., Ng, I. H. Y., Cheng, M. M. Y., Wong, T. K. C., & Tong, M. C. F. (2012). Evaluation of the ClearVoice strategy in adults using hiresolution fidelity 120 sound processing. *Clinical and Experimental Otorhinolaryngology, 5*(SUPPL. 1), 89–92.

Katz, J. (2015). In J. Katz, M. Chasin, K. English, L. J. Hood, & K. L. Tillery (Eds.), *Handbook of clinical audiology* (7th ed.). Wolters Kluwer Health.

Kurz, A., Rak, K., & Hagen, R. (2022). Improved performance with automatic sound management 3 in the MED-EL SONNET 2 cochlear implant audio processor. *PLoS One, 17*(9 September), 1–23.

Maruthurkkara, S., Case, S., & Rottier, R. (2022). Evaluation of remote check: A clinical tool for asynchronous monitoring and triage of cochlear implant recipients. *Ear and Hearing, 43*(2), 495–506.

Mauger, S. J., Dawson, P. W., & Hersbach, A. A. (2012). Perceptually optimised gain function for cochlear implant signal-to-noise ratio based noise reduction. *The Journal of the Acoustical Society of America, 131*(1), 327–336.

Mauger, S. J., Warren, C. D., Knight, M. R., Goorevich, M., & Nel, E. (2014). Clinical evaluation of the Nucleus ® 6 cochlear implant system: Performance improvements with SmartSound iQ. *International Journal of Audiology, 53*, 564–576.

McDermott, H. J., Henshall, K. R., & McKay, C. M. (2002). Benefits of syllabic input compression for users of cochlear implants. *Journal of the American Academy of Audiology, 13*(1), 14–24.

Moore, G. E. (1998). Cramming more components onto integrated circuits. *Proceedings of the IEEE, 86*(1), 82–85.

Moore, B. C. J. (2003). Coding of sounds in the auditory system and its relevance to signal processing and coding in cochlear implants. *Otol Neurotol.* 24(2):243–54. https://doi.org/10.1097/00129492-200303000-00019.

Moore, B. C. J., Glasberg, B. R., & Stone, M. A. (1991). Optimisation of a slow-acting automatic gain control system for use in hearing aids. *British Journal of Audiology, 25*(3), 171–182.

Mueller, H. G., & Johnson, R. M. (1979). The effects of various front-to-back ratios on the performance of directional microphone hearing aids. *Journal of the American Auditory Society, 5*(1), 30–34.

Neben, N. (2015). Take-home experience with the TV streamer for the application in experienced cochlear implant recipients. *Journal of International Advanced Otology, 11*(May), 64.

Nielsen, H. B., & Ludvigsen, C. (1978). Effect of hearing aids with directional microphones in different acoustic environments. *Scandinavian Audiology, 7*(4), 217–224.

Schafer, E. C., Huynh, C., Romine, D., & Jimenez, R. (2013). Speech recognition and subjective perceptions of neck-loop FM receivers with cochlear implants. *American Journal of Audiology, 22*(1), 53–64.

Sivonen, V., Willberg, T., Aarnisalo, A. A., & Dietz, A. (2020). The efficacy of microphone directionality in improving speech recognition in noise for three commercial cochlear-implant systems. *Cochlear Implants International, 21*(3), 153–159.

Stöbich, B., Zierhofer, C. M., & Hochmair, E. S. (1999). Influence of automatic gain control parameter settings on speech understanding of cochlear implant users employing the continuous interleaved sampling strategy. *Ear and Hearing, 20*(2), 104–116.

Warren, C. D., Nel, E., & Boyd, P. J. (2019). Controlled comparative clinical trial of hearing benefit outcomes for users of the Cochlear™ Nucleus ® 7 Sound Processor with mobile connectivity. *Cochlear Implants International, 20*(3), 116–126.

WHO. (2021). World report on hearing. In *World report 2021*. https://doi.org/10.2307/j.ctvndv9bj

Wolfe, J., Schafer, E. C., Heldner, B., Mülder, H., Ward, E., & Vincent, B. (2009). Evaluation of speech recognition in noise with cochlear implants and dynamic FM. *Journal of the American Academy of Audiology, 20*(7), 409–421.

Wolfe, J., Parkinson, A., Schafer, E. C., Gilden, J., Rehwinkel, K., Mansanares, J., Coughlan, E., Wright, J., Torres, J., & Gannaway, S. (2012). Benefit of a commercially available cochlear implant processor with dual-microphone beamforming: A multi-center study. *Otology & Neurotology, 33*(4), 553–560.

Wolfe, J., Morais, M., & Schafer, E. (2015). Improving hearing performance for cochlear implant recipients with use of a digital, wireless, remote-microphone, audio-streaming accessory. *Journal of the American Academy of Audiology, 26*(6), 532–539. https://doi.org/10.3766/jaaa.15005

Chapter 17
Cochlear Implants: Psychophysical Measures from Activation to Long-Term Management

Saji Maruthurkkara

Abstract Cochlear implant aftercare is essential for optimal hearing outcomes, involving device programming, hearing optimization, contralateral hearing aid adjustment, goal setting, performance monitoring, and ongoing support. Initial activation focuses on audibility and acceptance using methods like ECAP-based, population mean-based, thresholds-based, and ESRT-based fitting. Innovations such as profile scaling and loudness acclimatization enhance the process. Follow-up sessions optimize outcomes using traditional psychophysical methods or innovative approaches like master volume bass and treble adjustments, all based on hearing aid fitting principles. Long-term management includes in-clinic, remote, and self-care to sustain outcomes and address unexpected issues, with innovations like remote check.

Keywords ECAP · Mapping · Input dynamic range · ESRT · T level · C level

Introduction

The audiological care after the surgery for cochlear implantation involves several steps which assist recipients achieve best possible outcome and sustain this over their lifetime. This includes device programming and instruction, hearing optimisation, goal setting and performance monitoring, and ongoing counselling and support. The cochlear implant (CI) recipient's hearing journey starts with an 'initial activation'—the day they receive their first implantable device. There is some programming involved to get them started on their hearing journey. In the early months, more program optimization and fine-tuning of the programs are required (also known as maps). Over time, the map matures, becoming relatively stable and requiring minimal changes. During this phase of their journey, the CI recipient's needs

S. Maruthurkkara (✉)
Cochlear Limited, Macquarie University, Sydney, NSW, Australia
e-mail: SMaruthurkkara@cochlear.com

P. Kumar et al. (eds.), *Advances in Implantation Otology*,
https://doi.org/10.1007/978-981-96-8671-1_17

change, and they may become interested in getting more out of real-world hearing. Clinicians may use different tools to help patients achieve real-world hearing during this stage, which could differ from the tools used to optimize the map. For example, clinicians may consider using wireless accessories. Eventually, when the map is optimized and recipients know how to use their device and associated accessories, they may seek ways to maximize their hearing performance. At this stage the clinician's role may involve habilitation activities or training in communication strategies. One might rely on different tools, such as the hearing tracker that monitors the time spent listening to speech. Ultimately, the long-term goal is to provide lifetime monitoring and support, and clinicians may use tools like Remote Check.

The recipients' needs to keep changing throughout their journey; consequently, the objective of sessions with the recipient also shifts, necessitating a change in the tools employed. As the goals of the recipient change, the knowledge, skills and tools required by the clinician also need to change and adapt accordingly. This chapter will review the process involved in the initial activation, follow-up appointments and long-term management of CI recipients.

Initial Activation

Initial activation is that moment when a CI recipient acquires new hearing, as well as a new sound processor. This process can be conducted as early as the next day, or more typically 1–2 weeks after surgery when any swelling has reduced and the CI recipient has fully recovered from the effects of the surgical procedure (Parker et al., 2024). The recipient's goals for that day are to hear and learn how to use their new sound processor. At initial activation, the primary goal is comfortable audibility of sound, and importantly, facilitate acceptance of the device to get started on the electric hearing journey. The clinician should first review any surgical report and intra-operative measurements (if available) and then check impedances to ensure that the electrodes have been placed successfully in the cochlea and are functional. After aligning expectations and objectives and instructing the CI recipient about the tasks involved, device activation can commence. An essential task for clinicians involves creating a customized program, often referred to as a 'map.' This map defines the Threshold (T) level, which represents the minimum levels necessary to produce auditory sensations for each electrode. In Medel CIs, this level is denoted as THR. Going forward, we will refer to it as the *T level*. Additionally, the map specifies the maximum comfortable loudness level for each electrode, known by various terms such as *M level*, *MCL*, or *C level*. In this chapter, we will use the term *C level* for this purpose. However, the map created at the initial activation is never the only map the recipients will ever have, and neither is it the most perfect map they will ever have. Initially, they may not be able to tolerate loud sounds and thus not tolerate higher C levels, but over time they will acquire tolerance to louder sounds and therefore higher C levels. Similarly, the recipients' responses to T levels in the early stages of their hearing journey may not be accurate, but over time as they learn the task better and with improved listening skills, the T levels will change. As their hearing keeps evolving, so will their map.

As indicated previously, the objective of the initial activation is not to make the perfect map. Instead, it is to allow the recipients to achieve some level of audibility and, more importantly, help them accept the device to get them started on their hearing journey. Thus, during initial activation, it is a good idea for the clinician to spend as little time obtaining an audible and acceptable map as necessary. The majority of their time should be spent training the recipient and their caregivers on the basic operations of the sound processor, including how to manage batteries, to ensure confident use of the device in the home environment.

The Creation of a New Map Involves Two Steps:

Step 1*: *The creation of the map profile. There are multiple methods for the first step of creating a map profile, namely Electrical Compound Action Potential (ECAP) based, Thresholds based (also known as streamlined fitting), Electrical Stapedius Reflex Threshold (ESRT) based, Population mean based, or based on intraoperative measures like ECAP or Electrical Auditory Brainstem Response (EABR). While the preferred method to create a map profile varies among clinicians, ECAP-based fitting is one of the most popular (Browning et al., 2020). However, clinicians may also alter their approach based on the needs and skills of the recipient.

Step 2: Regardless of the method used for the first step, the second step is always adjusting the map profile in live speech to ensure audibility and acceptance.

The following sections will describe each method in detail, including situations where they may be suitable.

ECAP-Based Fitting

ECAP is the response of the auditory system to electrical stimulation (Stypulkowski & van den Honert, 1984). It is very similar to other evoked potentials like Auditory Brainstem Response (ABR), differing only in the mode of stimulation and measurement methods. For evoked potential measurements, like ABR, electrodes are placed on the scalp to measure the responses evoked by acoustic stimulation to the ears. The resulting waveform has multiple peaks, and the origin of the first peak is known to be from the auditory nerve close to the cochlea. Unlike ABR, ECAP measurements utilise the surgically implanted electrode array to deliver electrically-generated stimulation pulses, which directly record neural responses from within the cochlea rather than via the scalp electrodes. In other words, ECAP is simply the good old ABR response that one gets to measure much more easily.

Most clinicians who have worked with a cochlear implant would have measured ECAP. ECAP measurements are very popular for several reasons: (1) in contrast to ABR or ESRT measurements, which require specialized equipment, ECAP only requires standard CI programming equipment; (2) skin preparation and scalp electrode placements are not needed for ECAP, enabling easy response acquisition from otherwise non-cooperative young children who do not cooperate with probe or surface electrode placement; (3) ECAPs have a higher response measurement possibility, allowing their measurements in 96% of recipients (Cafarelli Dees et al., 2005)—this compares favorably to other measurements like EABR and ESRT, where the response rate is only 71–91% (Kileny et al., 1994; Van den Borne et al., 1994) and 57–83% (Kosaner et al., 2009; Stephan & Welzl-Müller, 1994), respectively; (4) ECAP thresholds lend themselves to successful creation of MAPs, as shown by researchers and clinicians around the world (Botros et al., 2013; Brown et al., 2000; Craddock et al., 2003; Kaplan-Neeman et al., 2004; Pedley et al., 2007; Scorpecci et al., 2016 & Smoorenburg et al., 2002). Thus, ECAP based fitting is popular and often considered routine today.

Since the first measurement of ECAPs in cochlear implantees in the 1990s (Gantz et al., 1994), the ECAP measurement software and artifact reduction methods have improved. It is possible to automatically measure ECAP thresholds at a click of a button with Automatic Neural Response Telemetry (AutoNRT®) (Botros et al., 2007). The median difference between the ECAP responses identified by clinicians and AutoNRT was 3 current levels (CL) (van Dijk et al., 2007). In 93% of cases, when AutoNRT looked for a response, it found a response when clinicians also found a response. When clinicians identify ECAP thresholds visually, variability in the thresholds is seen across clinicians; however, the thresholds obtained with AutoNRT were close to the average NRT® thresholds from multiple clinicians (Botros et al., 2007).

ECAPs provide a simpler alternative to threshold-based methods for creating a new map during initial cochlear implant activation. Creation of an ECAP-based map at initial activation involves first the measurement of ECAP threshold (tECAP) at multiple electrodes across the electrode array. Next, the levels at the unmeasured electrodes are interpolated, and the shape of the tECAP profile is used to create the profiles for C and T levels. Rather than spending time measuring T levels with a new map, the T levels profile is set below C levels based on the average dynamic range (DR) of a large CI user population. The C and T level profile is then adjusted together using live speech to a point where conversational speech is loud but comfortable. In Cochlear™ Nucleus® CI, a control called Master Volume (MV) is used for making this adjustment. Similar controls exist for CIs from other manufacturers. The clinician can then further refine adjustments to emphasise or de-emphasise high and low-frequency information to improve sound quality. In Nucleus CIs, Bass and Treble (B&T) controls are used for this purpose. Similar controls exist for CIs from other manufacturers. In addition, a comfort sweep can be performed by stimulating across groups of electrodes along the array to balance loudness across the entire profile. Botros et al. (2013) had shown that maps created with tECAP based fitting with MVBT, with or without C and T level adjustments, provide similar speech perception scores in quiet and noise compared to the traditional threshold-based fitting method. This means it is possible to achieve an audible map that is acceptable for the recipient and is also on par with the threshold-based fitting method that many clinicians have been using for a long time, which is more time-consuming. Several other studies have replicated the same result (Gibasiewicz et al., 2014; Kiss et al., 2014; Müller-Deile et al., 2017 & Vroegop et al., 2017).

Recently, the speed of making AutoNRT measurements has been improved in Cochlear's Custom Sound® Pro software by adaptively changing the starting presentation level based on previous measurements. With these changes, the tECAP can be measured at nine electrodes in the same time it takes to measure at five electrodes using previous algorithms. Research shows that when a map is created using nine tECAPs, it has a better match to a map created using 22 tECAPs compared to the one created using five tECAPs (Maruthurkkara & Bennett, 2022a, b). Measuring tECAP at more than nine electrodes does not improve the accuracy of the profile match to 22 electrode tECAP beyond the test-retest difference of NRT, which is reported to be 4CL (Müller-Deile, 2009).

Intraoperative ECAP-Based Fitting

Impedance and ECAP measurements are routinely performed intraoperatively soon after placement of the electrodes in situ. These measurements help in confirming the integrity of the implant and the placement of the electrodes in the cochlea. In Medel and Advanced Bionics CIs, the measurement parameters used for intraoperative and postoperative ECAP measurements are similar (Gärtner et al., 2018; Van Den Abbeele et al., 2012). However, in Nucleus CIs, a faster stimulation rate (250 Hz) is employed for intraoperative ECAP measurements to expedite the process. It's worth noting that this faster stimulation rate is not typically used post-operatively, as it may be too loud for some recipients. The tECAPs obtained intraoperatively are higher than post-operative tECAPs due to the different stimulation parameters used and perhaps because the intraoperative environment is different. However, the shape of the tECAP profile is very similar to the postoperative tECAP (Spivak et al., 2011; Telmesani et al. 2016).

The most common approach for ECAP-based fitting is to use postoperative measurements because (1) that's what most of the studies have used; and (2) it is quick and easy to make postoperative NRT measurements. However, ECAP-based fitting does not rely on the overall level of the tECAP; rather, it relies on the shape of the profile. Since the shape of the intraoperative and postoperative tECAPs are similar, intraoperative tECAPs can be used to create new maps for recipients. The process of map creation remains consistent, with one key difference—during the initial activation, the first 5 minutes do not require ECAP measurements. Instead, you can create the map C and T levels profiles using the previously measured intraoperative tECAPs. Afterward, adjustment to the map is made in live-speech mode. For the recipient, this may provide a more positive experience because their initial sound encounter is based on hearing the voices of their loved ones, rather than the meaningless ECAP measurement beeps.

Population Mean-Based Fitting

Population mean represents the average C levels for a large population of CI recipients. The use of a population mean map enables the clinician to easily create an audible and comfortable map without needing to make any T and C level measurements in an initial activation. Just like using ECAP to create a starting profile, one can use the population mean C level to create the starting profile. The shape of the C and T level profiles is based on the average C levels of the population. Like other methods, the clinician increases the T and C levels till the sound perception is loud and comfortable for the recipient. The advantage of this method is that the recipient can start hearing live speech without any ECAP or T level measurements and may offer a better experience of initial activation.

One of the earliest attempts to use population mean values for setting C levels was made by Boyd (2010). In his study, he analyzed map data from 90 Medel Combi40+ implants, which appeared as a flat line. Consequently, he used a flat map to create MAP C levels for 12 Medel CI recipients. However, this approach resulted in significantly poorer speech perception. Subsequently, Kurz et al. (2019) also employed flat maps with newer models of Medel CIs, and once again, subjective sound quality ratings and speech perception were poor with flat maps. In the case of Advanced Bionics CI, Govaerts et al. (2010) developed a set of population-based map profiles called AutoMAPs using data from a large group of CI recipients. Studies have shown that these profiles allow a substantial proportion of CI recipients to achieve desired audibility, phoneme discrimination, loudness perception, and speech perception in quiet targets when AutoMAPs are used (Battmer et al., 2015; Buechner et al., 2015 and Meeuws et al., 2017). AutoMAPs developed for Nucleus cochlear implants (CIs) have been demonstrated to offer speech perception comparable to maps created through traditional programming methods (Zwolan et al., 2021).

With Nucleus CI, analysis of map C levels from over 24,000 Nucleus CI recipients showed that the C level profiles varied based on the type of the electrode array (Maruthurkkara & Bennett, 2024). In general, the C levels at the apical end of the cochlea are lower than those at the basal end. This tendency of higher levels at the basal end is also seen with tECAPs. The C level profile for implants with lateral wall electrodes, peri-modiolar (Contour®), and slim-modiolar electrodes have distinct shapes (Fig. 17.1).

A clinical study evaluating the performance of population mean maps showed no significant differences for speech perception in quiet and in noise between the population mean and the Threshold-based maps (Plasmans & Vanpoucke, 2015).

A population mean method may be preferred if the recipient is likely to be uncooperative for ECAP measurement or if the intraoperative or postoperative ECAP measurement showed no response or responses at a limited number of electrodes. The use of the population mean method is particularly valuable in cases where, despite significant time investment in obtaining ECAP or ESRT measurements, reliable responses cannot be obtained. In such situations, the population mean method

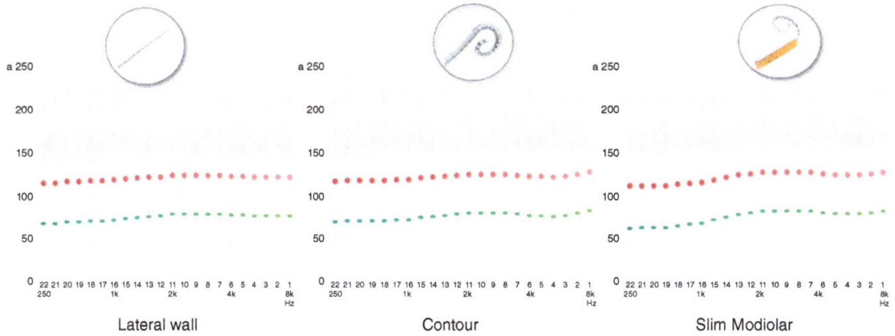

Fig. 17.1 Population means for lateral wall, contour and slim modiolar electrode arrays. Each panel displays channel numbers and their corresponding frequencies in Hz on the x-axis and current level on the y-axis. Red and green dots represent C and T levels, respectively. The shaded area indicates the expected range where approximately 66% of C levels are likely to fall. Insets above each panel show a visual representation of the respective electrode arrays. © Cochlear Limited 2025. Image courtesy of Cochlear Limited

can be employed without necessitating additional time investment during the initial activation. The improved success of population mean maps compared to flat maps can be attributed to their ability to restore the general tendency for higher levels in basal electrodes and also reinstate the array-specific tendencies for the levels.

Thus, the population mean can be used to create audible and acceptable maps during initial activation. As T and C levels typically change from what is created at initial activation, using this method is both time-efficient for the clinician and a less-taxing experience for the recipient. The population statistics can also be used as a guide to set C levels which will be discussed in the loudness acclimatisation section later in this chapter.

Threshold-Based Fitting

The traditional method for creating a starting map profile is by measurement of T levels across electrodes. For early-generation implants, threshold measurements were recommended to be measured across the entire array. However, as later generation implants introduced changes such as the use of monopolar stimulation modes that enabled greater uniformity in map profiles, a more streamlined fitting method is now recommended (Plant et al., 2005). This threshold-based fitting method involves obtaining threshold measurements at five different electrodes and has been shown to provide similar speech perception performance to the traditional method of measuring T levels across the 22-channel electrode array. T levels are typically measured on five electrodes across the electrode array. The T levels at unmeasured electrodes are interpolated. With this map creation method, once the T level profile has been established, the C levels are matched to the shape of this profile, and then the C level profile is raised using live speech until the map becomes comfortably loud for the CI recipient. The map profile is further optimised by performing loudness balancing across electrodes using a sweep at C levels. However, measuring thresholds can be challenging or unreliable with some young or uncooperative recipients. In such cases, the ECAP-based or population mean-based methods may be more suitable for initial activation.

ESRT-Based Fitting

A stapedius reflex is evoked in response to intense sounds in an intact auditory system, which is conventionally measured using tympanometry. The stapedius reflex can also be measured in response to electrical stimulation through the cochlear implant. The ESRT measurement can be utilised for the initial activation or troubleshooting of maps. The ESRT measurement requires two sets of equipment, the programming hardware to stimulate the cochlear implant and the tympanometer to measure the response on the contralateral ear. The process is as follows:

- Step 1 is to ensure an unobstructed external ear canal through otoscopy.
- Step 2 involves checking the middle ear through tympanometry. It is essential to obtain a type-A tympanogram to ensure that the mobility of the eardrum is not affected by any middle ear conditions.
- Step 3 is to obtain a good probe seal on the contralateral ear that can be maintained for a prolonged duration.
- Step 4 involves putting the tympanometer in reflex decay mode to start measuring the reflex. A higher frequency probe tone is recommended to be used, for example, 678 Hz or 1000 Hz to improve the success rate of the measurements (Wolfe et al., 2017).
- Step 5 is to place the sound processor on the implant and set up the programming equipment to send the stimulation.
- Step 6 involves measuring ESRT, where a stimulus is presented at an electrode at increasing levels till a stapedius reflex is observed on the tympanometer.

Once the ESRT measurements are complete, the C level profile is initially set equal to the ESRT profile shape. Subsequently, the C levels on the map are globally adjusted to ensure that live speech is perceived by the CI recipient as loud and comfortable.

While certain factors, such as middle ear issues and stapes removal during surgery, are known to cause an absence of ESRT, predicting who is likely to have ESRT present based on their history remains challenging. ESRT can only be successfully measured in approximately 57–83% of cochlear implant (CI) recipients (Kosaner et al., 2009; Stephan & Welzl-Müller, 1994) and obtaining a response can be challenging. The recipient needs to sit still for the entire measurement period. Sitting still can generally be problematic for children, and the intense stimulation required for ESRT measurements may make it more difficult with some children. Children with physical or mental disabilities, for whom objective measures are the most valuable, will find it challenging. One of the popular methods to keep children still is to let them watch a silent video. Handling multiple pieces of equipment can also be tricky, and often two clinicians are involved in completing the testing. The whole process can be very time consuming, and thus typically, measurements are completed only on 3–5 electrodes across the electrode array.

Other Objective Measures-Based Fitting

EABR was one of the first objective methods found clinically useful for CI fitting. Brown et al. (2000) demonstrated a statistically significant correlation (r = 0.56) between the threshold of EABR and C levels. They showed that the correlation could be improved (r = 0.77) by shifting the EABR profile using one measure C level. Thus research has shown that EABR can be used to obtain the shape of the map for initial activation. However, since the advent of ECAP, EABR has become less popular as its measurement requires both the CI stimulation equipment and a piece of separate equipment to make the EABR measurement. In addition, the two systems need to be synchronised before measures can be reliably made.

Wave I of EABR is obscured by the large electrical stimulus artifact, and one needs to develop considerable skill to perform such measurements. Cortical potentials have also been shown to have significant correlation (r = 0.93) with T levels (Visram et al., 2015). However, to make such measurements, one needs the recipient to be awake and still. Nonetheless, achieving this state with young children, who are the main focus of these objective measurements, can be quite challenging. Thus, although EABR and cortical measures can be used for initial activation for CI, they are seldom used in clinical practice.

EABR or cortical potentials help in advanced troubleshooting of CI recipients. Specifically, they are useful to confirm that the recipient is hearing when there are no detectable ECAPs and the recipient cannot reliably respond behaviorally. Additionally, these methods can help assess the overall integrity of the CI when other diagnostic approaches fall short.

Profile Scaling

Profile scaling is an algorithm that operates behind the scenes in Nucleus Custom Sound Pro fitting software. During live map adjustments, it subtly shapes and flattens the map profile. This adjustment accounts for the wider spread of neural excitation that occurs when stimulation levels are increased. To understand profile scaling, let's first review some basic concepts of electrical stimulation.

When electrical impulses are presented at CI electrodes, it stimulates the auditory nerve fibres and produces the sensation of sound. As the charge is increased, the

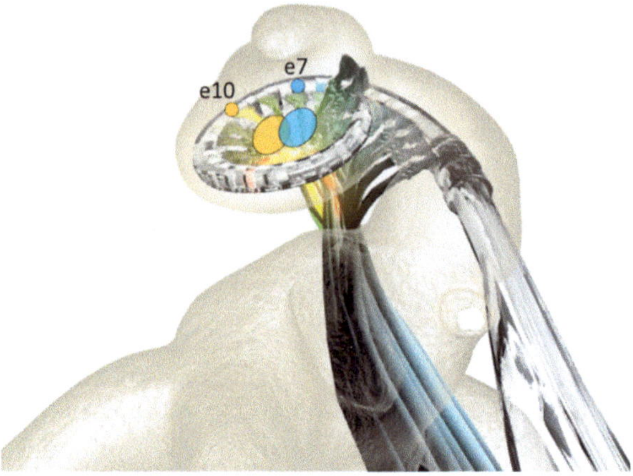

Fig. 17.2 Illustration of stimulation at T (small circle) and C levels (larger circle) at electrode 7 (blue) and electrode 10 (yellow). © Cochlear Limited 2025. Image courtesy of Cochlear Limited

loudness increases. The loudness perception for the recipient is determined by how many auditory nerve fibres are stimulated. When stimulation is presented at T levels, for example, on electrode 7, there is a discreet stimulation of very few auditory nerve fibres in the vicinity of the electrodes due to the low stimulation levels (Fig. 17.2). Likewise, when stimulation is presented at T levels at another electrode, for example, on electrode 10, it will produce a discreet stimulation at another set of nerve fibres. Thus, the T levels measured at neighbouring electrodes can be different, corresponding to the different nerve fibres that are stimulated. These subtle differences in T levels for adjacent electrodes produce a profile shape for T levels.

As the stimulation level is increased to stimulate at C levels, for example, at electrode 7, there will be a greater spread of excitation across multiple nerve fibres resulting in a larger neural response and increased loudness perception. Likewise, when there is C level stimulation at another electrode, for example, electrode 10, due to the larger spread of excitation, there may be some overlap in the region of nerve fibres that respond to C level stimulation of electrodes 7 and 10. Due to stimulation of common nerve fibres, the C levels at electrodes 7 and 10 might be similar, but they might not be the same. As T levels between electrodes can have greater differences than the C levels at the same electrodes, the profile shape for T levels may have more undulations, representing the differences in the stimulation of more localised nerve fibres. In contrast, the profile shape for C levels might be flatter compared to the shape of the T level profile.

The flattening effect of the levels may only be apparent if levels are measured on every electrode; however, if a map is created based on measurements from fewer electrodes, these flattening effects may be lost. As discussed above, in ECAP-based, threshold-based, and ESRT-based fitting approaches, the starting profile is created using a limited number of measurements. Once completed, the levels at the remaining electrodes are interpolated. Profile scaling is an algorithm that helps mimic

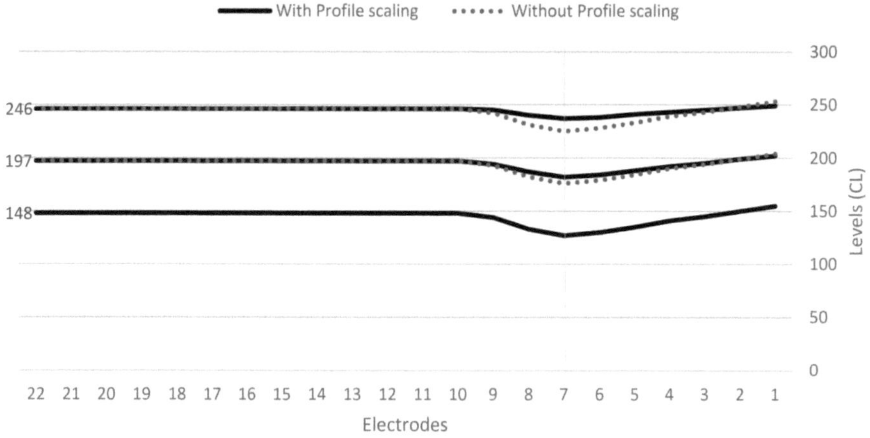

Fig. 17.3 Illustration of Profile scaling. The solid line depicts profile scaling, and the dotted line shows without profile scaling. © Cochlear Limited 2025. Image courtesy of Cochlear Limited

some natural flattening of C levels compared to T levels in maps created with limited number of measurements. Profile scaling progressively flattens the T and C level profile as the levels are increased globally.

Figure 17.3 illustrates the effect of profile scaling. The levels between electrodes 1 and 10 have a curve with maximum inflexion at electrode 7. The levels at electrodes 11 to 22 are shown as flat for this illustration. At the lowest level, electrode 7 is around 148 CL. As the loudness is increased on all channels such that electrode 7 is at 197CL, profile scaling (solid line) is applied to provide less curvature, or a subtle flattening, compared to no profile scaling (dotted line). Profile scaling is applied each time the levels are increased, thus producing a greater flattening effect at higher levels. The effect of profile scaling is more apparent at the higher level when electrode 7 is at 246 CL, where a slightly greater flattening of the profile curvature is applied on electrode 7. A suitable analogy to explain the effect of profile scaling is to compare it to ironing clothes to remove wrinkles. When one irons over a wrinkled shirt, the more times one moves the iron over the wrinkles, the more they become flattened and smoothed out. Likewise, profile scaling is applied to smooth out 'wrinkles' in the map profile. Profile scaling, however, does not completely flatten the map profile even at the maximum loudness levels; rather, it focuses on minimising the deviations of outliers on specific electrodes. It applies more to C levels than to T levels, and this effect is very subtle. Botros and Psarros (2010) found that maps created using ECAP thresholds with profile scaling achieved a significant improvement in approximating the profile shape of the maps created using psychophysical measurements of T and C levels. They reported that a significantly greater number of CI recipients, who assessed the sound quality of the maps while they were blinded to the method used for creating the maps, preferred the ECAP map with profile scaling compared to the maps created using ECAP only.

Loudness Acclimatisation

Many CI recipients delay cochlear implantation until they no longer receive sufficient benefit from hearing aids. As a result, they may have experienced many years of inadequate or distorted sound amplification. Since they are used to poor amplification, for many, their first experience of the sounds received from their implant during initial activation can be overwhelming. The phenomenon of poor acceptance of sounds is well-known among first-time hearing aid users (Arlinger et al., 1996), especially regarding the reintroduction of high-frequency sound and overall volume. Thus, the C levels at initial activation are set at a conservatively low level. Over time, recipients may tolerate and accept louder levels. Since this acclimatisation could happen in the first few days for some recipients, it is desirable for the recipients to have access to a series of progressively louder maps saved in their processor that they can use at home. Recipients can be encouraged to gradually shift to the louder maps over the first few weeks. One method to achieve this is to load the progressively louder maps to different program locations of the sound processor. Most sound processors offer four program locations, which means the clinician can create only three additional progressively louder maps for trial. If the difference in loudness between maps is relatively large, it might deter some recipients from trying the louder maps at home. However, using smaller differences in loudness between maps may lead to the recipient reaching a ceiling effect. Therefore, they may need to return to the clinic for further adjustment sooner or more frequently. In Nucleus sound processors, one can enable MVBT (Master Volume, Bass and Treble) control which allows the recipients to increase the loudness by up to +10CL or up to compliance limits in small loudness steps of 2CL. This allows the use of discreet steps of loudness and a greater range of loudness growth for the recipient. In some cases, the recipient may not like the raising of the global C levels or MV (Master Volume) because this may make the high pitches (i.e., treble) too loud. The additional BT (Bass and Treble) controls can help them increase the MV further while keeping the treble lower. Thus, MVBT adjustments enable recipients to make fine adjustments by themselves without needing to wait for their next clinic visit to make those adjustments.

Vroegop et al. (2017) asked recipients to adjust their maps in real-world environments using MVBT. They reported that the Speech Spatial Qualities Questionnaire - Comparative (SSQ-C) scores with the modified maps showed significant improvement in perceived auditory functioning; yet, there were no significant changes in speech perception or acceptable noise measures on average.

The population statistics of maps from established maps can be helpful in guiding this process. In the FOX fitting approach (Govaerts et al., 2010), progressively louder Automaps are created and loaded into multiple sound processors. The recipient is asked to progress from the softer maps to louder maps. In Custom Sound Pro fitting software, the average C levels from the population +/– 1 SD are used to create the expected range. This range, which represents the C levels at one year after implantation for 68% of the population, can be used as a target by the clinician to set the C levels for the map.

Training and Counselling

Important activities in the initial activation are device training on essential functions and counselling regarding what to expect and habilitation activities. The five areas that require training include:

1. Wearing the sound processor, in which getting the recipient to practice wearing and taking off the device is recommended
2. Switching the processor on and off
3. Changing or charging batteries, in which giving the recipient an estimate of the expected battery life would be helpful
4. Changing programs and volume, and
5. Care and maintenance of the device, for example, the use of the accessory provided to demoisturise while storing the sound processors at night such as the "dry and store".

The sound processor typically comes with a variety of accessories; however, one does not need to explain the use of each accessory in the initial activation session as the recipient may not be ready to take in all the information or may not need all options explained at this point. In any case, a separate session should be scheduled to explain the use of the accessories. In some cases, it may be useful to ask the recipients to try and figure out the use of the accessories by themselves before that session. Counselling should cover what to expect in terms of detecting sounds and comprehension of speech, considering their hearing history. Recipients should expect to detect a variety of sounds and should be advised to explore their environment to try and detect sounds. Maintaining a diary of sounds they heard may be a useful activity. Feedback on the type of sounds they heard and, more importantly, those they could not detect would provide valuable insights into the required steps for mapping in the following session. Although the recipients should expect to detect sounds, they should be counselled that they may not understand everything immediately, and that identifying the direction of sounds around them might be challenging.

Summary of Initial Activation

An initial activation is a significant event in the life of a CI recipient, and that day is remembered long after it has occurred. The clinicians should make every effort to ensure a positive experience for the recipients and their families at initial activation. An early activation soon after surgery can reduce the anxiety of the recipients and their families. One way to do it is, by reducing the duration between surgery and the initial activation as far as possible. The objective of the initial activation is to achieve some level of audibility and acceptance of the device and not to create the perfect map. To achieve an audible map, one may start by spending 5 minutes measuring

ECAPs, or spend 10 minutes measuring T levels, or spend no time in creating a population mean map, or if one has access to intraoperative ECAP, ESRT or EABR thresholds, one may use them as well. Regardless of the method used to create the starting profile, the key next step is to raise the levels overall in live speech such that speech is loud and comfortable. Research has shown that all these methods to create a starting profile can help achieve an audible and acceptable map; thus, one would be doing a service to the recipients by selecting a method that takes the least amount of time and effort for the recipient and so that time can be spent to show them the basic use of their new sound processor.

Follow-Up Sessions

CI recipients require a lifetime of support to maintain optimal hearing performance, and one needs to provide ongoing support to enable them to continue achieving their personalised hearing goals.

In a follow-up session, one wants to make sure that the map the recipients have is most optimal for them at any given time. At the initial activation, a map was developed that ensured audibility and acceptability for the recipient. Now one wants to optimise it further to provide them with the very best outcomes possible. One also wants to fine-tune it based on the feedback and experience of the recipients, and aim to make it even more acceptable for them to enjoy listening. Some of the auditory abilities a clinician wants for the recipients are detecting and discriminating sounds and speech, good perception of varying loudness, and, ultimately, good speech perception or understanding. In this context, it is worth considering applying insights from the hearing aid fitting process to CI fitting.

Hearing Aid vs. CI Fitting

Let us start by comparing the differences and commonalities between hearing aid fitting and CI fitting. The first step for hearing aid fitting is the measurement of the audiometric thresholds across multiple frequencies. The audiogram informs us on the amount of hearing loss the individual has. Using the audiogram as the starting point, specific rules are applied to obtain the target gain. When a hearing aid is fitted based on the target gains, one expects that the user will achieve detection, discrimination, and good speech perception, and further fine-tuning can be made based on their feedback. Some of the most popular prescriptive formulae for the creation of target gains to aid hearing aid fitting are Desired Sensation Level (DSL) and the methods developed by National Acoustics Laboratory (NAL). The fundamental principle behind DSL is "to make all frequencies comfortably loud", and the fundamental rule behind NAL is "equal loudness across all frequencies" (Dillon, 2012). Prescriptive formulae will also have to take into account factors like the upward spread of masking to make sure that the low frequencies do not mask the high frequencies. Using an audiogram and applying the prescription rule is possible because one is using the natural hearing mechanism. It may be impaired, but the way the natural hearing mechanism works is predictable. So, one can apply some of the rules and thereby get prescriptions. However, there is no prescription with CI fitting because the stimulation is not like the natural hearing mechanism and is thus not predictable.

In stimulating the cochlear implant, different electrodes have varied current paths across the cochlea (Nogueira et al., 2016). The routes taken by the electric current at each electrode varies and is not predictable. Additionally, the current paths may change from one recipient to another for many reasons such as (1) variations in tissue properties (due to inflammation, fibrosis, or individual differences) that affect the electric field, (2) the angle at which each electrode is inserted and (3) variability in the cochlear anatomy (for example, cochlear size, shape, and orientation). Secondly, one is dealing with CI recipients with poor neuronal survival who have greater degrees of hearing loss (Nadol, 1997). There might be some portions of the cochlea where the neural survival is reduced and must be compensated for. Even with hearing aid fitting, if some areas have poor neural survival, the so-called dead regions, our ability to use some of the prescriptive formulae is undermined. With CI, one is dealing with an even greater proportion of people with such poor neuronal survival. Looking on the bright side, with CI, there are fewer interactions between low and high frequencies, so there is no need to cater to the upward spread of masking, as may be the case for acoustic amplification.

Even though we cannot predict the targets, we can use some of the fundamental rules that we use for hearing aid fitting. For example, making all frequencies comfortably loud, as would be the objective with DSL, is possible by measuring C levels and ensuring that all the C levels are comfortably loud. Making equal loudness perception across all frequencies, as would be the case with NAL, is achieved by sequentially stimulating across all electrodes using the "sweep" function and adjusting the levels to ensure that the loudness from one electrode to another is the same. Such an approach has been shown to achieve good outcomes (Shapiro & Bradham, 2012).

Evolution of CI Fitting Approaches

Cochlear implant devices and their fitting strategies have evolved since the first commercial implants were released in 1982. Early generation devices, such as the Nucleus 22 series of implants, did not have extracochlear electrodes and were programmed using bipolar modes or common ground stimulation modes. These intracochlear stimulation modes typically had less predictable and non-uniform map profiles across the array, requiring measurements to be made across all available electrodes. So, one had to measure T and all C levels for each electrode individually.

In contrast, recent generation implants have one or more extracochlear electrodes, enabling the use of monopolar stimulation modes.

With monopolar stimulation, map profiles tend to be lower and more uniform in nature. The advantage of this is that measurements can be made on a subset of electrodes allowing interpolation to be used for setting the levels on the remaining, unmeasured electrodes. Therefore, one can measure fewer electrodes and then interpolate the unmeasured electrodes to achieve equal loudness across all electrodes and ensure that they are comfortably loud. Therefore, most CI fitting software enables global adjustments to T or C levels as the overall C levels seem to be quite similar, and it is not necessary to make those individual adjustments. The fitting software from Advanced Bionics, Medel and Cochlear also allow the clinician to change the shape of the T and C level profiles using various functions, such as tilt. In Cochlear's Custom Sound Pro fitting software, global changes using MV for C or T levels, one can also make bass and treble changes.

Adjusting Map Levels Using Master Volume, Bass and Treble (MVBT)

MVBT was born out of some fundamental research in CI programming. To understand this, let us start with an analogy. In science, we would like to look at the basic ingredients of everything. For example, we would like to know "What is everything around us made of?" The answer is "atoms". The subsequent question would be "What are atoms made of?" and the answer would be "protons, neutrons and electrons". We often examine basic ingredients, and understanding these fundamental components enhances our scientific work. A similar inquiry arises when contemplating the essential ingredients that shape a map. To answer these questions, Smoorenburg et al. (2002) performed principal component analysis on a substantial collection of maps to identify the principal components that give the shape for a map. The three main components identified were: *Shift*, *Tilt* and *Curvature*. *Shift* pertains to the amount of loudness increase needed in T and C levels within a MAP; *Tilt* represents the difference in low and high frequency emphasis; and the *Curvature* describes the overall contour of the profile.

When one combines these three components in various ways, one can create any map. This is like the concept of the three primary colours, and if one combines the three primary colours, one can make any colour. But each of the components are not equal in importance. Let us look at another analogy. If we want to make a cake, we might use 30% flour, another 30% maybe sugar, and then we need baking powder. We only need a sliver of the baking powder, although it is an essential component. Without baking powder, probably one will not get a good cake; despite that we only need a tiny amount of it. Similarly, one can look at the relative importance of these three components and their contribution to a map. The shift contributes to 93.7%, and it is by far the most important component of the whole map. The tilt contributes about 3.7% and curvature another 1.5%. The fact that the sum of the three components is 99% implies that combining shift + tilt + curvature enables one to create 99% of the maps. Other components make up the final 1%. Smoorenburg et al. (2002) took an original map and tried to recreate it with just one component, the shift. The error between the measured and the created map was up to 9 current units (CU) at the extremities. The error reduced when they combined shift and tilt, which brought it down to around 6 CU. When they combined all three components, the overall error reduced to about 3 CU. Thus, theoretically, it is possible to create maps based on just these three components.

Practically, shift is something one uses all the time, and there is already a button function for applying shift to increase and decrease stimulation levels within most fitting software. If one starts with a map of 100CL, a slight increase in the shift will slightly increase the loudness percept for the recipient. Continuing to apply further increases in the shift will result in corresponding increases in loudness for the recipient (Fig. 17.4a). These global loudness adjustments are easy for clinicians to make using the software and only require the CI recipient to make judgements and give feedback about volume and comfort, a concept that is already familiar to them.

As far as tilt is concerned, a small adjustment reduces the low-frequency emphasis while simultaneously increasing the high-frequency emphasis (Fig. 17.4b). Increasing amounts of tilt will result in a corresponding increase in low-frequency reduction (with simultaneous high-frequency increase). However, change to tilt is less commonly used than shift (Vaerenberg et al., 2014), probably because its

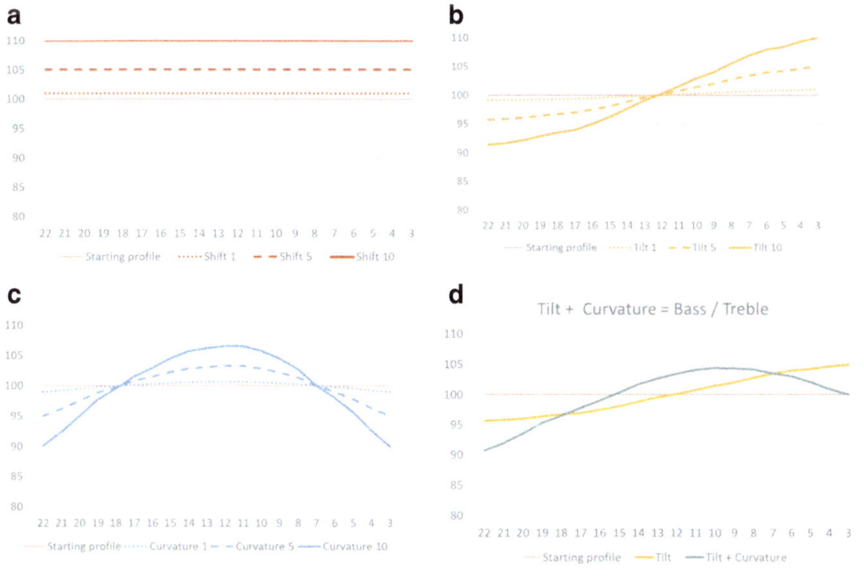

Fig. 17.4 Effects of change in various components on the shape of the map profile - (**a**) Shift, (**b**) Tilt, (**c**) Curvature and (**d**) Bass & Treble. © Cochlear Limited 2025. Image courtesy of Cochlear Limited

clinical effects may not be as straightforward. The simultaneous increase in high frequencies while attempting to reduce low frequencies may introduce new sound quality issues with the high frequencies during the process of resolving those associated with the low frequencies. Nevertheless, we do have the tilt button function available in some fitting software.

A button function that one hardly ever finds in fitting software is the curvature button. This is because such a button will simply curve the whole profile (Fig. 17.4c). Clinicians typically use buttons in fitting software to address sound quality issues reported by CI recipients. However, instances where the clinician needs to simultaneously reduce low and high frequencies while increasing mid-frequencies are inconceivable. One can view it in a way similar to the baking powder analogy—while the baking powder is indispensable for making a good cake, by itself does not taste good. Similarly, while the curvature is also an important component of a map yet, on its own, has limited clinical application.

While the component curvature alone has direct clinical applications, a combination of tilt and curvature can lead to a reduction in emphasis on low frequencies, accompanied by a slight change in the high-frequency region of the MAP. In the Custom Sound Pro software developed by the Cochlear Ltd. Australia, there is a *bass* control that applies this combination of curvature and tilt. Similarly, the software features a *treble* control that combines tilt and curvature to specifically impact high frequencies, with minimal impact on the low-frequency area of the map. (Fig. 17.4d). Making bass and treble adjustments during fitting is also a concept familiar to most CI recipients, being a common function in use with stereo and audio systems for many years.

Shift or MV is an essential part of what we do in programming. In the initial activation section, four methods for creating new maps were described. In all four methods, the way one creates the shape of the map is different but what is common to them all is that once the shape is obtained, one goes on air (i.e., live speech mode) and raises all the C levels, which is akin to using shift. The volume, bass and treble controls used for global adjustment are closer to the language used by the CI recipient to describe the sound quality issues as they experience them. The recipients will not say that they have a problem with a particular electrode; however, they may say things like “it’s all too loud”, “too soft”, “too low pitched”, or “too high pitched”. They typically give qualitative feedback. The MVBT controls allow the clinician to act on the qualitative feedback. The clinician can adjust C and T levels at individual electrodes, when global adjustments are not enough, to go down one level and perform finer adjustments. Too much focus on adjusting/measuring levels at individual electrodes and inadequate focus on global adjustments may lead to underfitting. This was demonstrated in a study where researchers reviewed the maps from 161 implanted children (Incerti et al., 2018). The children were divided into two groups of later implanted older children and early implanted younger children. For the later implanted children, the electrical dynamic range (DR) at six months after CI, 3 years, and 5 years of age, showed no significant difference. Similarly, for the early implanted children, the DR at 3 years and 5 years was stable. But, for the early implanted children, the DR at six months after CI was significantly lower than the

DR observed for the same children at 3 years of age. This is because the C levels were set conservatively lower, and the T level was set higher than where they should be, giving them a smaller DR. The authors of the study conclude that we should be using a less conservative approach in setting T and C levels, especially for early implanted children, which may result in an early more optimised map. It is worthwhile to focus more on global adjustments, not just to raise them indiscriminately. Instead, it is about spending time in carefully adjusting the T and C levels to create the most optimal DR required for those recipients.

Comfort Level Adjustments

As discussed in the section comparing hearing aid fitting to the CI fitting, the two fundamental principles, (1) making all frequencies comfortably loud, and (2) equal loudness across all frequencies, used for hearing aid fitting are also applicable to CI fitting. One can meet these two requirements by ensuring comfortably loud and balanced C levels. The traditional method for achieving this is by measuring C levels using the psychophysical method, which involves the following five steps:

- Step 1 is to present beeps on one electrode and ask the recipient to rate the loudness of the beep using a loudness rating chart like that shown in Fig. 17.5 (Rasetshwane et al., 2015). The C level is raised till they are at a loud but comfortable level. Similar psychophysical C level measurements are made at multiple electrodes across the electrode array.
- Step 2 is to interpolate C levels at all the unmeasured electrodes, which will yield a profile shape. The C levels set using the psychophysical method only ensures that beeps at individual electrodes are loud and at comfortable level. If live speech is presented to the map at this stage, the stimulation of electrodes across the electrode array will cause loudness summation, and the speech will sound too loud for the recipient.
- Step 3 involves a global reduction of the C levels to a lower level in preparation to go live on the map. The degree to which C levels are lowered differs from clinician to clinician.
- Step 4 is to present live speech stimulation to the map.
- Step 5 is to increase the C levels globally till the speech is loud and comfortable.

In steps 1 and 2, C levels were meticulously measured at multiple electrodes for providing the shape of the profile as well as the overall level. The profile shape is retained, but the loudness level, when beeps are loud but comfortable, is discarded. Recipients do not listen to beeps; rather, they listen to live speech through the map. The level at which the beeps are loud and comfortable is not important, rather the level at which 'speech' is loud and comfortable should be the point of focus.

In steps 4 and 5, the C levels of the map are set based on the loudness of live speech. Measuring the psychophysical C levels is time-consuming and can be a

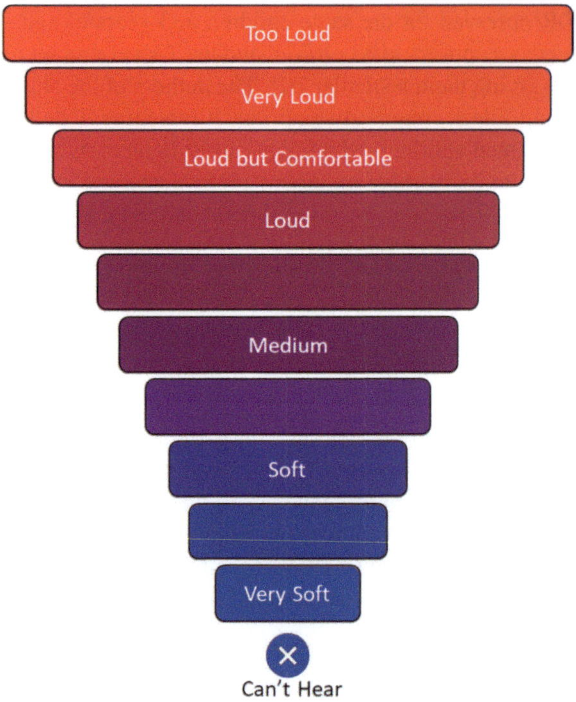

Fig. 17.5 Loudness rating chart. © Cochlear Limited 2025. Image courtesy of Cochlear Limited

difficult task for recipients (Shapiro & Bradham, 2012). Overall, we only utilise the shape of the profile and the loudness rating of the map is done in live speech.

In Cochlear's Custom Sound Pro software, a newer approach to set C levels is employed (Botros et al., 2013), where the order of the measurements is reversed. The first step is to start with a probable profile shape for the map and make global adjustments, such that the overall loudness of live speech is loud and comfortable. The sound quality may not be optimal at that stage, but the levels would have been set in the presence of the loudness summation due to live speech. The second step is to play beeps in bands of electrodes or at single electrodes to ensure that the beeps are of equal loudness; this step ensures that the shape of the profile is optimised. Every time a beep is played, it is preceded and followed by live stimulation, thus ensuring that the C levels are set by considering the loudness summation at every stage. A three-channel beep, which has greater loudness summation than a single channel beep, is played for the loudness balancing task. The map profiles created with the monopolar mode of stimulation are generally smooth, and adjustment of the profile using a three-channel control allows a good balance of C levels across the array. There may be instances when one channel may be an outlier from its neighbouring electrodes in terms of C levels; in such instances, a single channel control may be required to adjust the C levels for one channel alone. The new approach has fewer and easier steps for both the clinician and the recipient and can be completed in less time than the traditional psychophysical C level method.

Threshold Level Adjustments

T levels are measured using standard threshold measurement techniques like the Hughson-Westlake (1944) method. Typically, the measurement commences at a level loud enough for the recipient to hear, and the level is decreased using large step sizes till the stimulus is no longer heard. Subsequently, the stimulus is increased using a small step size to establish the threshold. The stimulus consists of a pulse train delivered at the same rate as the map's per-channel stimulation rate, applied to a single electrode for a duration of 500 msec. Adult recipients are typically asked to indicate that they heard the sound. Clinicians vary in their preferred methods for eliciting responses from CI recipients. Some clinicians instruct recipients to raise their finger, while others prompt them to say 'yes.' Yet another approach involves asking recipients to tap on the table using a pen each time they hear a beep. With children, conditioned play audiometry techniques are often used. Unlike pure tone audiometry, where the target is the point at which 50% of the stimulus is heard, the target here is to reach the 100% point in T level measurement. This is because the T level is usually the point where the stimulation is intended for the softest sound.

In an ideal situation, sound loudness would steadily rise from T levels to C levels. However, for certain recipients, there might be electrodes where this monotonic increase does not strictly occur, resulting in a phenomenon known as *T-tails*. These T-tails represent a situation where, as the current level increases from the threshold, the loudness initially rises slowly up to a certain point, and then it grows more rapidly. To address this, it is advisable to identify electrodes exhibiting T-tails and set the T levels to a point where there is a consistent rise in loudness. A sweep at the midpoint between T and C levels (50% of DR) may be useful in detecting and correcting for T-tails. The process involves playing beeps at successive electrodes at 50% of DR and asking the recipient to rate the loudness of the beeps. The T levels are adjusted such that there is equal loudness across the electrode array for the beeps at 50% of the DR. Table 17.1 and Table 17.2 lists scenarios where the sweep and balance at C levels and at 50% of DR may be useful.

Some fitting software may allow sweeping at T levels, but it is not recommended to ask recipients to rate the loudness at T levels as it may be too hard for recipients. Like C levels, loudness summation also occurs at T levels. Smoorenburg et al. (2002) showed that when T levels were set using live stimulation, the live T levels were 25–30 CL lower than the T levels measured using the single-channel beeps. Thus, to address sound quality issues, it may be necessary to globally adjust the T levels despite them being measured meticulously. Tables 17.1 and 17.2 gives scenarios such as 'soft sounds too soft' or 'too soft in background noise' where global T level adjustments may be useful.

Table 17.1 Recommended actions to resolve issues with loudness and with soft sounds

Parameter	Symptom	Recommendation
Loudness	Own voice loud, others soft	Sweep and balance at Cs and at 50% of DR Decrease Cs and increase sensitivity Counsel recipient Check gain and Maximum Power Output (MPO) Check for occlusion effect
	Sounds always too soft, regardless of C-level	Ensure electrodes are in compliance Optimise power Turn off affected electrodes Check microphone and microphone cover Verify receiver and hearing aid function Check residual hearing in both ears Confirm and/or change acoustic settings
	Too loud	Check sensitivity Sweep and balance at C levels Decrease all Cs Decrease all Ts and Cs Check volume control Check acoustic loudness Check gain and MPO, conduct real ear measurements
Soft sounds	Cannot detect Ling's sounds/cannot discriminate Ling's sounds	Check microphone and microphone cover Check sensitivity Check Ts are audible Increase relevant Ts Increase relevant Cs Increase sensitivity Verify receiver and hearing aid function Check residual hearing in both ears
	Soft sounds too soft	Check microphone and microphone cover Sweep and balance at 50% of DR Increase all Ts Decrease loudness growth Check for loose contacts Try Wide Dynamic Range Compression (WDRC) Check residual hearing in both ears
	Soft sounds too loud	Sweep and balance at 50% of DR Decrease all Ts Increase loudness growth Try linear prescription
	Too soft	Check sensitivity Check microphone and microphone cover Increase master volume Check Ts are audible Increase all Ts Ensure electrodes are in compliance Optimise power Check for wax in the hybrid receiver and hearing aid Check gain and MPO, conduct real ear measurements Check for loose contacts Verify receiver and hearing aid function Check residual hearing in both ears

Table 17.2 Recommended actions to resolve sound quality issues and issues with background noise

Parameter	Symptom	Recommendation
Sound quality	All sounds flat/all sounds sound the same	Counsel recipient Sweep and balance at C levels Sweep to check tonotopicity Check microphone and microphone cover Check residual hearing in both ears Verify receiver and hearing aid function
	Boomy/echoic/hollow/roaring	Sweep and balance at Cs and at 50% of DR Decrease all Cs Decrease bass Check microphone and microphone cover Counsel recipient Check for occlusion effect Reduce acoustic gain Ask about tinnitus, or environments where roaring occurs Check for acoustic feedback
	Crackling	Check microphone and microphone cover Check for loose contacts Perform otoscopy/tympanometry
	Crashing/popping/gurgling	Sweep and balance at Cs and at 50% of DR Check for sharp differences between C levels Check microphone and microphone cover Ensure electrodes are in compliance Optimise power Check hardware Counsel recipient Check for loose contacts
	Fuzzy/humming	Sweep and balance at Cs and 50% of DR Decrease all Ts Decrease all Cs Decrease bass Check microphone and microphone cover Counsel recipient Verify receiver and hearing aid function Check for acoustic feedback
	High pitched/metallic/tinny/ screeching/sharp	Sweep and balance at Cs and at 50% of DR Decrease treble Use more apical electrodes Turn off high-frequency electrodes Check microphone and microphone cover Counsel recipient Recheck gain/MPO Check vent size
	Ringing/pinging/whistling	Sweep and balance at high frequencies Decrease treble Check microphone and microphone cover Check for acoustic feedback
	Too low pitched	Sweep and balance at Cs and 50% of DR Decrease bass Check microphone and microphone cover Counsel recipient Check for occlusion effect
	Unbalanced/distorted/rough	Sweep and balance at Cs and at 50% of DR Decrease all Cs Check for sharp differences between C levels Check microphone and microphone cover Ensure electrodes are in compliance Optimise power Check hardware Counsel recipient Check acoustic hardware Balance loudness
	Unpleasant/painful/annoying electrodes	Decrease relevant Cs Turn off affected electrodes Check hardware Check that the four most basal electrodes are turned off

Table 17.2 (continued)

Parameter	Symptom	Recommendation
Background noise	Background noise too loud	Sweep and balance at 50% of DR Enable zoom and/or BEAM in the sound processor Use SCAN Use Signal-to-Noise Ratio - Noise Reduction (SNR-NR) Use ForwardFocus Decrease sensitivity Unselect "less" for "soften loud sounds [Auto Snsitivity Control (ASC)]" Increase base level Use ASC/volume control Use Adaptive Dynamic Range Optimizer (ADRO) Increase TSPL
	Too soft in background noise	Sweep and balance at Cs and at 50% of DR Select 'less' for soften loud sounds (ASC) Check prescription method
	Sounds intermittent	Ensure electrodes are in compliance Optimise power Try different coil type Try stronger magnet Check hardware Verify receiver and hearing aid function
	Tinnitus with implant use	Decrease all Cs Decrease stimulation rate Turn off affected electrodes Check acoustic loudness Check residual hearing in both ears Conduct a tinnitus evaluation

Contralateral Hearing Aid

Bimodal hearing refers to hearing with a combination of an electrical input with a CI in one ear and acoustic input with a hearing aid on the contralateral ear. The use of a hearing aid on the non-implanted ear provides the recipient access to binaural hearing cues by reducing head shadow effect, binaural redundancy and complementarity.

Reducing the head shadow effect enhances the listener's ability to hear the speech from the ear closer to the signal when the speech and noise come from different directions by improving the signal to noise ratio for the ear closer to the source of speech. Binaural redundancy is the improvement in the listener's ability to hear the speech when the speech and noise come from the same direction. The advantage lies in the brain's remarkable ability to integrate correlated duplicate copies of a sound signal from both ears centrally, while simultaneously filtering out uncorrelated noise from each ear. Complementarity (Ching et al., 2007) is the improvement in the listener's ability to segregate competing voices, discriminate between voiced and voiceless sounds and identify stress and intonation in tonal and non-tonal languages. The advantage comes from utilising the complementary low-frequency information containing voice fundamental frequencies, which conveys voice onset time and suprasegmental information. The voice onset time helps in distinguishing between voiced and voiceless consonants. Suprasegmental information helps identify stress, intonation as well as identifying the speaker in a competing voice situation. These binaural cues help in improved localisation (Ching et al., 2007; Potts et al., 2009), speech perception in quiet (Ching et al., 2001; Potts et al., 2009), speech perception in noise (Ching et al., 2005; Kong et al., 2005), enhanced sound quality and music perception (Gfeller et al., 2008; Giannantonio et al., 2015; Kong et al., 2005; Sucher & McDermott, 2009) for CI recipients using bimodal hearing. The use of the hearing aid on the non-implanted ear also helps avoid auditory deprivation (Ching et al., 2007).

Most CI recipients may have some level of hearing on their non-implanted ear and could benefit from bimodal hearing, especially when the unaided thresholds at 250 Hz and 500 Hz are less than 80 dB HL (Illg et al., 2014). CI recipients with a poorer hearing on the contralateral non-implanted ear might benefit more from a second implant than a hearing aid. Bilateral CIs may offer better outcomes for hearing speech in noise and localisation due to more symmetry in the available binaural cues.

Individuals with hearing loss are encouraged to wear their hearing devices, be it hearing aids, bone conduction implants, or a CI, consistently every day to obtain maximum benefit and to avoid auditory deprivation. This advice does not change just because they had a CI surgery. Recipients should be advised to continue to use their hearing aid on the contralateral ear even before the initial activation of their CI and continue to use the contralateral aid even after initial activation. This will help them acclimatise to the novel bimodal hearing and derive the bimodal benefits sooner.

Now let us look at the steps involved in fitting the contralateral hearing aid.

- Step 1 is to optimise the fitting for the CI in monaural condition as described in sections above.
- Step 2 involves fitting and verifying the chosen prescription in the contralateral hearing aid. English et al. (2016) have shown that using the NAL-NL2 prescription leads to a good loudness balance between the Hearing aid and CI. However, if the recipient has had significant experience with a different prescription, such as DSL, they may prefer to continue with a familiar fitting prescription. In all cases, it is recommended that the hearing aid fitting be verified using real ear measurements.
- Step 3 is to perform a loudness balance between the CI and hearing aid such that sounds are perceived to be in the middle of the head and not lateralise to either ear. This can be achieved by presenting continuous live or recorded speech at conversational levels (65 dB SPL) and adjusting the hearing aid gain till equal loudness is achieved between both ears. It is recommended to test if loud real-world sounds cause discomfort in the bimodal condition and adjust accordingly.
- Step 4 is to match the hearing aid program settings to that of the CI so that similar accessory mixing ratios and noise reduction features are used in both devices.
- Step 5 is to pair the hearing aid and CI to wireless accessories and smartphones so that they can derive the benefits of bimodal audio streaming.

Effects of Map Levels on Speech Perception

The most common activities in a follow-up appointment are threshold and comfort level measurement (Vaerenberg et al., 2014). The signal processing in the sound processor is such that the soft sounds are presented at T levels, and the loud sounds are presented at C levels. Figure 17.6 shows the loudness growth function for Nucleus sound processors. The softest sound presented at T level is 25 dBN (N weighted sound pressure level), which is determined by the TSPL setting of the map. Any sound below the TSPL is inaudible. As the loudness of the input sounds increases from 25 dBN to 65 dBN, the loudness of the electrical output from the sound processor is increased, according to a loudness growth function. Loud sounds at 65 dBN are presented at C levels, and any sound louder than 65 dBN is compressed and presented at C levels. Similarly, in MED-EL and Advanced Bionics CIs, as the loudness of the input sounds increases, the loudness of the electrical output from the sound processor is also increased. (Fig. 17.6).

Once T and C levels are set appropriately, the soft sounds presented at T levels are audible and the loud sounds presented at C levels are comfortably loud. We expect a properly fitted map to help the recipient in detection, discrimination, loudness perception, and speech perception tasks. Let us look at the relative importance of setting T and C levels accurately. Figure 17.7a shows the histogram of electrical stimulation at electrode 21 when speech was presented at conversational loudness level (65 dB SPL) to a Nucleus CI. The sound processor, programmed with a map

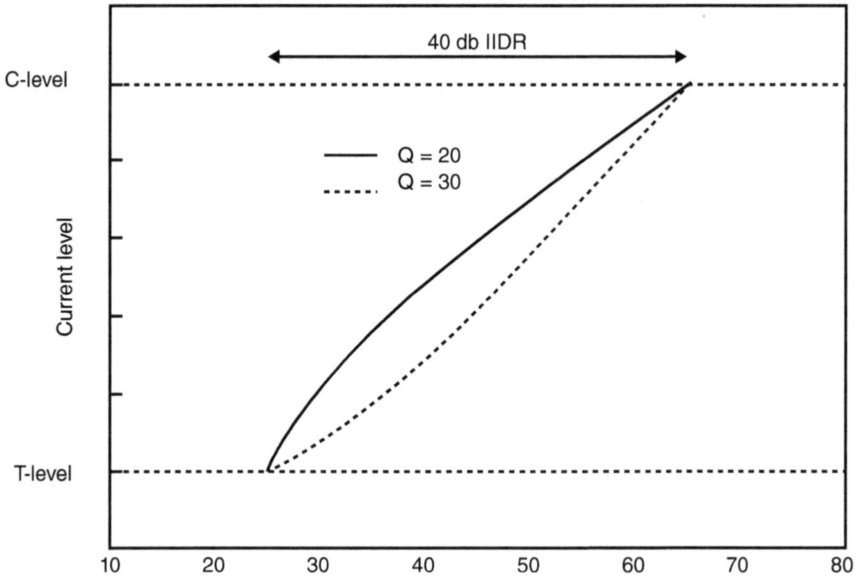

Fig. 17.6 Loudness growth function in Nucleus Sound processors. © Cochlear Limited 2025. Image courtesy of Cochlear Limited

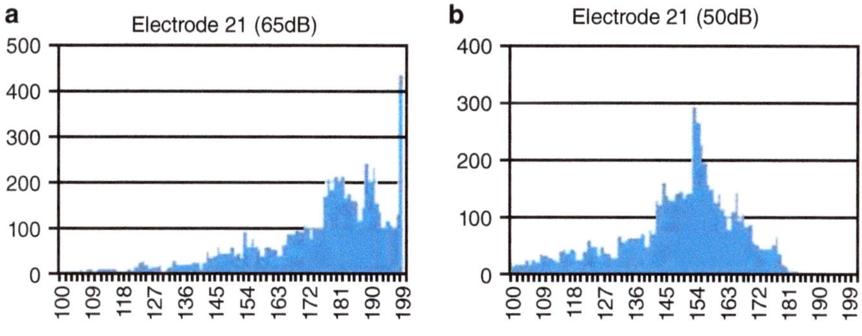

Fig. 17.7 Histogram of T and C level stimulation for (**a**) conversational speech (65 dB SPL) and (**b**) speech at 3 meters away (50 dB SPL). © Cochlear Limited 2025. Image courtesy of Cochlear Limited

where the T and C levels set at 100 CL and 200 CL, respectively, was positioned in a free field. The highest point of stimulation occurs at 200 CL (C level); this is because all speech above the CSPL (65 dBN) is compressed and presented at C levels. Most stimulation is presented somewhere close to C levels, and very little stimulation occurs at T levels. Thus, one can conclude that the C level is where most of the stimulation occurs. Figure 17.7b shows the histogram of electrical stimulation at electrode 21 when speech was presented at 50 dB SPL.

In the real-world, speech at 50 dB SPL is akin to someone talking at a conversational level at a distance of about 5–6 meters from the listener. For example, when the teacher speaks at a normal conversational level in the front of the classroom, the child at the back receives speech at around 50 dB SPL. In this case, the stimulation has shifted to the middle of the DR, but most of the stimulation is still towards the upper half of the DR, i.e., towards C levels. In both cases, there is much more stimulation occurring towards the C level than towards T levels. If the C levels are set incorrectly to a lower than required level, all the stimulation will sound softer and impact the CI recipient's speech perception. However, if T levels are set too low, it will make the very soft sounds inaudible without significantly impacting speech perception in day-to-day life. Thus, the accurate setting of C levels should have a greater effect on speech perception than for the accurate setting of T levels. Willeboer (2008) reported that speech perception for words in quiet was significantly poorer when the C levels were lowered. Most CI recipients can typically notice the impact of a single step change in the volume setting. This corresponds to approximately a 2% change in C levels for Nucleus devices, 3.5% for Advanced Bionics, and 1.5% for MED-EL sound processors.

Busby and Arora (2016) assessed the effect of inaccurately setting T levels on speech perception in quiet and in noise. When T levels were raised to a level higher than the measured T levels, soft sounds became more audible, and speech perception for words in quiet (50 dB) was not affected compared to the original map. However, high T levels also made the background noise loud, significantly impacting speech perception in noise. When the T levels were dropped below where they should have been, soft sounds became inaudible, and recipients started missing out on certain sounds. Consequently, the perception of soft speech in quiet (50 dB SPL) was significantly poorer than the baseline map. However, as low T levels also resulted in making the background noise inaudible, it did not affect speech perception in noise. The interesting finding in their study was that the effects mentioned above occurred only when the T levels were increased or decreased more than 30% of DR. When the inaccuracies in the T levels were within 30% of DR, there was no effect on speech perception or in the subjective feedback from the recipients. A combination of findings of Willeboer (2008) and Busby and Arora (2016) demonstrate that the accuracy of setting C levels has a greater effect on the speech perception where a 2% of DR change is perceivable. In contrast, inaccurate T levels have a weak effect on speech perception, where inaccuracy of 30% of DR or higher change leads to perceivable differences. Therefore, one can conclude that the clinician should be spending more time getting the C levels right in the map than measuring T levels at each session.

Map Levels Over Time

Several studies have looked at how T and C levels change over time. Hughes et al. (2001) showed that T levels in the map remained stable in adults 24 months post-implant. Children showed a significant increase in T level in the first 12 months after the initial activation but no significant increase beyond the first year. Henkin et al. (2003) reported that for prelingually deaf implanted children, T levels and DR increased in the first three months, and C levels increased in the first six months. However, the levels stabilised by one-year post-implant. Incerti et al. (2018) analysed T and C level trends six months after CI in children aged 3 to 5 years. They found that T levels and the C levels stabilise at age 3 with no significant changes at the age of 5 years. Gajadeera et al. (2017) reviewed the T and C levels changes in terms of percentage of DR in a period between 8 and 10 years after initial activation in adults. The median change in T and C levels was only about 3% of DR, suggesting that even after 8 to 10 years of implantation, there is only a minuscule change in T and C levels. The maximum change in T level was less than 12% of DR, and such a change is unlikely to influence speech perception as it is below 30% of DR (see discussion in an earlier section). For C levels, the maximum change over time was also less than 12% of DR. When recipients, using Nucleus sound processors, changed the volume using the volume control from maximum to the minimum level, the C levels were reduced by 20% of the DR. Thus, the maximum change in C levels brought about by repeated programming sessions was less than the degree to which recipients could change their C levels by themselves using the volume control. These studies suggest that once T and C levels have been established, they may not require repeat measurements at every follow-up appointment unless the need to do so is clinically indicated. There may be circumstances where the T and C levels change significantly, and one might need to remeasure them, but in most cases, one does not need to adjust them. Let us pause and think about what this means. CI recipients take time and effort to visit their clinics, which tells us that they derive some value from visiting the clinic. Mapping is considered the clinician's primary activity, although several other clinical activities are performed in the session. If map levels are not significantly impacting the recipient's hearing, why are they visiting the clinic? Surely it cannot be just for the mapping. We may conclude that the other activities performed in the clinic provide value, which motivates the recipient to visit their clinic for follow-up appointments. In other words, an appointment is more than just programming.

An Appointment Is More Than Mapping

It takes time and effort for CI recipients to visit the clinic. When asked about the reason the recipients visit the clinic, the first thing that comes to mind for most clinicians and recipients is the word mapping. It is also common to name the appointments as *mapping session*, which makes it seem like mapping is the only thing that happens in a follow-up appointment. The reality is that there is much more happening in an appointment. In two clinical studies conducted in 4 clinics from the United Kingdom and one clinic in Australia, 28 clinicians were asked what activities they performed in 93 recipient appointments (Maruthurkkara et al. 2022a, b). Only 22% of the activities involved mapping, and the remaining activities included counselling, training, ENT referral, replacing parts, rehabilitation, fitting a new sound processor or accessory and hearing performance measurements. The term counselling is used to cover a variety of activities like (1) helping recipients feel empowered to have greater ownership of their hearing health; (2) helping them improve social engagement using technology; (3) helping them with communication strategies and training; (4) putting them in touch with other peers and professional groups which can give them further support; and (5) giving them emotional support (Bennett et al., 2021). There is a whole lot of other activities unrelated to mapping, but equally important, that clinicians perform for their patients to deliver holistic patient-centred care. The value derived from these activities is likely to motivate recipients to continue visiting their clinic for follow-up sessions.

The question "why do recipients visit their clinic?" can be answered using the 5 Whys approach (Ohno, 2006): (1) Why do recipients seek help? They seek help because they have hearing loss. (2) Why is having hearing loss a problem? Hearing loss is a problem because it leads to a communication problem. (3) Why is poor communication ability a problem? Poor communication ability is a problem because it prevents forming new relationships. Recipients might find ways to communicate with people they know but forming new relationships is a problem (Broese van Groenou et al., 2013). (4) Why is the inability to form new relationships a problem? Inability to form new relationships is a problem because it leads to withdraw from social situations. (5) Why is withdrawal from social situations a problem? Withdrawal from social situations is a problem because it leads to loneliness and depression. So, we have hearing loss, ultimately leading to loneliness and depression. One might think that the clinicians are just treating hearing loss and communication ability, but the motivating factor for recipients stems from far more basic needs in their life. According to the American Speech-Language-Hearing Association (ASHA) (n.d.), creating an individualised plan of care involves identification, assessment, and documentation. It is about looking at all the treatment options, about managing and maintaining therapeutic relationships with the recipient. It is about looking into cultural, linguistic, financial considerations; into medical, physical, cognitive, social and emotional factors, making sure that there is a quality of care and making sure that there is a personal support system. Thus, there are a wide variety of activities performed in an appointment, and these have very little to do with mapping.

The CI recipients' hearing journey with their implant starts at the initial activation, which requires mapping, and there is a focus on mapping in the early months for map optimisation. However, as their journey continues, their needs might change; they may want more help with real-world hearing, which may be supported by giving them appropriate tools, for example, wireless accessories. They might want to maximise their performance, and one might want to provide them rehabilitation support. A range of rehabilitation materials are available on CI manufacturers' websites. Several smartphone apps are available for rehabilitation. These include BabyBeats and WordSuccess from Advanced Bionics for auditory training, Meludia from Medel for music training, and the Hearing Tracker functionality in Cochlear's Nucleus Smart App. The Hearing Tracker aims to improve exposure to speech based on data logs. In the long term, the recipients need lifetime monitoring of their hearing device and support as and when issues arise, and yet other tools like remote monitoring tools such as Remote Check or Remote fitting tools may be necessary. Throughout their journey, the recipients' needs will change, and while mapping is an important part, it is not the only activity that can be used to support them. As the name suggests, patient-focused care is about focussing on the recipient and not the computer screen.

Goals

As discussed in the previous section, there are a variety of valuable activities, in addition to mapping, that the clinicians can perform during follow up appointments. However, as the activities are often performed based on the need at that moment, they may sometimes be completed in unstructured ways and may not be documented sufficiently to enable follow up in future appointments or can be continued by another clinician. The Client-oriented scale of improvement (COSI) is a great tool to provide a structure and guide the activities required based on the recipients' motivations and goals captured by it.

COSI was originally developed for hearing aid users (Dillon et al., 1997) and has been widely used during hearing aid fitting. One starts by making a note of all the specific needs for the recipient before hearing aid fitting. Next, goals are established collaboratively, focusing on specific needs and hearing aid features are selected based on the goals. During the first follow up session, the goals are reviewed, and the level of improvement using the hearing aid is documented against each goal. As no hearing device is perfect, while aiming to address some or most of the client's hearing needs expressed pre-fitting, often the client will report new problems that have emerged after commencing with hearing aids. For example, they might have feedback problems, battery life issues, comfort issues etc., not present before they used hearing aids. Documenting goals and the improvement has helped demonstrate the value of hearing aids to the client. It helps to focus on the positives and motivate them to persevere with their hearing aids.

With CI recipients, COSI can be used on an ongoing basis rather than just before and after fitting the device. It can help document any progress made on existing challenges and record new challenges that require action and ongoing attention across multiple sessions. To address the issues, the clinician might perform some activities, like fit an assistive listening device, change some settings, perform mapping; but there may also be activities that the recipient needs to perform. This could include continuing rehabilitation activities at home or using the prescribed setting or a device in a challenging environment. In other words, there might be some homework for the recipients. In the Custom Sound Pro software (Cochlear Ltd. Australia), an agreed action plan can be documented along with the desired goals. It can help make it clear to the recipient what their homework is and can be used to follow up on in the next session. Questionnaires are a very popular way of assessing subjectively perceived outcomes for a recipient. Questionnaires contain standard questions, and recipients rate how well they perform in the listed scenarios; however, the scenarios in the questionnaires need not be relevant or the most important for the recipient. COSI is a highly customised questionnaire, where the question is set based on what is relevant and most important to the recipient. A historical record of their goals that are already deemed achieved or where significant progress has been made can be valuable insights for counselling. On a day when the recipient is frustrated with a lack of progress, their historical records may help remind them of how much progress has already been made and how far they have come in their journey.

Setting Goals

Next, let us look at how to set goals. They involve the following steps:

1. *Open-ended question:* The very first step is to start with an open-ended question. The question could be, "In which environment do you have the most difficulty in listening?", "What are the biggest listening challenges that you encounter?" etc. The recipient might need a moment to reflect and think about this question. Then, the clinician should encourage them to freely express everything that comes to mind and note the emerging themes. Typically, the most important issues are the first that come to their mind.

2. *Explore:* Once some level of unstructured information is obtained, then it is time to explore and elicit all areas of difficulties. The clinician can probe further to clarify what the recipient reported to determine the specific situations where the hearing difficulty is experienced. Some recipients, who are not very good at recognising the issues they encounter, can be prompted using the list of issue categories such as conversation in noise /quiet/on the phone /at a seminar, awareness of doorbell/traffic noise/phone ring or understanding while watching television etc.
3. *Identify top issues:* The next step is to identify the top 3–5 issues. As soon as they start talking, the first thing they say is usually the top-of-mind issues. It is recommended that a maximum of 5 goals are set at any one time, as more might be overwhelming for the recipient.
4. *Write SMART goals:* The next step is to write the goals based on the top issues. The COSI provides broad categories to select; however, it is beneficial to write down SMART (specific, measurable, attainable, relevant and time-bound) goals. It is very important that the goals are specific so that appropriate action plans can be set. The specific goals will also ensure ease of reviewing in the next session. These specific goals should also be measurable. In addition, only attainable goals must be selected. For unattainable goals, the clinician's role is to counsel and help the recipients understand the limitations and arrive at realistic expectations. By design, the goals set will be relevant to the recipients as they are based on their top 3 to 5 concerns and suitable to be time-bound.
5. *Rate ability:* The next step is to ask the recipients to rate their current ability to hear in the specified environment on a five-point scale "Hardly ever able", "occasionally able", "able half the time", "Able most of the time", and "Almost always able". When the goal is specific, it makes it easier for the recipient to give an accurate rating before and after they tried the steps in the action plan.
6. *Set action plan:* The final step is to develop an action plan that is likely to help the recipients attain their goals. This requires knowledge and information on the best ways to resolve issues. Tables 17.1, 17.2 and 17.3 list the recommended actions to take in response to issues commonly reported by CI recipients. For example, they may already have specific programs or accessories that could help them towards their goals, but they might not be using them consistently. A review of datalogs can help uncover any issues in how they are using the programs or accessories. The clinician might also need to know when a problem cannot be solved. Finally, the clinician ought to guide the recipients in mentally envisioning themselves implementing the action plan within their real-life, everyday contexts. This visualization process enables them to openly discuss any potential challenges they may encounter while executing the plan.

Let us imagine we have a recipient who has a complaint related to difficulty understanding speech in noisy environments. If only the COSI category label "conversation with a group in noise" is documented, then it would be difficult for the clinician to remember all the details of the discussion in the next session. A poor example for writing the goal is "to hear easily in a noisy environment". As it does

Table 17.3 Recommended actions to resolve issues at specific situations and other issues

	Symptom	Recommendation
Specific situations	Cannot hear well on telephone	Try audio streaming with a smartphone Try wireless phone clip Try a hearing aid on the other ear Try Telecoil Try portable phone cable
	Cannot hear the television well	Try TV streamer Try mini mic placed near the TV speaker Try mains isolation cable
	Cannot hear well at seminars	Try wireless mini microphones Try Telecoil
	Cannot hear well at meetings	Try increasing sensitivity Try wireless mini microphones Try lapel mic
	Cannot hear well in the car	Try wireless mini microphones Try lapel mic
	Unable to hear other people's speech when using streaming through Mini mic/TV streamer/telecoil	Change mixing ratio
Other issues	Facial nerve stimulation	Decrease relevant C-levels Increase pulse widths Turn off affected electrodes Reduce master volume Try a different stimulation mode Confirm electrode array placement
	Sounds intermittent	Ensure electrodes are in compliance Optimise power Try different coil type Try stronger magnet Check hardware Verify receiver and hearing aid function
	Tinnitus with implant use	Decrease all Cs Decrease stimulation rate Turn off affected electrodes Check acoustic loudness Check residual hearing in both ears Conduct a tinnitus evaluation

not give more information than the category label, it is not specific and not measurable. A better way to capture the goal would be, for example, "I want to be able to understand my group of four friends when I am sitting in my school cafeteria". The key difference is that it describes the specific environment and the specific group of people the recipient wants to communicate with. When the goal is detailed and specific, the recipients can also more easily think back to the situation and give a more accurate rating for their current hearing ability. In this example, the recipient may be advised to: (a) try using a noise reduction program, (b) try a wireless accessory, or (c) try communication strategies, all of which can be recorded in the action plan.

The clinician might need to help the recipients with specific steps in acquiring the additional accessories they might need. When the recipients come back for an annual follow-up session one year after the previous session, the clinician can open the recorded goals and be reminded of that conversation they had last year and pick it up where they left off.

Goal setting is also applicable for children, who likely face more significant hearing challenges than do the adults. Children go to schools that inherently have a very noisy and challenging listening environment. Even if it is a child using the best technology, children being children, may not be using them to their highest potential. For example, when the teacher is teaching in a classroom, it is pretty common for children to have fun among themselves when the teacher is not looking. This creates a challenging listening environment as the child's attention is divided between the teacher and his/her friends. While a child with normal hearing might cope very well, such distractions are likely detrimental for children with hearing loss. The solution might lie not just in the use of technological solutions, like FM systems, but also in requiring tactical, non-technological solutions, such as greater oversight from teachers. We should let children be children, but it is essential to identify issues affecting the outcome. Goal-setting might help in uncovering such complex issues and could help families find solutions jointly with the professionals.

By regularly having goal-setting conversations, which can help build trust, recipients may feel comfortable opening up more and engaging in deeper conversations. Goal setting using COSI is a collaborative process where the recipient and the clinician are joined together to make the goals. It increases client engagement in the process, is very quick, and is relevant for the client. It helps to evaluate the functional hearing and evaluate how the recipients are doing in their real-world situations, and ultimately it can improve the outcomes in all those areas which a speech perception test cannot measure. It is about personalised patient care and is beyond fitting. Overall, it increases the focus on outcomes and patient focussed care.

Recommended Workflow

The best practice for any clinical session involves three steps: (1) assessment, (2) treatment, and (3) follow up. Figure 17.8 shows a checklist of activities that can be followed in a follow-up fitting session.

Assessment The first step in assessment is a discussion with the recipient regarding the reasons for the visit to the clinic. Documenting the top concerns can help plan the session, evaluate the session's success, and determine the next steps after the session. Obtaining relevant details in the case history and a review of data already available on file is useful in determining the root cause of the concerns. In addition, they help uncover issues that the recipient has not reported. Inspection of the implant site, area behind the pinna and the ear canal can reveal the medical

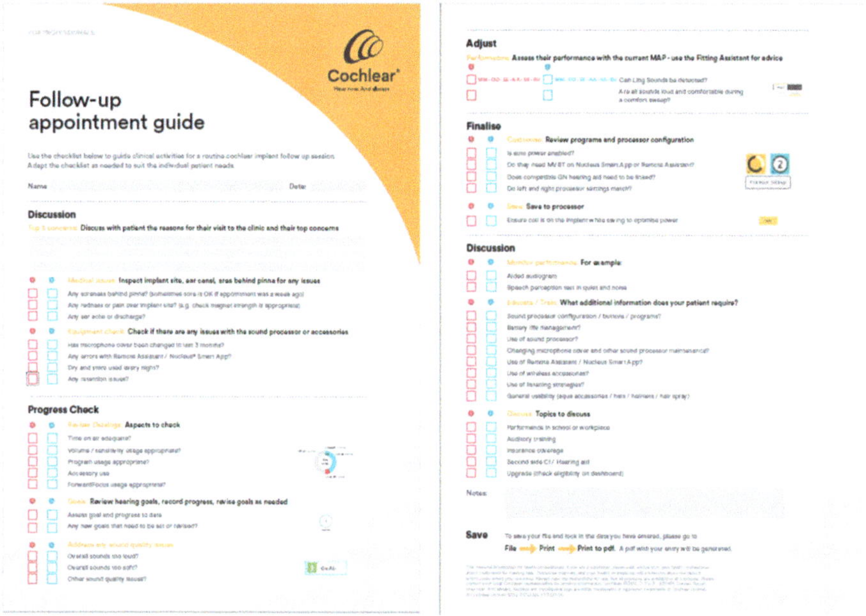

Fig. 17.8 Nucleus Follow-up appointment guide (Cochlear Ltd., 2020). © Cochlear Limited 2025. Image courtesy of Cochlear Limited

issues requiring intervention. Although the best practice is to empower recipients to take responsibility of taking care of their sound processor, it is helpful to check whether they are changing mic covers and using the dehumidifiers at night. The review of the datalog can help uncover any issues pertaining the way the recipients use their devices or their communication environments. Review of goals previously set or setting new goals is also an essential part of the diagnostic process. In the discussion, any hearing-related issues may emerge; however, if they do not, it is useful to enquire if they have had any sound quality issues. The assessment may also include speech perception tests or tests of audibility using an aided audiogram or the Ling's six sound tests (Ling, 1989). A sweep at C levels can also uncover the possibility of some sounds being too loud for the recipient.

Treatment The treatment for the recipient should be determined based on the issues identified in the assessments and should be aligned with the top concerns voiced by the recipient. A common fallacy is that with CI mapping is synonymous with treatment. As discussed in the earlier section, mapping may not be required in all sessions if the assessments did not reveal a need for mapping. Issues may be resolved by adjusting the program or processor settings, adjusting the hearing aid on the contralateral ear, adjusting the power levels, or providing training on the proper use of the technology or communication strategies. Explanation of the test results to help them understand their hearing ability and performing counselling to set realistic expectations are also important parts of the treatment. Tables 17.1, 17.2 and 17.3

lists the recommended actions to take in response to some issues commonly reported by CI recipients, and many of the treatment options do not involve mapping. Therefore, the clinician should always be guided by what they find in their assessment to decide how to structure their appointments. As Steve Jobs has famously said, “deciding what not to do is as important as deciding what to do”.

Follow up Sometimes, the recipients will need to play an active role in overcoming the issues they face. For example, they might need to use a unique program or accessory in the real-world environment, or they might need to use MVBT to make subtle adjustments to their maps, or they might have to try the strategies to improve device usage, or tactics to help them cope better in challenging listening environments. Once the potential action plans are identified, the clinician might need to help the recipients tailor it further to suit their own environment and lifestyle. This might require the clinician and the recipients to jointly brainstorm ways to adopt the action plans, all of which involve in-depth conversations. The recipients and the clinician will need to agree on the appropriate time frame when the outcomes of the action plans can be reviewed, and the date for the next follow-up appointment can be determined based on it. The clinician also has a duty to get recipients thinking about larger/longer-term projects that can potentially have a lasting impact on the recipients’ life, like having the second CI or getting a hearing aid on the other ear, upgrading the sound processor or getting an insurance plan to cover upgrade or loss of their sound processor etc.

Example Scenarios Now, let us look at a couple of case scenarios to see how this may look in practice. Let us imagine we have a (fictitious) recipient ‘Peter Jones’ who has come to a clinical session and had his implant for 18 months. Peter tells the clinician that everything is going well apart from some difficulty understanding speech in noisy situations. Session A in Fig. 17.9 shows one way to conduct the session. The session starts at 9:00 AM; the clinician’s first five minutes are spent reviewing the prior session notes. Then the clinician begins by measuring T levels at three electrodes. There was about 1–2 CL change in the T levels, and the process takes about 10 minutes. Then the clinician measures C levels at several electrodes for 15 minutes, and there is about 1CL change in 2 electrodes across the electrode array whereas no change is found in all the other electrodes. This has taken the session to 9:30. The clinician spends 5 minutes performing a C level sweep to check the loudness levels, and everything was quite well balanced, and no adjustment was required. Then the clinician does an equipment check using the listening earphones and asks Peter when he changed the mic cover. Peter reports that he has not changed it for months. So, the clinician changes it for him. The final 5 minutes are spent talking about the next appointment, and they find a suitable time for the next appointment. This is one example of how a session could be run. Can this session be done differently? What are some actions of the clinician that could be changed?

Session B in Fig. 17.9 shows an alternative method of conducting the session. The session starts at 9:00 AM; the clinician views the previous session history,

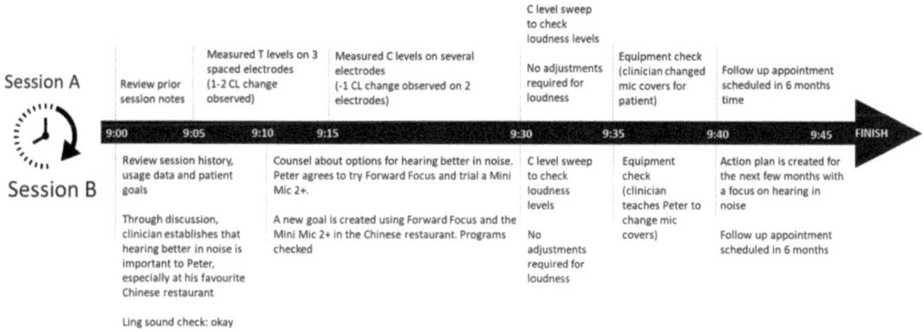

Fig. 17.9 Illustration of two distinct approaches for conducting a CI follow-up appointment. Session A, a predefined set of activities are adhered to. Session B activities are tailored based on the specific needs expressed by the patient. © Cochlear Limited 2025. Image courtesy of Cochlear Limited

looks at the usage data, looks at the patient goals, and enters into a discussion with Peter. The clinician delves deeper to understand what Peter means by having problems in a noisy situation. When the clinician probes further, Peter explains that he struggled to hear the conversation in his favourite Chinese restaurant. The clinician performs a quick Ling sound check and confirms that soft sounds are audible; all these activities are completed in the first 10 minutes. The clinician spends the next 20 minutes discussing the different options for hearing better in noise. Of all the options, Peter agrees to try ForwardFocus and agrees to try the Minimic 2+. The clinician records the goal and describes the action plan to use the Minimic 2+ in that Chinese restaurant. Then the clinician goes to processor settings in the software to ensure that ForwardFocus is enabled. The clinician spends 5 minutes performing a quick C level sweep to ensure that C levels are equal in loudness and finds that no adjustments are required. The clinician asks Peter when he changed the mic cover and finds out that the mic cover was not changed for months. The clinician hands over the mic cover to Peter and asks him to change it by himself, guiding him through the process so that he can do it by himself at home the next time. And in the last five minutes, the clinician reviews the action plan once again and reminds Peter that in the next six months, he should try the Minimic and ForwardFocus. They decide to meet again after six months, and at this point, it is obvious both to Peter and his clinician what they will be doing at the next visit; they will be reviewing how many times he tried ForwardFocus and the Minimic, and they will discuss what progress he has made. The key difference was that in session A, there was a lot of focus on mapping and measuring T levels and C levels, although there was not a lot of change in the map levels. In session B, the clinician went directly to the primary issue reported by the recipient instead of T and C level measurements and the first 30 minutes was spent on that. In both sessions, a C level sweep was done, and it was seen that it required no adjustment. In session B, the clinician taught the recipient how to change the mic cover rather than changing it for him so that he would be able to do it by himself the next time. Finally, in the last 5 minutes, in session B, both the recipient and the clinician were very clear about what they will be doing in the next session. The goal of that next session was very clear in session B, whereas in session A it might have been a bit vague for both of them as to what was going to happen, and perhaps the next session would be a repeat of much that occurred in the current session. Ultimately, it is up to the clinician to choose the kind of session they want to conduct. The key questions are what kind of session would benefit more for the recipient? What kind of session will motivate the recipient to continue to engage with the clinic and reduce the risk of being lost to follow up?

Summary of Follow Up Sessions

One of the goals of a follow-up appointment is to optimise the map to provide the best performance for the recipient. CI mapping methods have been inspired by hearing aid fitting principles but have evolved over time with modern methods that lay emphasis on beginning with global adjustments and then proceed to adjustment at the individual electrode level only if warranted by the outcomes measured. Traditionally, it was considered that follow up appointment was just for mapping; however, there are many more activities that a clinician can be performing in the follow-up session based on the goals and needs of the recipient.

Long Term Management

Remote Programming

The necessity of traveling to the clinic for follow-up appointments can be particularly challenging for recipients, especially those residing far from the clinic. Reports indicate that some recipients are lost to follow-up due to the difficulties associated with clinic visits (Rooth et al., 2017). The inconvenience of scheduling sessions and commuting to the clinic may discourage seeking help for seemingly minor issues, leading some recipients to endure problems rather than seeking timely assistance. Clinicians often schedule follow-up sessions to assess progress with strategies provided earlier, and this can be effectively accomplished through video calls without necessitating in-person visits.

Remote programming represents a telehealth solution that effectively tackles the challenges associated with traveling to the clinic for appointments (Slager et al., 2019). Figure 17.10 shows the schematic diagram for remote programming. Amidst the Covid-19 pandemic, there was a noticeable surge in the adoption of remote programming as an alternative when traveling to the clinic posed health and safety risks (Kim et al., 2021). Existing methods for remotely programming cochlear implants require specialized computer hardware and proprietary programming software to be installed on a personal computer (PC) at the remote location. While remote

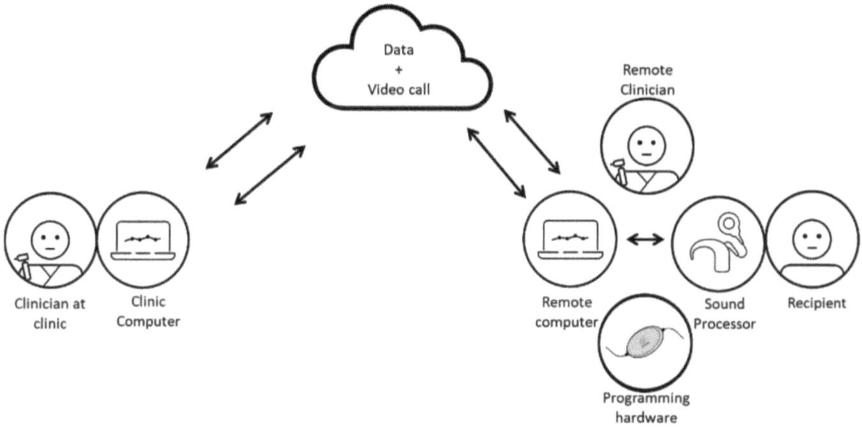

Fig. 17.10 Schematic diagram of Remote programming. © Cochlear Limited 2025. Image courtesy of Cochlear Limited

programming reduces travel burdens for certain recipients, it imposes significant administrative efforts and costs on clinics. These tasks involve preparing, sending, retrieving, and maintaining the remote programming hardware and software. Unfortunately, this administrative overhead may also result in delays when scheduling remote programming appointments due to the time required for equipment exchange.

Remote programming for CI recipients has been reported in several studies in the last decade (Takano et al., 2021; Luryi et al., 2020; Schepers et al., 2019; Slager et al., 2019; Hughes et al., 2018; Goehring & Hughes, 2017, Samuel et al., 2014; Kuzovkov et al., 2014; Eikelboom et al., 2014; Hughes et al., 2012; Wesarg et al., 2010; McElveen et al. 2010 and Ramos et al., 2009). A range of networking software packages are used to control the CI fitting software remotely. The audio-visual software used for communication has proved to be reasonably reliable with only occasional loss of connection or delays. The studies report that remote programming provides equivalent listening benefits as compared with in-clinic appointments. Both clinicians and recipients have provided highly positive feedback on the experience of remote programming. The majority of the studies were conducted with a local facilitator in the same room as the recipient to assist the recipient during the session. Such sessions are conducted at a clinic/facility that is local to the recipient. The local facilitator takes responsibility for the upkeep and connecting of programming hardware. Although the remote programming via the local clinic reduces the travel for recipients, it incurs costs to the clinic for the additional space and personnel involved. A better approach may be to send the programming equipment and computer to the recipient's home (Slager et al., 2019). However, sending the remote programming to home incurs additional costs for shipping, and the clinic has to spend additional time preparing the devices and repurposing the kit for different recipients, which involves cleaning and repacking. Additionally, the recipient needs to be sufficiently technically savvy and have a good internet connection.

Recently, remote programming has been made possible via smartphone apps, eliminating the need to physically mail programming hardware to recipients. These app-based solutions effectively address technical challenges associated with traditional remote programming methods. *Remote Assist*, an app-based technology for programming Nucleus cochlear implants, has been reported as easy to use and reliable. When combined with sending replacements by post, it is capable of addressing 80% of the issues observed during typical follow-up sessions (Maruthurkkara, 2024).

Remote Check

As discussed above, follow-up appointments for CI recipients should be guided by assessing any issues the recipient faces. The majority of long-term CI recipients have stable maps and are likely to have minimal, if any, issues with their devices. However, there may be some issues where the clinician can help them. The current clinical practice is to schedule annual appointments for all CI recipients and assess if there are issues to resolve. Thus, a clinic visit would have assessments that guide the interventions. Although the evaluations would uncover that some recipients need help, some people may not need any help. For such recipients, the travel to the clinic and time spent by the clinician for assessments may have been avoided. Remote Check is an asynchronous recipient assessment tool that allows the CI recipients to complete a series of tests at home using just their smartphone connected to their sound processor. The results are sent to the clinician via the internet, and it enables the clinician to determine if the recipient requires a clinic visit. Remote Check would save the recipient an unnecessary trip to the clinic. It may also help the clinician prioritise their time for recipients who may need their help or on candidates who are yet to receive the gift of hearing.

Figure 17.11 shows the flow diagram and screens in Remote Check. The first step is for the clinician to enrol a recipient to Remote Check via a web-based professional portal. The recipient receives a notification on the Nucleus Smart App on their smartphone that the remote check is due. There are four tasks that the recipient needs to complete: three implant site photos, a two-part questionnaire, an aided threshold test (ATT), and a speech in noise test called the digit triplet test (DTT) (Smits et al., 2004). The questionnaire includes the adult and parent versions of the Speech, Spatial and Qualities questionnaire (Galvin & Noble, 2013; Noble et al., 2013) and has questions on medical, fitting, training and sound quality-related aspects. In the ATT, pure tones are streamed via Bluetooth to the sound processor, and the recipient presses a button to respond. Recipients are asked to indicate if they heard the sound by swiping towards "yes" and swiping to "no" if no sound is heard. The ATT provides an aided audiogram across audiometric frequencies. In DTT, sets of digit triplets are presented in speech shaped noise, and the recipients are asked to

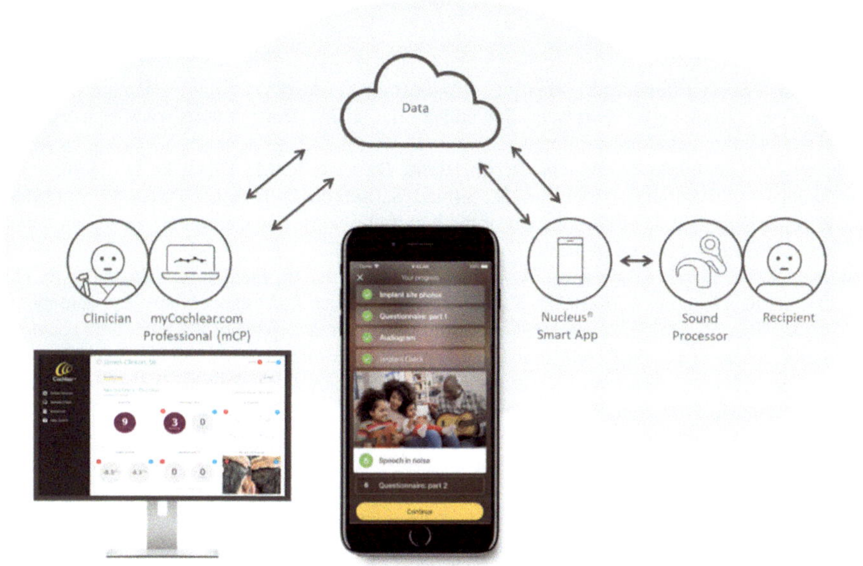

Fig. 17.11 Flow diagram and screens in Remote Check, an app-based tele-health solution for CI recipients. © Cochlear Limited 2025. Image courtesy of Cochlear Limited

respond by selecting the numbers on the screen. The DTT determines the speech reception threshold. In addition to the recipient driven tasks outlined above, Remote Check also includes an automated impedance check and extraction of usage data from the sound processor. The Remote Check results are packaged and sent securely via the internet for the clinician to review offline. A couple of proof-of-concept studies (Maruthurkkara et al., 2022a, b) showed that Remote Check provides sufficient information to determine the need for clinical intervention, agreeing with clinical observation on the need for a clinic visit for 99% of recipients. A remote check completed soon after a clinical appointment could be used as a baseline check, and any subsequent remote check is compared against the baseline check. In clinical studies (Maruthurkkara et al. 2022a, b), Remote Check tests were shown to have high test-retest reliability enabling within recipient comparison of test results. A large majority of recipients found remote check easy to use and felt that they would be cared for by their clinician while using the Remote Check service. The data collection for the study was completed before COVID-19, and thus the high acceptance of Remote Check with recipients was independent of the impact of the global pandemic and imposed restrictions that made travel to the clinic difficult. Rather, it indicated that the concept of remote check in itself was welcomed by most CI recipients and helped build confidence in the access and level of care made remotely.

References

American Speech-Language Hearing Association (ASHA) (n.d.) Person-Centered Care in Audiology Retrieved September 1, 2021 from https://www.asha.org/aud/person-centered-care-in-audiology/

Arlinger, S., Gatehouse, S., Bentler, R. A., Byrne, D., Cox, R. M., Dirks, D. D., Humes, L., Neuman, A., Ponton, C., Robinson, K., Silman, S., Summerfield, A. Q., Turner, C. W., Tyler, R. S., & Willott, J. F. (1996). Report of the Eriksholm workshop on auditory deprivation and acclimatization. *Ear and Hearing, 17*(3 Suppl), 87S–98S.

Battmer, R. D., Borel, S., Brendel, M., Buchner, A., Cooper, H., Fielden, C., Gazibegovic, D., Goetze, R., Govaerts, P., Kelleher, K., Lenartz, T., Mosnier, I., Muff, J., Nunn, T., Vaerenberg, B., & Vanat, Z. (2015). Assessment of 'fitting to outcomes expert' FOX™ with new cochlear implant users in a multi-Centre study. *Cochlear Implants International, 16*(2), 100–109.

Bennett, R. J., Barr, C., Montano, J., Eikelboom, R. H., Saunders, G. H., Pronk, M., Preminger, J. E., Ferguson, M., Weinstein, B., Heffernan, E., van Leeuwen, L., Hickson, L., Timmer, B. H. B., Singh, G., Gerace, D., Cortis, A., & Bellekom, S. R. (2021). Identifying the approaches used by audiologists to address the psychosocial needs of their adult clients. *International Journal of Audiology, 60*(2), 104–114.

Botros, A., & Psarros, C. (2010). Neural response telemetry reconsidered: I. The relevance of ECAP threshold profiles and scaled profiles to cochlear implant fitting. *Ear and Hearing, 31*(3), 367–379.

Botros, A., van Dijk, B., & Killian, M. (2007). AutoNR: An automated system that measures ECAP thresholds with the nucleus freedom cochlear implant via machine intelligence. *Artificial Intelligence in Medicine, 40*(1), 15–28.

Botros, A., Banna, R., & Maruthurkkara, S. (2013). The next generation of Nucleus(®) fitting: A multiplatform approach towards universal cochlear implant management. *International Journal of Audiology, 52*(7), 485–494.

Boyd, P. J. (2010). Evaluation of simplified programs using the MED-EL C40+ cochlear implant. *International Journal of Audiology, 49*(7), 527–534.

Broese van Groenou, M., Hoogendijk, E. O., & van Tilburg, T. G. (2013). Continued and new personal relationships in later life: Differential effects of health. *Journal of Aging and Health, 25*(2), 274–295.

Brown, C. J., Hughes, M. L., Luk, B., Abbas, P. J., Wolaver, A., & Gervais, J. (2000). The relationship between EAP and EABR thresholds and levels used to program the nucleus 24 speech processor: Data from adults. *Ear and Hearing, 21*(2), 151–163.

Browning, L. M., Nie, Y., Rout, A., & Heiner, M. (2020). Audiologists' preferences in programming cochlear implants: A preliminary report. *Cochlear Implants International, 21*(4), 179–191.

Buechner, A., Vaerenberg, B., Gazibegovic, D., Brendel, M., De Ceulaer, G., Govaerts, P., & Lenarz, T. (2015). Evaluation of the 'fitting to outcomes eXpert' (FOX®) with established cochlear implant users. *Cochlear Implants International, 16*(1), 39–46.

Busby, P. A., & Arora, K. (2016). Effects of threshold adjustment on speech perception in nucleus cochlear implant recipients. *Ear and Hearing, 37*(3), 303–311.

Cafarelli Dees, D., Dillier, N., Lai, W. K., von Wallenberg, E., van Dijk, B., Akdas, F., Aksit, M., Batman, C., Beynon, A., Burdo, S., Chanal, J. M., Collet, L., Conway, M., Coudert, C., Craddock, L., Cullington, H., Deggouj, N., Fraysse, B., Grabel, S., Kiefer, J., et al. (2005). Normative findings of electrically evoked compound action potential measurements using the neural response telemetry of the nucleus CI24M cochlear implant system. *Audiology & Neuro-Otology, 10*(2), 105–116.

Ching, T. Y., Psarros, C., Hill, M., Dillon, H., & Incerti, P. (2001). Should children who use cochlear implants wear hearing aids in the opposite ear? *Ear and Hearing, 22*(5), 365–380.

Ching, T. Y., Hill, M., Brew, J., Incerti, P., Priolo, S., Rushbrook, E., & Forsythe, L. (2005). The effect of auditory experience on speech perception, localization, and functional performance of children who use a cochlear implant and a hearing aid in opposite ears. *International Journal of Audiology, 44*(12), 677–690.

Ching, T. Y., van Wanrooy, E., & Dillon, H. (2007). Binaural-bimodal fitting or bilateral implantation for managing severe to profound deafness: A review. *Trends in Amplification, 11*(3), 161–192.

Craddock, L., Cooper, H., van de Heyning, P., Vermeire, K., Davies, M., Patel, J., Cullington, H., Ricaud, R., Brunelli, T., Knight, M., Plant, K., Dees, D. C., & Murray, B. (2003). Comparison between NRT-based MAPs and behaviourally measured MAPs at different stimulation rates—A multicentre investigation. *Cochlear Implants International, 4*(4), 161–170.

Dillon, H. (2012). *Hearing aids*. Boomerang Press.

Dillon, H., James, A., & Ginis, J. (1997). Client Oriented Scale of Improvement (COSI) and its relationship to several other measures of benefit and satisfaction provided by hearing aids. *Journal of the American Academy of Audiology, 8*(1), 27–43.

Eikelboom, R. H., Jayakody, D. M., Swanepoel, D. W., Chang, S., & Atlas, M. D. (2014). Validation of remote mapping of cochlear implants. *Journal of Telemedicine and Telecare, 20*(4), 171–177.

English, R., Plant, K., Maciejczyk, M., & Cowan, R. (2016). Fitting recommendations and clinical benefit associated with use of the NAL-NL2 hearing-aid prescription in Nucleus cochlear implant recipients. *International Journal of Audiology, 55*(Suppl 2), S45–S50.

Gajadeera, E. A., Galvin, K. L., Dowell, R. C., & Busby, P. A. (2017). Investigation of electrical stimulation levels over 8 to 10 years postimplantation for a large cohort of adults using cochlear implants. *Ear and Hearing, 38*(6), 736–745.

Galvin, K. L., & Noble, W. (2013). Adaptation of the speech, spatial, and qualities of hearing scale for use with children, parents, and teachers. *Cochlear Implants International, 14*(3), 135–141.

Gantz, B. J., Brown, C. J., & Abbas, P. J. (1994). Intraoperative measures of electrically evoked auditory nerve compound action potential. *The American Journal of Otology, 15*(2), 137–144.

Gärtner, L., Lenarz, T., & Büchner, A. (2018). Fine-grain recordings of the electrically evoked compound action potential amplitude growth function in cochlear implant recipients. *Biomedical Engineering Online, 17*(1), 140.

Gfeller, K., Oleson, J., Knutson, J. F., Breheny, P., Driscoll, V., & Olszewski, C. (2008). Multivariate predictors of music perception and appraisal by adult cochlear implant users. *Journal of the American Academy of Audiology, 19*(2), 120–134.

Giannantonio, S., Polonenko, M. J., Papsin, B. C., Paludetti, G., & Gordon, K. A. (2015). Experience changes how emotion in music is judged: Evidence from children listening with bilateral cochlear implants, bimodal devices, and normal hearing. *PLoS One, 10*(8), e0136685.

Gibasiewicz, Stieler, Stainsby, et al. (2014). Pilot evaluation of NFS for hybrid fitting. In *Müller (ed.). Abstracts of the 13th International Conference on Cochlear Implants and Other Implantable Auditory Technologies* (p. 771).

Goehring, J. L., & Hughes, M. L. (2017). Measuring sound-processor threshold levels for pediatric Cochlear implant recipients using conditioned play audiometry via telepractice. *Journal of Speech, Language, And Hearing Research: JSLHR, 60*(3), 732–740.

Govaerts, P. J., Vaerenberg, B., De Ceulaer, G., Daemers, K., De Beukelaer, C., & Schauwers, K. (2010). Development of a software tool using deterministic logic for the optimization of cochlear implant processor programming. *Otology & neurotology: Official publication of the American Otological Society, American Neurotology Society [and] European Academy of Otology and Neurotology, 31*(6), 908–918.

Henkin, Y., Kaplan-Neeman, R., Muchnik, C., Kronenberg, J., & Hildesheimer, M. (2003). Changes over time in electrical stimulation levels and electrode impedance values in children using the Nucleus 24M cochlear implant. *International Journal of Pediatric Otorhinolaryngology, 67*(8), 873–880.

Hughes, M. L., Vander Werff, K. R., Brown, C. J., Abbas, P. J., Kelsay, D. M., Teagle, H. F., & Lowder, M. W. (2001). A longitudinal study of electrode impedance, the electrically evoked compound action potential, and behavioral measures in nucleus 24 cochlear implant users. *Ear and Hearing, 22*(6), 471–486.

Hughes, M. L., Goehring, J. L., Baudhuin, J. L., Diaz, G. R., Sanford, T., Harpster, R., & Valente, D. L. (2012). Use of telehealth for research and clinical measures in cochlear implant recipients: A validation study. *Journal of Speech, Language, And Hearing Research: JSLHR, 55*(4), 1112–1127.

Hughes, M. L., Goehring, J. L., Sevier, J. D., & Choi, S. (2018). Measuring sound-processor thresholds for pediatric Cochlear implant recipients using visual reinforcement audiometry via telepractice. *Journal of Speech, Language, And Hearing Research: JSLHR, 61*(8), 2115–2125.

Hughson, W., & Westlake, H. (1944). Manual for program outline for rehabilitation of aural casualties both military and civilian. *Trans Am Acad Ophthalmol Otolaryngol, 48*, 1–15.

Illg, A., Bojanowicz, M., Lesinski-Schiedat, A., Lenarz, T., & Büchner, A. (2014). Evaluation of the bimodal benefit in a large cohort of cochlear implant subjects using a contralateral hearing aid. *Otology & neurotology: Official publication of the American Otological Society, American Neurotology Society [and] European Academy of Otology and Neurotology, 35*(9), e240–e244.

Incerti, P. V., Ching, T. Y. C., Hou, S., Van Buynder, P., Flynn, C., & Cowan, R. (2018). Programming characteristics of cochlear implants in children: Effects of aetiology and age at implantation. *International Journal of Audiology, 57*(sup2), S27–S40.

Kaplan-Neeman, R., Henkin, Y., Yakir, Z., Bloch, F., Berlin, M., Kronenberg, J., Migirov, L., Hildesheimer, M., & Muchnik, C. (2004). NRT-based versus behavioral-based MAP: A comparison of parameters and speech perception in young children. *Journal of Basic and Clinical Physiology and Pharmacology, 15*(1–2), 57–69.

Kileny, P. R., Zwolan, T. A., Zimmerman-Phillips, S., & Telian, S. A. (1994). Electrically evoked auditory brain-stem response in pediatric patients with cochlear implants. *Archives of Otolaryngology--Head & Neck Surgery, 120*(10), 1083–1090.

Kim, J., Jeon, S., Kim, D., & Shin, Y. (2021). A review of contemporary teleaudiology: Literature review, technology, and considerations for practicing. *Journal of Audiology & Otology, 25*(1), 1–7.

Kiss, Tóth, Lajkó, et al. (2014). In Gordon & Papsin (Eds.), *Speech processor fitting using Nucleus Fitting Software (NFS)* (p. 62). Abstracts of the 8th International Symposium on Objective Measures in Auditory Implants.

Kong, Y. Y., Stickney, G. S., & Zeng, F. G. (2005). Speech and melody recognition in binaurally combined acoustic and electric hearing. *The Journal of the Acoustical Society of America, 117*(3 Pt 1), 1351–1361.

Kosaner, J., Anderson, I., Turan, Z., & Deibl, M. (2009). The use of ESRT in fitting children with cochlear implants. *The Journal of International Advanced Otology, 5*(1), 62–71.

Kurz, A., Hagen, R., Van de Heyning, P., & Mertens, G. (2019). Flat-based fitting: The evaluation and usefulness of a new strategy-based fitting approach for cochlear implants. *European Archives of Oto-Rhino-Laryngology, 276*, 3239–3245.

Kuzovkov, V., Yanov, Y., Levin, S., Bovo, R., Rosignoli, M., Eskilsson, G., & Willbas, S. (2014). Remote programming of MED-EL cochlear implants: Users' and professionals' evaluation of the remote programming experience. *Acta Oto-Laryngologica, 134*(7), 709–716.

Ling, D. (1989). *Foundations of spoken language for hearing-impaired children* (Vol. 11). Alexander Graham Bell Association for the Deaf, Inc.

Luryi, A. L., Tower, J. I., Preston, J., Burkland, A., Trueheart, C. E., & Hildrew, D. M. (2020). Cochlear implant mapping through telemedicine-a feasibility study. *Otology & neurotology: Official publication of the American Otological Society, American Neurotology Society [and] European Academy of Otology and Neurotology, 41*(3), e330–e333.

Maruthurkkara, S. (2024). Cochlear implant remote assist: Clinical and real-world evaluation. *International Journal of Audiology*, 1–11. Advance online publication.

Maruthurkkara, S., & Bennett, C. (2024). Development of custom sound® pro software utilising big data and its clinical evaluation. *International Journal of Audiology, 63*(2), 87–98.

Maruthurkkara, S., Allen, A., Cullington, H., Muff, J., Arora, K., & Johnson, S. (2022a). Remote check test battery for cochlear implant recipients: Proof of concept study. *International Journal of Audiology, 61*(6), 443–452.

Maruthurkkara, S., Case, S., & Rottier, R. (2022b). Evaluation of remote check: A clinical tool for asynchronous monitoring and triage of Cochlear implant recipients. *Ear and Hearing, 43*(2), 495–506.

McElveen, J. T., Jr., Blackburn, E. L., Green, J. D., Jr., McLear, P. W., Thimsen, D. J., & Wilson, B. S. (2010). Remote programming of cochlear implants: A telecommunications model. *Otology & neurotology: Official publication of the American Otological Society, American Neurotology Society [and] European Academy of Otology and Neurotology, 31*(7), 1035–1040.

Meeuws, M., Pascoal, D., Bermejo, I., Artaso, M., De Ceulaer, G., & Govaerts, P. J. (2017). Computer-assisted CI fitting: Is the learning capacity of the intelligent agent FOX beneficial for speech understanding? *Cochlear Implants International, 18*(4), 198–206.

Müller-Deile, J. (Ed.). (2009). *Verfahren zur Anpassung und Evaluation von Cochlear Implant Sprachprozessoren* (1st ed., pp. 40–69). Median Verlag von Killisch-Horn GmbH. ISBN 978-3-941146-01-3.

Müller-Deile, Dillier, Buchner, et al. (2017). In Arenberg & McAlpine (Eds.), *Prospective multicenter evaluation of a partially automated CI fitting method compared to the clinically established procedure* (p. 266). Abstracts of the 2017 Conference on Implantable Auditory Prostheses.

Nadol, J. B., Jr. (1997). Patterns of neural degeneration in the human cochlea and auditory nerve: Implications for cochlear implantation. *Otolaryngology—head and neck surgery: official journal of American Academy of Otolaryngology-Head and Neck Surgery, 117*(3 Pt 1), 220–228.

Noble, W., Jensen, N. S., Naylor, G., Bhullar, N., & Akeroyd, M. A. (2013). A short form of the speech, spatial and qualities of hearing scale suitable for clinical use: The SSQ12. *International Journal of Audiology, 52*(6), 409–412.

Nogueira, W., Schurzig, D., Büchner, A., Penninger, R. T., & Würfel, W. (2016). Validation of a Cochlear implant patient-specific model of the voltage distribution in a clinical setting. *Frontiers in Bioengineering and Biotechnology, 4*, 84.

Ohno, T. (2006). Ask 'why' five times about every matter. https://www.toyota-myanmar.com/about-toyota/toyota-traditions/quality/ask-why-five-times-about-every-matter. Retrieved August, 2021

Parker, R., Muzaffar, J., AuD, M. A., & Brassington, W. (2024). Early activation of cochlear implants: A systematic review and narrative synthesis. *Cochlear Implants International, 25*(1), 81–92.

Pedley, K., Psarros, C., Gardner-Berry, K., Parker, A., Purdy, S. C., Dawson, P., & Plant, K. (2007). Evaluation of NRT and behavioral measures for MAPping elderly cochlear implant users. *International Journal of Audiology, 46*(5), 254–262.

Plant, K., Law, M. A., Whitford, L., Knight, M., Tari, S., Leigh, J., Pedley, K., & Nel, E. (2005). Evaluation of streamlined programming procedures for the nucleus cochlear implant with the contour electrode array. *Ear and Hearing, 26*(6), 651–668.

Plasmans, A., & Vanpoucke, F. (2015). *How well are hearing targets met during NFS streamlined fitting?* D755960 Cochlear Ltd Clinical Investigation Report.

Potts, L. G., Skinner, M. W., Litovsky, R. A., Strube, M. J., & Kuk, F. (2009). Recognition and localization of speech by adult cochlear implant recipients wearing a digital hearing aid in the nonimplanted ear (bimodal hearing). *Journal of the American Academy of Audiology, 20*(6), 353–373.

Ramos, A., Rodriguez, C., Martinez-Beneyto, P., Perez, D., Gault, A., Falcon, J. C., & Boyle, P. (2009). Use of telemedicine in the remote programming of cochlear implants. *Acta Oto-Laryngologica, 129*(5), 533–540.

Rasetshwane, D. M., Trevino, A. C., Gombert, J. N., Liebig-Trehearn, L., Kopun, J. G., Jesteadt, W., Neely, S. T., & Gorga, M. P. (2015). Categorical loudness scaling and equal-loudness contours in listeners with normal hearing and hearing loss. *The Journal of the Acoustical Society of America, 137*(4), 1899–1913.
Rooth, M., King, E. R., Dillon, M., & Pillsbury, H. (2017). Management considerations for Cochlear implant recipients in their 80s and 90s. Hearing Review, (Aug).
Samuel, P. A., Goffi-Gomez, M. V., Bittencourt, A. G., Tsuji, R. K., & Brito, R. D. (2014). Remote programming of cochlear implants. *CoDAS, 26*(6), 481–486.
Schepers, K., Steinhoff, H. J., Ebenhoch, H., Böck, K., Bauer, K., Rupprecht, L., Möltner, A., Morettini, S., & Hagen, R. (2019). Remote programming of cochlear implants in users of all ages. *Acta Oto-Laryngologica, 139*(3), 251–257.
Scorpecci, A., D'Elia, A., Malerba, P., Cantore, I., Consolino, P., Trabalzini, F., Paludetti, G., & Quaranta, N. (2016). Maps created using a new objective procedure (C-NRT) correlate with behavioral, loudness-balanced maps: a study in adult cochlear implant users. *European archives of oto-rhino-laryngology: official journal of the European Federation of Oto-Rhino-Laryngological Societies (EUFOS) : affiliated with the German Society for Oto-Rhino-Laryngology—Head and Neck Surgery, 273(12)*, 4167–4173.
Shapiro, W. H., & Bradham, T. S. (2012). Cochlear implant programming. *Otolaryngologic Clinics of North America, 45*(1), 111–127.
Slager, H. K., Jensen, J., Kozlowski, K., Teagle, H., Park, L. R., Biever, A., & Mears, M. (2019). Remote programming of Cochlear implants. *Otology & neurotology: Official publication of the American Otological Society, American Neurotology Society [and] European Academy of Otology and Neurotology, 40*(3), e260–e266.
Smits, C., Kapteyn, T. S., & Houtgast, T. (2004). Development and validation of an automatic speech-in-noise screening test by telephone. *International Journal of Audiology, 43*(1), 15–28.
Smoorenburg, G. F., Willeboer, C., & van Dijk, J. E. (2002). Speech perception in nucleus CI24M cochlear implant users with processor settings based on electrically evoked compound action potential thresholds. *Audiology & Neuro-Otology, 7*(6), 335–347.
Spivak, L., Auerbach, C., Vambutas, A., Geshkovich, S., Wexler, L., & Popecki, B. (2011). Electrical compound action potentials recorded with automated neural response telemetry: Threshold changes as a function of time and electrode position. *Ear and Hearing, 32*(1), 104–113.
Stephan, K., & Welzl-Müller, K. (1994). Effect of stimulus duration on stapedius reflex threshold in electrical stimulation via cochlear implant. *Audiology, 33*(3), 143–151.
Stypulkowski, P. H., & van den Honert, C. (1984). Physiological properties of the electrically stimulated auditory nerve. I. Compound action potential recordings. *Hearing Research, 14*(3), 205–223.
Sucher, C. M., & McDermott, H. J. (2009). Bimodal stimulation: Benefits for music perception and sound quality. *Cochlear Implants International, 10*(Suppl 1), 96–99.
Takano, K., Kaizaki, A., Kimura, A., Nomura, K., Yamazaki, N., Shintani, T., & Himi, T. (2021). Telefitting of nucleus Cochlear implants: A feasibility study. *American Journal of Audiology, 30*(1), 16–21.
Telmesani, L. M., & Said, N. M. (2016). Electrically evoked compound action potential (ECAP) in cochlear implant children: Changes in auditory nerve response in first year of cochlear implant use. *International Journal of Pediatric Otorhinolaryngology, 82*, 28–33.
Vaerenberg, B., Smits, C., De Ceulaer, G., Zir, E., Harman, S., Jaspers, N., Tam, Y., Dillon, M., Wesarg, T., Martin-Bonniot, D., Gärtner, L., Cozma, S., Kosaner, J., Prentiss, S., Sasidharan, P., Briaire, J. J., Bradley, J., Debruyne, J., Hollow, R., Patadia, R., et al. (2014). Cochlear implant programming: A global survey on the state of the art. *TheScientific World Journal, 2014*, 501738.
Van Den Abbeele, T., Noël-Petroff, N., Akin, I., Caner, G., Olgun, L., Guiraud, J., Truy, E., Attias, J., Raveh, E., Belgin, E., Sennaroglu, G., Basta, D., Ernst, A., Martini, A., Rosignoli, M., Levi, H., Elidan, J., Benghalem, A., Amstutz-Montadert, I., Lerosey, Y., et al. (2012). Multicentre

investigation on electrically evoked compound action potential and stapedius reflex: How do these objective measures relate to implant programming parameters? *Cochlear Implants International, 13*(1), 26–34.

Van den Borne, B., Mens, L. H., Snik, A. F., Spies, T. H., & Van den Broek, P. (1994). Stapedius reflex and EABR thresholds in experienced users of the nucleus cochlear implant. *Acta Oto-Laryngologica, 114*(2), 141–143.

van Dijk, B., Botros, A. M., Battmer, R. D., Begall, K., Dillier, N., Hey, M., Lai, W. K., Lenarz, T., Laszig, R., Morsnowski, A., Müller-Deile, J., Psarros, C., Shallop, J., Weber, B., Wesarg, T., Zarowski, A., & Offeciers, E. (2007). Clinical results of AutoNRT, a completely automatic ECAP recording system for cochlear implants. *Ear and Hearing, 28*(4), 558–570.

Visram, A. S., Innes-Brown, H., El-Deredy, W., & McKay, C. M. (2015). Cortical auditory evoked potentials as an objective measure of behavioral thresholds in cochlear implant users. *Hearing Research, 327*, 35–42.

Vroegop, J. L., Dingemanse, J. G., van der Schroeff, M. P., Metselaar, R. M., & Goedegebure, A. (2017). Self-adjustment of upper electrical stimulation levels in CI programming and the effect on auditory functioning. *Ear and Hearing, 38*(4), e232–e240.

Wesarg, T., Wasowski, A., Skarzynski, H., Ramos, A., Falcon Gonzalez, J. C., Kyriafinis, G., Junge, F., Novakovich, A., Mauch, H., & Laszig, R. (2010). Remote fitting in nucleus cochlear implant recipients. *Acta Oto-Laryngologica, 130*(12), 1379–1388.

Willeboer, C. (2008). *Simplifying cochlear implant speech processor fitting*. PhD thesis, University of Utrecht, Universal Press.

Wolfe, J., Gilbert, M., Schafer, E., Litvak, L. M., Spahr, A. J., Saoji, A., & Finley, C. (2017). Optimizations for the electrically-evoked Stapedial reflex threshold measurement in Cochlear implant recipients. *Ear and Hearing, 38*(2), 255–261.

Zwolan, T. A., Presley, R., Chenier, L., & Buck, B. (2021). Investigation of an outcomes-driven, computer-assisted approach to CI fitting in newly implanted patients. *Ear and Hearing, 42*(3), 558–564.

Chapter 18
Cochlear Implants: Objective Measures in Mapping

Chandan Saha and Krithika Iyengar Saha

Abstract A cochlear implant (CI) helps create the sensation of sound through electrical signals. Various parameters are measured and set to ensure the electrical patterns produced by the device correspond to sounds that help maximize speech intelligibility. MAP of a CI can be considered as the software program that codes the acoustic information in the environment to electrical codes that stimulate the auditory nerve. The primary goal of the MAP or the Cochlear Implant listening program includes providing optimal audibility and speech understanding as well as comfort even in complex listening environments. This chapter deals with objective measures such as electrically evoked compound action potential, electrically evoked stapedial reflex threshold, electrically evoked auditory brainstem response, and electrically evoked cortical potential used for the assessment of appropriateness of a MAP among cochlear implant users.

Keywords Cochlear implant · eSRT · Mapping · eCAP · Electrically evoked auditory brainstem response (eABR)

Introduction

Cochlear implant (CI) helps create sensation of sound through electrical signals. For optimal function, CI processors need to be programmed and tailored for each user (Nunn et al., 2019; Ciprut & Adıgu, 2020). Various parameters are measured and set to ensure the electrical patterns produced by the device correspond to sounds that help maximize speech intelligibility. Every CI user is given a MAP, which is a unique configuration of settings that defines the operational range of their implant. MAP of a CI can be considered as the software program that codes the acoustic information in the environment to electrical codes that stimulate the auditory nerve. The MAP, therefore, is very important as it codes the acoustic dynamic range into

C. Saha · K. I. Saha (✉)
Decibel Audiology and Speech Clinic Pvt Ltd, Kolkata, India

P. Kumar et al. (eds.), *Advances in Implantation Otology*,
https://doi.org/10.1007/978-981-96-8671-1_18

an equivalent electric dynamic range for an individual. The MAP includes setting of the minimum electrical stimulation that generates a percept (threshold or T-level) and maximum comfortable stimulation (C- or M-level). This method of ascertaining the optimal values for a particular recipient is popularly called Mapping. It is accomplished using a company specific proprietary software and hardware interface coupled to the speech processor and depends on the behavioural responses from the cochlear implantee.

The primary goal of the MAP or the Cochlear Implant listening programme includes providing optimal audibility and speech understanding as well as comfort even in complex listening environments. MAP parameters contribute significantly to each recipient's listening and speech perception abilities (Nunn et al., 2019), in particular the psychophysical limits of intensity scaling the lower Threshold (T-Level) and the upper limit of Comfort (C-level). Inappropriately set C or M levels may lead to reduced speech understanding whereas very high C or M levels can lead to painful stimulation (Ciprut & Adıgu, 2020; Spivak & Chute, 1994). Several factors influence the parametric values of the MAPs. Some are related to the electro-neural interphase, such as the position of the implanted electrodes, density of the spiral ganglions, and electrolytic composition of the scalar fluid. However, some factors are related to the subject or the measurement procedure, such as listening experience, listening attention, judgement related to signal detection, and responsiveness (the ability to perform a conditioning task).

A typical CI mapping is done through subjective fine-tuning, wherein parameters are adjusted using psychophysical loudness scaling procedures (Mittal et al., 2015; Vaerenberg et al., 2014). The subjective mapping method requires active participation from the recipient, with the outcome depending heavily on the recipients' attributes of attention, patience, and cognitive-linguistic skills needed to complete the required tasks with reliability and repeatability (Andrade et al., 2014; Bresnihan et al., 2001). This method of programming may not be suitable for some CI subgroups, which include very young children, individuals with severe deficits in speech and language, or those with low cognitive abilities. In such cases, typical subjective CI programming can create a suboptimal MAP that may give preference to comfort over speech perception which can cause issues in understanding speech as well as delay in language development in children (Kosaner et al., 2018). As in the case of establishing hearing thresholds, reliable and objective measures are preferred for establishing an appropriate dynamic range for speech perception in these sub-groups who are limited in their ability to provide clear subjective loudness judgements (Andrade et al., 2014; Kosaner et al., 2018).

Objective measurements can be achieved without any active feedback from the patient. These methods, which rely on neural or physiological responses elicited via electrical stimuli generated from CI electrodes, are thus proposed for obtaining valuable information for programming the speech processor (Bayat et al., 2018; Bergeron & Hotton, 2015). Currently, the objective measurements are used for verifying the device function, identifying possible malfunctioning electrodes, and verifying the integrity and function of the auditory pathways. They also assist in programming the speech processor and obtaining a baseline of neural function for tracking potential changes over time, monitoring changes in electro-neural interphase over time, measuring discrimination of different stimuli, estimating plasticity of the auditory system, and optimizing electrode position for appropriate frequency allocation.

Over the years, electrophysiology based objective methods have been used to estimate the electrical dynamic range, thereby minimizing the effects of various factors on the MAP. Apart from estimating the dynamic range, these electrophysiological measures have also been used to validate the MAP. These measures have also been used to evaluate the maturation of the auditory system post Cochlear Implantation which can be considered as a measure of the outcome. Electrophysiological measures are used to estimate, validate and measure the effectiveness of the MAP in achieving the maturational milestones of the auditory neural pathway. The commonly used electrophysiological methods -- eCAP, eSRT, eABR, and cortically evoked auditory potentials (CAEP) have been discussed here.

Electrically-Evoked Compound Action Potential (eCAP)

The physiological event of importance in eCAP measurement is the action potential from the first-order neurons in the cochlea. These action potentials are evoked using electrical stimulation presented via the electrodes implanted in the cochlea. These electric stimulations, when presented in the cochlear fluids, stimulate a group of nerve cell bodies (spiral ganglions). Each nerve cell in the vicinity of the stimulation field generates an action potential. As the recorded potential is the summation of action potentials generated by a group of nerve fibres, it is termed as Compound Action Potential (CAP). In Cochlear Implants, these CAPs are evoked using electrical stimulation and hence they are called electrically-evoked compound action potential (eCAP).

Principle of eCAP

Like any evoked potential measurement, eCAP requires specific stimulation and recording parameters. Present day cochlear implants use a set of electrodes from the implanted array to deliver the electrical stimulation and another set of electrodes to record the response. A tiny electrical voltage is delivered through the stimulating electrodes. As a response to this stimulation, the spiral ganglions generate an electrical potential with a very short latency (within 1 ms). This potential, called eCAP, is recorded as a negative potential (N1) at about 0.2–0.4 ms after the stimulus onset. This negative peak is often followed by a considerably smaller positive potential (P2) or a plateau occurring at about 0.6–0.8 ms (Abbas et al., 1999; Brown et al., 1998; Cullington et al., 2000). The amplitude of the eCAP can be as large as 1–2 mV. This is essentially the Wave I of the ABR but is comparatively more robust and stable than the electrically evoked ABR (Brown et al., 1998), as eCAP is recorded closer to the generator site than the scalp-recorded ABR. The eCAPs also have a clear edge over the cortical potentials. They require a far smaller test duration and are prominently visible inside the first year of life, making them less susceptible to the maturational effects than the cortical potentials (Hughes, 2012). The Basic principle behind the recording of eCAP is shown in Fig. 18.1.

The most challenging aspect in eCAP recording is removing stimulus artifact since the stimuli as well as the responses are electrical in nature, and both are present spatially and temporally in close proximity to each other inside the cochlea. The problem is worsened by the fact that the stimulus is several times (about 1000 times) bigger than the response. Alternating polarity stimulation, forward masking paradigm, and triphasic pulse rejection are the most commonly used methods for artifact reduction.

When using alternating polarity, the responses to "anodic first" and "Cathodic first" stimuli are stored in two separate buffers. When the responses in these two buffers are added, they cancel the remnant charge from the stimulus artifact. The forward masking subtraction paradigm uses four sets of stimulus patterns and the responses for each are recorded in separate buffers. These responses are then subtracted from the other in a way to cancel the stimulus related artifacts. This approach uses the concept of temporal masking i.e. forward masking, wherein a masker stimulus is delivered first, and following a short delay called 'Masker Probe Interval' (MPI), the probe is delivered. Let us understand how this works with an illustration. Let us assume that the four buffers arc four sets --Set A to Set D,with each set storing responses to specific stimulation conditions, as shown below:

Set A: Probe (stimulus) pulse
Set B: Masker pulse + Probe (stimulus) pulse
Set C: Masker Pulse
Set D: no pulseonly recording amplifier set on and off

For stimulation Set B, the presentation of the "masker stimulus" puts the nerves into refractory phase and the MPI is set such that the "probe pulse" is presented while

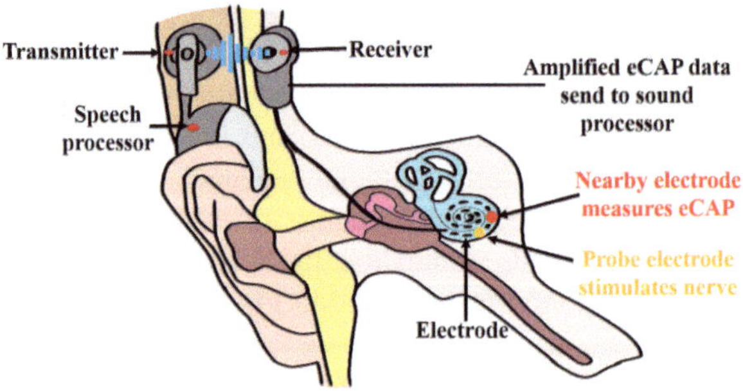

Fig. 18.1 Basic principle behind the recording of eCAPs: (1) the electrical impulses from a probe electrode stimulates the nerve fibres; (2) an electrode in the vicinity of the stimulating electrode records the response created by the stimulation; (3) the recorded eCAP is amplified and transmitted to the PC via the sound processor for analysis; [Image Courtesy of MED-EL Company]

the nerve fibres are still in refractory phase, which leads to no response generation for the "probe" and the buffer, therefore, records only the neural response to the masker stimulus. Stimulation set D is presented to record the switch on artifact of the amplifier or any other incidental artifacts. So, the responses recorded in each buffer would be in a way shown in Table 18.1.

The subtraction is done in a way that the difference of Set C and Set D is subtracted from Set B, and the obtained outcome is subtracted from Set A, and we get the final response [A- {B- (C-D)}]. See Table 18.2 for an illustration of this process to achieve the resultant response to only the probe pulse. So, at the end we have only the response elicited by the probe stimulus. Success of this approach, however, is dependent on the ability of the masker to put majority of nerve fibres into refractory phase and setting the MPI shorter than the recovery time of the nerves.

The triphasic pulse rejection is another method of reducing the artifacts from an eCAP recording. To cancel the remnant charge from the biphasic stimulation charge, a third phase of negative charge (usually 10% of the first phase) is added to the biphasic pulse.

Equipment Needed for Obtaining eCAP

The most essential component of the eCAP measurement hardware is a cochlear implant with capability to perform Bi-directional Telemetry. This measurement does not require any other equipment and can be completed using the

Table 18.1 Stimulation and the corresponding responses recorded in each of the four buffers when using a forward masking subtraction paradigm

Set (Buffer)	Stimulation	Response recorded
A	P	$R_p + A_P + A_{AMP}$
B	M–P	$R_M + A_M + A_P + A_{AMP}$
C	M	$R_M + A_M + A_{AMP}$
D	–	A_{AMP}

Note: Alphabets 'A' to 'D'—various sets (buffers); 'P'—probe pulse; 'M'—masker pulse; 'R_P'—response to probe pulse; 'A_P'—pulse artifact; 'A_{AMP}'—amplifier switch-on artifact; 'R_M'—response to masker pulse; 'A_M'—masker artifact

Table 18.2 A step-by-step illustration of how the response to only the probe pulse is preserved while cancelling the artifacts

Process	Response	Result
C-D	$R_M + A_M + A_{AMP} - A_{AMP}$	$R_M + A_M$
B- (C-D)	$R_M + A_M + A_P + A_{AMP} - R_M - A_M$	$A_P + A_{AMP}$
A- {B- (C-D)}	$R_p + A_P + A_{AMP} - A_P - A_{AMP}$	R_p

Note. Alphabets 'A' to 'D'—various sets (buffers); 'P'—probe pulse; 'M'—masker pulse; 'R_P' response to probe pulse; 'A_P'—pulse artifact; 'A_{AMP}'—amplifier switch-on artifact; 'R_M'—response to masker pulse; 'A_M'—masker artifact

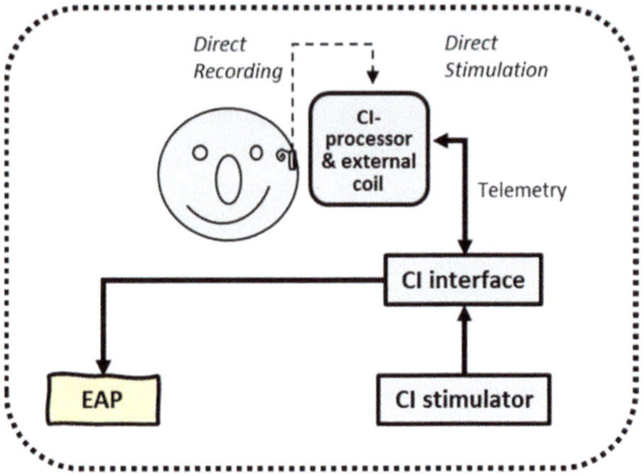

Fig. 18.2 Schematic diagram of hardware connectivity for recording eCAP

manufacturer's designated programming or telemetry software. This Bi-directional Telemetry was first introduced commercially in 1998, and since then it has undergone several refinements and automation at multiple layers. Presently, most of the FDA-approved CI manufacturers have this capability with different names -- eCAP recording in Cochlear Ltd. devices is called Neural Response Telemetry (NRT), in MED-EL devices it is named Auditory Response Telemetry (ART), and it is named as Neural Response Imaging (NRI) in Advanced Bionic devices.

Ideal Measuring Conditions for eCAP

Best outcomes in eCAP measurement requires a host of factors to be aligned in a way to complement each other. The major factors that affect eCAP measurements and constitute ideal conditions for recording them are appropriately placed electrode array in working condition within the scala tympani, functional spiral ganglion cells in the cochlea, acceptable electrical impedance, absence of radiofrequency or electrical interference, and stable connectivity between the external sound processor and the components of the implant. While several other factors might also contribute to the final recording, their influence would have less of a bearing than the once just mentioned.

Procedure for Obtaining eCAP

The connections of various external hardware components should be established in way shown in the schematic diagram in Fig. 18.2. The connectivity with the internal implant components is then established using appropriate transmitting coil placed over the receiver stimulator of the implant. A vital step in ensuring best outcomes is

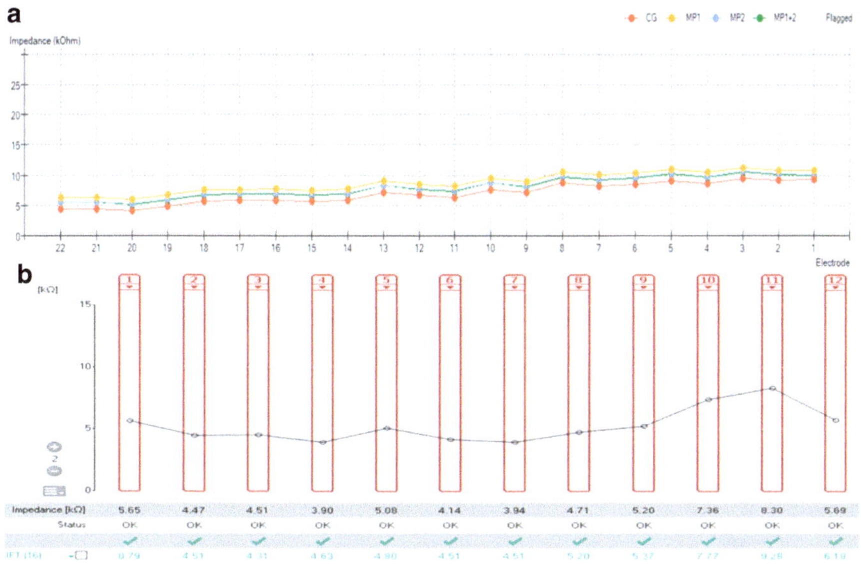

Fig. 18.3 Screenshots of electrode impedance measurement from two leading cochlear implant manufacturers (A) Cochlear Ltd., (B) MED-EL

electrode impedance measurement. Fig. 18.3 shows screenshots of measured electrode impedance from two leading manufacturers of cochlear implants. Once all the above steps are accomplished, the eCAP measurement can begin by choosing the electrode(s) for which the measurement is desired. All present-day software's optimize most of the measurement parameters and perform automatic recording of the responses.

An eCAP finding is commonly described using the terms "Threshold of the eCAP"(T-eCAP) and "Amplitude Growth function" (AGF). The slope and threshold are the two commonly derived measures from the AGF. The slope represents the growth of the eCAP response as a function of the stimulus level and threshold refers to the level needed to elicit a minimal neural response. T-eCAP is defined as the zero crossing on the thus calculated regression line. T-eCAP levels are clinically used to estimate behavioural levels during mapping. Figure 18.4 shows the screenshots of eCAP recording from two leading manufacturers.

Applications of eCAP

1. One of the best applications of the eCAP lies in its ability to predict a stimulus level that assures audibility to the recipient. This allows us to use the information from eCAP for setting the psychophysical parameters of the MAP when it is not possible to garner reliable behavioural responses.

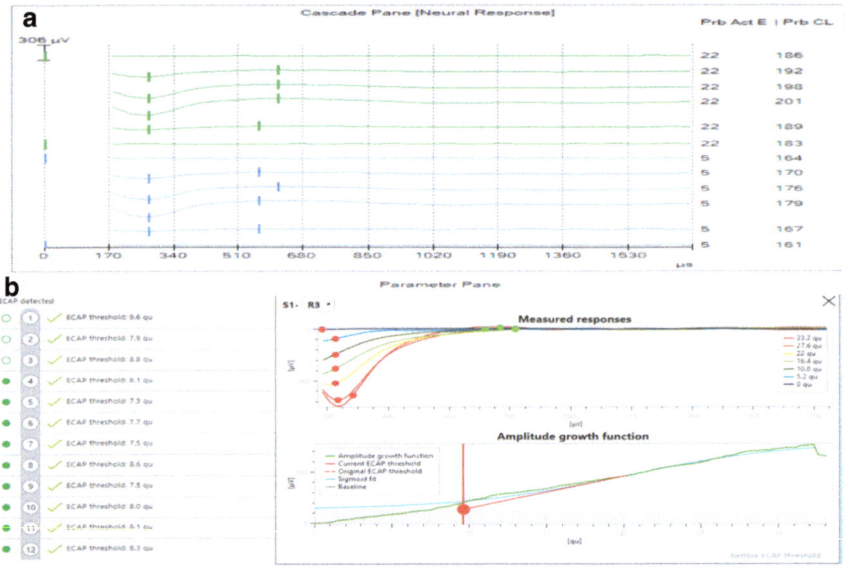

Fig. 18.4 Screenshots of (**a**) eCAP recording in the software of Cochlear Ltd., (**b**) CAP and AGF recording in the MED-EL software

2. Presence of eCAP affirms response of the auditory nerve to electrical stimulation and provides insights into the neural health through measures like *Recovery function* and *Amplitude growth function*. It also provides information about the positioning of electrode by measuring the spread of excitation.
3. The eCAP helps to ascertain functioning of the electroneural interface. It allows to assess functioning of electrodes, functioning of neural fibres, the electrodes' proximity to the neural fibres, and thus its ability to stimulate them.
4. It can also be used as an objective baseline to which subsequent measurements can be compared.

As stated above, one of the major applications of eCAP is that it provides information about the stimulus intensity sufficient to stimulate the nerve fibers, thereby allowing us to adjust MAP parameters in the clinical settings. There are two clinical methods for setting up MAP parameters using eCAP: *eCAP contour method and T-C offset method*. These are delineated below:

The eCAP Contour Method for Obtaining eCAP

This method, also called eCAP profile method, was suggested by Smoorenberg et al. (2002). In this method, eCAP is measured from all possible electrodes. In Advanced Bionics and MED-EL systems, "M" levels are set following the contour of the eCAP thresholds. The "M" level in all electrodes is set in "Live Mode" to a level where satisfactory auditory responses are observed without signs of discomfort. The "T" levels are traditionally set as a percentage (8–10%) of the M levels. In the Cochlear Ltd. systems, the T and C levels follow the eCAP contour. After the eCAP measures are performed, keeping the eCAP contour information intact, both T and C levels are dropped to inaudible levels (typically below 100 current level). A dynamic range of 5–10 current level is set and levels are gradually increased in Live Mode until the signs of audibility are observed. Beyond this only the C levels are increased maintaining the contour until the signs of discomfort start appearing.

The T/C Offset Method for Obtaining eCAP

This method is used when minimal amount of behavioural responses are possible. This method was given by Hughes et al 2000. eCAP is measured in as many electrodes as possible, but in no less than 5 electrodes. In fact, in the typical clinical setting, most clinicians choose exactly five electrodes for eCAP measurement, unless there is an indication to use a higher number. The finding of unusually high eCAP for one of the five chosen electrodes necessitates acquisition of eCAPs from additional electrodes on either side of the electrode with an aberrant finding. Nonetheless, choice of just five electrodes to begin with is not mandatory. A centrally located electrode where eCAP is present is chosen and the T and C levels are measured. The difference between the eCAP and the psychoacoustic levels are called the "T" offset or "C" offset. The T and C levels are set for all electrodes using the same T and C offsets.

Most studies have reported a weak to moderate correlation of eCAP to Threshold (T-levels) and upper-stimulation levels (C-levels), and it has a tendency to overestimate comfort levels, thereby causing over-stimulation in many cases (Brown et al., 2000; Lorens et al., 2003). Clinicians have been using eCAP-based information as a guide to determine stimulation levels for cochlear implantees from whom reliable feedback about the loudness of the signals is difficult to obtain. However, several studies have suggested that the electrically-evoked stapedial reflex thresholds (eSRT) more accurately predict the T and C levels than do eCAP, and therefore eSRT should be considered a more sensitive alternative to eCAP for predicting the T and C levels (Polak et al., 2005; Scorpecci et al., 2016).

Electrically-Evoked Stapedial Reflex Test (eSRT)

The stapedial reflex is typically produced in response to an intense acoustic stimulation of the ear, which leads to a change in static admittance at the level of tympanic membrane. However, using the same principle and pathway, even an intense electric current from the cochlear implant can elicit stapedius muscle contraction, and its threshold is called the eSRT (Messersmith et al., 2018). It is possible to directly visualize stapedial contraction intraoperatively. Alternatively, the eSRT can be intraoperatively recorded using a standard immittance measure or an electromyographic measure. It is also possible to use the standard immittance measure to obtain postoperative eSRTs (Bergeron & Hotton, 2015; Guida et al., 2019).

Principle of eSRT

Any intense stimulus triggers the afferent fibres of vestibulocochlear nerve originating in the cochlea. This triggered response travels to the motor nuclei of the facial nerve on ipsilateral as well as contralateral side via the ipsilateral cochlear nucleus. The efferent pathway from the motor nuclei to the facial nerve finally helps complete this reflex arc. Since the facial nerve transcends its fibers to the stapedius muscles on both sides, the resultant contraction of the stapedial muscles takes place on both sides. This action of the stapedius muscles pulls the ossicular chain backwards, leading to an increase in stiffness at the tympanic membrane (Hughes, 2012).

Equipment Needed for eSRT

The software used for CI fitting procedures is used to accomplish eSRT measurements. Various parameter settings in the software, such as pulse duration, repetition rate, etc. are replicas of the ones used for finding the psychophysical behavioural levels, such as the T and C levels, during mapping. An immittance meter with a 226-Hz probe tone, along with facility for reflex decay measurement, is required for recording the change in the stiffness created by the stapedial muscle contraction.

Ideal Measuring Conditions for Obtaining eSRT

Several things must fall in place to accomplish a successful eSRT measurement. The first and foremost is the middle ear condition. It is imperative to have a normally functioning middle ear, which can be ascertained by the evidence of a normal tympanogram, at least to some extent. It is also necessary to have a speech processor in the best working condition. We all know that cooperation from the subject is a must for successful recording of the stapedial reflex threshold; therefore, a cooperative calmly seated CI recipient is also a must.

Procedure for Obtaining eSRT

For recording the stapedius reflex, a contralateral reflex measurement is needed. Therefore, the probe is placed in the ear contralateral to the implanted ear, ensuring a hermetic seal, to record changes in admittance at the tympanic membrane due to the stapedius muscle reflex. As mentioned before, the reflexive contraction of the stapedial muscle is a bilateral phenomenon, thus the decrease in admittance can also be observed in the ear contralateral to the cochlear implant, despite the stimulation in the implanted ear. Once the stapedius reflex is detected, an ascending-descending technique is used, beginning with an initial high current level and gradually descending until the stapedius reflex disappears. To decide on the amount of reduction in stimulus level, the cues from the reflex amplitude in response to the previous stimulus level are used. The lowest electrical stimulus level producing a recordable stapedial reflex with a minimum change in static admittance of 0.02 ml is termed as the threshold of the stapedius reflex or eSRT (Hernandez et al., 2019). To measure the acoustic reflex, the reflex decay recording window is selected. In the presence of a continuous probe tone of 226 Hz, the biphasic pulses from the cochlear implant are presented, beginning with a low, tolerable stimulus level and progressively increasing in small steps until a time-locked decrease in admittance is observed. The eSRT is then used to obtain an eSRT-based objective map in a manner shown Fig. 18.5.

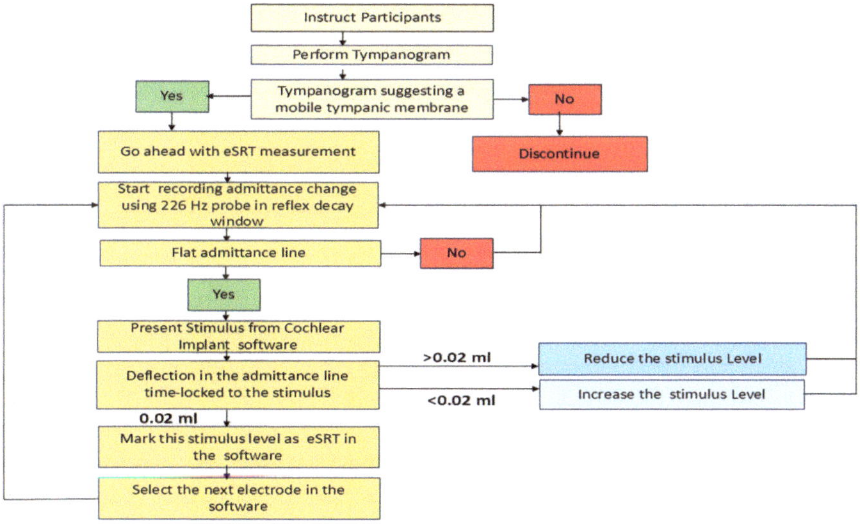

Fig. 18.5 Schematic representation of the typical mapping procedure using the electrically-evoked stapedial reflex threshold (eSRT)

Advantages of Using eSRT for Mapping

In comparison with the eCAP, an eSRT requires lesser electrode threshold recording time. When using it on a typical cochlear implant recipient, an eSRT takes a mean time of about 35 s as opposed to the mean time of 120 s needed for an eCAP-based threshold measurement (Kosaner et al., 2018). A further advantage of eSRT is that it requires minimal cooperation from the recipient and is not affected by state of arousal. It is therefore gaining importance while working with difficult to test population (Carson et al., 2018). To cap it all, eSRT thresholds remain stable over time (Bergeron & Hotton, 2015; Kosaner, 2010).

Numerous studies in adults have shown a high degree of correlation of eSRT with the upper stimulation level (Polak et al., 2006; Spivak et al., 1994). Also, eSRT produces equal loudness judgement across the electrodes within the electrode array, which leads to perceptual benefits such as an optimum sound quality and speech identification. In fact, the speech identification performance with eSRT-based programs have been found to be on par with those obtained using psychophysical methods of programming. The studies using eSRT-based estimation of the upper stimulation level in paediatric population suggest that such children used their cochlear implants for longer time periods and rarely reported discomfort to sounds around them, including speech (Gordon et al., 2004). The use of eSRT has also been instrumental in identifying poor performers due to irregular device use arising out of discomfort associated with excessively high upper stimulation levels.

Electrically-evoked Auditory Brainstem Response (eABR)

An acoustically-evoked Auditory Brainstem Response (ABR) typically has 5 peaks, which arise from various levels in the ascending auditory pathway, beginning with the first two (waves I and II) from the auditory nerve, the third (wave III) from the cochlear nucleus with some contributions from the superior olivary complex, and the final two (waves IV and V) from the innervations in the lateral lemniscus and inferior colliculus. On the basis of the difference in latencies between any two peaks, one can estimate the neural conduction time between the generators of the peaks in question (Moller & Jannetta, 1982a, b; Pontonet al., 1996). An eABR waveform has a similar appearance and consists of the same peaks as their acoustic counterparts, with an exception of wave I, which is obscured due to the presence of a large stimulus artifact. Further, the latencies of each of the visible eABR peaks is 1–2 ms shorter than the corresponding peaks in the acoustic ABR (Wang et al., 2009). This is because the stimulus delivered via the implant bypasses the conduction delay of the peripheral auditory system to directly stimulate the spiral ganglion cells. The generators in the mid-brainstem are believed to be responsible for eABR wave III whereas the eABR wave V is thought to have its origin in the upper brainstem (Van den Honert & Stypulkowski, 1986). CI patients exhibit more neural synchronicity to electrical stimulation than do the normal hearing individuals to acoustic stimulation, which again could be related to the direct stimulation of the auditory nerve with an instantaneous-onset electrical pulse (Gordan et al., 2002).

Principle of eABR

eABR can be recorded using a needle electrode at the round window niche or by using surface electrodes. Several researchers have investigated presence of electrical responses to stimulation using needle electrode before CI surgery (Alfelasi et al., 2013; Kileny et al., 1992; Nikolopoulos et al., 2000; Pau et al., 2006). eABR can also be recorded by electrical stimulation of the inner ear or spiral ganglions using the intra-cochlear electrode array of the CI and measuring the responses using surface electrodes (like in conventional acoustic ABR). A company-specific programming software produces the desired stimulus levels to stimulate individual electrodes, one at a time. An external trigger cable, which connects the stimulating unit to the EP measuring unit, ensures that the EP measuring unit, with the help of surface electrodes, records time-locked responses to the electrical stimulation of the brainstem via the auditory nerve. The radio frequency (RF) of the CI system may need to be switched off during the recording to avoid interference of high frequency artifacts. In order to minimize the effects of signal artifacts, an eABR waveform is typically obtained by averaging response to 1000-2000 individual pulses.

Equipment Needed for eABR

The setup needed for an eABR recording is shown in Fig. 18.6. This set-up requires a personal computer (PC) installed with the software for recording evoked potentials (EP), another PC installed with the CI programming software, and a trigger

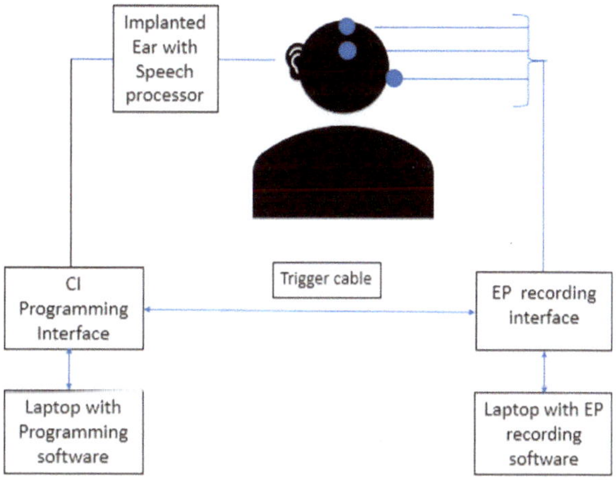

Fig. 18.6 Electrode montage and setup for recording eABR. The Ground electrode is placed at the high forehead (Fz), reference on the lower forehead (Fpz) and active on the mastoid (A1/A2) contralateral to the ear with CI

cable connecting the CI programming interface to the EP recording software. The speech processor and transmitting coil of the implant are connected to the CI programming interface, which is in turn connected to a PC with CI programming and stimulation software. The CI programming interface triggers the EP recording system. After the stimulus onset in the programming software, the transmitting coil of the speech processor is turned-off for 10 ms to allow a short window for RF-free recording. The surface electrodes on the recipient's head (Fz, Fpz, A1/A2) can pick up the responses generated from various generator sites, apply pre-amplification to them and transfer them to the EP system for further processing.

Procedure of Obtaining eABR

The eABR recording is begun by presenting the electrical stimulus just below the C levels or at levels that the recipient can comfortably tolerate. Most often, a visual inspection method is used to identify waves III and V of eABR to label them manually. During eABR recording, the current level is increased in steps of 10 and reduced by 5, depending upon the presence or absence of wave V. Typically, two or three runs of a minimum 1000 sweeps each are used to examine replication to ensure accurate identification of eABR peaks. The minimum current level at which wave V is recorded in at least two waveforms is marked as the threshold of eABR (tEABR) (Fig. 18.7).

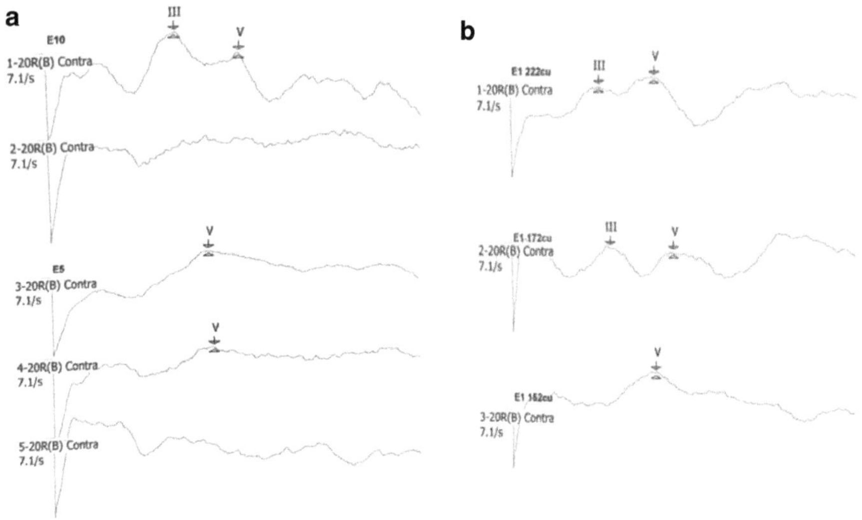

Fig. 18.7 Waveforms of eABR: (**a**) typical eABR waveform on electrode 10 and electrode 5; (**b**) recording of eABRs to obtain tEABR for the electrode number 1 with decreasing stimulus levels

Ideal Recording Conditions for eABR

The best recordings of eABR are achieved when a calm and quiet recipient is lying in a bed in a silent testing room. There is no dire need to sedate, even if the recipient is a child. In young children, who may not otherwise cooperate when awake, recordings are best obtained with natural sleep; older children may be instructed to stay calm and avoid movements during testing. Non-cooperative children can be sedated with a paediatrician-recommended sedative. Adequate electrical grounding ensures reduced electrical interference.

Advantages of eABR

Preoperatively, eABR has been used as a tool to assess the ability of the auditory pathway to respond to electrical stimulation. eABR has also been used as a tool to predict outcomes of CI surgeries in ears with inner ear malformations (Zhang et al., 2010). It also helps in making a decision between cochlear implantation and auditory brainstem implantation.

Intraoperatively, eABR recordings have been used to assess the electrode placement and functioning of the CI system. eABR responses provide evidence that the auditory nerve of the recipient is responding to electrical stimulation and these responses vary depending on the underlying malformation (Nashwa et al., 2022).

Post-operatively, eABR has an important use as an objective measure for CI programming, especially in children. The eABR detection threshold can be used to estimate the T levels of a patient. The eABR thresholds show better correlation with T levels than do they with C levels (Nashwa et al., 2022).

Apart from its use in establishing T and C levels, eABR has also been used to confirm auditory functioning in special populations of children, especially in children with Auditory Neuropathy Spectrum Disorder (ANSD). The presence of eABR confirms the usefulness of cochlear implantation in synchronous firing of the neural elements at the brainstem. Children with ANSD exhibiting normal eABR tend to show better speech perception outcomes than do those with absent or abnormal eABR (Nashwa et al., 2022). Therefore, the presence of eABR helps in providing reassurance to the patient or the family.

eABR has also been used as a measure to evaluate auditory brainstem development and plasticity postoperatively. It has been used in the functional evaluation of the auditory system in the period between the initial implant activation and at a later point after the continued cochlear implant use (Nashwa et al., 2022). The quality of the eABR waveform has been reported to correlate well with postoperative speech perception. eABR can be used as a tool to measure the developed and enhanced central auditory plasticity caused by long-term electric stimulation (Nada et al., 2022).

Electrically-evoked Cortical Auditory Evoked Potential (eCAEP)

Numerous studies have been carried out to study the effect of auditory stimulation on the presence and maturation of the Electrically-evoked Cortical Auditory Evoked Potentials (eCAEP), especially the P1-N1-P2 complex. Though objective measures help us estimate threshold, comfortable levels, and binaural integration at the brainstem level (Gordon et al., 2012), these methods fail to provide information about higher cortical regions along the central auditory pathway. eCAEPs provide information about the central auditory development and the functioning of higher centres of the central auditory pathway (Stapells, 2002). eCAEPs can measure and predict thresholds in CI users more accurately than do eCAPs (Abbas & Brown, 2015). After cochlear implantation and device activation, the P1 peak of eCAEP follows the normal sequence of development, whereas the P2 peak appears later. In cases with longer auditory deprivation, P2 takes a very long time to mature. P1 shows high degree of sensitivity for changes in auditory function after cochlear implantation in children with congenital profound hearing loss; however, it is essentially normal in children who acquired profound deafness after acquiring normal speech-language development (Ponton et al., 2000). Studies have reported significant changes in N1 and enhanced P3 amplitudes after implantation in adult cochlear implant recipients (Jordan et al., 1997; Kaga et al., 1991).

In the last few years, presence of P1-N1-P2 complex has been shown to be associated with speech detection in both children and adults using amplification (Tavora-Vieira et al., 2022; Sarvanan et al., 2024). Presence of repeatable eCAEP for speech stimulus indicates that speech is audible to the individual and it indicates detection and perception of speech at higher auditory centres (Tavora-Vieira et al., 2022). eCAEPs are present and the amplitudes and latencies of N1-P2 complex in CI users with good speech understanding are comparable to normal hearing individuals (Oviatt & Kilnery, 1991). Furthermore, many studies have also demonstrated the benefit of using eCAEP as an objective measure to verify CI performance, with some studies suggesting a strong correlation between eCAEP thresholds to behavioural thresholds (Tavora-Vieira et al., 2022), giving significance to the presence or absence of eCAEP during CI mapping or map verification. Sarvanan and colleagues studied electrically evoked late latency response with single electrode stimulation in the apical, middle, and basal regions in cochlear implant users and also evaluated their relationship with speech perception (Sarvanan et al., 2024). They reported no significant differences in P1 and N1 latencies, and P1 amplitude across electrode sites. However, significantly larger N1 and P1-N1 amplitude were observed for apical stimulation compared to basal stimulation. A moderate positive correlation was reported between speech recognition scores in quiet and both N1, and P1-N1 amplitudes for apical stimulation. A typical eCAEP recording in the free field setup is shown in Fig. 18.8.

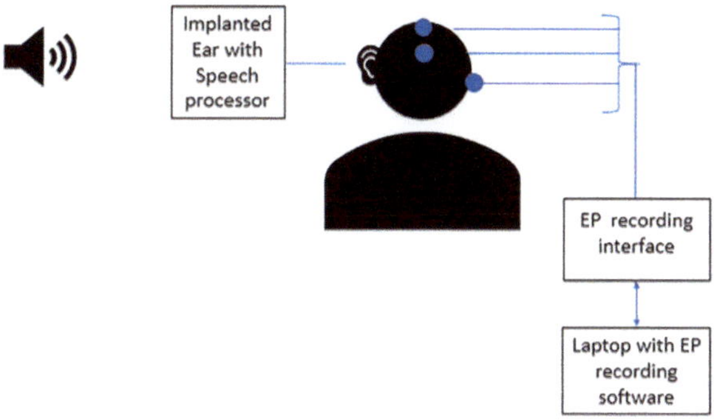

Fig. 18.8 A typical setup for recording eCAEP in free field

Equipment Needed for Obtaining eCAEP in Free Field

A free field, often also referred as sound filed, setup requires impedance-matched loud speakers to be used for stimulus delivery. Additionally, electrophysiological testing hardware and software with facility to record CAEP, and recording electrodes to pick-up surface potentials are needed.

Procedure and Recording Conditions

The recipient should be awake during the procedure and produce as little movements as possible. eCAEPs are elicited using speech stimuli with different frequencies and levels. Electrode impedance is ideal if kept under 3–5 kΩ with residual noise below 3 μV. The number of epochs can vary from 150–500. The stimulus at an intensity of 60 dB nHL is presented through a loud speaker placed at a 0° azimuth. The eCAEPs are identified by visual detection or using automated statistical detection of the responses using the software-specific algorithm. eCAEPs can also be recorded using direct stimulation through the processor using the CI programming software, which in turn triggers the EP recording software to record potentials using surface electrodes (Fig. 18.9).

Evidence that eCAEP measures can be used to monitor the maturation of the central auditory pathways in CI recipients (Sharma et al., 2002), estimate hearing thresholds (Cardon & Sharma, 2021; Hoppe et al., 2001; Lightfoot & Kennedy, 2006), and evaluating auditory refractory effects (Cowper-Smith et al., 2013) are steadily increasing. Additionally, post-implantation speech perception has been found to have positive correlation with eCAEP measures as studied using the P2 latency (Kelly et al., 2005; Liebscher et al., 2018), and with N1 and N1-P2 amplitudes (Makhdoum et al., 1998; Zhang et al., 2010). More details on the utility of eCAEPs are available in chapter 22.

In this overview, we have provided examples of the current clinical objective measures and advances which have the potential to optimize outcomes from cochlear

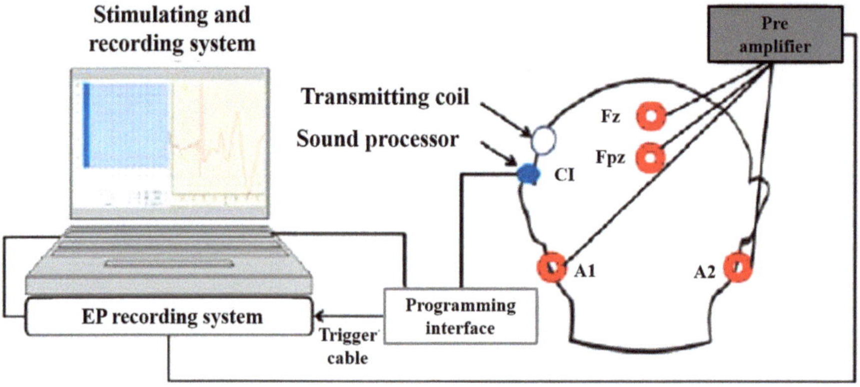

Fig. 18.9 A typical setup and electrode montage used for recording eCAEP. The active electrode is placed at the vertex (Cz), reference on the mastoid contralateral to the CI ear, and the ground at the forehead

implantation. We have broadly covered how objective measures can help understand sound transmission through the auditory pathway and provide optimized hearing to CI users.

References

Abbas, P. J., & Brown, C. J. (2015). Assessment of responses to cochlear implant stimulation at different levels of the auditory pathway. *Hearing Research, 322*, 67–76.

Abbas, P. J., Brown, C. J., Shallop, J. K., Firszt, J. B., Hughes, M. L., Hong, S. H., & Staller, S. J. (1999). Summary of results using the nucleus CI24M implant to record the electrically evoked compound action potential. *Ear and Hearing, 20*(1), 45–59.

Alfelasi, M., Piron, J. P., Mathiolon, C., Lenel, N., Mondain, M., Uziel, A., & Venail, F. (2013). The transtympanic promontory stimulation test in patients with auditory deprivation: Correlations with electrical dynamics of cochlear implant and speech perception. *European Archives of Oto-Rhino-Laryngology, 270*(6), 1809–1815.

Andrade, K. C., Leal, M. d. C., Muniz, L. F., Menezes, P. d. L., Albuquerque, K. M., & Carnaúba, A. T. (2014). The importance of electrically evoked stapedial reflex in cochlear implant. *Brazilian Journal of Otorhinolaryngology, 80*(1), 68–77.

Bergeron, F., & Hotton, M. (2015). Comparison of eSRTs and comfort levels in users of Digisonic SP cochlear implants. *Cochlear Implants International, 16*(2), 110–114.

Bresnihan, M., Norman, G., Scott, F., & Viani, L. (2001). Measurement of comfort levels by means of electrical stapedial reflex in children. *Archives of Otolaryngology—Head & Neck Surgery, 127*(8), 963–966.

Brown, C. J., Abbas, P. J., & Gantz, B. J. (1998). Preliminary experience with neural response telemetry in the nucleus CI24M cochlear implant. *The American Journal of Otology, 19*(3), 320–327.

Brown, C. J., Hughes, M. L., Luk, B., Abbas, P. J., Wolaver, A., & Gervais, J. (2000). The relationship between EAP and EABR thresholds and levels used to program the nucleus 24 speech processor: Data from adults. *Ear and Hearing, 21*(2), 151–163.

Cardon, G., & Sharma, A. (2021). Cortical neurophysiologic correlates of auditory threshold in adults and children with normal hearing and auditory neuropathy Spectrum disorder. *American Journal of Audiology, 30*(1), 28–42.
Carson, N., Leach, L., & Murphy, K. J. (2018). A re-examination of Montreal cognitive assessment (MoCA) cutoff scores. *International Journal of Geriatric Psychiatry, 33*(2), 379–388.
Çiprut, A., & Adıgül, Ç. (2020). The relationship between electrical stapedius reflex thresholds and behaviorally most comfortable levels in experienced Cochlear implant users. *The Journal of International Advanced Otology, 16*(1), 8–12.
Cowper-Smith, C. D., Green, J., Maessen, H., Bance, M., & Newman, A. J. (2013). Refractory effects of the N1 event-related potential in experienced cochlear implant patients. *International Journal of Audiology, 52*(2), 104–112.
Cullington, H., Hodges, A. V., Butts, S. L., Dolan-Ash, S., & Balkany, T. J. (2000). Comparison of language ability in children with cochlear implants placed in oral and total communication educational settings. *The Annals of Otology, Rhinology & Laryngology, Supplement, 185*, 121–123.
Gordon, K. A., Papsin, B. C., & Harrison, R. V. (2002). Auditory brain stem and midbrain development after cochlear implantation in children. The annals of otology, rhinology & laryngology. *Supplement, 189*, 32–37.
Gordon, K. A., Papsin, B. C., & Harrison, R. V. (2004). Toward a battery of behavioral and objective measures to achieve optimal cochlear implant stimulation levels in children. *Ear and Hearing, 25*(5), 447–463.
Gordon, K. A., Salloum, C., Toor, G. S., van Hoesel, R., & Papsin, B. C. (2012). Binaural interactions develop in the auditory brainstem of children who are deaf: Effects of place and level of bilateral electrical stimulation. *The Journal of Neuroscience, 32*(12), 4212–4223.
Guida, M., Falcioni, M., Di Lella, F., Negri, M., Fagnani, E., & Vincenti, V. (2019). Multi-electrode sequential versus single electrode stimulation to elicit the stapedial reflex during cochlear implantation: Correlation with maximum comfort level. *European Annals of Otorhinolaryngology, Head and Neck Diseases, 136*(3), 169–172.
Hernandez, L. C., Sánchez, L. C., Olivares, M. C., Rodríguez, C., Finley, C. C., & Saoji, A. A. (2019). Effect of probe-tone frequency on ipsilateral and contralateral electrical stapedius reflex measurement in children with cochlear implants. *Ear and Hearing, 40*(3), 732–740.
Hoppe, U., Rosanowski, F., Iro, H., & Eysholdt, U. (2001). Loudness perception and late auditory evoked potentials in adult cochlear implant users. *Scandinavian Audiology, 30*(2), 119–125.
Hughes, M. (2012). *Objective measures in cochlear implants*. Plural publishing.
Hughes, M. L., Brown, C. J., Abbas, P. J., Wolaver, A. A., & Gervais, J. P. (2000). Comparison of EAP thresholds with MAP levels in the nucleus 24 cochlear implant: Data from children. *Ear and Hearing, 21*(2), 164–174.
Jordan, K., Schmidt, A., Plotz, K., von Specht, H., Begall, K., Roth, N., & Scheich, H. (1997). Auditory event-related potentials in post- and prelingually deaf cochlear implant recipients. *The American Journal of Otology, 18*(6), S116–S117.
Kaga, K., Kodera, K., Hirota, E., & Tsuzuku, T. (1991). P300 response to tones and speech sounds after cochlear implant: A case report. *The Laryngoscope, 101*(8), 905–907.
Kelly, A. S., Purdy, S. C., & Thorne, P. R. (2005). Electrophysiological and speech perception measures of auditory processing in experienced adult cochlear implant users. *Clinical Neurophysiology, 116*(6), 1235–1246.
Kileny, P. R., Miller, J. M., Kemink, J. L., & Shallop, J. K. (1992). Prediction of auditory nerve survival in humans using the electrical auditory brainstem response. *The American Journal of Otology, 13*(4), 381–382.
Kosaner, J. (2010). Generating speech processor programmes for children using ESRT measurements. *Cochlear Implants International, 11*(sup2), 20–24.
Kosaner, J., Spitzer, P., Bayguzina, S., Gultekin, M., & Behar, L. A. (2018). Comparing eSRT and eCAP measurements in pediatric MED-EL cochlear implant users. *Cochlear Implants International, 19*(3), 153–161.

Liebscher, T., Alberter, K., & Hoppe, U. (2018). Cortical auditory evoked potentials in cochlear implant listeners via single electrode stimulation in relation to speech perception. *International Journal of Audiology, 57*(12), 933–940.

Lightfoot, G., & Kennedy, V. (2006). Cortical electric response audiometry hearing threshold estimation: Accuracy, speed, and the effects of stimulus presentation features. *Ear and Hearing, 27*(5), 443–456.

Lorens, A., Skarżyński, H., Piotrowska, A., Walkowiak, A., Śliwa, L., & Kochanek, K. (Eds.). (2003). *Objective methods of postoperative tests in cochlear implant patients. International Congress Series*. Elsevier.

Makhdoum, M. J., Groenen, P. A., Snik, A. F., & van den Broek, P. (1998). Intra- and interindividual correlations between auditory evoked potentials and speech perception in cochlear implant users. *Scandinavian Audiology, 27*(1), 13–20.

Messersmith, J. J., Entwisle, L., & Stout, A. (2018). Electrically evoked Stapedial reflex threshold: A procedure. *Perspectives of the ASHA Special Interest Groups, 3*(9), 4–12.

Mittal, R., Ramesh, A. V., Panwar, S. S., Nilkanthan, A., Sinha, V. R., Nair, S., & Raj, P. (2015). Mapping of pediatric cochlear implant recipients using electrical auditory brainstem responses as a tool. *Indian Journal of Otology, 21*(1), 14–18.

Møller, A. R., & Jannetta, P. J. (1982a). Auditory evoked potentials recorded intracranially from the brain stem in man. *Experimental Neurology, 78*(1), 144–157.

Møller, A. R., & Jannetta, P. J. (1982b). Evoked potentials from the inferior colliculus in man. *Electroencephalography and Clinical Neurophysiology, 53*(6), 612–620.

Nada, N., Kolkaila, E., Schendzielorz, P., & El Mahallawi, T. (2022). Electrically evoked auditory brainstem response in cochlear implantation: What you need to know (short review). *The Egyptian Journal of Otolaryngology, 38*(1), 67.

Nikolopoulos, T. P., Mason, S. M., Gibbin, K. P., & O'Donoghue, G. M. (2000). The prognostic value of promontory electric auditory brain stem response in pediatric cochlear implantation. *Ear and Hearing, 21*(3), 236–241.

Nunn, T. B., Jiang, D., Green, T., Boyle, P. J., & Vickers, D. A. (2019). A systematic review of the impact of adjusting input dynamic range (IDR), electrical threshold (T) level and rate of stimulation on speech perception ability in cochlear implant users. *International Journal of Audiology, 58*(6), 317–325.

Oviatt, D. L., & Kileny, P. R. (1991). Auditory event-related potentials elicited from Cochlear implant recipients and hearing subjects. *American Journal of Audiology, 1*(1), 48–55.

Pau, H., Gibson, W. P., & Sanli, H. (2006). Trans-tympanic electric auditory brainstem response (TT-EABR): The importance of the positioning of the stimulating electrode. *Cochlear Implants International, 7*(4), 183–187.

Polak, M., Hodges, A. V., King, J. E., Payne, S. L., & Balkany, T. J. (2006). Objective methods in postlingually and prelingually deafened adults for programming cochlear implants: ESR and NRT. *Cochlear Implants International, 7*(3), 125–141.

Polak, M., Hodges, A., & Balkany, T. (2005). ECAP, ESR and subjective levels for two different nucleus 24 electrode arrays. *Otology and Neurotology, 26*(4), 639–645. https://doi.org/10.1097/01.mao.0000178145.14010.25

Ponton, C. W., Eggermont, J. J., Kwong, B., & Don, M. (2000). Maturation of human central auditory system activity: Evidence from multi-channel evoked potentials. *Clinical Neurophysiology, 111*(2), 220–236.

Ponton, C. W., Moore, J. K., & Eggermont, J. J. (1996). Auditory brain stem response generation by parallel pathways: Differential maturation of axonal conduction time and synaptic transmission. *Ear and Hearing, 17*(5), 402–410.

Bayat, A. (2018). Comparison of neural response telemetry and electrical stapedius reflexes with behavioral thresholds in Cochlear implant users. *Asian Journal of Pharmaceutics (AJP), 12*(03).

Saravanan, P., Devi, N., & Geetha, C. (2024). Electrically evoked late latency response using single electrode stimulation and its relation to speech perception among paediatric cochlear implant users. *Frontiers in Human Neuroscience, 18*, 1441854.

Scorpecci, A., D'Elia, A., Malerba, P., Cantore, I., Consolino, P., Trabalzini, F., et al. (2016). Maps created using a new objective procedure (C-NRT) correlate with behavioral, loudness-balanced maps: A study in adult cochlear implant users. *European Archives of Oto-Rhino-Laryngology, 273*, 4167–4173.

Sharma, A., Dorman, M. F., & Spahr, A. J. (2002). A sensitive period for the development of the central auditory system in children with cochlear implants: Implications for age of implantation. *Ear and Hearing, 23*(6), 532–539.

Smoorenburg, G. F., Willeboer, C., & van Dijk, J. E. (2002). Speech perception in nucleus CI24M cochlear implant users with processor settings based on electrically evoked compound action potential thresholds. *Audiology & Neuro-Otology, 7*(6), 335–347.

Spivak, L. G., & Chute, P. M. (1994). The relationship between electrical acoustic reflex thresholds and behavioral comfort levels in children and adult cochlear implant patients. *Ear and Hearing, 15*(2), 184–192.

Spivak, L. G., Chute, P. M., Popp, A. L., & Parisier, S. C. (1994). Programming the cochlear implant based on electrical acoustic reflex thresholds: Patient performance. *The Laryngoscope, 104*(10), 1225–1230.

Stapells, D. (2002). *Cortical event-related potentials to auditory stimuli*. Lippincott Williams & Wilkins.

Távora-Vieira, D., Wedekind, A., Ffoulkes, E., Voola, M., & Marino, R. (2022). Cortical auditory evoked potential in cochlear implant users: An objective method to improve speech perception. *PLoS One, 17*(10), e0274643.

Vaerenberg, B., Smits, C., De Ceulaer, G., Zir, E., Harman, S., Jaspers, N., Tam, Y., Dillon, M., Wesarg, T., Martin-Bonniot, D., Gärtner, L., Cozma, S., Kosaner, J., Prentiss, S., Sasidharan, P., Briaire, J. J., Bradley, J., Debruyne, J., Hollow, R., Patadia, R., et al. (2014). Cochlear implant programming: A global survey on the state of the art. *The Scientific World Journal, 2014*, 501738.

Van den Honert, C., & Stypulkowski, P. H. (1986). Characterization of the electrically evoked auditory brainstem response (ABR) in cats and humans. *Hearing Research, 21*(2), 109–126.

Wang, L., Zhang, Q., Wang, Q., Dong, M., & Zeng, Y. (2009). Functional evaluation of auditory system in patients with cochlear implant using electrically evoked auditory brainstem responses. *Acoustical Physics, 55*, 857–865.

Zhang, F., Anderson, J., Samy, R., & Houston, L. (2010). The adaptive pattern of the late auditory evoked potential elicited by repeated stimuli in cochlear implant users. *International Journal of Audiology, 49*(4), 277–285.

Chapter 19
Cochlear Implants: (Re)Habilitation

Sandy Magallan

Abstract The advancement of medical technologies has made hearing possible for those with limited hearing aid benefit through cochlear implantation. Aural habilitation refers to therapy focused on congenital and early childhood hearing loss in pre-lingually deafened children with the intent of obtaining auditory-oral skills for communication. Aural rehabilitation refers to therapy aimed at post-lingually deaf and hard of hearing adults, who are regaining auditory skills. This chapter aims to provide the reader tools for baselining and tracking progress with aural (re)habilitation, resources for aural (re)habilitation offered at little-to-no cost, and considerations to ponder while navigating the journey to functional auditory-oral communication.

Keywords Auditory verbal therapy · Listening skills · Speech language skills
Habilitation · Auditory comprehension · Auditory training

Introduction

This chapter will begin by distinguishing between aural habilitation and rehabilitation. Aural habilitation is focus of teaching auditory skills to those with little to no auditory experience, generally children with congenital or early childhood hearing loss. Aural rehabilitation is the teaching of compensatory skills to those that have vast auditory and language skills, but have acquired their hearing loss, mainly adults.

This chapter will also focus on spoken language and speech understanding as the ultimate goals of aural (re)habilitation. When beginning the process of aural (re)

S. Magallan (✉)
Doctor's Hospital at Renaissance, Ear Nose & Throat Institute, McAllen, TX, USA
e-mail: Sandy.Magallan@dhr-rgv.com

P. Kumar et al. (eds.), *Advances in Implantation Otology*,
https://doi.org/10.1007/978-981-96-8671-1_19

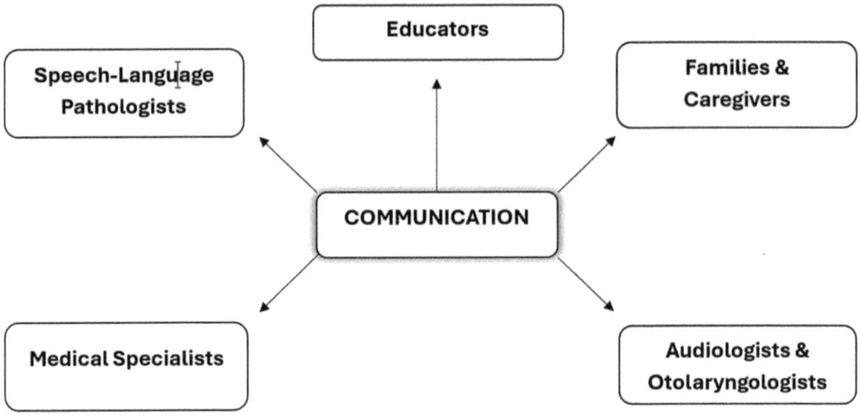

Fig. 19.1 An example of interprofessional collaboration

habilitation, many professionals work together to successfully achieve language goals and do not solely rely on one profession. The outcomes for children and adults are highly variable and are dependent on the intrinsic motivation and ability of the patient, availability/ease of access to local resources available, family or caregiver support, and more. Below you will find Fig. 19.1, which represents some of the specialties that may be involved in the hearing journey.

Speech-language pathologists (SLPs) can be involved prior to cochlear implantation but their role is emphasized in post-implantation intervention. This is particularly true when talking about children, who have experienced hearing difficulty prelingually, meaning they could not gain the receptive language skills needed for spoken language acquisition. SLPs not only expand learning in this area and evaluate progress toward language goals but can also be instrumental in teaching families how to create language-rich environments in the home setting, utilize repair strategies for effective communication, and help parents or caregivers reinforce therapeutic instruction. SLPs frequently report back to audiologists and other members of the interprofessional team to inform them of the child's progress. Though the emphasis on expressive language skills is highly valued by families and caregivers, SLPs can also assist in further developing other areas of language such as reading and writing skills, pragmatic skills, and teaching self-advocacy to children. In adults, speech-language pathologists can offer compensatory communication techniques to improve speech understanding in noisy environments or teach family members communication strategies for optimal communication with their deaf or hard of hearing loved ones. However, SLPs do not have a heavy presence in the rehabilitation of adults.

Educators often work closely with SLPs and audiologists in children. In early identified hearing loss, early childhood educators work with families and caregivers to develop language-rich environments and increase language opportunities primarily in the home setting. In the United States, this traditionally occurs before the age of 3, when many children can qualify for early educational opportunities locally. As the child grows older, they often require accommodations and other support for cognitive, linguistic and social-emotional development in the classroom. Some children may begin their educational journey in self-contained classrooms, or classrooms where children with similar hearing and communication abilities are receiving training from a teacher with specialized training. When starting in the self-contained classroom, if the child is capable of expanding communication significantly, they will transition into mainstream classrooms with their normal hearing peers at a later point. The use of hearing assistive technology (e.g. remote microphone for the teacher to wear on the lapel) and acoustic modifications of the classroom (e.g. adding rugs to floors) can offer optimum learning opportunities by significantly reducing background noise and reverberation and prioritizing the teacher's voice. Schools typically purchase and maintain hearing assistive technology to improve speech-in-noise ratios in the classroom and allow the students to borrow this technology during school hours. Additional services, such as supplemental teachings in the area(s) of weak academic performance, may also be offered to meet the educational goals of the child.

Perhaps the most influential factor in the aural (re)habilitation process is the involvement of family or caregivers. With children, family, and caregivers provide added support in the home setting and ensure proper support is being provided in the educational setting. Also, decisions on which language(s) will be targeted in aural (re)habilitation are often made for the child by family and caregivers. It is not uncommon to see that many families decide to choose a language model that resembles their communication mode. Rarely do families choose a different language model than their own (e.g. sign language). This is because over 90% of deaf infants are born to parents who can hear in the United States and figures may be similar in other countries (Mitchell & Karchmer, 2004). Familial cultural factors, parental/caregiver's educational experience and their perspectives on intervention, and socioeconomic status all play major roles in the experience of the child. Regarding adults, who are typically post-lingually deafened, family and friends are frequent communication partners in which sources of communication breakdowns occur. Difficulty in this area affects quality-of-life measures as this difficulty is experienced daily. Breakdowns in interpersonal interactions may appear in the form of in-person conversation(s), telephone communication, and difficulty with access to entertainment (i.e. television, music, and social events) which all rely on one's hearing sensitivity to participate and consists of complex auditory stimuli. The main goal of aural rehabilitation for adults is to offer adequate auditory access through cochlear implants and couple that with compensatory techniques to reintegrate the individual into their pre-hearing loss daily functions as much as possible. When effective reintegration is not possible, a new "sense of normalcy" will have to be established.

Many individuals with severe hearing loss will require the involvement of other medical specialists. Approximately 30–40% of children with congenital hearing loss also have at least one other disability (Hashemi & Monshizadeh, 2016). This means that hearing loss is not the only difficulty experienced by the child and this can make progress with aural habilitation slow or difficult. Similarly, adults may need to see a psychologist or psychiatrist to overcome the effects of depression and/

or anxiety caused by pre-implantation isolation. Moreover, interprofessional members who are a part of the post-implantation process will find that knowledge of behavioral techniques can be extremely important. Verbal behavior has been defined as a set of behaviors that are reinforced through the reaction of the communication partner (Cooper et al., 2007). Simply put, when a child uses verbal behaviors successfully and can get what they want in their environment, they are more likely to use that same verbal behavior or a similar one to achieve the same result. For example, if a toddler says, "milk" and the caregiver give the toddler milk, the child will continue to say "milk" to get more of that substance. Consequently, if a toddler uses "milk" to ask for a rubber ball, the caregiver may not make the correlation between the vocalization of "milk" and the rubber ball, and the child does not get the rubber ball and thus will not likely use the word "milk" for the rubber ball as this was an unsuccessful attempt. Also, behavioral techniques can be utilized to help children and adults' bond with their cochlear processors. In children, the author emphasizes the use of positive reinforcement and distraction techniques when working with caregivers as some may resort to punishment techniques first. For adults, the benefits of consistent use of the cochlear processor will often create intrinsic positive reinforcement when sound access is able to aid them communicate effectively. These are only a couple of examples of many behavioral techniques available to professionals to aid them in the aural (re)habilitation process.

Subsequently, it goes without saying that audiologists and otolaryngologists play a major role in the medical management of hearing loss. As discussed in a previous chapter (Chap. 12), otolaryngologists will verify medical candidacy and be involved in the surgical implantation of cochlear implants. Audiologists are involved in audiological candidacy determination, providing patient-specific counseling, and educating patients and their families on realistic post-surgical linguistic expectations. After the cochlear implant surgery, audiologists are largely involved in cochlear processor programming appointments, which are more frequent in the first year, validation and verification of the programming, educating patients and their families on the cleaning and maintenance of the devices, and more.

There are certain members of the interprofessional team that spend many hours every day with the child, such as parents and educators, and who can provide detailed feedback whereas the audiologist may only see the child a couple of hours every few months and only experience a restricted view of the patient's progress. The importance of regular interprofessional communication is emphasized because pre-lingually implanted children are unaware of auditory stimuli missing from their repertoire and are not effective reporters of their auditory experience. They simply cannot fill in the gaps of auditory information missed as one can with advanced language skills. On the other hand, adults are getting implanted post-lingually and are aware of distortions in speech or in the auditory stimuli that are lacking and are often able to "fill in the gaps" when auditory information is missed. They may also report to the audiologists regarding the difficulties they are experiencing, thus the need for interprofessional collaboration is a less common occurrence.

Finally, a change in the typical cochlear implant surgery and activation process is actively being investigated by many researchers around the world. Cochlear implant activation normally occurs between 4 to 6 weeks post-surgically to allow for the healing of the postauricular incision and reduction in edema (Alahmadi et al., 2023; Parker et al., 2024). However, emerging studies in the last few years have shown that early activation of the cochlear implant, even as early as hours after surgery, have resulted in no complications with the postauricular incision or skin flap and similar hearing outcomes when compared to the traditional activation timeline (Alahmadi et al., 2023; Parker et al., 2024). These studies aim to reduce economic strain on the families and individuals by reducing the number of days away from work or school, and reducing travel expenses as the surgery and activation appointments can occur on the same day and allow sooner access to auditory stimuli (Alahmadi et al., 2023). After the activation, the auditory-verbal focus of language acquisition can begin.

Erber's Hierarchy of Auditory Skills

Auditory skills development has been consistently classified into the following categories described by Erber: auditory detection/awareness, identification, discrimination, and comprehension. This is not to say that one level must be mastered before reaching the next. It is possible to experience growth in one level while simultaneously experiencing growth in another.

Erber's hierarchy of auditory skills is displayed (Fig. 19.2) as an inverted triangle to show basic skills at the point or bottom of the triangle and advanced skills at the triangular base or the top part of the illustration. The discussion on Erber's auditory skills development and top -down and bottom -up processing will be concurrently discussed in this section.

With prelingually deafened children, basic auditory skills may not be present at all. Interventionalists work with building basic auditory skills, such as auditory detection/awareness up to auditory comprehension. This process is termed bottom-up processing. This process may look like an SLP teaching a child to produce phonemes and later assist the child in producing syllables and words to sentences and

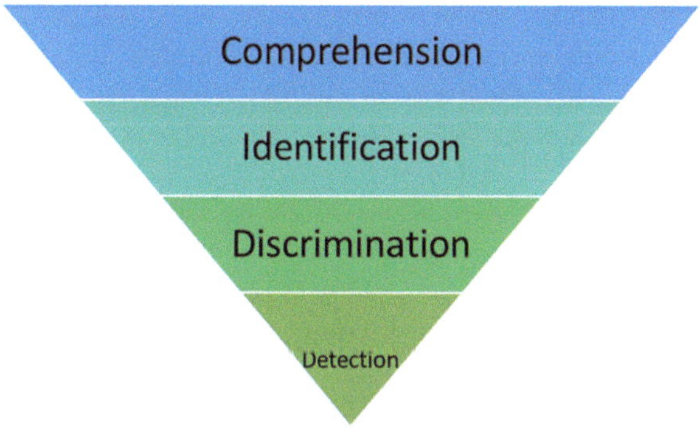

Fig. 19.2 Eber's hierarchy of auditory skill development

discourse. Verbal language, as heard by the child with normal hearing sensitivity, is acquired spontaneously with language-rich homes (i.e., homes with family members that converse often and may have books they read to their children). These children are not sitting down for therapeutic language sessions and learning phonemes one by one. The importance of mentioning this is to say that both bottom-up and top- down processes (which will be mentioned later) are happening simultaneously with children and adults. This being said, children still primarily learn verbal language with bottom -up approaches, particularly in speech-language therapy.

After cochlear implant activation in children, the first skill to develop is auditory awareness or auditory perception/detection. This skill represents the ability of the listener to know whether a sound is present in the environment or not (Erber, 1982). Another way to use auditory awareness is the practice of using the Ling- 6 Sound Test. This test is comprised of 6 phonemes: /m/, /a/, /u/, /i/, /ʃ/, and /s/. Audiologists can obtain aided detection in sound field through the speech awareness threshold (SAT) to infer access to speech. Access to speech and sound will build the foundation to obtain advanced auditory skills. In early programming appointments, not all speech and sounds will be heard. Audiologists can offer progressive programming, increasing in volume and clarity, to allow for comfortable acclimation to sound. This means that on activation day, 100% access to speech and sound is not available through the programming offered in the cochlear device.

The next complex level of auditory skills is called auditory discrimination. Auditory discrimination is a more advanced skill for a patient who is consistently wearing their cochlear processor. With this skill, the child practices distinguishing sounds using different sound experiences (Erber, 1982). For example, a child may learn the difference between hearing a cat meow and a dog's bark by observing these sounds in their environment while wearing their hearing devices. One way to use auditory discrimination in the clinical setting is to verify access to high-frequency sounds. The audiologist can limit the Ling-6 sound test to phonemes /s/ and /ʃ/. First, the audiologist can check for understanding of the task by informally testing, with visuals, to confirm the child can differentiate these two sounds by pointing to the correct card with its correlating grapheme or by producing the sounds through repeating. If the child can comprehend the task and distinguish the phonemes with visuals, then randomized presentations of both phonemes are tested in sound field in the sound booth by the audiologist. This is a challenging task as both /s/ and /ʃ/ are high-frequency sounds. The child patient must then be able to detect differences in the phoneme's formants to distinguish both phonemes using auditory information alone during testing. An easier discrimination task could involve a similar task to the one above, but with highly contrasted phonemes such as /s/ and /a/.

The third most complex auditory skill is called auditory identification. The patient has a great wealth of auditory experience at this point and has learned patterns to recognize and categorize auditory information (Erber, 1982). For example, a child may be presented with various farm animal toys such as a cow, a pig, and a horse. When presented with the auditory sound of a 'neigh', the patient is to select the correct animal from this closed set (i.e., the horse).

Finally, the most advanced skill is auditory comprehension. During auditory comprehension, basic and advanced language and auditory skills are in the child's repertoire. To evaluate this skill, the child may be questioned with open-response questions and the appropriateness of the response is evaluated by the audiologist or other professionals (Erber, 1982). A simple evaluation can focus on concrete subject matters such as items visualized in the room. An SLP can set up a situation in the therapy room and ask, "what happened to the book (on the floor)?" A more complex skill can also be evaluated by using more abstract concepts such as questioning the child on emotions, memories, and other topics. An example of this is a parent asking the child, "What happened yesterday? Why is your knee bruised?"

Adults with cochlear implants have had normal hearing at one point earlier in their life and many have advanced language, and some level of auditory comprehension is already in the adult's skillset. It makes sense that bottom-up processing may not be the best method in helping an adult with hearing difficulty. Top-down methodologies are implemented as part of aural rehabilitation, meaning we look at the "big picture" to derive meaning in what was heard. An example of this can look like an SLP teaching an adult compensatory strategy such as "filling in the blank" for a word not heard clearly in a sentence of a discourse. The SLP may instruct the adult to pay attention to the topic of the discourse and through deductive strategies and language experience, conclude what word was missed in the sentence is or what the meaning of the sentence was. This can be taught along with other strategies such as having the adult insist on always facing the speaker and lip-reading.

Aural Habilitation of Children

Cochlear implant technology has come a long way over the decades to provide access to spoken language in infants and young children who would have not otherwise had the opportunity to develop auditory-verbal skills. Technology has increased the diagnostic potential for newborns and infants and made early intervention possible for the mediation of hearing loss' effects. Medical advancements have also allowed micro preemie and premature newborns to thrive with fewer medical complications. However, it is widely known that preemies, micro preemies, and infants born with certain risk factors for hearing loss are estimated to be at a 10 times greater risk for hearing loss, with some studies showing up to 4 in 100 infants who are diagnosed with hearing loss, when compared to full-term healthy infants which have up to 3 in 1000 births resulting in hearing loss (Clark-Gambelunghe & Clark, 2015; Wroblewska-Seniuk et al., 2017). This portion of the chapter will discuss aural habilitation in typically developing children, that is children without medical and cognitive complexities, and who are acquiring at least one spoken language.

Auditory development begins at a gestational age of approximately 25 weeks (Clark-Gambelunghe & Clark, 2015). Research has historically shown that the fluid surrounding the embryo during the later stages of development allows for the mother's voice and other low-frequency sounds to be received while dampening high-frequency sounds (Clark-Gambelunghe & Clark, 2015; Estabrooks et al., 2016). Vibratory sound stimulation studies are being performed to investigate diagnostic and intervention capacity for embryos while in the womb. Current studies have shown that newborns can detect sounds to their left or right side, recognition of the mother's voice, cease activity when speech was presented at conversational levels, and perception of music pitch with frequencies below 4000 Hz while in the womb or shortly after birth (Estabrooks et al., 2016). In children, we focus on bottom-up strategies for spoken language development.

Implementing Aural Habilitation

Baseline Performance

To measure progress in a child, a baseline must be obtained to monitor progress towards language goals. This is typically obtained by a SLP who is a specialist in language development and language disorders. Not all SLPs have experience in aural habilitation. SLPs, teachers of the deaf, and even audiologists may seek certification in Listening and Spoken Language specialization, known as auditory-verbal therapist (AVT) certification, through the internationally available Alexander Graham Bell Academy to gain skills in aural habilitation techniques (AG Bell Academy 2024). AVT training is an extensive topic that can thoroughly explained in its own book, therefore the details of AVT training will not be discussed in this chapter. AVT-trained professionals are highly recommended in the aural habilitation of children.

Hearing Age

While the child is acquiring auditory skills, one can obtain the child's hearing age for baseline measurement. The hearing age is calculated when full-time use of the cochlear device after implantation occurs. Recall from earlier that full-time use is considered to use at least 80% of the time in all waking hours (Park et al., 2019). If the child has been implanted and their processor programmed, but datalogging consistently shows 3 hours of use on average per day for the last 6 months, the hearing age is zero (0). An average of 3 hours a day for the last six months for a child who is awake 10 hours is not sufficient for oral speech and language skills to develop and counseling on increasing device use is critical so that the child isn't further delayed. Discussion of pre-implantation language goals to gently remind parents or caregivers of the desired outcome will suffice. On the contrary, if a child was implanted and has an average of 8 hours on average of daily use with 10 hours of wakefulness for

1 year, the hearing age is 12 months. Hearing age together with Johnson's 1-to-1 Rule will assist professionals in tracking language progress.

Johnson's 1-to-1 Rule

In the last scenario, in the child with full-time device use, we would expect the child to speak their first word or pseudoword in the same amount of time as a child with normal hearing and typical language development (Estabrooks et al., 2016). This philosophy is based on Johnson's 1-to-1 Rule. Specifically, this rule states that auditory skills and expressive language growth, by minimum, should resemble the same growth rate as a typically developing child with sufficient auditory access (Estabrooks et al., 2016). If language growth rates are not meeting this expectation, factors influencing poor language outcomes must be quickly identified to take advantage of the critical period for language acquisition. With respect to audiology, poor programming by an inexperienced audiologist or lack of compliance with the audiologist's recommendations by families and caregivers can have serious negative long-term effects of language deprivation. Programming verification with behavioral testing, a quick assessment of access to the Ling-6 sounds, the measurement of auditory access and comfort levels through eSRT, and/or electrophysiological methods such as eCAP and eABR can be performed. ECAP and eABR will not be discussed in detail in this chapter (Chap. 18) as these are very specific tests available to audiologists only. Aided audiogram performance in the sound field can also assist an audiologist in ensuring access to the sounds across the speech frequency range (with heavier focus on 1000–4000 Hz). The sensitive period for language acquisition is short. This is why early intervention is such a hot topic. Most studies suggest that the sensitive period for deaf children is around 3.5 years of age because implantation after that age has been correlated with poor language outcomes, thereby invalidating pre-implantation language outcomes discussed with families (Marschark et al., 2019).

Table 19.1 Ling-6 sound test details (Estabrooks et al., 2016)

Sound	First formant	Second formant
/m/: a low-frequency sound	250–350 Hz	1000–1500 Hz
/a/: a low-frequency sound, back vowel	768–1030 Hz	1370–1551 Hz
/u/: a low-frequency sound, mid vowel	430–460 Hz	1105–1170 Hz
/e/: a low and high-frequency sound, front vowel	536–610 Hz	2530–2680 Hz
/ʃ/: a high-frequency sound	1500–2000 Hz	4500–5500 Hz
/s/: a high-frequency sound	5000–6000 Hz	

Ling 6 Sound Test

Earlier we mentioned the Ling- 6 Sound Test, which can be performed with speed, minimal training, and accuracy (Table 19.1). The Ling- 6 Sound Test is comprised of the following sounds in the English language:

The Ling-6 sound test is a quick and easy test that can be utilized in various settings (e.g., home, schools, therapy setting) and by various individuals (e.g. parents, educators, therapists). This test can be utilized in the following ways: to informally assess unaided speech access at a distance (i.e., at 6 feet), to assess aided speech access, and for daily checks of equipment function (Audiology Online, 2004). It is recommended that the Ling-6 sound test be taught to individuals involved in the aural habilitation of the child so that future appointments with the audiologist maximize programming efficiency. Sounds consistently missed and heard should be tracked to assist with programming modifications. Daily tracking of performance outcomes with the Ling-6 sound test can also provide the speech pathologist and audiologist with information on the device's function. Often, cochlear processor cables can cause intermittent connections, and dirty microphone covers muffle speech and sounds, and the need to review device integrity can be sooner detected when a sudden change is noticed in Ling-6 performance. (Advanced Bionics, 1990; Cochlear, 2018).

Table 19.2 Validation measures for children

Name	Ages for normative use	Languages available	Summary
Infant Toddler Meaningful Auditory Integration Scale (IT-MAIS)	Birth to 2 years of age	English, Spanish, and translated to many other languages	Parent interview questionnaire that assesses the areas of vocal behavioral, alerting to sounds, and deriving meaning from sound (Advance Bionics, n.d.).
Parent Evaluation of Aural/ Oral Performance of Children (PEACH)/+	Birth to 5 years of age	English, Chinese, Dutch, Italian, Malay, Norwegian, Sinhala, Hebrew, Spanish, Swedish, Thai, Turkish, Vietnamese, Portuguese, Finnish	Used by parents and professionals to check the child's hearing effectiveness in realistic settings (LOCHI Study, 2019)
Auditory Skills Checklist (ASC)	Any age	English, Spanish	Used by parents and professionals to track auditory development and set goals based on the Erber hierarchy of auditory development (Med-El, 2024).
Early Listening Function (ELF) for Infant and Toddlers	Birth to 3 years of age	English, Spanish	Questionnaire used by parents that contains 12 listening activities that can be completed by the parent in the home setting at varying distances (Success for Kids with Hearing Loss, 2023).

Validation Measures

Another way of tracking auditory skill development is the inclusion of validation measures. Questionnaires and checklists such as IT-MAIS, PEACH, ASC, and ELF can be utilized by any trained professional or parent (as indicated in Table 19.2) to document skills seen outside of the audiologist appointment. Below you will find general information about these validation measures for your reference. This list is not comprehensive and free downloadable content may be available as indicated in the reference list.

Levels of Complexity

In reference to Eber's Hierarchy of Auditory Development, SLPs will often start with achievable goals to build confidence and encouragement. As the child begins to incidentally learn sounds and speech around them with consistent device use, goals can start to become more complex, scaffolding the learning of new and more complex auditory skills. Figure 19.3 is an example of the spectrum of complexity for attaining auditory skills. The professional can target one level of complexity at a time or mix several complex situations for harder goals. For example, a child beginning therapy can practice learning phonemes, with visualization of the professional's mouth, in a quiet therapy room. As the child can quickly move through initial goals, the child can begin to work at the level of short utterances and learning

EASY →	HARD
Quiet	Loud
Visuals	No Visuals
Familiar	Unfamiliar
One Speaker	Multiple Speakers
Concrete Concepts	Abstract Concepts
Close Speaker	Distant Listener
Clear Speech	Distorted Speech
Phoneme	Discourse
Closed Set of Responses	Open Set of Responses
Context	No Context
Structured Responses	Spontaneous Responses

Fig. 19.3 Spectrum of complexity

other components critical to spoken language, while practicing in the quiet therapy room. If a child has succeeded with other mid-level speech and language goals, the child can produce more complex, realistic scenarios such as speech comprehension with multiple speakers in an environment with low environmental noise (to simulate a classroom). Some children may continue to struggle with complex language skills and will need continued support from technology (remote microphone) or visuals, until they reach a more independent level.

Varying difficulties of each auditory skill can be examined. Many children, for example, experience speech in noisy classroom settings with varying speech-to-noise ratios. The educational audiologist may want to uncover whether the child is having difficulty detecting speech in a noisy classroom by utilizing Ling-6 sound testing with varying speech-to-noise ratios and asking the child to repeat the test sentence heard. More examples of how to structure speech and sound goals with varying difficulty are included above in Fig. 19.3.

Educational Setting

The goal of aural habilitation or AVT is to build auditory skills as closely as possible to the child's chronological age when compared to typically developing children. As the child approaches those speech and language targets, children who may have been placed in self-inclusive classrooms may be evaluated for readiness in the mainstream classroom setting. There are many factors determining whether the child should mainstream or not. Some of these are external factors relate to the educational support the school can offer in the mainstream classroom, including hearing assistive technology such as remote microphones or sign language interpreters. Other times, intrinsic factors, such as the child's ability to successfully interact with their peers, may play a role in this determination. The Placement and Readiness Checklist (PARC) is a tool that can be used to determine readiness at different points in the child's educational journey and can be found in the reference list at the end of this chapter (Success for Kids with Hearing Loss, 2023). The PARC battery offers insight into what support looks like in the educational setting from primary to secondary school settings and much more.

Collectively, those involved in aural rehabilitation need to be aware that auditory skills development depends on various factors, including cognition. Early intervention is the goal of any child navigating the aural habilitation process to shorten the length of time between lack of auditory awareness to spoken language development. The sensitivity period for language acquisition is short, and therefore, strong attempts must be made early in the process to ensure the optimal spoken language outcomes for the child. Many individuals are involved in the training of children in a multitude of settings, however, because young infants are primarily in the home setting, the participation and training of parents and caregivers plays a major role in the early stages. Professionals, in this early stage, are tracking auditory and verbal development to ensure that skills are being obtained consistent with the amount of intervention the child receives, the accuracy of cochlear processor programming, and what is revealed on device use through datalogging. Aural rehabilitation for the deaf or hard of hearing child should consider the individualized preferences and needs of the child, family unit, and desired communication outcome.

Factors Affecting Cochlear Implantation Outcomes Post Activation

Medical Factors

Advances in minimally invasive surgical techniques have resulted in cochlear implantation surgeries in infants that carry no greater surgical risk when compared with older children (Naik et al., 2021). The surgical timing of cochlear implantation will naturally have an influence on auditory and language development. Some surgical centers and surgeons opt to implant sequentially, or one ear at a time, while others choose to implant simultaneously, or both ears at the same time. When choosing sequential implantation, bonding of the child with the contralateral side's implant is best achieved when the timing between both implants is minimal. Largely, studies have shown that bilateral cochlear implantation can provide acoustic benefits such as equal access to speech and sound to the right and left of the patient, binaural summation, better speech understanding in noise, and accuracy in sound localization (Sharma et al., 2020). Some families choose to implant unilaterally regardless of bilateral candidacy and may aid the contralateral side with a high-powered hearing aid to result in a bimodal hearing solution. Different options for cochlear implant electrode arrays may allow surgeons to retain low-frequency residual hearing for activation of a hybrid processor, which allows simultaneous stimulation of the auditory system via acoustic and electrical methods. Candidacy for cochlear implantation has expanded in many countries to allow for single-sided deafness implantation to occur. In the past, single-sided deafness (SSD) implantation was contraindicated by arguments of access to CROS hearing aids and bone conduction hearing devices. Naturally, the binaural auditory benefits are not wholly experienced with these methods of hearing. Bimodal, SSD, and hybrid implants will not be discussed extensively in this chapter due to the high variability in outcomes but rather mentioned for consideration during the family's counseling of options.

Early Intervention

Newborn hearing screenings are becoming widely implemented on the global scale as researchers and professionals are realizing the importance of the early detection and intervention of hearing loss in infants and young children. The philosophy of

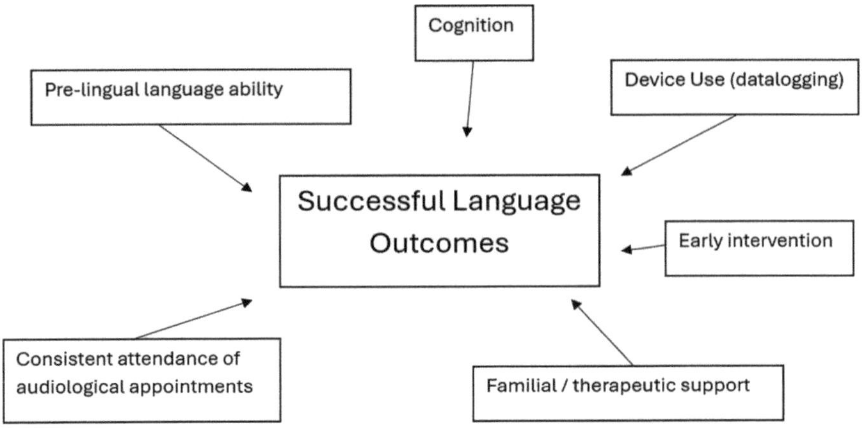

Fig. 19.4 A list of factors leading to successful language outcomes

"the earlier the intervention the better," has quickly become a mantra in our field. Cochlear implants are widely recognized as an acceptable form of intervention in infants 9 months of age and younger. Largely, studies have shown that research supporting cochlear implantation under 1 year of age is limited due to limited measurements of prelingual auditory skills required for speech and language acquisition, the lack of controlled variables, and inconsistent definitions of early and late intervention, all clouding the results of existing long-term language outcomes studies (Marschark et al., 2019).

It is nearly impossible to list every possible influence on the success of aural habilitation in children, with some influences depicted in Fig. 19.4, but some topics warrant being included in this section. Prelingual communication capacity and cognitive ability, both contributing factors in linguistic outcomes, have not largely been included or detailed in recent cochlear implant research thereby further obscuring correlates of successful outcomes in cochlear implant patients (Marschark et al., 2019). Furthermore, some children can experience intermittent auditory access or progressive hearing loss, such as those with auditory neuropathy spectrum disorder and congenital cytomegalovirus respectively and may show better long-term language outcomes due to prior language exposure, also skewing the long terms analysis of language acquisition in implanted children. To add to the complexities of studying language outcomes, many aural habilitation procedures discuss the consistent use of cochlear processors (i.e. daily average of hours used) as another factor for successful outcomes. In the past, consistent use was defined as a minimum of 8 hours of use per day on average, but recent recommendations suggest that attaining 80% use during waking hours, when all waking hours cannot be achieved, shows promise in infants who are awake less hours in the day than older children (Gagnon et al., 2021; Park et al., 2019). Finally, other factors contributing to low success in aural habilitation are low maternal education, low socioeconomic status, larger family size, late identification of hearing loss and/or implantation, and limited time spent in aural habilitation (Quittner et al., 2013).

Spoken language acquisition in children with hearing loss is the primary goal of post-cochlear implantation. Successful outcomes have been identified in children implanted early, especially by one year of age. Early implantation reduces the time spent without auditory stimulation and approximates auditory development in children with normal hearing. Medical advancements have made it possible for infants to seek cochlear implantation below 12 months of age with minor differences in surgical and postsurgical medical management and equal auditory outcomes when compared to standard timelines. Despite this, several studies report that there are not a lot of recordable data to quantify prelingual auditory development in infants below 1 year of age which makes candidacy determination with high-powered hearing aids and post-cochlear implant activation auditory skill growth data difficult to measure in infants (Marschark et al., 2019). Numerous factors, such as low device use and improper maintenance of microphone covers in the processor, can negatively influence progress in attaining spoken language, therefore professionals involved should track speech and language development and continue the counseling process to encourage families to continue the journey towards their chosen communication goal.

Aural Rehabilitation of Adults

Adults who have little to no perceived speech understanding benefit with power hearing aids may also be cochlear implant candidates. The focus of this section will be on post-lingual deafness in adults. Adults already have many years of language experience and can "fill in the gaps" when distorted speech or competing noise is present, and the hearing loss negatively affects speech comprehension. However, this increases cognitive load and causes fatigue. Moreover, children and adults require hearing for communication, occupational, social, environmental and safety purposes. When undergoing the cochlear implant candidacy process with an adult, the determination of which ear to implant may vary by recommendations made by the clinic's audiologist and/or surgeon. One point of view is that implanting the ear with poorer speech understanding offers the patient "less to lose" and the possibly of significant auditory access to gain. If the implant is unsuccessful or offers very limited success, very little functional hearing is lost by implanting this ear. Another point of view focuses on giving the patient "the best chance of speech understanding" by implanting the better performing ear first. The thought behind this concept is that this ear has been receiving auditory stimulation consistently and therefore, may offer quick access to meaningful auditory input. However, should little to no auditory benefit be received, the patient will be left with a poorer hearing binaurally (i.e., poor speech understanding in the implanted ear and contralateral hearing aid-aided ear). These decisions are important to consider because many adults choose to implant only one ear, despite bilateral candidacy.

Because normal hearing has typically been experienced at an earlier point in an adult's life, auditory input from cochlear implants may not align with the patient's expectation of outcomes. Listening through a cochlear implant is not the same as natural hearing. A couple of patients of this author have described the listening experience as robotic and unnatural during the first few months of use. Moreover, adult patients are expected to participate in aural rehabilitation, which is primarily performed in the home setting. Therapy in the comfort of one's home where the environment can be largely controlled, such as the ability to turn down the television, is useful to encourage the adult patient. Other settings, such as restaurants, where the patient cannot control the volume of the patrons or music in that establishment may cause frustration and disappointment in this process. The timing and duration of the therapy can also offer convenience in the home setting. Finally, many resources have been offered online and for free for adults, which makes the home setting ideal for aural habilitation. More online resources can be found in the cochlear implant manufacturer's website free of cost.

Most resources for adults focus on compensation techniques for oral communication. Again, the cochlear implant does not offer normal hearing, and some patients may experience a degree of deterioration of auditory input in quiet and especially in noisy environments. Adults who are active socially and have occupations will have more communication needs in complex environments than an adult living with their spouse in a quiet home with little visitors. Tailored aural rehabilitation goals will focus on what the patient finds to be important to make large impacts.

Table 19.3 Validation measures for adults

Name	Languages available	Summary
Cochlear Implant Quality of Life (CIQOL-35)	English, and translated to French, German, Arabic	Patient questionnaire that assesses expectations in the following domains: Communication, emotional, entertainment, environment, listening effort, and social. Patients should have 12 months of CI experience. Not normed for single-sided deafness recipients. Is offered at no cost at: https://medicine.musc.edu/departments/otolaryngology/research/cochlear-implant (MUSC Foundation for Research Development, 2019).
Comprehensive Cochlear Implant Questionnaire (CCIQ)	English	Self-assessment of physical, psychological, and social benefits of cochlear implantation developed by the New York Eye and Ear Infirmary and can be found here: https://cdn-links.lww.com/permalink/mao/a/mao_2013_10_14_king_on-13-181r2_sdc1.pdf (New York Eye and Ear Infirmary, n.d.)
Client Oriented Scale of Improvement (COSI)	More than 20 languages	For professional use. An open-ended patient questionnaire for patient goal-tracking within a pre-determined time frame, available for free here: https://www.nal.gov.au/nal_products/cosi/ (Cochlear, 2024)

Validation Measures

One way of finding out what is important to the patient is by using validation measures. In Table 19.3, you will find common questionnaires to assist the professional in targeting relevant goals for the adult undergoing aural rehabilitation.

Adults can make meaningful progress, however, become discouraged with the slow pace of stabilization of auditory skill set. This is where the SLP and/or audiologist can use the validation measures to baseline and document progress.

Implementing Aural Rehabilitation

Aural rehabilitation can begin in many ways. As mentioned earlier in the pediatric section, bilateral implantation, when indicated, provides far superior results than unilateral implantation in bilaterally qualified candidates. Device wear time, duration of deafness, cognitive status, socioeconomic factors, and family support largely impacts communication outcomes in the adult as well. One special consideration for adults is dexterity and limited range of motion for arm movement. Adults can develop arthritis and other conditions, making the placement of a cochlear processor on the head challenging. In these cases, aural rehabilitation may also focus on adapting and teaching the patient how to use their cochlear processors with modifications. Low vision may also be experienced by patients and special considerations should be made with patients experiencing this as well. Listening training in quiet at the beginning of aural rehabilitation is important to retrain the brain by isolating auditory stimuli but can quickly move into top-down approaches given the typical adult's language experience.

One resource for aural rehabilitation is Angel Sound offered by Tiger Speech. Angel Sound was developed as a free resource (https://angelsound.tigerspeech.com/) where patients can access many auditory stimuli of varying complexities at their own pace while tracking progress (Emily Fu Foundation, n.d.). Though there are pediatric-oriented graphics on this website, don't be fooled. There are complex auditory tasks that can be very challenging, even for adults with normal hearing sensitivity. Additionally, many cochlear implant manufacturers also offer resources on their patient portals to assist with refining auditory skills. Specifically, Cochlear offers Telephone with Confidence, a phone call-based task to improve speech understanding in phone conversations where lip-reading cannot occur. Every day, the patient calls the free phone number and a recording is played while the patient follows along a written script (Cochlear, n.d.). Aside from these resources, the professional can offer simple recommendations to teach patients to advocate for slower speech and rephrasing in their communication partners when the original message was not heard. Reducing background noise (when possible) or putting one's back towards the main sources of noise (to reduce background noise utilizing sophisticated microphone algorithims) can also be offered as a quick tip. Occasionally, adult patients will need the assistance of SLPs for added support and/or the use of hearing assistive technology (i.e. remote microphones) for difficult listening environments.

Aural rehabilitation in adults often occurs with self-guided methods and produces strong communication outcomes. This is because adults already have a strong foundation for auditory-oral language. There are many resources available to adults that can be accessed in the comfort of their home. Adult's auditory needs differ from children's in that performance in an educational setting is not a typical area of concern, they are starting their auditory journeys with a strong language foundation, and have the ability to self-navigate their therapy. However, performance in occupational and social settings take precedence along with concerns of regaining auditory skills that were lost.

Teletherapy in Children and Adults

The study on outcomes of aural (re)habilitation services by means of teletherapy has been talked about extensively in recent years. The COVID-19 pandemic's influence on this topic has expanded research with many studies being performed between 2021 and 2022 as per a PubMed search performed by this author. Despite the need for social isolation during the pandemic, the needs of cochlear implant patients did not change, and professionals had to seek innovative ways to reach their patients. Teletherapy has been regarded as a low-cost and convenient alternative for patients receiving services and professionals alike. Approximately 80% of individuals needing hearing health care services are in low- and middle-income countries, and disparities are greater in regional areas of Africa, the Eastern Mediterranean, and South Asia (Lin & Chen, 2024). Implementation of this method of treatment removes travel restrictions (particularly for those living hours away from specialty services or are limited in their physical mobility), decreases the amount of time required in the patient's schedule (as travel time is now eliminated), can utilize various types of accessible equipment (e.g., such as cell phones, tablets or computers) thereby having the potential to increase the patient's access to services and satisfaction (Lin & Chen, 2024). From the provider's perspective, equipment is also readily available on both the patient and professional's end, but there are more considerations before providing teletherapy. For example, patient confidentiality and security can be difficult to maintain through electronic communication. Ensuring confidentiality and security can be costly for the provider (Lin & Chen, 2024). Additionally, the patient's comfort with technology can hinder progress and poor reliability of internet services for patients in rural areas can negatively affect the quality of the appointment. Moreover, teletherapy can create situations in which the provider loses control during the appointment (e.g., such as noisy children and other distractions being present in the background in the middle of a session), thereby reducing effectiveness. As for the cochlear processors themselves, programming can occur through remote programming sessions via implant manufacturer's apps and has shown efficiency. Another consideration is the status of the cochlear equipment itself. The audiologist must ensure that the microphone covers have been changed as per each manufacturer's guidelines and that other components are functional before modifying the programming. This can be difficult to achieve during an appointment with a new user who is unfamiliar with their processor and hard of hearing. Despite some of these challenges, positive feedback has been received from patients and professionals alike and most studies support implementing teletherapy for adults (Claridge & Kroll, 2021; Verma et al. 2022a, b; Lin & Chen, 2024). The consensus is that more research is needed to evaluate patient language and auditory outcomes when receiving teletherapy aural (re)habilitation services.

On the contrary, fewer studies reported the efficacy of aural habilitation in children. Ling and Chen (2024) discussed their findings to be safe and comparable when utilizing teletherapy (compared to in person services), with no significant differences when obtaining telemetry, obtaining the upper and lower limits of the dynamic range in cochlear implant programming, and speech outcomes in children and adults. Verma et al. (2022) discussed that adults have adopted positive views on teletherapy but pointed out that the parents of children with cochlear implants much prefer in-person therapy. Moreover, their pilot study involving 27 prelingual children with unilateral cochlear implants with significant speech and language delays was divided into two groups based on the mode of therapy they received, traditional in-person therapy or teletherapy. Their results show that both delivery modes showed increased speech, language, and hearing skills, but the in-person group had greater growth in all three areas than the teletherapy group (Verma et al. 2022a, b). The authors speculate that this may be attributed to the difficulty of providing pediatric aural habilitation services through teletherapy for both clinicians and families. For parents, less familiarity with cochlear processors and the aural habilitation process coupled with behavioral management and limited attention in their child proved to be too challenging (Claridge & Kroll, 2021). On the other hand, parents also reported that more feedback from the professional was received, and additional parent-coaching was given when compared with in-person sessions (Claridge & Kroll, 2021).

The efficacy of teletherapy has been investigated with many studies occurring in the last 5 years. The COVID-19 pandemic has forced researchers to gain multiple perspectives on the services in adults and children. It is not surprising to find that studies have shown that over 90% of parents of deaf and hard of hearing children have positive feedback with teletherapy sessions and reports that they are confident in the ability of the therapist to provide this service (Constantinescu et al., 2014). In the adult's experience, many reported favorable perspectives as patients were able to save time and money while getting access to quality care (Lin & Chen, 2024).

References

Advanced Bionics. (1990). *Tools for toddlers: The Ling 6 sound check.* https://www.advancedbionics.com/content/dam/advancedbionics/Documents/libraries/Tools-for-Toddlers/tools-for-parents/The-Ling-Six-Sound-Check.pdf

Advanced Bionics. (n.d.) *IT-MAIS: Infant-toddler meaningful auditory integrated scale.* https://www.advancedbionics.com/content/dam/advancedbionics/Documents/Regional/VN/Libraries/Tools-for-Schools/Educational_Support/Assessment-Tools/ITMAIS-ResourceBrochure.pdf

AG Bell Academy. (n.d.). *About the LSL specialist certification.* https://agbellacademy.org/certification/

Alahmadi, A., Abdelsamad, Y., Alothman, N. I., Alshalan, A., Almuhawas, F., Alamari, N. A., Allyousef, M. Y., Alhabib, S. F., & Hagr, A. (2023). A literature review on cochlear implant activation: From weeks to hours. *Ear Nose & Throat Journal.*

Audiology Online. (2004). *Using the Ling 6 sound test everyday.* https://www.audiologyonline.com/articles/using-ling-6-sound-test-1087.

Claridge, R., & Kroll, N. (2021). Aural rehabilitation via telepractice during COVID-19: A global perspective on evolving early intervention practices. *International Journal of Telerehabilitation, 13*(1), e6362.

Clark-Gambelunghe, M. B., & Clark, D. A. (2015). Sensory development. *Pediatric Clinics, 62*(2), 367–384.

Cochlear. (2018). *Ling 6 sound flash cards.* https://mss-p-007-delivery.sitecorecontenthub.cloud/api/public/content/17b77f153c114d0d87a51aa2198a78bd?v=b4a7c42d

Cochlear. (2024). *Cochlear implant evaluation toolbox: Incentives and obstacles to the routine use.* https://pronews.cochlear.com/cochlear-implant-evaluation-toolbox-outcomes-measures/

Cochlear. (n.d.) *Telephone with confidence.* https://www.cochlear.com/us/en/home/ongoing-care-and-support/rehabilitation-resources/resources-for-adults/telephone-with-confidence

Constantinescu, G., Waite, M., Dornan, D., Rushbrooke, E., Brown, J., McGovern, J., Ryan, M., & Hill, A. (2014). A pilot study of telepractice delivery for teaching listening and spoken language to children with hearing loss. *Journal of Telemedicine and Telecare, 20*(3), 135. https://doi.org/10.1177/1357633X14528443

Cooper, J. O., Heron, T. E., & Heward, W. L. (2007). *Applied behavioral analysis* (2nd ed.). Pearson Education.

Emily Fu Foundation. (n.d.). *Angel Sound TM.* https://angelsound.tigerspeech.com/

Erber, N. P. (1982). *Auditory training.* Alexander Graham Bell Association for the Deaf and Hard of Hearing.

Estabrooks, W., MacIver-Lux, K., & Rhoades, E. A. (Eds.). (2016). *Auditory-verbal therapy: For young children with hearing loss and their families, and the practitioners who guide them.* Plural Publishing.

Gagnon, E. B., Eskridge, H., Brown, K. D., & Park, L. R. (2021). The impact of cumulative cochlear implant wear time on spoken language outcomes at age 3 years. *Journal of Speech, Language, and Hearing Research, 64*(4), 1369–1375.

Hashemi, S. B., & Monshizadeh, L. (2016). Comparison of auditory perception in cochlear implanted children with and without additional disabilities. *Iranian journal of medical sciences, 41*(3), 186–190.

Lin, M. J., & Chen, C. K. (2024). Breaking sound barriers: Exploring tele-audiology's impact on hearing healthcare. *Diagnostics, 14*(8), 856. https://doi.org/10.3390/diagnostics14080856

LOCHI Study. (2019). *The PEACH and PEACH +.* https://www.outcomes.nal.gov.au/peach

Marschark, M., Duchesne, L., & Pisoni, D. (2019). Effects of age at cochlear implantation on learning and cognition: A critical assessment. *American Journal of Speech-Language Pathology, 28*(3), 1318–1334. https://doi.org/10.1044/2019_AJSLP-18-0160

Med-El. (2024). *Auditory skills checklist 10/PK.* https://bridgestore.us.medel.com/product/auditory-skills-checklist-10-pk/

Mitchell, R. E., & Karchmer, M. (2004). Chasing the mythical ten percent: Parental hearing status of deaf and hard of hearing students in the United States. *Sign Language Studies, 4*(2), 138–163.

MUSC Foundation for Research Development. (2019). Adult cochlear implant expectations questionnaire. https://web.musc.edu/-/sm/medicine/departments/otolaryngology/cochlear-implant/f/instrument-downloads/ciqol-expectations-automated-outcome-measure-scoring.ashx

Naik, A. N., Varadarajan, V. V., & Malhotra, P. S. (2021). Early pediatric Cochlear implantation: An update. *Laryngoscope Investigative Otolaryngology, 6*(3), 512–521.

New York Eye and Ear Infirmary. (n.d.). *Comprehensive cochlear implant questionnaire.* https://cdn-links.lww.com/permalink/mao/a/mao_2013_10_14_king_on-13-181r2_sdc1.pdf

Park, L. R., Gagnon, E. B., Thompson, E., & Brown, K. D. (2019). Age at full-time use predicts language outcomes better than age of surgery in children who use cochlear implants. *American Journal of Audiology, 28*(4), 986–992.

Parker, R., Muzaffar, J., AuD, M. A., & Brassington, W. (2024). Early activation of cochlear implants: A systematic review and narrative synthesis. *Cochlear Implants International, 25*(1), 81–92.

Quittner, A. L., Cruz, I., Barker, D. H., Tobey, E., Eisenberg, L. S., Niparko, J. K., & Childhood Development after Cochlear Implantation Investigative Team. (2013). Effects of maternal sensitivity and cognitive and linguistic stimulation on cochlear implant users' language development over four years. *The Journal of Pediatrics, 162*(2), 343–348.

Sharma, S. D., Cushing, S. L., Papsin, B. C., & Gordon, K. A. (2020). Hearing and speech benefits of cochlear implantation in children: A review of the literature. *International Journal of Pediatric Otorhinolaryngology, 133*, 109984.

Success for Kids with Hearing Loss. (2023). *Tests: Informal assessments for parents, students, teachers.* https://successforkidswithhearingloss.com/tests-informal-assessments-for-parents-students-teachers/.

Verma, H., Banumathy, N., Mishra, R., & Panda, N. K. (2022a). Outcome measures following tele-rehabilitation and conventional face to face rehabilitation in paediatric cochlear implant users during COVID-19 pandemic: A pilot study in a tertiary care setup. *Journal of Otology, 17*(1), 31–38.

Verma, H., Banumathy, N., Mishra, R., & Panda, N. K. (2022b). Outcome measures following tele-rehabilitation and conventional face to face rehabilitation in paediatric cochlear implant users during COVID-19 pandemic: A pilot study in a tertiary care setup. *Journal of otology, 17*(1), 31–38.

Wroblewska-Seniuk, K., Greczka, G., Dabrowski, P., Szyfter-Harris, J., & Mazela, J. (2017). Hearing impairment in premature newborns—Analysis based on the national hearing screening database in Poland. *PLoS One, 12*(9), e0184359.

Chapter 20
Assessment of Outcomes in Paediatric Cochlear Implant Users

Banumathy Nagamani, Rashmi Deshpande, and Rupali Mathur

Abstract Early identification of hearing loss, timely diagnosis, and early access to sound stimuli play a crucial role in developing age-appropriate linguistic competence in children with congenital hearing loss. Assessing the efficacy of aural rehabilitation is key to a successful rehabilitation program. This chapter explores the assessment of outcomes in paediatric cochlear implant users, emphasizing the importance of early identification and intervention for children with hearing loss. The authors discuss the dynamic process of habilitation and rehabilitation, highlighting the need for a comprehensive and individualized approach to address the unique challenges faced by each child. The chapter provides a detailed overview of assessment tools and techniques, covering various domains such as listening, speech, language, pragmatics, cognition, voice, music perception, literacy skills, play, and quality of life. Tracking them at regular intervals across these domains is a must. The authors also discuss the challenges faced in outcome audits, including variability in performance due to factors such as age at implantation, duration of implant use, associated disorders, and linguistic and cultural considerations.

Keywords Cochlear implants · Aural rehabilitation · Assessment tools · Speech-language · Music perception · Literacy · Cognition · Pragmatics · Play

---

B. Nagamani (✉)
Department of Otolaryngology-Head and Neck Surgery, Post Graduate Institute of Medical Education and Research (PGIMER), Chandigarh, Punjab and Haryana, India

R. Deshpande
Listen Learn and Communicate, HSLS (Hearing Speech and Language Services), Bengaluru, Karnataka, India

R. Mathur
Shabda Brahma Speech and Hearing Clinic and Cochlear Implant Centre, Ahmedabad, Gujarat, India

P. Kumar et al. (eds.), *Advances in Implantation Otology*,
https://doi.org/10.1007/978-981-96-8671-1_20

Introduction

Hearing loss identified at birth is estimated to be 1–3 per 1000 infants. Although Universal newborn hearing screening (UNHS) has been implemented in all countries, it has not been very successful in developing and underdeveloped countries either due to failure in following the UNHS protocol or loss to follow up following the failed screenings. However, with advances in hearing technology that have greatly improved over the last two decades, an increasing number of children with hearing loss are now serving as candidates for cochlear implants (CI), thereby enrolling themselves for rehabilitation. Since children with hearing loss are not a homogenous group, a single communication mode is not appropriate for all children diagnosed with hearing loss. Many children with hearing loss are born to parents with normal hearing. Considering this, an increasing number of parents of young children with hearing loss are now opting for learning to listen through an auditory-only mode for communication. Listening and spoken language intervention is mandatory for all children with hearing loss as significant delays in speech, language, and auditory development has a greater impact on many factors like psychosocial, literacy, academic and employment. There is a significant amount of literature regarding therapy post-cochlear implantation, but the same cannot be said regarding the assessment of speech and language skills following cochlear implantation, especially in multilingual countries. In this chapter, the authors will discuss the outcome measures in various domains in auditory rehabilitation. While authors discuss assessing intervention outcomes following implantation, terms such as habilitation and rehabilitation need to be clearly understood by all professionals involved in the team approach (Reader can refer to Chap. 19 for further details related to Rehabilitation).

Rehabilitation/Habilitation

For those planning to opt for CI, it is imperative to remember that there is an ongoing dynamic process of rehabilitation/or "habilitation", which is applicable for those who have had no access to auditory stimulation prior to CI surgery. Dettman et al. (1996) define habilitation in young children as a teaching or learning process during which the clinician facilitates the acquisition of auditory, speech, and language skills in a normal developmental pattern. This differs from the process of rehabilitation, which is typically followed in adults, who reacquire their lost communication skills after restoring their auditory sense through cochlear implantation. The process of intervening patients who have never heard before is referred to as intensive individualized habilitation; On the other hand, rehabilitation refers to intervening patients who are learning to hear again.

Children who may have had significant benefits with hearing aids till a particular age may not have adequate benefits when the language becomes more complex or even in strenuous listening conditions and hence may have undergone a cochlear implant surgery for improving their listening, speech, and language skills. Also, children with progressive hearing loss may have attained skills premorbid, but post-implantation they may need to relearn listening skills. Hence, the need for rehabilitation arises and the terminology (Re)habilitation may be appropriately used in some scenarios.

This process of habilitation/rehabilitation always involves an inter- or multi- disciplinary endeavour as children with cochlear implants may have associated issues and they would require specialized attention. Even otherwise, as professionals focus on holistic development there needs to be a larger interdisciplinary team approach to work with paediatric cochlear implantees. Not all team members may be involved with every child but they can be approached on a need basis. The team members include Audiologist, Speech Language Pathologist, Otolaryngologist, Paediatrician, Neurologist, Occupational therapist, Sensory integration therapist, Physiotherapist, Vision therapist, Psychologist, Education counsellor, and School administration. An effective collaboration between all these team members will allow professionals to have a patient and family-centered focus in rehabilitation.

Components of Rehabilitation

Habilitation programs must be comprehensive to enable a cochlear implantee with an early utilization of various sound stimuli and also integrate the various domains for effective communication. The components of rehabilitation ideally include effective counseling, managing the sensory deficit with appropriate technology, and a custom-made intervention plan for developing age-appropriate communication, which will focus on domains such as listening, speech, language, literacy, pragmatics, and cognition. The habilitation sessions should always integrate the goals focusing on all these domains. Addressing each domain as a separate goal will hinder the child's unified phenomenon of communication. Hence, professionals should always levy their focus on the "hybrid" approach to intervention, thereby establishing a balance between structured intervention and naturalistic interactions (Van Kleeck, 1986).

Overall, components of Aural (Re)habilitation post-CI comprise parental guidance for selecting the appropriate therapy program (depending on the presence of associated issues, age of cochlear implantation, availability of support services and resources), communication skill development focusing on various domains (auditory, speech and language, pragmatics) and literacy development (cognition, reading, and writing). The goals in therapy need to cover all the above aspects for a successful rehabilitation program. Regardless of the intervention method for an infant, toddler, or child, difficulties that may be faced by the recipient, the following factors should be considered during rehabilitation and addressed appropriately: options for mode of communication (aural, oral, aural-oral, & manual), auditory perception, higher/advanced language skills, education and vocational placement, psychosocial factors, scholastic performance, family and societal considerations. All these issues need to be addressed dynamically, as and when required, in the due course of therapy.

Bringing Sounds to Life

Early identification of hearing loss, timely diagnosis, and early access to sound stimuli play a very crucial role in developing age-appropriate linguistic competence in children with congenital hearing loss (Geers et al., 2003). As and when a child is activated/switched on with the cochlear implant, the brain starts receiving auditory stimuli. However, it may not be able to develop connections to associate meaning with what is being heard by the brain. To pursue an effective (Re)habilitation program, children opting for CI should first have adequate (sufficient) auditory access to various codes of respective languages, viz., the segmental (vowels & consonants) and supra-segmental (intonation, stress, & rhythm) aspects. Once the child has adequate access to various patterns and rules of language, the second critical condition is to associate meaning to the sounds heard, thereby bringing sounds to life (Robbins, 2018). Children cannot demonstrate functional benefits from CI unless they associate meaning with sounds. Associating meaning to sounds is a challenging task for CI children since a pre-lingual child needs to develop the novel code while a post-lingual child needs to re-map the novel signal onto an existing linguistic code (Robbins, 2018). Although digital technology may offer access to auditory stimuli, it is the intensive and didactic habilitation, along with a very well-nurtured auditory and spoken language environment at home and school, and the child's cognitive development/abilities that facilitate the opportunities for sounds heard to be more meaningful. For older children with CI, the re-learning process is referred to as rehabilitation. Akin to this, it is very clear that aural (re) habilitation is to be initiated at an early age for the most successful development of communicative competence in the future.

Aural Rehabilitation-Initiation

Aural rehabilitation is defined as 'any device, procedure, information, interaction, or therapy which lessens the communicative and psychosocial consequences of a hearing loss (Bally & Bakke, 2007). Aural rehabilitation may help to reduce participation limitations and facilitate better personal and environmental strategies to minimize the disabling effects of hearing loss (WHO, 2001). Considering the neural plasticity of the brain, children with hearing loss need a professional architect to build the child's brain during their early years. This will, in turn, enhance the connections and tune the neural networking. As the brain is one of the only organs which is not fully developed at birth, it needs to be built. Through auditory exposure, the brain starts to prune. In other words, those connections that are used get strengthened and those that are not, get pruned. This is the process through which the brain is shaped by neural wiring. Also, there is always an interdependence of audition, spoken language, and brain. Auditory performance refers to adaptive use of hearing for speech perception and production, while auditory capacity refers to integrity of the auditory system; and auditory experience refers to events that activate the auditory system. Congenital hearing loss restricts and reduces access to auditory experiences. The quality and quantity of auditory experience matter a lot as it eliminates, reduces, or distorts the speech cues sent to the brain. So, it hampers the rewiring of the brain. Still, a child with hearing loss should be taught spoken language through listening as speech is an acoustic event. Current digital technology can provide early auditory access to the sounds of speech and non-speech stimuli thereby optimizing the auditory brain development for most children with hearing loss.

Proficiency in spoken language at an early age is possible for most children with hearing loss, irrespective of the degree of hearing loss, provided they are identified early, fitted with appropriate hearing technology and offered early intervention services by qualified, trained professionals. Thus, the process of identifying, and diagnosing hearing loss, and providing different types of intervention after prescribing appropriate amplification devices, defines the term aural rehabilitation.

Aural rehabilitation, thus involves various strategies right from orienting parents or caregivers to the appropriate digital technology, guiding for selecting appropriate therapy program, early intervention program, communication skill development, which may involve all of the following domains, viz, audition, speech, language, literacy development, cognition and pragmatics.

Efficacy of Aural Rehabilitation

The International Classification of Functioning, Disability, and Health (ICF) is a framework for describing and organizing information on functioning and disability. The ICF conceptualizes a person's level of functioning as a dynamic interaction between her or his health conditions, environmental factors, and personal factors. It is a biopsychosocial model of disability, based on an integration of the social and medical models of disability. The Biopsychosocial model encompasses the entire journey of CI from candidacy to rehabilitation and outcomes need to be measured not only for listening, speech and language skills but other aspects like cognition, quality of life, play skills, etc. giving it a more holistic perspective.

Hedge and Pomaville (2008) refer to assessment as "a flexible but systematic process of testing hypotheses and evaluating the quality of learners' developmental progress". Assessing a child's access to any sound stimulus after implantation at regular intervals, making it more of a dynamic assessment during rehabilitation, enables the Speech-Language Pathologist (SLP)/interventionist to understand the child's progress right from baseline. It is a mode of tracking the child's growth on different domains, namely, speech, language, audition, pragmatics and cognition. The timeline that is generally recommended is 3 months interval from baseline till one-year post-switch-on, followed by 6 months interval. It also means to assess a family's understanding of forming goals for their child to access sound and language, to understand various communication options, and to finally identify tools that would assess the progress of the child on all the above-mentioned domains.

A detailed assessment plays a crucial role in evaluating the outcome of any cochlear implant program. It gives us an insight into the anticipated outcome in children with cochlear implants. Various kinds of assessment tools are there to measure the skills of children with cochlear implants. However, professionals must first understand the instrument they are using, before administering them with respect to its purpose, skills assessed, age group and type (formal or informal). Formal (standardized) and informal assessment are the two types of assessment procedures used as tools for measuring outcomes in children with cochlear implants. However, SLPs generally use more formal assessment tools. There are different types of assessments as discussed below:

(a) **Formal assessment**: these are mostly data-based and systematic tests to assess various skills. Formal assessments are usually carried out to make comparisons between the group of learners, monitor progress and to provide accountability. The following are the types of formal assessment:

   (i) Norm-referenced assessment:

   Norm-referenced assessments are used to compare a child's performance to that of a group of same-age peers (norm group). They help us determine whether a child's performance is delayed or at par with that of a sample of his/her peers. They usually assess the broad skill sets.

   (ii) Criterion-referenced assessment

   Criterion-referenced assessments are designed to measure mastery of certain skill sets without reference to the performance of other children (Popham & Husek, 1969). A child's performance on a criterion-referenced item or group of items should indicate mastery of a set of skills (Popham & Husek, 1969). These types of tests can be used to monitor progress.

(b) **Informal assessments**: these are spontaneous forms of assessment, which are content and performance-driven and not data-driven. They are less structured and non-standardized methods of evaluation.

   (i) Observation
   (ii) Checklists or rating scale
   (iii) Questionnaire/parental interviews
   (iv) Language sampling

   All the above informal assessments can be used to supplement data obtained from the formal test (Fujiki & Willbrand, 1982). There are various factors which need to be considered while deciding appropriate test instruments. Specifically, the two measures i.e. validity and reliability which play a significant role in deciding the selection of test instruments. According to Field (2005) 'Validity' refers to measuring what it is intended to measure; While 'Reliability' indicates how consistent are the findings of any assessment tool over time. Another important factor that needs to be considered is the standardization of assessment tools. A standardized tool is one that warrants all participants to respond to the items/questions in a similar manner and are scored in a consistent way, thereby making it possible for the clinician to compare an individual's performance to other individuals or groups of individuals. Whereas, a non-standardized tool measures the performance of an individual and does not focus on obtaining scores in order to compare one's performance to another's.

Assessment of Basic Skills

There are certain basic building blocks that need to be understood while we step into the rehabilitation of children with hearing loss. For an effective development and acquisition of above-mentioned building blocks, these assessments should also be specific, hierarchical, and measurable on various domains, viz., audition, language, speech, pragmatics and cognition. In addition to these, a special focus will be levied on voice, music perception, literacy skills and play. These domains play a vital role in the long-term progress of children with CI with respect to their scholastic performance and day-to-day functional life skills. Each domain will be discussed in the following sections:

Assessment of Listening/Auditory Skills

There is a need to assess the functional listening skills which will include assessing a child's acoustic and phonemic access to sounds. In young children, listening skills can be assessed in a hierarchical manner so as to be able to monitor child progress e.g. assessing auditory detection, discrimination, identification and comprehension. Speech recognition, also called speech perception, refers to how well individuals use auditory and/or visual information to understand spoken messages. Speech recognition testing involves assessing how well someone can recognize speech units such as phonemes, words, and sentences (Tye-Murray, 2020). Speech perception defines how complex, auditory patterns are processed by the central nervous system (CNS) of the CI user. Assessment of these skills need to be performed in quiet as well as in presence of noise.

Materials/Tools for Assessing Listening Skills

The following section enlists various tools to assess listening skills in children with hearing loss following an appropriate management.

- **Functional Auditory Performance Indicators** (FAPI): The Functional Auditory Performance Indicators (FAPI) is a comprehensive assessment tool designed to evaluate and track auditory development and listening skills in children, particularly those with hearing impairments, including cochlear implant users (Stredler-Brown & Johnson, 2001, 2003). Developed to provide a holistic view of auditory performance, the FAPI assesses various aspects of auditory function that are critical for effective communication and learning: sound detection, sound discrimination, sound localization, and auditory comprehension.
- **Infant-Toddler Meaningful Auditory Integration Scale** (IT-MAIS): The Infant-Toddler Meaningful Auditory Integration Scale (IT-MAIS) is a specialized assessment tool designed to evaluate auditory performance and integration in young children, specifically those under the age of 2 years. Developed by Zimmerman-Phillips et al. (2001), this scale focuses on understanding how well infants and toddlers use auditory information in their daily interactions.
- **Meaningful Auditory Integration Scale** (MAIS): The Meaningful Auditory Integration Scale (MAIS), developed by Robbins et al. (1991), is a specialized assessment tool designed to evaluate auditory development and integration in children, particularly those with hearing impairments, including those who use cochlear implants. The MAIS is intended for use with children older than 5 years of age. The MAIS is designed to assess how well older children integrate auditory information into meaningful and functional communication. It focuses on evaluating the practical use of auditory skills in daily life and interactions, providing insights into how effectively children with hearing loss are utilizing their hearing abilities.
- **Categories of Auditory Performance** (CAP): The Categories of Auditory Performance (CAP- Archbold et al., 1995) is a structured assessment tool designed to evaluate the auditory abilities of children with hearing impairments, including those using cochlear implants. CAP provides a comprehensive framework for categorizing and tracking auditory performance across different levels

of auditory skill. The CAP is used to assess and categorize the auditory performance of children based on their ability to detect, discriminate, and understand sounds. It provides a standardized way to evaluate the effectiveness of auditory interventions and track progress over time.

- **Auditory Skills Assessment**: screen children as young as 3 years 6 months for early auditory and phonological skills in the age range of 3.6–6:11 years (Geffner & Goldman, 2010).
- **Early Speech Perception** (ESP) in English (Moog & Geers, 1990): The ESP Test in English is designed to assess the auditory and speech perception abilities of young children, specifically those aged 2–5 years. This test evaluates various aspects of speech perception, including the ability to detect and discriminate speech sounds and to understand simple spoken words and sentences. It is used to gauge early speech development in children with hearing impairments and those using cochlear implants.
- The adaptation of ESP has been carried out for Hindi (Bhimte & Rangasayee, 2018), Tamil (Tamilmani & Gore, 2002), Malayalam (Jijo & Yathiraj, 2010) & Marathi (Kuruvilla and Sarda (2012) -speaking children, providing culturally and linguistically appropriate assessment.
- **Parents' Evaluation of Aural/Oral Performance of Children** (PEACH) (Ching & Hill, 2005) (age of 5 years and below): It is a questionnaire to assess a child's behaviour in everyday situations.
- Parents' Evaluation of Aural/Oral Performance of Children and Ease of Listening (PEACH+) – Ching & Hill, 2007; Age group: children below 5 years
- SCAN 3- C (Keith, 2009): It is a valid and reliable battery of tests to help identify auditory processing disorders in children.; Age group; 5:0–11:11 years.
- The APCEI-scale (Acceptation, Perception, Comprehension, oral Expression, speech Intelligibility)—(Noel Petroff et al., 2006). It assesses the overall performance of child using CI and it covers 5 domains and rate them on 1–5 scale: acceptance (A) of the hearing aid or implant, aided auditory perception (P), comprehension (C) of perceived oral message (without lip-reading), oral expression (E) and voice-use (syntax), and the child's intelligibility (I) Items suited to preschool up to 7 years. Table 20.1 enlists all the above tools and Table 20.2 enlists the Indian tools for assessing listening skills.

Table 20.1 List of tests to assess listening skills

S. No	Test	Author/year	Age range	Domains
1.	Functional Auditory Performance Indicators (FAPI)	Stredler-Brown and Johnson (2001), 2003)	All ages	Sound detection Sound discrimination Sound localization Auditory comprehension
2.	The Infant-Toddler Meaningful Auditory Integration Scale (IT-MAIS)	Zimmerman-Phillips et al. (2001)	Infants and toddlers (0–3 years)	Evaluate auditory behaviour in hearing-impaired children in everyday interactions.
3.	The Meaningful Auditory Integration Scale (MAIS)	Robbins et al. (1991)	Children (typically 5+ years)	Evaluate auditory behaviour in hearing-impaired children in everyday interactions.
4.	The Categories of Auditory Performance (CAP)	Archbold et al. (1995)	Below the age of 3	Evaluate auditory abilities in children with cochlear implants
5.	Auditory Skills Assessment	Geffner and Goldman (2010)	Ages 3:6–6:11	Assess following Auditory skills: Speech Discrimination in noise, Mimicry, Blending, Rhyming, Tonal discrimination Tonal patterning
6.	Early Speech Perception (ESP) in English	Moog and Geers (1990)	2–5 years	Assess the auditory and speech perception abilities of young children. Also adapted in various languages including: Hindi (Bhimte & Rangasayee, 2018) Tamil (Tamilmani & Gore, 2002), Malayalam (Jijo & Yathiraj, 2010) Marathi (Kuruvilla & Sarda, 2012)
7.	Parents' Evaluation of Aural/Oral Performance of Children (P.E.A.C.H.)	Ching and Hill (2005)	Infants to school-aged children	Questionnaire to assess child's behaviour in everyday situation.
8.	Parents' Evaluation of Aural/Oral Performance of Children and Ease of Listening (PEACH +)	Ching and Hill (2007)	Children below 5 years	Questionnaire to assess the effectiveness of hearing devices in young children.
9	The Auditory Processing of Complex Environmental Information Scale (APCEI)	Noel Petroff et al. (2006)	Preschool up to 7 years	Acceptation, Perception, Comprehension, Oral expression, Speech intelligibility

Table 20.2 List of tests to assess speech perception in Indian context

S. No	Test	Authour/year
1.	Speech identification test for children in Kannada	Vandana (1998)
2.	Speech in noise test in Marathi	Anjusha and Sarda (2008)
3.	Speech in noise test in Indian English (SPIN-IE)	Yathiraj et al. (2010)
4.	Speech in noise test in Kannada	Vaidyanath and Yathiraj (2012)
5.	English monosyllabic word identification test for children	Rout (1996)
6.	Picture speech identification test for children in Hindi	Chaudhary and Yathiraj (2003)
7.	Lexical neighbourhood test for Indian-English children	Patro and Yathiraj (2010).

Assessment of Language Skills

Language skills are usually described in two domains: receptive (understanding) and expressive (expression; speaking) skills. Children with severe to profound sensorineural hearing loss (SNHL) face innumerable challenges in developing spoken language. This is due to their inability to detect acoustic-phonetic cues which are very essential for speech perception (Bradham & Jones, 2008; Niparko, 2010). Learning language through listening is reported to serve as an effective marker for scholastic performance in future for children with normal hearing (Geers et al., 2008). There is a strong association delineated between cochlear implantation and improvement in receptive and expressive language skills (Niparko, 2010).

There is also a strong correlation between the development of age-appropriate linguistic competence to the development of literacy (Geers et al., 2003). Hence assessing language skills is of paramount importance in children with CI. Research indicates that the language abilities of children with CI improve significantly especially if they are implanted early age (Quittner et al., 2016; Ruben, 2018).

Materials/Tools for Assessing Language Skills

(a) **Receptive-Expressive; Semantics; Syntax**

1. Scales for Early Communication Skills (SECS) (Moog & Geers, 1975): It assesses the language skills of children with hearing impairment (HI). It assesses both receptive and expressive language skills. It includes a section on verbal and nonverbal communication in receptive and expressive language skills. Age range: 2–8.11 years.
2. Integrated Scales of Development (ISD) (Cochlear Ltd., 2010): it outlines typical stages of development in the areas of listening, receptive and expressive language, speech, cognition and social communication. It is a developmental scale and should be used as a guide only. Age range: 0–48 months.

3. Cottage Acquisition Scales for Listening and Spoken Language (CASSLS) (by Elisabeth Wilkes Sunshine Cottage School for Deaf Children, San Antonio, USA, 1999): It is a criterion-referenced based assessment tool to monitor language acquisition skills of children with hearing loss. There are five parts of CASSLS which are receptive and expressive language, social skills, listening, play, cognition and speech; Age range: Birth to 8 years
4. ABFW Child Language Test-Part B–Vocabulary (Andrade et al., 2004): It assesses expressive vocabulary qualitatively and quantitatively. It evaluates vocabulary in nine areas that are clothing, animals, foods, means of transportation, furniture and utensils, professions, places, shapes and colours, toys and musical instruments. Age range: 0–5 years.
5. MacArthur Communicative Development Inventories (MCDI): Fenson et al. (1993): It is used to assess language and communication skills. It evaluates the parent's knowledge of their child's emerging language skills. It includes measures for three age ranges- word and gestures form (8–18 months), words and sentence forms (16–30 months) and communication developmental inventory III (30–37 months). Age range: 8–37 months.
6. Meaningful Use of Speech Scale (MUSS): This questionnaire was created by Robbins and Osberger in 1990. It assesses the use of oral language in children presenting with hearing impairment. The parent report questionnaire assesses the child's use of everyday situations. Age range: It can be used with children of all ages.
7. Preschool Language Scale (PLS-5) (Zimmerman et al., 2011): It is a standardized language test which has two scales- auditory comprehension and expressive language. Age range: Birth to 7.11 years.
8. Assessment of language development (ALD): Lakkanna et al. (2008): It is a criterion-referenced tool to measure the development of receptive and language skills in children in India. It assesses various areas such as vocabulary, syntax, semantics and higher linguistic skills. The test material includes questionnaires and standardized pictures. Age range: Birth to 7.11 years.
9. Peabody picture vocabulary test (Dunn & Dunn, 1997); Age group: 2.6–90+ years; It assesses listening and understanding of single-word vocabulary.
10. Reynell Developmental Language Scales (RDLS—Reynell & Gruber, 1990); Age range 1–6 years; It measures receptive and expressive language.
11. Clinical Evaluation of Language Fundamentals (CELF-4); Semel et al. (2003); Age group: 5–21.11 years; It includes 47 items. It measures lan-

guage ability. Individuals aged 5–8 years complete items 1–28 and individuals aged 9–21 complete items 14–47.

12. The CELF-Preschool, Second Edition (Wiig et al., 2004): Age range: 3–6 years; It identifies and diagnoses language deficits.
13. North Western Syntax Screening Test (NWSST—Lee, 1970): 3–7.11 years; It measures receptive and expressive syntax.
14. Linguistic Profile test in regional languages such as Kannada (Suchitra & Karanth, 1990), Hindi (Monica, 1995), Malayalam (Asha, 1997), Telugu (Suhasini, 1997), Picturized version for young children (3–7 years) was developed in seven other Indian languages (including Kannada and Hindi, Tamil, Oriya, Gujarathi, Marathi and Bengali) by UNICEF funded joint project at RRTC, Madras and NIHH, Bombay; The Linguistic Profile Test assesses Phonology, Syntax and Semantic. Age range: 3–7 years or 6–15 years
15. Malayalam language test (Rukmini (1994): Age range: 3–7 years: this test assesses semantics and syntax; Kannada Language Test (Shyamala et al., 2003); Age range: 5–8 years): This test assesses receptive and expressive skills in semantics and syntax.
16. Test for Acquisition of Syntax in Kannada (TASK) (Basavaraj, 1981). it assesses syntax. Age range: 1–5 years.
17. Screening test for the acquisition of syntax in Kannada (Basavaraj, 1981): It assesses syntax. Age range: 1–5 years.
18. A syntax screening test in Tamil (SSTT) (Sudha, 1981): It assesses Syntax; Age range: 2–5 years.

Tables 20.3 and 20.4 lists the above tools to assess Language Skills in Paediatric Cochlear Implantees.

(b) Pragmatics

Pragmatics is the study of the use of language in communicative interactions. Pragmatic behaviours are situation-based and environment-specific; therefore, it is helpful to assess pragmatic skills in a variety of situations (Shipley & McAfee, 2016). Language and pragmatics are very important domains for social communication. Pragmatics entails development of communicative functions, child's response to communication, and the way the child participates in interaction and conversation (Dewart & Summers, 1995).

Materials to Assess Pragmatic Skills: Table 20.5 lists the Pragmatic assessment tools.

Table 20.3 Tools to assess language skills in CI children

S.No	Test name	Author and year	Age range	Domain
1	Scales for early communication skills (SECS)	Moog and Geers (1975)	2–8.11 years	Receptive and expressive language skills; verbal and nonverbal communication
2	St. Gabriel's curriculum for the development of audition, language, speech and cognition.	Tuhoy et al. (2005)	0–6 years	Audition, speech, cognition, social interaction, fine and gross motor skills
3	Integrated scales of development (ISD)	Cochlear Ltd. (2010)	0–48 months	Listening, receptive and expressive language, speech, cognition and social communication
4	Cottage acquisition scales for listening and spoken language (CASSLS)	Wilkes (2001)	Birth to 8 years	Receptive and expressive language, social skills, listening, play, cognition and speech
5	ABFW child language test-part B	Andrade et al. (2004)	0–5 years	Expressive vocabulary qualitatively and quantitatively;
6	MacArthur communicative development inventories (MCDI)	Fenson et al. (1993)	8–37 months	Language and communication skills.
7	Meaningful use of speech scale (MUSS)	Robbins and Osberger (1990)	Children of all ages	Use of oral language
8	Preschool language scale (PLS-5)	Zimmerman et al. (2011)	Birth to 7.11 years	Auditory comprehension and expressive language
9	Assessment of language development (ALD)	Lakkanna et al. (2008)	Birth to 7.11 years	Vocabulary, syntax, semantics and higher linguistic skills
10	Peabody picture vocabulary test	Dunn and Dunn (1997)	2.6 to 90+ years	Listening and understanding of single word vocabulary
11	Reynell developmental language scales (RDLS)	Reynell and Gruber (1990)	1–6 years	Receptive and expressive language
12	Clinical evaluation of language fundamentals (CELF-4)	Semel et al. (2003)	5–21.118 years	Language ability
13	The clinical evaluation of language fundamentals (CELF)-preschool, second edition	Wiig et al. (2004)	3–6 years	Identifies and diagnoses language deficit
14	North Western syntax screening test (NWSST)	Lee (1970)	3–7.11 years	Receptive and expressive syntax

Table 20.4 Indian tests to assess language skills in CI children

S.No	Test name	Author and year	Age range	Domains
1	Malayalam language test	Rukmini (1994)	3–7 years	Semantics and syntax
2	Kannada language test	Shyamala et al. (2003)	5–8 years	Receptive and expressive skills in semantics and syntax
3	Linguistic profile test in Kannada	Suchitra and Karanth (1990)	6–15 years	Phonology, syntax and semantics
4	Linguistic profile test in Hindi	Monica (1995)		
5	Linguistic profile test in Malayalam	Asha (1997)		
6	Linguistic profile test in Telugu	Suhasini (1997)		
7	Linguistic profile test- picturised version for young children -in seven other Indian language (including Kannada and Hindi, Tamil, Oriya, Gujarati, Marathi and Bengali)	UNICEF funded joint project at RRTC, Madras and NIHH, Bombay.	3–7 years	
8	Screening test for the acquisition of syntax in Kannada	Basavaraj (1981)	1–5 years	Syntax
9	A syntax screening test in Tamil (SSTT)	Sudha (1981)	2–5 years	Syntax

Table 20.5 Tools for pragmatic assessment

S. No	Test	Author/year	Age-range	Domains
1.	Test of pragmatic skills	Shulman (1985)	3–8 years	Assess pragmatic language skills on six dimensions of pragmatic language: Physical setting Audience Topic Purpose Visual-gestural cues Abstraction
2.	Pragmatic language skills inventory (PLSI)	Gilliam and Miller (2006)	5 to 12.11 years	Assess children's pragmatic language abilities on these three subscales: Personal interaction skills, Social interaction skills Classroom interaction skills
3.	Pragmatic protocol age	Prutting and Kirchner (1987)	Greater than 5 years	Assess the pragmatic aspects of language including: Verbal aspect Paralinguistic aspect Non-verbal aspects

(continued)

Table 20.5 (continued)

S. No	Test	Author/year	Age-range	Domains
4.	Children communication checklist 2	Bishop (2006)	4:0–16:11 years	Questionnaire screens for communication problems in children two domains: 1. Language: Speech, Syntax, Semantics, Coherence 2. Pragmatics: Initiation, Scripted language, Context, Nonverbal communication, Social relations Interests
5.	Test of pragmatic language –2	Phelps-Terasaki and Phelps-Gunn (2007)	6–18 years.	Assess the six core subcomponents of pragmatic language: Physical setting Audience, Topic Purpose (speech acts) Visual-gestural cues Abstraction
6.	Developmental protocol for pragmatics in Indian context kannada speaking children	Dheepa and Shyamala (2005)	1–8 years	Pragmatics in Kannada speaking children

Assessment of Speech

Speech production requires highly complex and coarticulatory movements of the articulators involved. During assessment, both the articulation and phonological process assessment needs to be done. The primary purposes of an assessment of articulation and phonological processes should include describing the articulatory or phonological development and status of the child, evaluating the presence of deviations in the development to warrant concern or intervention, analyzing if the errors are due to articulation or phonological process.

Analysis should include number of errors and its types (substitutions, omissions, distortions, & additions), form of errors (distinctive features, & phonological processes), consistency of errors, stimulability, Intelligibility, rate of Speech, prosody and orofacial examination (Shipley & McAfee, 2016).

Materials/Tools for Assessing Speech Skills

1. Speech Intelligibility Rating scale: developed at Ali Yavar Jung National Institute of Speech and Hearing Disabilities (AYJNISHD), Mumbai (2003).
2. Brown's stages of Mean length of utterance (MLU) assessment: A strong communication marker to understand language development in children.

   Table 20.6 summarizes the Indian tools and other Western tools that is commonly used to assess articulation in CI children.

All the above-mentioned tools for speech and language assessment should be carefully chosen based on domain-specific and age-specific measures. Although clinicians' focus is on outcome measures based on standardized tools, informal assessment also plays a major role in assessing their language behaviours. Speech and language sampling is one of the effective means of informal assessment for SLPs. The stepwise sampling procedure is explained in the next section.

Table 20.6 Tests to assess articulation in Indian languages

S. No	Test	Authour/year	Age-range
1	Hindi picture word articulation test	Kacker et al. (1989)	3–7 years
2	Gujarati articulation test, Kannada articulation test	Rathna and Bettageri (1972)	5–9 years
3	Malayalam articulation test	Maya (1990)	3–7 years
4	Marathi articulation test, Bengali articulation test	Banik (1988)	4–7 years
5	Deep test of articulation in Bengali—picture form	Barman and Savithri (1991)	4–7 years
6	Articulation test in Tamil	Maya (1990)	3–6 years
7	Articulation test in Telugu	Padmaja (1988)	2.6–4.6 years
8	Computerized assessment of phonological processes in Malayalam (CAPP-M)	Sreedevi et al. (2013)	2.0–3.6 years
9	Computer based assessment of phonological processes in Kannada (CAPP-K)	Sreedevi and Chandran (2014)	2–3.6 years
Other tools to assess articulation			
1	Goldman-Fristoe test of Articulation-2 (GFTA-2)	Goldman and Fristoe (2000)	2–21 years
2	Khan-Lewis phonological analysis, second edition (KLPA-2)	Khan and Lewis (2002)	2–21 years
3	Arizona articulation proficiency scale, third edition (AAPS-3)	Fudala (2000)	1.5–18 years

Speech and Language Sampling

Speech-language samples form a very focal part of the assessment of a child's communicative abilities. They can be the basis for determining whether a problem exists and, if so, identifying the child's specific deficiencies and needs. A speech-language sample should be long enough to obtain a truly representative sample of the child's speech and language. A minimum of 50–100 distinct utterances is needed for a language sample, 200 or more different utterances will provide a better sample. To obtain a reliable and valid speech-language sample one needs to build a rapport with the child and reduce the interruptions and distractions. The clinician will need to preselect materials and topics that will be interesting to the child and follow her lead in elaborating or changing topics. Samples in multiple environments (e.g., clinic, playground, home) is desirable. The contexts should be altered (e.g., conversation, narratives, responses to pictures) but rote numbers, alphabets or nursery rhymes etc. should be avoided. Instead of 'yes/no' questions, it is preferable to use questions that require lengthier responses. Careful consideration of a child's age, cultural background, language development for appropriate topics is required (Shipley & McAfee, 2016). Brown's stages of Mean length of utterance (MLU) assessment can be used as a strong communication marker to understand language development in children.

Assessment of Voice

Voice quality in children with severe to profound hearing loss is affected due to absence of auditory feedback. Hyper nasal resonance, deficits in fundamental frequency, intensity and duration of voice are the common voice deficits seen in children with severe to profound hearing loss. Use of cochlear implants leads to improvement in their voice quality. A study by Upadhyay et al. (2019), revealed voice quality of children with CI is poor and deviant from their control group (normal hearing children). Another study by Srividya et al. (2016) revealed that early intervention and training played a significant role in the quality of voice in children with CI. However, the range of variability was higher in children with CI than normal hearing children. Hence, it is very important to assess voice quality in children with CI due to variability in voice quality. The various parameters that need to be assessed are pitch, intensity (loudness), vocal quality, resonance, respiratory support and posture.

Materials/Tools for Assessing Voice

There are two modalities for assessing voice, viz., perceptual (subjective) and acoustical (Objective analysis):

Acoustic analysis can be performed with tools, such as VAGHMI, CSL(MDVP) and Dr. Speech. Perceptual analysis can be carried out with various rating scales, such as Consensus Auditory -Perceptual Evaluation of Voice (CAPE—V) (ASHA, 2002).

Assessment of Cognition

Cognition though not directly a component of language, is definitely inherently related to language. A child's cognitive abilities affect language development in all aspects. Mental processes for learning, remembering, and using knowledge are essential for normal language acquisition and use. During a language assessment, it is helpful to take note of the child's cognitive abilities, including his or her attention and focus, reasoning ability, perception, memory, organization of self and thoughts, and overall executive function (Shipley & McAfee, 2016).

Materials/Tools for Assessing Cognition

1. Test of Nonverbal Intelligence Fourth Edition (TONI-4) is a language-free test, ideal for evaluating those with questionable or limited language ability (Brown et al., 2010); Age range: 6 years to 89.11
2. St. Gabriel's Curriculum for the Development of Audition, Language, Speech and Cognition (Tuhoy et al., 2005): It assesses audition, speech, cognition, social interaction, fine and gross motor skills. It is a criterion-referenced test which uses direct observation, behaviour elicitation and parental report to elicit information. It is used for the age range of 0–6 years.

Table 20.7 summarizes the above tests used to assess Cognition.

Table 20.7 Tools to assess Cognition in CI children

S. No	Test name	Author and year	Age range	Domain
1	Test of nonverbal intelligence fourth edition (TONI-4)	Brown et al. (2010)	6 years to 89.11	Cognition
2	St. Gabriel's curriculum for the development of audition, language, speech and cognition.	Tuhoy et al. (2005)	0–6 years	Audition, speech, cognition, social interaction, fine and gross motor skills

Assessment of Music Perception

Research worldwide indicates that music is well appreciated by children with CI, which ranges to a degree that is qualitatively different from adults who are implanted with CI (Hsiao & Gfeller, 2012). Music should be an integral component of CI rehabilitation rather than a separate domain (Robbins, 2018).

Processing prosodic information involves similar skills to those required in Music perception (Sallat & Jentschke, 2015), and emerging evidence also supports a common cerebral network involved in both lexical/phonological and melodic processing (Schön et al., 2010). Music Perception may offer a useful universal non-verbal marker for language acquisition. An accurate, standardized assessment of Music perception skills would offer new opportunities to probe non-verbal auditory skills such as pitch, meter, and melodic contour; however, few tests, batteries, or scales have been developed for use in children under 10 years of age, a crucial neurodevelopmental period (Barros et al., 2017).

Materials Tools for Assessing Music Perception

1. Gordon's Primary Measures of Music Audiation (PMMA- Gordon, 1979): These are two aptitude tests designed to diagnose and measure music potential. Both tests have a similar design. The primary test is recommended for use with younger children (Kindergarten to Grade 3). The intermediate test is recommended for older children or younger children who find the primary test too easy. Age range: Kindergarten to Grade 3.
2. Music in Children With Cochlear Implants (MCCI) (Roy et al., 2014): The MCCI assesses rhythm, pitch, melody, harmony, and timbre perception. Age range: Younger than 9 years of age. Table 20.8 lists the tests used to assess Music Perception.

Table 20.8 Tests to assess Music Perception

Name of the test	Author/year	Age range
Gordon's primary measures of music Audiation (PMMA)	Gordon (1979)	Grade K to 3
Music in children with Cochlear implants (MCCI)	Roy et al. (2014)	<9 years

Assessment of Literacy Skills

Literacy is often described as an individual's ability to read and write. Research has indicated that literacy (reading and writing skills) is closely related to language ability of children with cochlear implant. Research has shown that children using CI have reached higher levels of reading and writing ability when compared to children using hearing aids (Spencer et al., 2003; Van Vermeulen et al., 2007). However, there is a lot of variability seen, some children with CI may do extremely well while some may lag (James et al., 2008; Spencer et al., 2003; Van Vermeulen et al., 2007). Phonics, phonemic awareness, vocabulary, fluency, reading comprehension and writing are the various domains which we need to consider while assessing the literacy skills in children with cochlear implant.

Materials Used for Assessing Literacy Skills

1. Early Reading Skills—(Rae & Potter, 1973): This test assesses visual perceptual skills and assessment of phonics and coding process. Age range: Grades 1–8
2. Reading readiness test in Kannada (Devaki, 1978): The test comprises three subtests. They are vocabulary, auditory discrimination and visual discrimination. Ears. The test of auditory discrimination was developed by Kumudavalli in 1973 and restandardised by Devaki in 1978. Age range: 3–6.6 years.
3. Test for examining expressive morphology (TEEM) (Shipley et al., 1983). The test assesses expressive morpheme development in children ages 3 through 7 years. It uses an assortment of morphemes and allomorphic variations in a sentence-complete format with pictures. The performance on individual items can be compared to the ages at which 75% and 90% of children achieve each item. The child's total score can be compared to the score ranges achieved by children tested in the sample. It's 54 items evaluate variations of six major morphemes in present progressives, plurals, possessives, past tenses, third-person singulars and derived adjectives. Age range: 3–7 years
4. Early identification of Language based Reading disabilities: A Checklist (Catts, 1997). Research and clinical practice display that many reading disabilities are language-based. As the language deficits associated with reading disabilities are often present during the preschool years, these language deficits can serve as early indicators/markers of risk for reading disabilities. Professionals can use this checklist for the early identification of reading disabilities. Age range: Kindergarten to Grade 1
5. Phonological Awareness Test in Marathi (PAM) (Waknis & Vanaja, 2024): This is a comprehensive test which consists of evaluation of phonological awareness at four levels i.e., sentence level, syllable level, rhyme level and phoneme level. The test can be used for assessment of phonological awareness of children from junior kindergarten to Grade II in Marathi medium schools. Age range: Junior Kindergarten to Grade 2

6. Checklist to Screen Children with Reading Difficulty (CSRD) for Classroom Teachers (Joshi & Vanaja, 2016). This checklist was administered on typically developing children and was found to be a useful tool for screening children with reading difficulties. Age range: 6–8 years
7. S.I.F.T.E.R. Screening Instrument for Targeting Educational Risk can be used for various age ranges.

   (a) Preschool S.I.F.T.E.R. (Screening Instrument for Targeting Educational Risk) in Preschool Children (Anderson & Matkin, 1996). It identifies those children who are at-risk for developmental or educational problems due to hearing problems and need further observation and investigation. This tool must be filled by teachers and assesses the domains of pre academics, attention, communication, class participation and social behaviour. Age range: 3 years – Kindergarten, 3–6 years.
   (b) Elementary S.I.F.T.E.R. (Elementary Grade Screening Instrument for Targeting Educational Risk (Anderson, 1989): it assesses academic, attention, communication, class participation and social behaviour in children with hearing loss Age range: Grade 1 to Grades 5 or 6
   (c) Secondary S.I.F.T.E.R (Screening Instrument for Targeting Educational Risk in Secondary Students) (Anderson, 2004) assesses academic, attention, communication, class participation and social behaviour in children with hearing loss in middle and high school. Age range: Middle and High school

8. Test of preschool early literacy (TOPEL) (Lonigan et al., 2007) Children starting kindergarten or first grade are required to have adequate knowledge of vocabulary, phonological awareness, and print knowledge. This test assesses the same and comprises three subtests i.e., print knowledge, definitional vocabulary and phonological awareness. This test identifies preschoolers who are at risk for literacy problems, hence paving the way for early intervention. Age range: 3–5.11 years
9. Comprehensive test of Phonological Processing (CTOPP- 2), (Wagner et al., 2013): This test assesses the phonological skills required for reading fluency. It provides scores for phonological awareness (including phoneme isolation), phonological memory, and rapid symbolic and non-symbolic naming. Age range: 4–24.11 years
10. The phonological Awareness Literacy screening assessment (Invernizzi et al., 2004) PALS consists of two instruments (PALS-K and PALS 1–3) that measures young children's knowledge of important literacy fundamentals of phonological awareness, alphabet awareness, letter sound knowledge, spelling, concept of word, word recognition in isolation, and oral passage reading. PALS helps to identify students who may be at risk for reading difficulties and require literacy intervention. PALS-K evaluates alphabet knowledge, phonological awareness, print concepts and writing. Age range: Kindergarten, Grades 1–3

11. Early Literacy Screening Tool (ELST) (Shanbal et al., 2011) is a screening tool to be used in school for children. Age range: 3–6 years)
12. Test for Pre- Academic Skills (T- PAS) (Singh & Malar, 2015). It assesses pre -reading, pre-writing and pre-number skills. Age range: Less than 6 years
13. An adaptation of early reading skills (ERS) in Hindi (ERS-H) (Priyadarshi et al., 2018): It has various subtests which include perceptual discrimination skills, phoneme/syllable, grapheme/letter correspondence, blending test, structural analysis test and reading passage. Age range: 6–13 years; Grades I–VIII.

Table 20.9 summarizes the tests used to assess Literacy Skills in CI Children.

Table 20.9 Tests to assess Literacy Skills

S. No	Name of the test	Author/year	Age range
1	Early Reading skills	Rae and Potter (1973)	Grades 1–8
2	Reading readiness test in Kannada	Devaki (1978)	3–6.6 years
3	Test for examining expressive morphology (TEEM)	Shipley et al. (1983)	3–7 years
4	Early identification of language based Reading disabilities: A checklist	Catts (1997)	Preschool
5	Phonological awareness test in Marathi (PAM)	Waknis and Vanaja (2018)	Junior K to Grade 2
6	Checklist to screen children with Reading difficulty (CSRD) for classroom teachers	Joshi and Vanaja (2016)	6–8 years
7	Screening instrument for targeting educational risk (S.I.F.T.E.R)		
7.a	Preschool S.I.F.T.E.R	Anderson and Matkin (1996)	(Age 3 years to Kindergarten), (3–6 years)
7.b	Elementary S.I.F.T.E.R	Anderson (1989)	Grades 1–5/6
7.c	Secondary S.I.F.T.E. R	Anderson (2004)	Middle and high school
8	Test of preschool early literacy (TOPEL)	Lonigan et al. (2007)	3–5.11 years
9	Comprehensive test of phonological processing (CTOPP- 2)	Wagner et al. (2013)	4–24.11 years
10	The phonological awareness literacy screening assessment (PALS-K and PALS 1–3)	Invernizzi et al. (2004)	Kindergarten to Grade 3
11	Early literacy screening tool (ELST)	Shanbal et al. (2011)	3–6 years
12	Test for pre- academic skills (T- PAS)	Singh and Malar (2015)	<6 years
13	Adaptation of early reading skills (ERS) in Hindi (ERS-H)	Priyadarshi et al. (2018)	6–13 years; Grades I–VIII

Assessment of Play

Westby (1980) investigated the child's cognitive level through play. A range of preverbal and early language structures can be built by choosing appropriate toys for rehabilitation, enabling natural interaction to be as open-ended as possible (Dettman et al., 1996). They state that young children can be exposed to several auditory contrasts while they are within the context of play (For e.g., while bathing a doll, the syllabic pattern, rub rub rub; wash wash wash; brush brush brush, gets used more repeatedly facilitating auditory bombardment). Also, language used in a play context always includes syntactically correct phrases, although the target word gets repeated very often.

Materials/Tools for Assessing Play

1. Play Assessment Scale (PAS): (Fewell, 1986): PAS assesses the development of play in young children and the 45-item scale is developmentally sequenced and is organized into eight age ranges. Age range: 2–36 months
2. The Play Assessment Questionnaire (PAQ) (Calhoun, 1987): There are 45 items in a parent-questionnaire format to assess children's symbolic play. This is based on PAS. Age range: 2–36 months
3. The Play in Early Childhood Evaluation System (PIECES) (Kelly-Vance et al., 1999): It is an assessment tool that can be used to identify strengths and weaknesses in the area of play skills and helps identify an area in need of intervention, to screen classrooms for general areas of need or to help determine eligibility. It provides information on three main types of play: exploratory play, simple pretend play and complex pretend play. Age range: birth to 5 years

   Table 20.10 summarizes the tests briefed above for assessing play.

Table 20.10 Tests to assess play skills in CI children

S. No	Name of the test	Author/year	Age range
1	Play assessment scale (PAS)	Fewell (1986)	2–36 months
2	The play assessment questionnaire. (PAQ)	Calhoun (1987)	2–36 months
3	The play in early childhood evaluation system (PIECES)	Kelly-Vance et al. (1999)	Birth to 5 years

Assessment of Communicative Competence & Quality of Life (QOL)

Cochlear implants in children with severe to profound hearing loss leads to significant improvement in their speech and language skills. It further leads to their greater participation in various social contexts and integration in normal school. One must include the social aspect to measure or assess a child's global development. Hence, quality of life assessment should be a part of an assessment protocol when assessing children with cochlear implant.

In the health literature, quality of life refers to the individual's ability to enjoy normal life activities, including the concepts of functional capacity and well-being (Guyatt, 1993). Literature describes two main areas while assessing QOL in children with CI; (1) first one includes the cost utility of the implant device and procedure, evaluating whether the audiological or language benefits justify the financial costs involved (Cheng et al., 2000; O'Neill et al., 2004) it includes individual subjective attitudes toward relative improvements in various aspects of the pediatric patient's life because of the cochlear implant, most often from the parents' perspective (Nicholas & Geers, 2003; O'Neill et al., 2004).

Materials/Tools for Assessing QOL

Table 20.11 enlists the tools used to assess QOL.

Table 20.11 Tests for assessing quality of life

S. No	Test name	Author and year	Age range	Domains
1	Hearing environments and reflection on quality of life (HEAR-QL)	Umansky et al. (2011)	7–12 years	Quality of life
2	The parenting stress index – 4 (PSI)	Abidin (2012)	0–12 years	Identifies parent child problem areas
3	Pediatric quality of life inventory (PedsQL™)	Varni et al. (2001); Varni et al. (2006)	2–18 years	Health-related quality of life (HRQOL) in healthy children and adolescents and those with acute and chronic health conditions.

Challenges Faced in Outcome Audit

The performance of children with cochlear implants varies widely due to multiple factors such as the onset of hearing loss, age at implantation, aetiology, inner ear malformations, number of active electrodes, choice of implant, duration of hearing loss (Blamey et al., 1992), associated problems/Comorbid disorders, socioeconomic status and multilingual considerations.

Recent research shows that learning more than one language is possible even in children with cochlear implants (Waltzman et al., 2003; Robbins et al., 2004; Thomas et al., 2008). However, bilingualism/multilingualism in children with cochlear implants is possible due to various factors such as early and bilateral implantation, no associated problems, exposure to various languages, fluent model of all the languages at home, regular rehabilitation and adequate social interaction in different languages. So, during case history, clinicians can gather information about the language that a child is exposed to from the language exposure log. Another important thing is to find out the language proficiency in each language at two levels i.e. Basic Interpersonal Communication Skills (BICS) and Cognitive Academic Language Proficiency (CALP). Language Proficiency checklist (Bernhard & Laura, 1992) and Bilingual Family Interview (Robbins, 2004) can also be used. Further, based on the language exposure log, clinicians can decide the language that needs to be assessed and choose to use a combination of formal and informal assessment tools. Another important factor to look into is the comorbid conditions along with hearing loss in children. It is reported that approximately 30–40% of the children with hearing loss have additional difficulties (Berretteni et al., 2008; Centers for Disease Control, 2012). These additional difficulties can be developmental delay, autism, cerebral palsy, physical and motor delays, vision disorders, attention deficit hyperactivity disorder, speech and language delays etc.

Due to additional difficulties, they might not be able to complete the standard test battery protocol as prescribed. Professionals need to modify the testing protocol according to the needs of children with special needs, as they have limited vision or motor skills or cognitive skills to perform the test. There are various factors which professionals need to consider while assessing children with special needs. First, tasks can be modified according to the needs of the child. Using informal assessment such as observation, interviews and scales (as it is possible that a child may not have enough language or uses more gestures) along with formal tools. All the domains such as oro-motor ability, communication intent, behaviour, and attitudes should be assessed. Referral to other team members such as neurologist, psychologist, physiotherapist, occupational therapist as needed.

Recent studies have focused more on the qualitative aspects to assess the outcomes in children with special needs. These can be quality of life, activities of daily living, adaptive behaviours or behavioural improvements etc. There is definitely a need to develop more standardized assessment protocols and also offer multidisciplinary services to children with special needs (Rebecca, 2009).

Third, distance from the rehabilitation centre is also a matter of consideration for many children with CI in developing countries. However, this can be successful only if parents are equipped with the necessary technology such as smartphones or laptops at home, as most parents of CI children in tertiary care setup belong to the rural background. Hence assessing children in virtual mode poses a major challenge for clinicians. Finally, there is no uniformity in assessment protocol across clinics and institutes nationally, which is an obstacle for clinicians and academicians with respect to clinical practice and research. Hence, the need of the hour is to develop a standard assessment protocol for CI children to widen the scope for valid and multicentric research/clinical practice across the world.

Clinical audit of outcomes in children with CI is mandatory post-implantation. All professionals agree that no one size fits all. Clinicians find it challenging right from appropriate selection of assessment tools, testing the children at appropriate time intervals for outcome measures to choosing the right approach for rehabilitation viz. top-down/synthetic, bottom-up/analytic and hybrid approach owing to many factors such as age at implantation, duration of implant use, associated/ comorbid disorders, linguistic and cultural considerations, lack of domain and language specific tools in a multilingual scenario as in India. Hence, SLP's have to make a cautious decision while choosing the assessment tools for measuring outcomes post implantation as the tests or tools listed in this chapter include norm- and criterion- referenced tests as well, which can be preferably used with a minimum of 6–12 months post implantation and not as a baseline assessment. This warrants development of a common assessment protocol for auditing the outcome measures post implantation which can be materialized with multicentric research across clinical centres and institutes across India.

References

Abidin RR. (2012). Parenting Stress Index, Fourth Ed. (PSI-4). Psychological Assessment Resources.

Ali Yavar Jung National Institute of Speech and Hearing Disabilities (AYJNISHD). (2003). *Speech intelligibility rating scale*. AYJNISHD.

Anderson, K. (1989). *SIFTER: Screening instrument for targeting educational risks in children identified by hearing screening or who have minimal hearing loss*. Educational Audiology Education.

Anderson, K. L. (2004). *Secondary SIFTER*. Supporting Success for Children with Hearing Loss.

Anderson, K. L., & Matkin, N. H. (1996). *Screening instrument for targeting educational risk (S.I.F.T.E.R)*. Educational Audiology Association.

Andrade, C. R., Befi-Lopes, D. M., Fernandes, F. D., & Wertzner, H. F. (2004). *ABFW-Teste de linguagem infantil nas áreas de fonologia, vocabulário, fluência e pragmática* (pp. 51–82). Pró-Fono R Atual Cient.

Anjusha, M., & Sarda, S. (2008). *Development of speech in noise test in Marathi for children between 3–6 years*. Unpublished masters dissertation. Bharati Vidyapeeth University.

Archbold, S., Lutman, M. E., & Marshall, D. H. (1995). Categories of auditory performance. *The Annals of Otology, Rhinology & Laryngology, 166*, 312–314.

Asha, M. M. (1997). *Linguistic profile test (LPT in Malayalam) normative data for children in Grades I to X*. Unpublished master's dissertation. University of Mysore.

American Speech-Language-Hearing Association. (2002). Consensus Auditory-Perceptual Evaluation of Voice (CAPE-V). ASHA Special Interest Division 3, Voice and Voice Disorders. Retrieved from http://www.asha.org/uploadedFiles/ASHA/SIG/03/CAPE-V-Procedures.pdf

Bally, S. J., & Bakke, M. H. (2007). A peer mentor training program for aural rehabilitation. *Trends in Amplification, 11*(2), 125–131.

Banik, A. (1988). *Articulation test in Bengali*. Unpublished masters dissertation. University of Mysore.

Barman, A., & Savithri, S. R. (1991). *Deep test of articulation in Bengali*. Unpublished masters dissertation. University of Mysore.

Barros CG, Swardfager W, Moreno S, Bortz G, Ilari B, Jackowski AP, Ploubidis G, Little TD, Lamont A, & Cogo-Moreira H. (2017). Assessing Music Perception in Young Children: Evidence for and Psychometric Features of the M-Factor. Frontiers in neuroscience, 11, 18. https://doi.org/10.3389/fnins.2017.00018.

Basavaraj, A. R. (1981). *Development of a test in Kannada for assessing language acquisition in children*. Unpublished doctoral thesis. University of Mysore.

Bernhard, M., & Laura, R. (1992). Language development in children with cochlear implants. *Journal of Speech and Hearing Research, 35*(3), 650–658.

Berretteni, S., Forli, F., Passetti, S., Rocchi, A., Pollina, L., Cecchetti, D., Mancuso, M., & Siciliano, G. (2008). Mitochondrial non-syndromic sensorineural hearing loss: A clinical, audiological and pathological study from Italy, and revision of the literature. *Bioscience Reports, 28*(1), 49–59.

Bhimte, S. L., & Rangasayee, R. (2018). Development of Hindi early speech perception test. *Global Journal of Otolaryngology, 17*(1).

Bishop, D. (2006). *Children communication checklist-2*. U.S. Edition. The Psychological Corporation.

Blamey, P., Dawson, P., Dettman, S., Rowland, L., Brown, A., Busby, P., Dowell, R., Rickards, F., & Clark, G. (1992). Speech perception, production and language results in a group of children using the 22-electrode cochlear implant. *Australian Journal of Otolaryngology, 1*(2).

Bradham, T., & Jones, J. (2008). Cochlear implant candidacy in the United States: Prevalence in children 12 months to 6 years of age. *International Journal of Paediatric Otorhinolaryngology, 72*(7), 1023–1028.

Brown, L., Sherbenou, R. J., & Johnsen, S. K. (2010). *Test of nonverbal intelligence* (4th ed. (TONI-4)). PRO-ED, Inc.

Calhoun, D. (1987). *A comparison of two methods of evaluating play in toddlers*. Unpublished master's thesis. Colorado State University.

Catts, H. W. (1997). The early identification of language-based reading disabilities. *Language, Speech, and Hearing Services in Schools, 28*, 86–89.

Centers for Disease Control and Prevention. (2012). *Hearing loss in children*. Retrieved from https://www.cdc.gov/hearing-loss-children/about/index.html

Chaudhary, B., & Yathiraj, A. (2003). *Picture speech identification test for Hindi speaking children*. Unpublished master's dissertation. University of Mysore.

Cheng, A. K., Rubin, H. R., Powe, N. R., Mellon, N. K., Francis, H. W., & Niparko, J. K. (2000). Cost-utility analysis of the cochlear implant in children. *Journal of the American Medical Association, 284*(7), 850–856. https://doi.org/10.1001/jama.284.7.850

Ching, T. Y., & Hill, M. (2005). The parents' evaluation of aural/oral performance of children (PEACH) scale: Normative data. *Journal of American Academy of Audiology, 18*, 220–235.

Ching, T. Y., & Hill, M. (2007). The parents' evaluation of aural/oral performance of children (PEACH) scale: Normative data. *Journal of the American Academy of Audiology, 18*(3), 220–235. https://doi.org/10.3766/jaaa.18.3.4

Cochlear Ltd. (2010). *Integrated scales of development (ISD): From listen, learn and talk*; pp. 16–31.

Dettman, S., Barker, Rance, G., Dowell, R., Galvin, K., Sarant, J., Cowan, R., Skok, Hollow, Larratt, & Clark. (1996). Components of a rehabilitation programme for young children using the multichannel cochlear implant. In *Cochlear implant rehabilitation in children and adults*.
Devaki, D. (1978). *A reading readiness test in Kannada: Its development and standardisation*. Unpublished master's dissertation. University of Mysore.
Dewart, H., & Summers, S. (1995). *The pragmatics profile of everyday communication skills in children*. Nfer-Nelson.
Dheepa, D., & Shyamala, K. C. (2005). A developmental protocol for pragmatics. *Journal of All India Institute of Speech and Hearing, 3*, 18–30.
Dunn, L. M., & Dunn, L. M. (1997). *Peabody picture vocabulary test*. third edition manual. American Guidance Service.
Fenson, L., Dale, P., Reznick, J. S., Thal, D., Bates, E., Hartung, J., Pethick, S., & Reilly, J. S. (1993). *The MacArthur communicative development inventories: User's guide and technical manual*. Singular Publishing Group.
Fewell, R. R. (1986). *Play assessment scale* (5th revision). University of Washington. CLAS: Play Assessment Scale. Retrieved September 15, 2024, from https://clas.illinois.edu/special/evaltools/cl00918.html
Field, A. (2005). *Discovering statistics using SPSS* (Vol. 1). Sage Publications.
Fudala, J. B. (2000). *Arizona articulation proficiency scale (AAPS-3)* (3rd revision). Western Psychological Services.
Fujiki, M., & Willbrand, M. L. (1982). A comparison of four informal methods of language evaluation. *Language Speech and Hearing Services in Schools, 13*(1), 42–52.
Geers, A., Tobey, E., Moog, J., & Brenner, C. (2008). Long-term outcomes of cochlear implantation in the preschool years: From elementary grades to high school. *International Journal of Audiology, 47*(Suppl 2), S21–S30.
Geers, A. E., Nicholas, J. G., & Sedey, A. L. (2003). Language skills of children with early cochlear implantation. *Ear and Hearing, 24*(1 Suppl), 46S–58S.
Geffner, D., & Goldman, R. (2010). *Auditory skills assessment*. Pearson Publishing.
Gilliam, J. E., & Miller, L. (2006). *PLSI: Pragmatic language skills inventory*. Pro-Ed.
Goldman, R., & Fristoe, M. (2000). Goldman-Fristoe test of articulation., second edition [Dataset]. In *PsycTESTS Dataset*.
Gordon, E. (1979). *GIA Publications—Primary Measures of Music Audiation—Complete Kit*. Retrieved September 12, 2024, from https://giamusic.com/resource/primary-measures-of-music-audiation-kgrade-3-complete-kit-pmma-instrumentaccessory-g2242k
Guyatt, G. H. (1993). Measuring health-related quality of life. *Annals of Internal Medicine, 118*(8), 622–629.
Hedge, M. N., & Pomaville, F. (2008). *Assessment of communication disorders in children*. Plural Publishing.
Hsiao, F., & Gfeller, K. (2012). Music perception of cochlear implant recipients with implications for music instruction: A review of the literature. *Update: Applications of Research in Music Education, 30*(2), 5–10.
Invernizzi, M., Meier, J., & Swank, L. (2004). Phonological awareness literacy screening for preschoolers [Dataset]. In *PsycTESTS dataset*.
James, D., Rajput, K., Brinton, J., & Goswami, U. (2008). Phonological awareness, vocabulary, and word reading in children who use cochlear implants: Does age of implantation explain individual variability in performance outcomes and growth? *Journal of Deaf Studies and Deaf Education, 13*(1), 117–137.
Jijo, P. M., & Yathiraj, A. (2010). *Early speech perception test development for Malayalam hearing impaired children* (pp. 105–119). A dissertation based articled published at AIISH.
Joshi, N., & Vanaja, C. S. (2016). Checklist to screen children with reading difficulty for classroom teachers. *Language in India, 16*(1), 185 199.
Kacker, S. K., Basavaraj, V., Thapar, A., Menon, N., & Vasudeva, R. (1989). *Hindi picture word articulation test development and standardization*. Staff'SAFA'project, AIIMS.

Keith, R. W. (2009). *SCAN-3 for children: Test for auditory processing disorders*. Pearson.

Kelly-Vance L, Ryalls B, & Cherney C. (1999). The Play in Early Childhood Evaluation System (PIECES) [Unpublished manuscript]. University of Nebraska-Lincoln.

Khan, L., & Lewis, N. (2002). *Khan-Lewis phonological analysis manual*. American Guidance Service.

Kumudavalli. (1973). Cited in Vatsala, S. N. (2018). *Improving Kannada reading performance of educable mentally retarded children ERIC (NCERT) project report*.

Kuruvilla, M., & Sarda, S. (2012). *Development of early speech perception test for Marathi-speaking children with hearing impairment*. Bharti Vidyapeeth University.

Lakkanna, S., Venkatesh, K., & Bhat, J. S. (2008). *Assessment of language development*. Omni Therapy Services.

Lee L. (1970). A screening test for syntax development. Journal of Speech and Hearing Disorders, 35, 103–112.

Lonigan, Wagner, Torgesen, & Rashotte. (2007). *TOPEL: Test of preschool early literacy* KIT Christopher J. Lonigan, Richard K. Wagner, Joseph K. Torgesen, Carol A. Rashotte: PRO-ED Inc. Official WebSite. Retrieved from https://www.proedinc.com/Products/12440/topel-test-of-preschool-early-literacy.aspx

Maya. (1990). *An articulation test battery in Malayalam*. Unpublished masters dissertation. University of Mysore.

Monica, S. (1995). *Linguistic profile test (LPT in Hindi)-normative data for children in Grades I to V*. Unpublished master's dissertation. University of Mysore.

Moog, J. S., & Geers, A. E. (1975). *Scales of early communication skills for hearing-impaired children*. Central Institute for the Deaf.

Moog, J. S., & Geers, A. E. (1990). *Early speech perception test for profoundly hearing impaired children*. Central Institute for the Deaf.

Nicholas, J. G., & Geers, A. E. (2003). Personal, social, and family adjustment in school-aged children with a cochlear implant. *Ear and Hearing, 24*(1 Suppl), 69S–81S.

Niparko, J. K. (2010). *Cochlear implants: Principles and practices* (2nd ed.). Lippincott Williams & Wilkins.

Noel Petroff, D. N., Dumont, A., & Busquet, D. D. (2006). The A.P.C.E.I: A method of displaying the audio-phonological performances of deaf children with hearing aids or implants. *Deaf knowledge, 17*, 19–27.

O'Neill, C., Lutman, M. E., Archbold, S. M., Gregory, S., & Nikolopoulos, T. P. (2004). Parents and their cochlear implanted child: Questionnaire development to assess parental views and experiences. *International Journal of Paediatric Otorhinolaryngology, 68*(2), 149–160.

Padmaja, S. (1988). *Test of articulation and discrimination in Telugu (TADT)*. Unpublished master's dissertation. University of Mysore.

Patro, C., & Yathiraj, A. (2010). *Lexical neighbourhood test: An Indian English version for children*. Unpublished master's dissertation. University of Mysore.

Phelps-Terasaki, D., & Phelps-Gunn, T. (2007). *Test of pragmatic language* (2nd ed.). Linguisystems.

Popham, W. J., & Husek, T. R. (1969). Implications of criterion-referenced measurement. *Journal of Educational Measurement, 6*(1), 1–9.

Priyadarshi, B., Goswami, S. P., Sen, M., & Krishnan, G. (2018). *An adaptation of early reading skills in Hindi (ERS-H)*. Unpublished AIISH Research funded project. All India Institute of Speech and Hearing.

Prutting, C. A., & Kirchner, D. M. (1987). A clinical appraisal of the pragmatic aspects of language. *The Journal of Speech and Hearing Disorders, 52*(2), 105–119.

Quittner, A. L., Cejas, I., Barnard, J., & Niparko, J. K. (2016). Benefits of cochlear implantation on the whole child: Longitudinal changes in cognition, behaviour, parenting, and health-related quality of life. In N. Young & K. Iler Kirk (Eds.), *Pediatric cochlear implantation*. Springer.

Rae, G., & Potter, T. (1973). *Informal reading diagnosis: A practical guide for the classroom teacher*. Prentice-Hall.

Rathna, N., & Bettageri, R. (1972). Tests of articulation in Kannada. *Journal of All India Institute of Speech and Hearing, 3*(1), 7–19.

Rebecca, S. (2009). The impact of early cochlear implantation on language development. *Journal of Paediatric Audiology, 13*(1), 45–53.

Reynell, J. K., & Gruber, C. P. (1990). *Reynell developmental language scales.*: U.S. Edition; Manual. Western Psychological Services.

Robbins, A. M., Koch, D. B., & Osberger, M. J. (2004). Speech perception and language development in children with cochlear implants. *Journal of Speech, Language, and Hearing Research, 47*(2), 279–290.

Robbins, A. M., & Osberger, M. J. (1990). *Meaningful use of speech scale (MUSS).* Indiana University School of Medicine.

Robbins, A. M., Renshaw, J. J., & Berry, S. W. (1991). Evaluating meaningful auditory integration in profoundly hearing-impaired children. *The American Journal of Otology, 12*(Suppl), 144–150.

Robbins, M. A. (2018). Twelve guiding premises of paediatric cochlear implant habilitation. *World Journal of Otorhinolaryngology and Head Neck Surgery, 3*(4), 235–239.

Roy, A. T., Scattergood-Keeper, L., Carver, C., Jiradejvong, P., Butler, C., & Limb, C. J. (2014). Evaluation of a test battery to assess perception of music in children with cochlear implants. *JAMA Otolaryngology – Head and Neck Surgery, 140*(6), 540–547.

Rout A. (1996). Monosyllabic speech identification Test in English for Indian children. Unpublished Dissertation submitted to the University of Mysore, Mysore, India

Ruben, R. J. (2018). Language development in the paediatric cochlear implant patient. *Laryngoscope Investigative Otolaryngology, 19*, 209–213. https://doi.org/10.1002/lio2.156

Rukmini, A. P. (1994). *Malayalam language test.* Unpublished doctoral thesis. University of Mysore.

Sallat, S., & Jentschke, S. (2015). Music perception influences language acquisition: Melodic and rhythmic-melodic perception in children with Specific Language Impairment. *Behavioural Neurology, 2015*(1), 606470.

Semel, E., Wiig, E. H., & Secord, W. A. (2003). *Clinical evaluation of language fundamentals.* fourth edition (CELF-4). The Psychological Corporation/A Harcourt Assessment Company.

Schön D, Gordon R, Campagne A, Magne C, Astésano C, Anton JL, et al. (2010). Similar cerebral networks in language, music and song perception. Neuroimage, 51, 450–461. https://doi.org/10.1016/j.neuroimage.2010.02.023.

Shanbal, J., Goswami, Prathima, & Chaithra. (2011). Cited in P Divya, N Kannan, S. P. & M. V. P. (2020). Effectiveness of phonological awareness skills test in Indian population. *The International Journal of Indian Psychology, 8*(3), 78–81.

Shipley, K. G., & McAfee, J. G. (2016). *Assessment in speech-language pathology: A resource manual* (5th ed.). Delmar Cengage Learning.

Shipley, K. G., Stone, T. A., & Sue, M. B. (1983). *TEEM: Test for examining expressive morphology.* KIT Kenneth G. Shipley, Terry A. Stone, Marlene B. Sue: PRO-ED Inc. Official WebSite. (n.d.). Retrieved September 13, 2024, from https://www.proedinc.com/Products/9925/teem-test-for-examining-expressive-morphology.aspx

Shulman, B. B. (1985). *Test of pragmatic skills.* Communication Skill Builders.

Shyamala, K. C., Vijayashree, & Jayaram, M. (2003). *Kannada language test. A project under AIISH research fund (ARF).* AIISH.

Singh, T., & Malar, G. (2015). *Study on influence of co-curricular training in visual arts on development of pre-academic skills in preschool children with hearing impairment.* Unpublished master's dissertation. University of Mysore.

Spencer, L. J., Barker, B. A., & Tomblin, J. B. (2003). Exploring the language and literacy outcomes of paediatric cochlear implant users. *Ear and Hearing, 24*(3), 236–247.

Sreedevi, N., & Chandran, S. (2014). *Computer based assessment of phonological processes in Kannada (CAPP-K).* Project under AIISH Research Fund (ARF), AIISH.

Sreedevi, N., John, M., & Chandran, S. (2013). Computerized assessment of phonological processes in Malayalam (CAPP-M). In *2013 IEEE Global Humanitarian Technology Conference: South Asia Satellite (GHTC-SAS)* (pp. 264–269). IEEE.

Srividya, A., Premalatha, B. S., & Gore, M. (2016). Comparison of acoustic analysis of voice parameters in children with cochlear implants and normal hearing. *Journal of Laryngology and Voice, 6*(2), 31–35.

Stredler-Brown, A., & Johnson, D. C. (2001, 2003). *Functional auditory performance indicators: An integrated approach to auditory development.* Retrieved from http://www.cde.state.co.us/cdesped/SpecificDisability-Hearing.htm

Suchithra, M. G., & Karanth, P. (1990). Linguistic profile test (LPT)-normative data for children in grades I–V. *Journal of the All India Institute of Speech and Hearing, 21*, 14–27.

Suchitra, T., & Karanth, P. (1990). Assessment of speech and language development in children with hearing impairments. *Indian Journal of Speech and Hearing, 5*(1), 15–23.

Sudha, K. M. (1981). *Syntax screening test in Tamil.* Unpublished master's dissertation. University of Mysore.

Suhasini, G. (1997). *Linguistic profile test (Telugu)-normative data for children in grades I to X.* Unpublished master's dissertation. University of Mysore.

Tamilmani, C. R. M., & Gore, M. (2002). *Speech perception test for Tamil speaking children with hearing impairment*, Unpublished master's dissertation. Dr. S. R Chandrasekhar Institute of Speech and Hearing.

Thomas, E., El-Kashlan, H., & Zwolan, T. A. (2008). Children with cochlear implants who live in monolingual and bilingual homes. *Otology & Neurotology, 29*(2), 230–234.

Tuhoy, J., Brown, J., & Mercer-Moseley, C. (2005). *St. Gabriel's curriculum for the development of audition, language, speech, cognition, early communication, social interaction, fine motor skills, and gross motor skills.*

Tye-Murray, N. (2020). *Foundations of aural rehabilitation: Children, adults, and their family members* (5th ed.). Plural Publishing.

Umansky, A. M., Jeffe, D. B., & Lieu, J. E. (2011). The HEAR-QL: Quality of life questionnaire for children with hearing loss. *Journal of American Academy Audiology, 22*(10), 644–653.

Upadhyay, V., Kumar, A., & Singh, P. (2019). Speech perception and language development in children with cochlear implants. *Journal of Paediatric Audiology, 15*(2), 112–120.

Van Kleeck, A. (1986). Language intervention with young children. Marc E. Fey. San Diego: College-Hill, 1986. Pp. xi + 358. *Applied PsychoLinguistics, 7*(4), 396–399.

Van Vermeulen, A. M., Bon, W., Schreuder, R., Knoors, H., & Snik, A. (2007). Reading comprehension of deaf children with cochlear implants. *The Journal of Deaf Studies and Deaf Education, 12*, 283–302.

Vandana S. (1998). The speech identification test for Kannada-speaking children [Unpublished independent project], University of Mysore, Mysore, India. http://192.168.100.20:8080/digitallibrary/AuthorT.do?jAuthor=Vandana,%20S

Varni, J. W., Seid, M., & Kurtin, P. S. (2001). The PedsQL™: Measurement model for the paediatric quality of life inventory. *Medical Care, 39*(8), 629–639.

Varni, J. W., Seid, M., & Kurtin, P. S. (2006). Pediatric quality of life inventory (PedsQL) version 4.0: Reliability and validity of the parent and child versions. *Health Quality of Life Outcomes, 4*(1), 1–9.

Wagner, T., Rashotte, & Pearson. (2013). *CTOPP-2: Comprehensive test of phonological processing*. Second Edition KIT.

Waknis A, & Vanaja CS. (2024). Copyright- Phonological Awareness in Marathi. https://doi.org/10.13140/RG.2.2.35884.68482

Waltzman, S. B., Robbins, A. M., Green, J. E., & Cohen, N. L. (2003). Second oral language capabilities in children with cochlear implants. *Otology & Neurotology, 24*(5), 757–763.

Westby, C. (1980). Language abilities through play. *Language, Speech, and Hearing Services in Schools, 11*(3), 154–161.

Wiig, E. H., Secord, W. A., & Semel, E. (2004). *Clinical evaluation of language fundamentals—Preschool.* second edition (CELF Preschool-2). The Psychological Corporation/A Harcourt Assessment Company.
Wilkes, E. M. (2001). Cottage acquisition scales for listening, language & speech [User's manual]. Sunshine Cottage School for Deaf Children.
World Health Organization. (2001). *International classification of functioning, disability and health.* Retrieved on November 20, 2022, from http://apps.who.int/iris/bitstream/10665/42407/7/9241545429_tha%2Beng.pdf
Yathiraj A, Vanaja CS, & Muthuselvi T. (2010). Speech in Noise Test in Indian English. Test material developed at the Department of Audiology, All India Institute of Speech and Hearing, Mysore, India. Available from: http://www.203.129.241.86:8080/digitallibrary/AuthorTitle.do?jAuthor=Asha%20Yathiraj%20and%20Vanaja,%20C.%20S. [Last accessed on 2017 May]
Zimmerman, I. L., Steiner, V. G., & Pond, R. E. (2011). *Preschool language scales* (5th ed.). The Psychological Corporation.
Zimmerman-Phillips, S., Osberger, M. J., & Robbins, A. M. (2001). *Infant-toddler meaningful auditory integration scale.* Advanced Bionics Corporation.

Further Reading

McConkey, R. A., Green, J. E., Waltzman, S. B. (2004). Bilingual oral language proficiency in children with cochlear implants. *Archives of Otolaryngology: Head and Neck Surgery, 130,* 644–647. https://doi.org/10.1001/archotol.130.5.644.

Chapter 21
Vestibular Function in Adult and Paediatric Cochlear Implant Recipients

Niraj Kumar Singh, Meghna Deepak, Akshay Kamath, Kumari Apeksha, Sachchidanand Sinha, Nirnay Kumar Keshree, and Prawin Kumar

Abstract Cochlear implantation, probably the best invention of the last century, has proved to be a boon for people with severe to profound hearing loss. However, the surgery performed for electrode insertion into the cochlea puts the surrounding structures within the temporal bone, vestibular system being one among them, at risk for iatrogenic damage. This chapter discusses the consequences of cochlear implantation on the vestibular health, and the consequences of post-implantation vestibular damage on various aspects of life, especially if ignored or not managed effectively.

Keywords Labyrinth · Cognition · Vertigo · Imbalance · Iatrogenic · Dizziness

---

N. K. Singh (✉) · A. Kamath · P. Kumar
Department of Audiology, All India Institute of Speech and Hearing, University of Mysore, Mysore, Karnataka, India

M. Deepak
All India Institute of Speech and Hearing, University of Mysore, Mysore, Karnataka, India

K. Apeksha
MarThoma College of Special Education, Kerala University of Health Sciences, Kasaragod, Kerala, India

S. Sinha
Pt. Jawaharlal Nehru Memorial Medical College and associated Dr. Bhim Rao Ambedkar Memorial Hospital, Pt. Deen Dayal Upadhyay Memorial Health Sciences and Ayush University of Chhattisgarh, Raipur, Chhattisgarh, India

N. K. Keshree
Sri Aurobindo Institute of Speech & Hearing, Sri Aurobindo University, Indore, Madhya Pradesh, India

P. Kumar et al. (eds.), *Advances in Implantation Otology*,
https://doi.org/10.1007/978-981-96-8671-1_21

Introduction

In Chapters 1 and 3, we have understood that cochlea and vestibule, the peripheral sensory organs of the auditory and vestibular system, respectively share close embryological, anatomical, and physiological relationship. This interrelatedness makes it logical to believe that disturbances in cochlear function may have a high probability of inducing a dysfunction in the vestibular system. It is apparent in congenital sensorineural hearing loss (Genovese et al., 2024) as well as acquired diseases of labyrinth, such as Meniere's disease (Young et al., 2003) and labyrinthitis (Kaya et al., 2017), to name a few.

Cochlear implant represents a successful neuroprosthesis offering rehabilitation for individuals with hearing impairment. As explained earlier in this book, cochlear implantation involves surgical insertion of an electrode array into the cochlea, which electrically stimulates the auditory nerve to offset the deficits in hearing. While the benefits of cochlear implantation on auditory function are manifold, questions have been raised about the procedure's impact on vestibular functioning. Vestibular deficits post-surgery are often overshadowed by the overwhelming success of auditory rehabilitation, but warrant attention.

The prime focus of this chapter is to describe the less-focused consequence of cochlear implantation, which is alteration in the vestibular status. This chapter will include the repercussions of cochlear implantation on vestibular functioning, histopathological changes in the vestibular apparatus following implantation, findings of various vestibular tests in adults and children post-implantation, as well as implications of these changes on the overall progress and quality of life of individuals with cochlear implantation.

How Does Cochlear Implantation Affect Vestibular Functioning?

As we begin to understand the effects of cochlear implantation on the vestibular system, we must know the mechanisms underlying these effects. It involves an interplay of surgical procedures, neurophysiological interactions, and adaptive responses.

Post-implantation, vertigo or dizziness is attributed primarily to the surgical trauma causing temporary or permanent end-organ damage (Clark et al., 1988). It is assumed to be by way of traumatic insertion of electrodes, increased labyrinthine pressure, perilymphatic gusher, or reaction with the foreign body. These in turn result in labyrinthine inflammation, bone formation or tissue changes, and hydrops (Handzel et al., 2006; Tien & Linthicum, 2002). Additionally, electrical stimulation can cause excitation of the vestibular nerve in addition to the auditory nerve (Black et al., 1980; Ito, 1998) which could further affect the vestibular function.

Apart from generalized dizziness and vertigo, the occurrence of endolymphatic hydrops presenting as Meniere's syndrome (Kubo et al., 2001) and otoconia displacement leading to Benign Paroxysmal Positional Vertigo (BPPV) have been observed post-implantation (Limb et al., 2005; Swain, 2022; Zanetti et al., 2007). Drilling related vibrational trauma leading to dislodgement of otoconia and bone dust entering the semicircular canals are amongst the assumed causes of BPPV. This is substantiated by studies showing increased incidence rate of BPPV by 2.2% post-implantation in adults (Limb et al., 2005).

The above-discussed factors put together can cause vestibular abnormalities post-surgery, whose prevalence ranges from 20% to 80% (Hänsel et al., 2018). The resulting manifestations represent a broad spectrum of symptoms and findings on the vestibular test battery discussed further in this chapter.

Post-implantation Histopathological Changes in Vestibular Apparatus

Despite significant advancements in surgical techniques, electrode arrays, and implant design aimed at minimizing trauma; literature highlights histopathological alterations in the inner ear, including the vestibular apparatus following implantation. Understanding these changes is crucial as they underpin shifts in residual hearing and, more significantly, balance. Having understood various reasons behind vestibular impairment subsequent to cochlear implantation in the previous section, let us shift our focus to the structural alterations that underscore these vestibular disturbances.

Post-implantation structural changes are pronounced in the Saccule due to its anatomical proximity and connections to the Cochlea. Alterations in Saccule were identified in 55% of the 11 examined bones; the specific alterations were distortions of the saccular membrane, fibrosis, vestibular ossification, and reactive neuromas post-implantation (Tien & Linthicum, 2002). The higher prevalence of the collapsed Saccule across diverse studies underscores its significance in the vestibular deficits experienced post-implantation (Handzel et al., 2006). Additionally, reports also show occurrences of new bone formation, tissue fibrosis, saccular membrane ruptures, sub-epithelial thickening, foreign body granuloma, and damage to the blood labyrinthine barrier (Li et al., 2021; Tien & Linthicum, 2002).

In order to comparatively analyse surgically induced hydrops across three distinct vestibular structures, Su-Velez et al. (2020) examined 15 human temporal bones. The most common finding observed in 88.2% of samples was saccular hydrops, which was followed by utricular hydrops in 47.0% and semicircular canal (SCC) hydrops in 23.5%. Although other investigations showed lower prevalence of saccular hydrops (~60%), it was still more prevalent than the utricular and SCC hydrops (Deng et al., 2022; Ishiyama et al., 2016; Richard et al., 2012). Nonetheless, lesser prevalence of SCC hydrops does not mean that the semicircular canals are not spared of structural damage. Su-Velez et al. (2020) noted changes in the sensory epithelial layer of the semicircular canals, including loss of hair cells, membrane flattening, damage to supporting structures crucial for cellular integrity, and thinning of the neuroepithelium of the Crista ampullaris. The former study also inferred that when hydrops include both Utricle and SCC, there is a heightened likelihood of the patient experiencing post-implantation vestibular symptoms such as vertigo and imbalance.

There are appreciable alterations in the vestibular end-organs following cochlear implant surgery. Investigations have looked beyond the end organs to determine post-surgical changes, if any, and equivocal findings have been reported. Handzel et al. (2006) found no evidence of deafferentation to the peripheral vestibular system or changes in Scarpa's ganglion cells after implantation. However, Tien and Linthicum (2002) reported the formation of reactive neuromas following cochlear implantation. Therefore, further evidence is required to reach a definitive conclusion regarding the extent of damage to the vestibular neurons. The above discussed changes are thought to be established due to the surgical damage because of direct trauma, associated infection, interruption of the endolymphatic system, blocking of ductus reunies, haemorrhage, or vascular changes produced by insertion of implant electrodes (Handzel et al., 2006). In addition, all discussed end organ changes are subject to variations in the surgical approach. Based on histopathological evidence, the Round window approach is favoured over Cochleostomy, whenever possible, to reduce the risk of endolymphatic hydrops (Richard et al., 2012; Su-Velez et al., 2020). This approach supports full scala tympani electrode insertion, aiming to minimize disruption and damage to the endosteum, which is a common occurrence in cochleostomy procedures (Danielian et al., 2021; Wanna et al., 2015).

The histopathological aspects discussed above provide insight into potential functional balance impairments in cochlear implant recipients as a consequence of structural alterations. While some changes may be asymptomatic (Handzel et al., 2006; Tien & Linthicum, 2002), others may induce symptoms of vertigo and imbalance, proving the need for a thorough evaluation to obtain a complete picture of the balance status of an individual and possible future manifestations. Moreover, these findings show that more research is warranted to evolve and refine surgical techniques and electrode designs to minimize damage to the vestibular periphery, especially Saccule.

Vestibular Function in Adult Cochlear Implantees

Though the cochlear implantation procedure and device remain considerably unaltered, the manifestation of vestibular deficits and the results on various tests employed for assessment vary considerably between adults and children. The role of congenital deficits in paediatrics, and varied etiology for hearing loss in adults, as well as the role of central compensation may cause this variability. Hence, this section specifically focuses on the vestibular consequences of cochlear implantation in adults.

Behavioural Manifestation of Vestibular Deficits Among Adult Cochlear Implantees

In the days following surgery, many adults experience episodes of vertigo, typically exhibiting a pattern of gradual recovery. These episodes can vary widely in terms of the nature of vertigo (rotatory, to-and-fro vertigo, and light-headedness), frequency of the episodes (continuous, daily, irregular), duration of episodes (continuous or lasting for seconds, minutes, or days), and triggering factors (motion). Other symptoms that might accompany dizziness include tinnitus, nausea, sweating, headache, and fear of fall. The variability can result from many patient-related factors like etiology, age, and study-related factors like method of sampling, criteria employed for defining abnormality, and so on.

The most frequently reported post-implantation symptom in adults is instability (González-Navarro et al., 2015; Zawawi et al., 2014). Other symptoms like dizziness, vertigo (true spinning sensation), light-headedness, and unsteadiness while walking are also evidenced (Buchman et al., 2004; Katsiari et al., 2013). Enticott et al. (2006) reported that the post-implantation vertigo in older and younger subjects are of equivalent severity on Dizziness Handicap Inventory (DHI) and Activity Balance Confidence (ABC). The other symptoms in their cohort were blurred vision, particularly during locomotion, and a greater risk of falling, in addition to dizziness, nausea, and instability. True vertigo is also present in a few adults immediately after the surgery, which they believed was possibly a BPPV episode (Filipo et al., 2006). Kubo et al. (2001) evaluated individuals with late-onset dizziness approximately a month after the implantation. The symptom complex in these patients aligned with those of Meniere's disease, suggesting hydrops of the labyrinth.

Rah et al. (2016) explored the etiology behind the nature of post-implantation vertigo. In their study, the patients with transient dizziness immediately after the Cochlear implantation (CI) surgery subsequently ended up with vestibular paresis (80%) or BPPV (20%). Among those with recurrent episodic dizziness, 75% were found to have endolymphatic hydrops whereas 25% had vestibular migraine. Apart from this, individuals with immediate, prolonged dizziness showed bilateral vestibular hypofunction (3/4) before surgery; the worsening of the already existing deficit (deteriorating after surgery) might have led to prolonged dizziness in these individuals. Therefore, the post-surgery presentations are in most likelihood the manifestations of the underlying etiologies.

Not merely the nature but the frequency and duration of vertigo also vary depending on the etiology. Krause et al. (2009, 2010) reported that for a majority of individuals, the vertigo episodes either occurred daily or were irregular in frequency, with the duration of single episodes lasting seconds to minutes to days. Motion was the triggering factor for majority of the adults reporting vertigo after CI surgery. Most adults reported vertigo to start within the first post-operative week. Half of the adults with vertigo recovered (became asymptomatic) within 2 months of the surgery, and the remaining took longer, sometimes necessitating additional vestibular rehabilitation.

Many adults with CI often report dizziness even before the CI surgery, suggesting significant pre-surgical vestibular impairment in adults with SNHL and persisting symptoms post-implantation suggest damage to the peripheral system (Katsiari et al., 2013). However, these deficits are further exacerbated after CI, as supported by various studies mentioned in this section. A clear understanding of this aspect can be had from the observations in a study on adults who underwent bilateral sequential cochlear implantation with the second side undergoing surgery after a gap of 7–96 months from the day of first implant (Wagner et al., 2010). In their study, pre-implantation DHI scores of 18–68 were reported in nearly 30% adults with post-lingual deafness, thereby confirming pre-implantation vestibular dysfunction in them. After the first side implantation, there was a significant increase in the DHI score (a significant increase was considered when the DHI scores increased by at least 6) in 5 patients, which included exacerbation of symptoms in one patient who already had a pre-implantation DHI score of 18. This confirms that a unilateral CI not only has a potential of making the already existing vestibular symptoms worse but also brings the risk of fresh onset vestibular symptoms in those who did not have them before the surgery. Interestingly though, one patient with a significantly high pre-implantation DHI score (68) showed a betterment of the condition after the unilateral cochlear implantation (post-surgical DHI score = 52). Even more interesting was the fact that this patient showed a DHI score of 0 (no dizziness) by the 23rd post-implantation month. While this was a rare occurrence, it suggests that vestibular function may even improve after cochlear implantation. While the improvement in the balance function after CI is not well documented in other studies, it can be posited that this was brought about by improved spatial orientation created by the aid of being able to hear again from one ear (Wagner et al., 2010). We believe that this might be caused by resumption of vestibular stimulation due to the spread of current to the ipsilateral vestibular neurons, making a bilateral vestibulopathy turn unilateral, thereby allowing for central compensation, as has been reported in several unilateral vestibular pathologies such as vestibular neuritis and labyrinthitis (Helmchen et al., 2009; Shupert, 2018; Zu Eulenburg et al., 2010). When the patients underwent cochlear implantation on the second side, 7 (35%) showed a significantly worse DHI score than the immediate pre-second surgery baseline (baseline taken just before the second implantation). Among these, 3 were those in whom the first implantation had already caused dizziness and the second one worsened it, whereas 4 were those in whom neither the first implantation had produced dizziness nor did they have dizziness before the first implantation. Another interesting aspect from this study was the findings of the assessment to measure the baseline DHI scores before implantation on the second side. Among those with a high DHI score soon after the first implantation ($n = 10$), 6 had significant reduction of the score, suggesting significant improvement in balance function over a 7–29 months gap between the two surgeries. Among the remaining four, 2 had no change whereas the other 2 had significant worsening over a 14–31 months period after the first implantation despite no significant change in the DHI scores soon after the first implantation. This suggests that the change in vestibular function could be immediately after the surgery or slowly progress over time, probably because of the inflammatory changes, cellular necrosis, and fibrosis over a long period of time after the surgery. Alternatively, it might also be caused by the current spread from the cochlear implant to the vestibule and vestibular neurons, especially if attention was not paid while adjusting the current levels during the device programming (mapping). While Wagner et al. (2010) conducted their study on merely 20 post-lingually deafened adults who underwent sequential bilateral cochlear implantation, the findings suggest that continuous monitoring of balance function over a long period of time after both surgeries is a must to pick up balance issues not only immediately after CI but also the possibility of delayed onset balance deficits months after the surgery. Assessing vestibular functions in adults before and after cochlear implantation is crucial for understanding the impact of implantation on their balance, spatial orientation, and overall quality of life.

Outcomes of the Behavioural Balance Assessment of Adult Cochlear Implantees

Behavioural balance assessment offers insights into the functional implications of vestibular dysfunction. A comprehensive battery of tests thoroughly assesses the balance function, gait, spatial orientation, and visual-vestibular-proprioceptive interaction. These tests may include various questionnaires, postural tests, tests of gait stability, nystagmus evaluation, and occulomotor function, among others. Static and dynamic postural control is likely to be poorer in adults post-implantation (Bozkurt et al., 2022).

Questionnaires

Questionnaires, such as the Dizziness Handicap Inventory (DHI) and Activities Balance Confidence (ABC), are administered frequently to assess the impact of vestibular symptoms. Similar to the presenting symptoms, the changes in pre- and post-test questionnaire scores are variable across individuals. Despite variability, it reflects a considerable change in functional balance in some individuals following surgery, some of which was described earlier in this chapter.

Post-surgical increase in DHI scores have been reported in up to 30% of individuals (Dagkiran et al., 2019; Enticott et al., 2006; Mikkelsen et al., 2017). Other reports indicate no significant change in DHI scores (le Nobel et al., 2016) except for significant reductions (improvements) in the emotional subcategory scores (Buchman et al., 2004). However, in general, DHI scores post-CI are found to be poorer than those of adults of the same age without CI (Bozkurt et al., 2022). In addition, DHI scores correlate with objective vestibular tests in the early and late post-operative periods (Dagkiran et al., 2019). Similar findings have been reported for the ABC questionnaire. While it reflected poorer performance in 30% of implantees pre- and post-implantation in one study (Enticott et al., 2006), another study reported high balance confidence 2 years post-CI (Murray et al., 2020).

Tests for Functional Balance and Posture

Various individual tests as well as scales consisting of several tests serve the purpose of assessing the postural control. Individual tests, such as the classical Romberg test, are reported to be normal pre- and post-operatively (Weinmann et al., 2021); however, these findings on the classical Romberg test could be because of the lack of sensitivity of this test in detecting subtle, less severe balance deficits (Jacobson et al., 2011; Straumann, 2016). The performance of cochlear implanted adults was found to be poorer than the non-CI adults on Berg's Balance Scale, which is a 14-item scale to assess behavioural balance in adults (Bozkurt et al., 2022). Baudhuin (2008) evaluated the patients on various measures like the Berg Balance Scale (BBS), Dynamic Gait Index (DGI), Timed up and Go (TUG), and four static balance tasks which were performed with the eyes open and with the eyes closed. In their study, changes in balance post-implantation were evident on specific tasks, such as the tandem Romberg with eyes closed and the parallel stance on foam with eyes closed (Baudhuin, 2008). Further, a significant decrease in at least one of the behavioural measures after CI was seen in around 36% of the adults. Therefore, it can be concluded that balance is affected after cochlear implantation, although not in every implantee. In fact, a majority of adults show no change in their balance function after cochlear implantation. Whether one finds balance deficits in them depends on the test used and its sensitivity. Tests with more complex demands on the vestibular function typically show more abnormal results and in a larger patient cohort than simple tasks involved in tests such as the classical Romberg test.

Static and Dynamic Posturography

Quantitative technical measures can measure and quantify postural control. Static and dynamic posturography can help quantify the lack of postural control after CI. On the static posturography test, which included sub-tests such as the Modified Clinical Test of Sensory Interaction and Balance, Limits of Stability test, Rhythmic Weight Shift test, Sit-to-stand test, Walk Across test, Tandem Walk test, and Forward Lunge test, the performance of cochlear implanted adults with at least 1 year of device use was poorer than that of the healthy adults (Bozkurt et al., 2022). Some of these findings were also found by Kluenter et al. (2009) who reported significant alteration of the composite score on the Clinical Test of Sensory Interaction and Balance, and some parameters such as step speed and step width on Walk Across and Tandem Walk tests after CI, irrespective of the surgery techniques. Stieger et al. (2018) observed that individuals under 60 years of age and with normal balance control before implantation showed poorer balance control index (BCI) and gait after the CI surgery. In contrast, those above 60 years of age or with pre-operative pathological BCI showed significantly improved performance on Tandem Walk test postoperatively. Therefore, it can be noted that the static posturography test outcomes after CI vary across studies with worsening (Stieger et al., 2018; Kluenter et al., 2009), no effects (Čakrt et al., 2024) and improvement (Stieger et al., 2018;

Kaczmarczyk et al., 2019; Wiszomirska et al., 2019) reported after cochlear implantation. However, in the absence of a study with a sizeable data pool, this area demands further exploration.

The computerized dynamic posturography (CDP) has inclusion of additional variables and test parameters in the testing module. Sensory organization test (SOT) is the most commonly used protocol of CDP test. It assesses a patient's performance in 6 different conditions with each condition progressively challenging the patient's ability to maintain balance. The conditions 1–3 are administered on a fixed platform under the patient's feet with differences in the availability of visual cues. The conditions 4–6 additionally include platform tilts to highten the difficulty by minimizing the availability of somatosensory (proprioceptive) cues. Figure 21.1 shows different conditions and Table 21.1 shows the interpretations of various possible findings.

Studies on SOT using CDP have shown no significant change in performance on conditions 5 and 6 after cochlear implantation in young and older adults as groups (Brey et al., 1995; Buchman et al., 2004). Nonetheless, Brey et al. (1995) reported significant post-implantation worsening of performance (from being within normative range pre-operatively to falling in the pathological range post-operatively) in

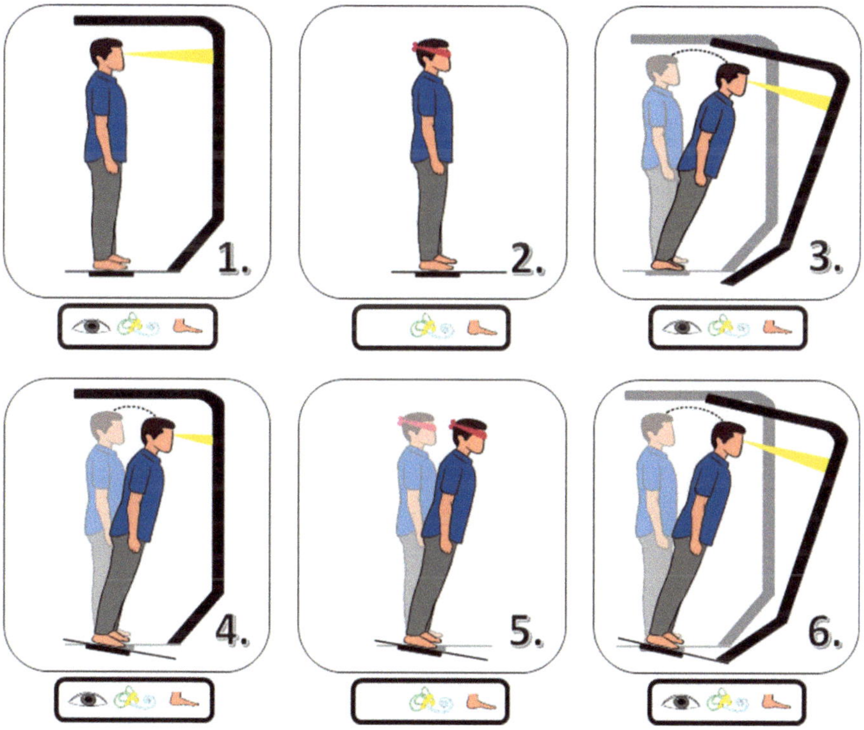

Fig. 21.1 Various test conditions of Sensory Organization Test (SOT) on Computerized Dynamic Posturography (CDP). Icons below each sketch indicate sensory conditions involved: vision, vestibular, and proprioception

Table 21.1 Sensory analysis using the outcomes from various conditions on Sensory Organization Test (SOT) on Computerized Dynamic Posturography (CDP)

Ratio of conditions	Name of the parameter assessed	Inference on functionality
$\frac{\text{Condition 2}}{\text{Condition 1}}$	SOM (somatosensory)	Assesses the ability to use the somatosensory (proprioceptive) input for maintaining balance.
$\frac{\text{Condition 4}}{\text{Condition 1}}$	VIS (visual)	Assesses the ability to use the visual input for maintaining balance.
$\frac{\text{Condition 5}}{\text{Condition 1}}$	VEST (vestibular)	Assesses the ability to use the vestibular input for maintaining balance.
$\frac{(\text{Condition 3} + \text{Condition 6})}{(\text{Condition 2} + \text{Condition 5})}$	PREF (preference)	Assesses the reliance on visual input for maintaining balance, despite the input being inappropriate.

one young adult below 60 years of age. On the contrary, the same study also reported significantly improved post-implantation performance on conditions 5 and 6 in one young and one older adult. In fact, some of the studies have shown clear evidence for substantial long-term improvements in the postural control in conditions 5 and 6 on SOT, probably indicating the role of central compensation (Buchman et al., 2004; Parietti-Winkler et al., 2015). Additionally, the performance in the CI switched-on condition in the presence of a stationary background music was reported to further improve the performance of cochlear implant recipients (Buchman et al., 2004). Guigou et al. (2018) went a step further and conducted dynamic posturography in silence and in the presence of a rotating sound. The rotating sound affected balance in unilateral and bilateral implantees but not the controls. Sensory preference varied across unilateral and bilateral implantees. The former depicted higher vestibular preference, while the latter showed higher vestibular and visual preference.

Subjective Visual Vertical

Subjective Visual Vertical (SVV) evaluates an individual's perception of verticality and is believed to assess the function of the otolith organs, specifically Utricle (Clarke et al., 2003). Several authors report no difference in SVV post-operatively (le Nobel et al., 2016; Čakrt et al., 2024). Transient SVV deviation away from the operated ear on day one, with retention up to a week, is reported by other researchers (Truong et al., 2022; Tan et al., 2023). This suggests that the SVV deficits are present post-implantation and likely to be temporary, but can be permanent in some cases. Tilts seen on SVV examination are more significant in individuals experiencing dizziness post-implantation (Truong et al., 2022). These deficits are exacerbated by visual tilts in the direction of their deficit (Gnanasegaram et al., 2016).

There is a view that cochlear stimulation potentially improves SVV results and hence the otolith functioning. This was supported by findings of a study where electric pulse trains delivered using the CI shifted the abnormal tilt from being tilted in the direction of the unoperated ear to towards the center (Gnanasegaram et al., 2016). However, another study following a similar paradigm reported no difference in verticality perception between the device-on and device-off conditions (le Nobel et al., 2016).

Other less Explored Behavioural Tests

In addition to postural control, various tests are administered to assess the ocular-motor system and nystagmus. The Head Impulse Test (HIT) assesses the vestibulo-ocular reflex, primarily during bedside assessment. A majority of the studies report no pre- and post-implantation compensatory eye movements on HIT in adults (Basta et al., 2008; Melvin et al., 2009). In contrast, Colin et al. (2018) reported abnormal HIT in 18% of adults before surgery, which increased to 59% after surgery. While HIT assesses the compensatory eye movements, the Dynamic Visual Acuity (DVA) is a test of gaze stability induced by the vestibulo-ocular reflex. Gaze instability during head movement is frequent and is reported in about 50% of adults with CI on computerized DVA (Murray et al., 2020). However, contradictory findings have also been reported. Melvin et al. (2009) observed no change in the performance on passive DVA task after cochlear implantation. The Head Shake Nystagmus test (HSN) is often included in the battery for assessing the velocity storage, which is likely to be affected in cases of a unilateral vestibular pathology. The studies using the HSN test report equivocal findings with some showing no significant alteration (Melvin et al., 2009; Colin et al., 2018) whereas others observing a positive result in a small sub-section post-operatively (Meli et al., 2016). Further, skull vibration-induced nystagmus is also an indication of a unilateral loss with the fast phase of the nystagmus beating in the direction of the ear with normal function (Dumas et al., 2008). Nearly one-third of adult CI recipients showed vibration-induced nystagmus with findings consistent with a vestibular pathology in the implanted ear (Colin et al., 2018). Presence of BPPV is also a possibility and its occurrence post-implantation was verified in a few individuals using the Dix-Hallpike test (Murray et al., 2020). Hence the positioning test battery consisting of the Dix-Hallpike test and the McClure-Pagnini test should be a part of the vestibular test battery in adults post-CI.

The variability in outcomes across different tests and studies underscore the need for a comprehensive approach to understanding the impact of implantation on balance and spatial orientation. This emphasizes the role of other objective measures to complement the subjective assessment.

Objective Vestibular Assessment

An array of diagnostic tests are employed to obtain a detailed picture of the vestibular function in adults with cochlear implants before and after surgery. It comprises of objective measures like Vestibular-Evoked Myogenic Potentials (VEMP), Caloric testing, and Video Head Impulse Test (vHIT) alongside subjective assessments. The aim is to provide an understanding of the individual's vestibular status, specific to end organs of balance, to understand its potential impact on their activities of daily living and quality of life.

Vestibular-Evoked Myogenic Potential

VEMP is a vital tool to assess the functioning of the otolith organs and the vestibular nerve. The two major VEMP sub-types, cervical and ocular VEMPs (cVEMP and oVEMP), are among the most extensively researched tests to study the effect of cochlear implantation on the vestibular periphery. Given the changes the VEMP test has itself undergone over the past two decades, in this section we will focus on the studies done after the year 2000. In general, the results of studies in this regard are in alignment with each other and report significant post-implantation deterioration of VEMP responses in a majority of the adult cochlear implant recipients (Imai et al., 2019; Krause et al., 2010; Parkes et al., 2017; West et al., 2021; de Castro Vaz et al., 2022). While, different studies have shown different proportions of affected VEMPs on the implant side, several of them show affected cVEMPs and/or oVEMPs in nearly 50% of implanted ears. In case of unilateral adult cochlear implantees, the VEMP responses on the non-implanted side are usually unaffected (Robard et al., 2015; Chen et al., 2016; West et al., 2021). Although rarely, bilateral altered responses, and even more rarely, unaltered VEMP responses on the cochlear implant side and altered one on the contralateral side have also been observed (Rasmussen et al., 2021). A few studies have also shown contradictory findings of no change in VEMP results after implantation (Katsiari et al., 2013). However, no one-to-one correlation is established between the VEMP responses and factors like age, gender, and symptoms (Bogle, 2010; Chen et al., 2016). This could possibly be attributed to each test assessing only one of the five end-organs which makes findings on just one test inaccurate in explaining the presence of symptoms. Alternatively, central compensation might have alleviated the symptoms whereas the test results remain deficient, thereby causing a mismatch between the test results and the symptomatology.

A question regarding which end-organ has a higher likelihood of damage during cochlear implantation is pertinent, especially the comparison between the two otolith organs, given their proximity to the Cochlea. One group of researchers believe that the Saccule is relatively more prone to damage than the Utricle, with semicircular canals' damage assuming the bottom place in the likelihood of cochlear implantation-associated damage (Handzel et al., 2006; Tien & Linthicum, 2002). Sosna-Duranowska et al. (2021) found absence of cVEMP and oVEMP responses in 19.2% and 17.4%, respectively. Further, all individuals with a loss of oVEMP post-operatively also had an absent cVEMP. However, not all with an absent cVEMP had an absent oVEMP. Therefore, Saccule seems to have more vulnerability than Utricule, even though the difference could be only slight (Basta et al., 2008; Krause et al., 2009; Chen et al., 2016). Damage to Saccule is likely a consequence of the insertion trauma due to its anatomical proximity to the Cochlea (Basta et al., 2008).

This is well supported by histopathological evidence showing the presence of saccular hydrops and collapsed saccular membrane in nearly 59% samples; however, the Scarpa's ganglion cell count and hair cell densities was found to be similar between the implanted and the non-implanted sides. It appears that the hydropic Cochlea could probably be the result of obstruction of endolymphatic flow in the Ductus reuniens (Handzel et al., 2006). These factors in combination can affect post-implantation cVEMP responses.

Not all studies comparing the utricular and saccular functioning comply with the above discussed results. Imai et al. (2019) found significantly higher abnormal findings on oVEMP (91%) than cVEMP (56%) post-operatively. While the precise reason for this aberrant finding is not well understood, a study posited that the presence of air in the vestibule caused by the perilymphatic fistula during the CI surgery could be the reason for more utricular abnormality than saccular (Kusuma et al., 2005).

Most of the above discussed studies have shown affected post-implantation VEMPs within days to a few weeks after the cochlear implantation. However, massive drilling and surgical procedure could also lead to long term effects that need not necessarily be picked on the short-term follow-ups. Therefore, long-term effects of implantation on otolith function are also of interest. In this regard, Rasmussen et al. (2021) reported a loss of 50% (5/10) VEMPs on the implanted side 14 weeks after implantation compared to the fourth month, confirming a possibility of otolith function deterioration several months after the implantation.

The results of the studies employing VEMPs should be interpreted cautiously, as a vast majority of these studies have used air conduction stimulation. Significant alterations in middle ear mechanics can hamper the effective transfer of air-conducted stimuli to the inner ear, leading to insufficient energy reaching the otolith organs, which in turn could cause overestimation of the otolith damage. These assumptions were confirmed by the finding of significantly higher VEMP response rates for bone conduction (BC) stimulation, consistent with a reduced low-frequency absorbance in WBT, affecting air conduction VEMPs (AC-VEMPs) (Merchant et al., 2020). Hence, BC-VEMPs can predict post-CI otolith damage better than the AC-VEMPs, and therefore, BC-VEMPs make a better choice than the AC-VEMPs. Nonetheless, BC VEMPs have their own set of challenges, none more so than the insufficient stimulus output from the typical commercially available bone vibrators such as the Radioear B71. Hence, one should use bone vibrators that give higher outputs and are compatible with the VEMP equipment. Radioear B81 and B250 could be possible options, but a Minishaker could also make a fine choice to overcome the barrier of insufficient stimulus output clouding the inferences.

Electrical Co-stimulation of Saccule

Facial nerve stimulation due to the current spread from the cochlear implant electrode is a well-understood phenomenon. In a way similar to the Facial nerve stimulation, the Inferior vestibular nerve (IVN) or Saccule could be co-stimulated during cochlear implant's functioning for auditory nerve stimulation. In fact, evidence supports the hypothesis that electrical stimulation via CI can stimulate the vestibular apparatus, causing sound-induced vertigo. Coordes et al. (2012) reported this phenomenon in 18% of their patients. VEMPs were elicited in four of the 26 participants in response to an acoustic stimulus via the CI processor. In addition, there was no effect on utricular function and postural stability, indicating primarily co-stimulation of the saccular macula or IVN. This co-stimulation is not necessarily a disadvantage and can occasionally compensate for the surgical damage. This was confirmed by a study that found significant improvements in cVEMP responses with CI turned-on compared to it being turned-off (Miwa et al., 2019). Therefore, electrical co-stimulation of the Saccule and IVN via CI can sometimes lead to sound-induced vertigo but may also provide compensation for the surgical damage.

Assessing the Vestibulo-Ocular Reflex

Assessing the Vestibulo-ocular Reflex (VOR) through tests such as Video Head Impulse Test (vHIT), Caloric testing, and Rotational Chair Test (RCT), provides insights into the status of the semicircular canals. Traditionally, the scleral search coil technique was used to assess VOR. Using this technique, one study found a low post-operative VOR gain in up to 30% of individuals for horizontal and 50% for vertical semicircular canals. Several studies have documented significant abnormality in the caloric response and the vHIT response among adults following implantation (Bittar et al., 2019; Colin et al., 2018; Jang et al., 2023; Wagner et al., 2010; West et al., 2021). However, semicircular canals remain the least affected end organs after CI surgery (Handzel et al., 2006; Tien & Linthicum, 2002).

Video Head Impulse Test

vHIT is frequently employed to assess the VOR in response to high-frequency simulation (head jerks), offering an assessment of all three semicircular canals. The presence of refixation (also called corrective) saccades and reduction of the VOR gain on this test are two major indicators for the presence of VOR deficits in a person. Several researchers have investigated the effects of CI on the vHIT response parameters in adults.

West et al. (2021) showed decreased mean post-implantation VOR gain in adults with CI. In their study, the lateral canal VOR gain decreased from 0.92 pre-operatively to 0.84 post-operatively. They also observed an increase in the refixation saccades; however, the difference was statistically not significant. Rasmussen et al. (2021) also reported a lowering of the mean VOR gain from 0.93 pre-operatively to 0.89 post-operatively; however, the change was statistically not significant. Nonetheless, when analysing the individual participants' data, they observed presence of corrective saccades in seven individuals, and abnormal gain in one individual post-operatively, who otherwise had normal vHIT responses before the surgery.

Other studies also report a minimal or no post-implantation change in the VOR gain (Carmona et al., 2018; Guan et al., 2021); however, some others found appearance of refixation saccades post-operatively despite there being no evidence for these in the pre-operative evaluation in various proportions of participants in their study (Migliaccio et al., 2005; Batuecas-Caletrio et al., 2015; Janky & Patterson, 2020). Therefore, vHIT post-implantation should be interpreted with a combination of gain and corrective saccades (Janky & Patterson, 2020). Among the three semicircular canals, responses of the lateral canal is more affected than the vertical canals, and the posterior canal shows the least impact of cochlear implantation on vHIT responses (Kardooni et al., 2022).

Caloric Test

The Caloric test uses the temperature gradient induced low frequency fluid movement to assess the lateral semicircular canal's function. This test assesses the lateral semicircular canal of one side independent of the other. Several studies have investigated the changes in caloric response parameters, such as slow phase velocity (SPV), stimulability in response to caloric stimuli (reduced or absent stimulation amounting to hyporeflexia or areflexia, respectively), and unilateral weakness (canal paresis), in adult cochlear implantees.

West et al. (2021) reported a mean post-implantation increase in unilateral weakness by about 22% (change from 20.5% preoperatively to 42.9% post-operatively) on the bithermal caloric test. Although demonstrated using a different caloric response parameter, Krause et al. (2010) also observed a significant deterioration in the caloric response in their study participants. In their study, the mean SPV on the implanted side dipped from 39.2° per second pre-operatively to 23.9° per second post-operatively. Several later studies confirmed the findings of reduced SPV and abnormal or hypofunctional caloric responses post-implantation (Buchman et al., 2004; Kuang et al., 2015; Rasmussen et al., 2021; Guan et al., 2021; Quimby et al., 2024). Although less explored, age has been found to be associated with post-implantation change in caloric responses. A study observed higher odds of poorer post-implantation caloric results among older adults than the young adults (Enticott et al., 2006). While most of the above discussed findings on the caloric test are on the expected lines, at least a few studies have reported the interesting finding of improved post-implantation caloric responses in a few individuals (Kubo et al., 2001; Szirmai et al., 2001). Even more interesting was the finding of significantly higher responses or greater SPV to caloric stimulation in patients complaining of delayed dizziness (Kubo et al., 2001). The presenting symptoms in these patients with greater post-implantation SPV than pre-implantation were similar to those of Meniere's disease, indicating post-implantation labyrinthine hydrops. Generally, the abnormal caloric responses can range from unilateral hyporeflexia to bilateral areflexia. Individuals with caloric responses suggestive of a bilateral vestibular loss post-operatively typically show persistent dizziness, while a majority of adults with other caloric abnormalities show improvement in dizziness (Abramides et al.,

2015). However, these findings require more studies before they can be generalized. Some researchers consider pre- and post-implantation caloric responses to be predictors of performance with CI (Quimby et al., 2024), whereas other researchers have found results against the same (Bodmer et al., 2007; Yang et al., 2016).

Several adults with a concomitant hearing and vestibular dysfunction also undergo cochlear implantation to experience better hearing. When evaluating changes in caloric responses among such individuals, Colin et al. (2018) observed a post-implantation increase of caloric abnormality and areflexia rate by 8% each in adults who had at least one episode of vertigo with a balance disorder pre-operatively. While several studies have reported significantly abnormal pre-operative caloric responses in some adults, they have specifically not discussed how the post-operative caloric responses of these specific individuals were. Therefore, there is not enough evidence to generalize the information in this regard.

Some studies have also performed caloric test and vHIT before and after implantation in the same group of subjects to better understand the sensitivity of each of these tests in investigating the post-implantation change in VOR. While the results of vHIT are variable across studies, caloric test shows relatively consistent findings. Bittar et al. (2019) reported that caloric test is more sensitive in detecting hypofunction in the lateral semicircular canal than vHIT. In their study, the pre-operative abnormal caloric test findings were found in 32% and abnormal vHIT in 18% of the adults. The sensitivity in detecting vestibular impairment among caloric tests and vHIT tests was found to be 1.8:1 among the adult implantees. While it does indicate the dominance of the caloric test over vHIT in detecting vestibular abnormalities among cochlear implantees, one needs to remember that the two tests assess entirely different frequencies and hair cell types. While caloric test investigates low frequencies and tests for the functioning of Type II hair cells, vHIT is a test of high-frequency VOR originating from Type I hair cells (Leng & Liu, 2020). Hence, they cannot be treated as replacements for each other.

Rotational Chair Test

The Rotational Chair Test (RCT) assesses the low-frequency response of the lateral semicircular canal. Sinusoidal Harmonic Acceleration (SHA) test is the most commonly used sub-test of RCT. The response parameters recorded on this sub-test are VOR gain (ratio of the eye velocity to the chair velocity), phase (time shift of the eye velocity with reference to the chair velocity), and symmetry (comparison of VOR gain between leftward and rightward chair rotations). These measurements are typically done for chair oscillations at 0.01, 0.02, 0.04, 0.08, 0.16, 0.32, and 0.64 Hz. Buchman et al. (2004) observed no significant change in VOR gain, phase, or symmetry at post-implantation measurements performed 1 month, 4 months, 1 year, and 2 years after cochlear implantation. However, when they further sub-categorised groups on the basis of the pre-implant caloric test outcomes, they found substantial phase differences between the groups at the 4-months post-implantation stage for sinusoidal frequencies of 0.08 and 0.16 Hz. This difference continued to exist even at the measurement points of 1 year and 2 years. This is suggestive of a post-implantation labyrinthine effect in those who had a pre-implantation caloric weakness in the implanted ear. They also reported post-implantation decrease in the total caloric response of 21°/s greater in 29% of individuals with an intact caloric response pre-implantation, which persisted throughout the study period. Recently, Piker et al. (2020) found no significant post-implantation change in the gain or phase on SHA using RCT in a group of 10 adult cochlear implantees. However, when the pre- and post-implantation results of each patient was compared against the normative data, 20% (2 out of 10) participants showed an increase in the phase lead after implantation. While both these participants had phase leads in the extreme low frequencies (below 0.08 Hz) pre-operatively, the phase leads outside the laboratory norms involved more frequencies (up to 0.32 Hz) at the three-month follow-up point. However, this study did not investigate its participating patients in the period between cochlear implantation and the 3-month follow-up point. Therefore, one cannot accurately estimate the precise number of patients with a post-implantation effect on SHA test of RCT.

Oculomotor Function Assessment in Adult Cochlear Implantees

Oculomotor examination evaluates the functioning of vital visual systems such as the Gaze system, Saccade system, Optokinetic system and Smooth pursuit system. These tests are typically conducted using videonystagmography techniques. The cochlear implantees who experienced post-operative vertigo had poorer saccadic accuracy and latency (Sarac et al., 2020). On the other hand, optokinetic tests in such individuals show no abnormality (Weinmann et al., 2021). However, literature in this area is scanty, making it challenging to draw definitive conclusions.

Quality of Life

The above-mentioned vestibular deficits on various tests impact the daily living of affected adults. Andries et al. (2022) evaluated health-related quality of life in adults over 55 years of age. They found that the Health Utilities Index (HUI)-3 multi-attribute scale and the HUI-3 emotion scale remained poorer, with vestibular loss significantly contributing to the findings.

From the above discussion of findings in adult cochlear implantees, one can conclude that cochlear implantation can significantly affect the vestibular system, leading to balance issues and an increased risk of falls. The exact nature and extent of these effects vary among individuals. However, all balance outcomes among adult cochlear implantees are not gloomy. Several individuals with pre-implantation vestibular dysfunction, especially bilateral vestibular hypofunction/dysfunction, may experience improved balance after cochlear implantation in the long run. However, it is essential for professionals to be aware of these effects and to provide appropriate rehabilitation to cochlear implant recipients to minimize negative impacts on cognition and overall quality of life. A holistic approach combining subjective and objective measures is essential for a comprehensive assessment of vestibular functions in adults undergoing cochlear implantation, before as well as for a substantial duration after implantation.

Vestibular Function in Children with Cochlear Implants

Children are not always mini models of the adults. While they might show similar results to adults on some aspects, higher plasticity and possibility of further developmental changes should make us view them from a different lens. This is no different for changes in vestibular function after CI. An additional factor that makes this group different from the adults is the difference in coaffection of auditory and vestibular systems between congenital hearing loss in children and acquired hearing loss in adults. Several studies have shown that children with congenital hearing loss requiring cochlear implantation also have a coexisting vestibular dysfunction (Cushing et al., 2008, 2013). While the percentage of such coexisting congenital hearing and vestibular dysfunction varies from 30% to 70% across the studies (Arnvig, 1955; Jafari & Asad Malayeri, 2011; Cushing et al., 2013), these percentages are substantially higher than the comorbidity of hearing loss and vestibular dysfunction in adults with acquired hearing loss who are cochlear implant candidates. The vestibular problems, however, could be exacerbated after cochlear implantation, and the histopathological evidences confirm these findings (Deng et al., 2022; Jacot et al., 2009). A young child's limited communication abilities makes it challenging to express the complex symptoms associated with imbalance or vertigo, emphasizing the need to assess the prevalence of such issues and provide appropriate rehabilitation. This section will elaborate on the vestibular functioning in children with cochlear implants.

Behavioural Symptoms

Unlike adults, children with cochlear implants typically exhibit fewer reports of dizziness, vertigo, falls, nausea, imbalance, or related symptoms compared, possibly due to their inability to express themselves. Hence, vestibular deficits are underestimated or ignored most often. An addition to this is the role of rapid compensation and sensory integration in children (Valente & McCaslin, 2011). Children reporting such symptoms often recover quickly, suggesting recovery from acute surgical trauma. Additionally, the symptoms are difficult to distinguish from other disorders or mere clumsiness. These complexities in children make studying the symptoms a problematic area. Studies comparing the symptoms across different patients, surgical procedures, and methodologies have yielded variable and inconsistent results. While some show an increase or novel occurrence of vestibular symptoms post-cochlear implantation, others indicate reduced symptoms or no change in frequency.

Commonly reported symptoms in children include vertigo and unsteadiness (Birman et al., 2015; Jacot et al., 2009). Birman et al. (2015) assessed vertigo in children aged 1 year and 7 months to 13 years and 6 months after 1 week of surgery. None of the children exhibited significant dizziness or instability. However, 8% reported slight unsteadiness during this period. Two children with slight unsteadiness had Large Vestibular Aqueduct Syndrome (LVAS). This indicates the presence of subtle post-implantation deficits in some children, especially those with congenital anomalies. In our experience, the manifestations of vestibular damage are evident during activities. The children with a post-implantation vestibular damage could be frequently colliding with objects around them, show imbalance or increased frequency of falls on uneven surfaces or surfaces with higher compliance like muddy pools, sandy beaches etc. However, a typical case history hardly explores such questions and therefore obscures the possibility of discovering balance related issues in challenging tasks and environments in a child's self-report. Another important piece of information is the delay in the acquisition of motor milestones, especially related to walking among those implanted within 12 months of age. De Kegel et al. (2015) tracked the motor development of children with congenital hearing loss at time points between 6 and 24 months at a 6-month interval each. The CI group showed a drop in gross motor performance in the span following implantation (6–18 months) compared to the group not receiving CI. Nonetheless, even in the CI group, there was a tendency towards recovery by the end of 2 years.

The typical symptoms associated with a vestibular deficit, like dizziness and vertigo following implantation in children, have been reported inconsistently, with rates ranging from 0.4% to 8.2% (Ajallouyean et al., 2011; Birman et al., 2015; Hansen et al., 2010; Psillas et al., 2014). Lin et al. (2006) found no variation in dizziness symptoms in around 2.4% of children, pre- and post-operatively. However, Chadha et al. (2009) observed a higher post-operative dizziness rate of approximately 30% in children aged 1–3 years with congenital inner ear abnormalities. This suggests that inner ear anomalies predispose a child to a heightened risk of vestibular issues post-implantation.

The variable symptoms discussed above are due to diverse underlying aetiologies or structural alterations. While in most children, it is difficult to associate the label of a condition, others exhibit symptoms typical of a few disorders post-implantation. Numerous case reports and prospective studies have documented trigger-evoked dizziness or motion-induced dizziness similar to paroxysmal positional vertigo (Zanetti et al., 2007), perilymphatic fistula (Kusuma et al., 2005), and vestibular migraine (Rah et al., 2016) among children in their post-operative period. However, a majority of studies have primarily focussed on post-implantation paroxysmal positional vertigo in children. In a study by Zanetti et al. (2007), paroxysmal positional vertigo was examined in 30 children and 32 adults with cochlear implants, revealing an overall 12.5% increase in its incidence compared to the general incidence, with relapses occurring on the same side after 3 months despite liberatory manoeuvres. Shetye (2012) reported a case of a 13-year-old female diagnosed with paroxysmal positional vertigo 2 years after surgery, attributed to vibrational trauma to the labyrinth.

Similar to adults, some children exhibit instability and prolonged dizziness, while others might have triggered vertigo. However, owing to the lack of communication abilities, especially among those implanted at a very young age, the symptoms might not be overtly explained. Keen observation during activities and motor development can reveal subtle manifestations of the deficits. Given the lack of consistent findings on the nature and duration of behavioural symptoms, utilizing subjective and objective tests for diagnosis of post-implantation vestibular deficits in children is essential. The test of choice depends on the development of children, as various levels of cooperation may be desired in each one of them.

Behavioural Balance Assessment

Conducting functional assessment of balance aids in evaluating a child's ability to maintain balance in real-world or daily life scenarios. This assessment is crucial for rehabilitation, symptomatic treatment, and enhancing the child's quality of life. It encompasses questionnaires, positional tests, nystagmus evaluation, and gaze stability tests amongst several others. These evaluations provide insight into a child's visual, vestibular, and proprioceptive abilities, as well as their interconnectedness, given the challenges in comprehending the child's symptoms in absence of these tests.

Questionnaires

The Dizziness Handicap Inventory (DHI) and Paediatric Vestibular Symptom Questionnaire (PVSQ) are commonly used to assess the impact of vestibular issues (Guan et al., 2021; Mohamed et al., 2024). PVSQ is specifically designed for children aged 6–17 years and includes 11 questions. Since several children might be unable to directly understand and answer the questions, parents can be used as communication partners for a better accuracy of response. In a study investigating vertigo symptoms following cochlear implantation, no significant difference in pre-and post-implantation PVSQ scores was observed in children with unilateral CI. However, among children with bilateral CI, PVSQ scores increased on post-implantation day 3 and exhibited a decreasing trend towards day 30, suggesting that these changes may be transient reactions to the surgical trauma to the inner ear structures (Guan et al., 2021). Alternatively, it could even indicate changes due to central compensation after a peripheral vestibular damage.

In a similar study, DHI was administered by taking the responses of parents and caregivers regarding the symptoms of their children. The authors reported a significant post-implantation change in the responses to question four that read, "Does your child feel discomfort when playing roller coaster?" (Mohamed et al., 2024). The finding from this study brings us back to an earlier point about observing a child's behaviour during complex and more demanding activities. If the right questions are asked about the right tasks/activities, the identification of the obscured balance issues can be identified.

Generally, the questionnaires currently available for paediatric patientss barely reflect changes in balance following implantation, probably attributed to subtle nature of the symptoms and speedier recovery from the insult than adult implantees. However, these results have a dearth of validity and consistency as they are yet to be replicated.

Tests for Functional Balance Skills and Posture

The Paediatric Balance Scale (PBS) is a modified version of the Berg Balance Scale for children, featuring 14 tasks scored from 0 to 4 each. This scale offers age-based norms for comparison, aiding in the assessment of functional balance. Shah (2013) utilized PBS to assess balance function before and after intervention in children, with and without cochlear implants. Their findings revealed improved gross motor skills and postural control post-intervention. However, the initial PBS scores were below the normative average (35.5), indicating poorer balance in children with congenital hearing loss with or without cochlear implantation.

We have observed that children with cochlear implants who have unilateral or bilateral vestibular dysfunction often exhibit poorer performance on specific items of PBS. Notably, scores of ≤ 3 are commonly observed on items 8 (tandem stance), 9 (single leg stance), and 14 (limits of stability). The children may demonstrate increased sway during tasks with eyes closed, struggle with tandem gait positions resulting in greater sway, exhibit change of locus when asked to turn 360°, and show signs of clumsiness while stepping. The signs mentioned above are the subjective observations made in children with balance deficits; however, a corresponding reduced scores on individual tasks is not always encountered. Additionally, other studies also confirm that tasks performed with closed eyes are highly sensitive in identifying subtle balance deficits in children with total bilateral vestibular loss (TBVL). Among these tasks, one-foot standing with eyes closed demonstrated the best performance as a screening tool for TBVL, using a timed cut-off of 4 seconds (Oyewumi et al., 2016).

To check the effect of age at implantation on balance function, Mujdeci et al. (2021) examined PBS scores of two age groups and found no difference between them. The participants in two groups in their study had the mean age of 8.72 and 10.17 years. It is worth noting that the performance on PBS demonstrates a ceiling by approximately 8 years, which may have contributed to the lack of difference between the groups. Hence, PBS scores must be interpreted with caution. To overcome the age barrier in PBS, other tests should be chosen for assessing older children, one of them being the Bruininks-Oseretsky Test of Motor Proficiency Second Edition (BOT-2) or Third Edition (BOT-3).

The Bruininks-Oseretsky Test of Motor Proficiency (BOT) is a standardized clinical assessment tool designed to evaluate motor proficiency, including functional balance. It covers four subcategories namely fine manual control, manual coordination, body coordination, and strength and agility, and can be administered to individuals aged 4–21 years, following age and gender norms. The Third Edition has an upper age extension up to 25 years. The findings inliterature consistently indicate that children after cochlear implantation score below established norms on the BOT test (Cushing et al., 2008; Ebrahimi et al., 2016; Eustaquio et al., 2011; Janky et al., 2022, 2023; Oyewumi et al., 2016; Wu et al., 2022). To compare the effect of bilateral implantation and unilateral implantation on functional balance against non-implanted children, Eustaquio et al. (2011) employed the BOT-2 test. They reported no significant difference in performance based on mean scores among the groups. However, the scores of all three groups were lower than the normative and in alignment with the other studies (Cushing et al., 2008; Ebrahimi et al., 2016). Some researchers used BOT-2 to explore the effect of the device condition (cochlear implants switched-on versus switched-off) on balance. In a meta-analysis, Wu et al. (2022) observed significantly worse results on BOT-2 in children with SNHL who received CI than the children with typical hearing. However, they did note a slight improvement in balance when the implant was switched-on than when it was switched-off.

Standard clinical tests of posture and equilibrium, such as Fukuda stepping test and Romberg test, have also been administered on children with cochlear implants. In the Fukuda Stepping test, approximately 20% of children with unilateral cochlear implants showed affected results, with sway towards the implanted side or occasionally both sides indicative of bilateral hypofunction in some cases (Salem et al., 2021). Baudhuin (2008) reported notable alterations in the tandem stance Romberg test (also called the Sharpened Romberg test) and parallel stance on foam with eyes closed, following cochlear implantation. Another study, found no differences between early and late implant recipients in the tandem stance Romberg test (eyes open), Single Leg Stand (eyes open), and Timed Up and Go (TUG) score. However, the Early CI Group exhibited longer balance sustenance durations in tests with eyes closed and certain positions of the Postural-Computerized Integration and Balance (P-CTSIB) (Mujdeci et al., 2021).The authors concluded that Romberg test can detect balance deficits easily by reducing the proprioceptive and visual cues, but slight changes might go unnoticed on this test. Hence, P-CTSIB was superior in depicting balance deficit.

From the findings of studies in this sub-section, it is apparent that behavioral assessment tools like the Fukuda stepping and Romberg tests offer quick screening of post-implantation balance function, especially the Romberg on foam with eyes closed. Nonetheless, they lack objectivity. Both PBS and BOT-2 are sensitive and feasible tools to identify balance deficits after cochlear implantation. Though they tap into different age groups, both have established normative as well as independent tasks to identify the presence of deficits. However, all these tests can be performed on older children, typically over the age of 4 years.

Static Posturography

Static posturography, as discussed earlier in this chapter in the section on adults, encompasses various subtests and is highly sensitive in detecting performance variations. Literature strongly supports its effectiveness in assessing children post-implantation, particularly in identifying vestibular deficits when visual and somatosensory cues are compromised (Kelly et al., 2018; Nair et al., 2017; Situkho et al., 2023; Suarez et al., 2021). However, as with other tests, chronological age has effects on the posturography results, which limits its usability and value in case of young children undergoing cochlear implantation. In children with cochlear implants, Situkho et al. (2023) observed difficulties during the eyes closed condition, similar to other postural tests. However, the authors reported that a significant difference in findings on static posturography was observed for children under 8 years of age, not above it (Situkho et al., 2023).

A group of researchers investigated the center of pressure (COP) and sway velocity (SV) in children with cochlear implants. They found that children with CI and vestibular dysfunction exhibited higher COP and SV values than the typically hearing peers (Oikawa et al., 2018; Suarez et al., 2007). Additionally, Oikawa et al. (2018) noted that COP displacement in the mediolateral direction with sound was similar to that without sound. Several other studies though have reported better performance in posturography assessments when the CI was on than when it was off (Cushing et al., 2008; Schwab et al., 2010; Suarez et al., 2021). Overall, these findings suggest that static posturography could serve as a rapid evaluation tool for assessing vestibular dysfunction in children post-implantation and show tendency for better functional balance with the implant switched-on than when it is switched-off.

Gaze and Vision During Motion

Static visual acuity (SVA), Dynamic Visual Acuity (DVA), and the Gaze Stabilization Test (GST) tap on the oculomotor system under vestibular influences. There are equivocal findings on DVA results as some studies report significant differences in DVA post-implantation (Janky & Givens, 2015), whereas others report no significant difference between children with normal hearing, and those with unilateral or bilateral cochlear implantation (McSweeny et al., 2021). Janky and Givens (2015) evaluated SVA, DVA and GST in children post-CI and compared their performance against children with hearing sensitivity within normal limits. They found no correlation of vestibular loss with the performance on SVA and GST; however, DVA exhibited significant correlation with vestibular functioning. Although the study did not provide an explanation for this inconsistency, it is deemed significant as it could address issues such as blurred vision, which might impact a child's academic performance in terms of reading and writing abilities. However, there is no consensus on these results post-implantation owing to limited investigations and varied presentations.

Some researchers have investigated the efficacy of the clinical Head Impulse test (HIT) in evaluating the VOR of children after cochlear implantation (Verrecchia et al., 2020). The authors noted that 21 (60%) children exhibited normal responses on both sides, 6 (17.15%) showed unilateral abnormal HIT responses, and another 6 (17.15%) showed bilateral abnormal responses, albeit in a younger age range (4 – 46 months). They reported significant correlation between the findings on HIT and vHIT among cochlear implantees. However, using HIT below 6 months could be questionable due to underdeveloped VOR and poor neck control (Verrecchia et al., 2020).

Subjective Visual Vertical

Research on the findings of SVV test post-implantation is limited in children. A study by Gnanasegaram et al. (2016) revealed a similar pattern of findings between children and adult cochlear implantees. They showed that 45% of children showed asymmetrical spatial orientation, which worsened by visual tilts. In addition, electric pulse trains via the CI improved abnormal perception, regardless of stimulation ear. However, the generalisation of this finding should be cautiously done due to a scarcity of studies in this area.

Based on our clinical experience, we believe that methodological adjustments to enhance children's comprehension would ensure consistent results on SVV. For instance, replacing the vertical line inside the bucket in Bucket test with a clown drawing can simplify the task, prompting the child to make it stand upright. Similarly, a drawing of a pot-bellied man sleeping in a supine position for the subjective visual horizontal test can elicit more valid responses from the child. Nonetheless, these ideas need clinical validation before they can be incorporated clinically.

Objective Vestibular Assessments in Children with Cochlear Implantation

In contrast to behavioural responses, objective vestibular assessments in children are considered more reliable and resistant to clinician bias. These tests are favoured for their directness and reliability, and are frequently employed alongside behavioural tests to validate the diagnoses and obtain direction for interventions. The typical objective tests encompass VEMP, caloric testing, vHIT, RCT, and CDP, each exhibiting considerable correlations with histopathological evidence. In this section we will discuss the research findings concerning each objective vestibular test and share our experiences of evaluating children with sensorineural hearing loss before and after cochlear implantation.

VEMP in Cochlear Implantees

A characteristic that makes VEMP, especially cVEMP, an appropriate test for assessing very young prospective cochlear implantees is its presence in even neonates and infants (Sheykholesami et al., 2005). This is probably the reason cVEMPs are the most explored vestibular test to study the effects of cochlear implantation in children.

Numerous studies have investigated VEMPs in children with cochlear implants both before and after implantation, aiming to understand the impact on the otolithic organs (Jin et al., 2006; Li & Gong, 2020; Licameli et al., 2009; Psillas et al., 2014; Xu et al., 2015). These studies consistently show a deterioration in VEMP responses (absent or reduced amplitude) post-implantation in the implanted ear (Abdelghaffar

& Elshazly, 2011; Bayat et al., 2020; Devroede et al., 2016; Gerdsen et al., 2022; Guan et al., 2021; Imai et al., 2019; Jin et al., 2006, 2008, 2009; Khalil, 2017; Koyama et al., 2021; Li & Gong, 2020; Licameli et al., 2009; Merchant et al., 2020; Parkes et al., 2017; Psillas et al., 2014; Thierry et al., 2015; Wang et al., 2022; Xu et al., 2015). However, contradictory findings also exist. Ajalloueyan et al. (2017) reported no signifcant poost-implantation change in VEMP amplitude in the implanted ear. Interestingly, deterioration of the VEMP response in non-implanted ear, in addition to the implanted ears, has also been reported (Psillas et al., 2014).

Pre-implantation assessment is crucial in children, particularly those with congenital deafness, as they may have a high likelihood of concurrent vestibular issues even before undergoing the surgery for cochlear implantation. The comorbidity of vestibular problems in children with congenital severe to profound sensorineural hearing loss ranges from 30% to 74% (Arnvig, 1955; Buchman et al., 2004; Jafari & Asad Malayeri, 2011). Among various peripheral structures, Utricle is more often affected than Saccule, despite Saccule's close association with the Cochlea, in children with congenital sensorineural hearing loss (Tanyeri et al., 2020). This finding highlights a key difference between pre-existing vestibular pathology more often linked to Utricle whereas the post-implantation vestibular issues are more often linked to saccular damage. Nonetheless, these group trends hardly matter when assessing a single child. Therefore, it is pertinent that pre-implantation status is examined in order to make meaningful inferences on the changes post-implantation.

Post-implantation, abnormal VEMP results were frequently observed across most studies. Nevertheless, the inconsistency among the studies was primarily related to the definition of a reduced VEMP response. Many studies focused solely on VEMP amplitude and employed varying criteria for defining a reduced response (Bayat et al., 2020; Li & Gong, 2020). Conversely, other studies used VEMP thresholds or a combination of different VEMP parameters (such as threshold, amplitude, latency, and inter-peak latency) to identify a reduced response (Abdelghaffar & Elshazly, 2011; Ajalloueyan et al., 2017; Dhondt et al., 2022). While several studies applied specific threshold values to determine the presence or absence of the VEMP response, the precise cut off value was often not specified in a majority of them (Abdelghaffar & Elshazly, 2011).

The first study to examine VEMP responses in children with CI was conducted by Jin et al. (2006). They used VEMPs to assess vestibular function in 12 children with CI before and after implantation. The authors reported that 58% (7/12) had abnormal VEMP responses pre-implantation, while 91.6% (11/12) showed abnormal responses post-implantation. However, the post-implantation data mentioned above was in the CI switched-off condition. In the CI switched-on condition, 4 children showed presence of VEMPs. These findings have been replicated in many subsequent studies, which showed post-implantation VEMP abnormality in 50–80% children (Licameli et al., 2009; Psillas et al., 2014; Xu et al., 2015; Jacot et al., 2009).

Post-implantation histopathological evidence indicates that Saccule is the most commonly affected structure, possibly due to its proximity to the Cochlea (Handzel et al., 2006; Tien & Linthicum, 2002). The histopathological findings have been supported by numerous studies which showed post-implantation changes more often in cVEMPs than oVEMPs (Bayat et al., 2020; Jin et al., 2006; Mohamed et al., 2024; Parkes et al., 2017; Wang et al., 2022; Xu et al., 2015; Imai et al., 2019).

Another area of concern is whether the current spread to the vestibular structures could interfere with the vestibular function when the implant is operational. In order to find evidence for this, a few studies have investigated VEMPs when the cochlear implant is switched-on and compared the findings against the findings when the cochlear implant was switched-off. They have consistently reported increased response rates, reduced asymmetry ratios, and higher amplitudes in the CI switched-on condition than the CI switched-off condition. The device switched-on condition witnesses an improvement of 30–50% over the device switched-off condition (Jin et al., 2008; Li & Gong, 2020). However, high variability in these results was observed in follow-up studies (Li & Gong, 2020).

Following cochlear implantation, acute surgical trauma may lead to initial vestibular symptoms that typically resolve after a few days. Numerous studies have investigated the recovery time of vestibular function post-implantation, yielding varied results (Ajalloueyan et al., 2017; Dhondt et al., 2022; Guan et al., 2021; Li & Gong, 2020; Psillas et al., 2014; Thierry et al., 2015). In a comprehensive study, Li and Gong (2020) investigated the recovery of post-implantation VEMPs over a period of 2 months, with intervention points being 5 days, 1 month, and 2 months after cochlear implantation. The pre-implantation response rates of oVEMP and cVEMP were 81.4% and 91.4%, respectively. At the 5-days post-implantation point, the response rates of oVEMPs decreased to 37.1% whereas cVEMP's response rates plummeted to 68.6%. After 1 month, oVEMPs were observed in 34.6% while cVEMPs were found in 72% of ears. At the 2 months post-CI follow up, oVEMPs were identified in 36% while cVEMPs were seen in 80% of ears. The authors concluded that a minimum recovery period of 2 months is necessary to stabilize vestibular responses post-implantation. More recent studies have found no discernible post-implantation change in VEMPs in children aged 6–11 months (Gerdsen et al., 2022; Mohamed et al., 2024). Our experience in this regard has the largest post-implant follow-up duration over a 7 years period, including the pre-implantation assessment. We followed-up 29 children, all of whom had a bilaterally present cVEMP preoperatively, thereby showing a 100% response rate before undergoing unilateral cochlear implantation. The post-implantation intervention points were post-implantation day 21, day 120–130 (about 4 months after the device activation) and day 2190–2300 (6–6.5 years after implantation), which yielded response rates of 59%, 52% and 66% respectively in the implant ears and 97%, 90% and 90% respectively in the non-implant ears. We would like to share some interesting findings that came along the way during these 7 years. In nearly 40% children, cVEMPs in the implant ears disappeared at some point before the first post-implantation follow-up investigation, most probably immediately after the surgery, and never reappeared in majority of them. A small percentage of these patients showed recovery of VEMP responses by 4 months or somewhere down the line before the 6-years follow-up point. Among those with the post-implantation presence of cVEMP, these potentials were lost by 4 months in a few and even a smaller minority after 4 months post-implantation. This suggests that the loss of VEMPs is not necessarily an immediate effect of a surgical trauma. Post-implantation inflammatory changes, and in a much longer run, the fibrosis within the Saccule may influence cVEMPs. Interestingly though, nearly 10% of children lost cVEMPs in their non-implant ears, especially in the period between 4 months and 6 years, despite only 3% losing them by post-implantation day 21. While we do not know the precise reasons for such late onset changes in the non-implant ears, we speculate that slow degenerative changes may have been initiated by massive drilling of the skull, and the strong vibrations were probably efficiently transmitted to the non-implant side's inner ear, leading to degenerative changes in a few non-implant ears over time. Alternatively, it might even be due to unknown progressive inner ear conditions, which probably may have occurred even if these children were not implanted.

While a majority of studies on post-implantation cVEMP have focussed on response prevalence (response rate) and amplitude, a few sporadic studies have also investigated the effect of cochlear implantation on the thresholds of VEMP. Abdelghaffar and Elshazly (2011) reported a post-implantation response rate of about 22%, and in those with a present cVEMP, its threshold ranged between 90 and 100 dBnHL. Later, Xu et al. (2015) reported a post-CI increase in cVEMP threshold by up to 8 dB SPL.

Comparison of Post-implantation VEMP Between Various Surgical Approaches

As you will recall from Chapter 13, cochlear implantation is done using two major approaches, one involving mastoidectomy to reach the middle ear (mastoidectomy approach) and the other using canal wall lifting to approach the middle ear (Veria technique). Slight variations of these, for example, use of cochleostomy for electrode insertion in to scala tympani or insertion through the round window following mastoidectomy, do exist. Different surgical techniques could be associated with different degrees of risk for damage to the surrounding structures, vestibular system being one among them. Therefore, developing knowledge base to understand the differences in impact of cochlear implantation on the vestibular periphery is crucial. Singh et al. (2021) compared the effects of the mastoidectomy (mastoidectomy followed by posterior tympanotomy and cochleostomy) approach and Veria technique on cVEMP in children aged 3–8 years. Post-implantation loss of cVEMP was found in nearly 40%, irrespective of the surgery technique, despite the presence of bilateral cVEMP preoperatively in all of them. Among those with the presence of cVEMP in the post-implantation evaluation, amplitudes were notably lower during switch-on and at the 4-month follow-up, again irrespective of the technique of surgery. Nonetheless, participants undergoing CI using mastoidectomy had significantly larger post-surgery cVEMP amplitudes than those using the Veria technique. This suggests that the mastoidectomy technique may better preserve saccular responses during CI surgery compared to the veria technique. Similarly, several studies suggest that the round window technique may be more effective in preserving otolithic function compared to the cochleostomy technique (Todt et al., 2008;

Krause et al., 2009). Although the above studies show alarming rates of abnormality after cochlear implantation, a common pitfall in all these studies is the use of air-conduction stimuli to elicit VEMPs. It is well known that the middle ear dynamics changes during and after cochlear implantation, some emanating from the surgical exploration of the middle with potential contribution from the increase in mechanical impedance due to electrode insertion within the cochlea (Hartl et al., 2016; Koka et al., 2017). This can lead to an increase in the air-bone gap, demonstrable even on the post-implantation audiogram (Hartl et al., 2016; Koka et al., 2017). Given the small dynamic range (115–125 dB peSPL) within which the air-conduction VEMPs operate (Janky & Shepard, 2009; Rodriguez et al., 2019), especially due to concerns with stimulus level safety (Singh et al., 2019; Krause et al., 2013; Strömberg et al., 2016), the increase in the air-bone gap by as little as 5–10 dB could obscure the VEMP responses. This could cloud the drawn inferences, making them error prone, despite an intact otolith system. Therefore, special caution is advised when evaluating VEMPs due to potential iatrogenic changes in middle ear structures post-implantation (Merchant et al., 2020). The higher frequency of cVEMP impact may stem from the surgical changes in the middle ear post-implantation that might cause conductive hearing loss (Melvin et al., 2009; Merchant et al., 2020). Hence, bone-conduction, which though has its own set of associated difficulties due to insufficient stimulus outputs from the commercially available bone vibrators, should be a more reliable option to predict the actual changes in saccular or utricular function after cochlear implantation.

Effect of the Mode of Stimulation on VEMP Findings After Cochlear Implantation

Owing to the above-discussed concerns about the use of air conduction VEMPs, recent studies have employed BC-VEMPs to evaluate otolithic damage following implantation. In their study of 73 CI ears, Dhondt et al. (2022) observed no significant impact of cochlear implantation on the amplitudes of bone conduction cVEMP (BC-cVEMP) but noted a significant reduction in ipsilateral N1 latency. In contrast, Kamath and Singh (2024) observed lower response rates and amplitudes of BC-cVEMP and BC-oVEMP in the implant ears than the non-implant ears after cochlear implantation. The response rates and amplitudes in the implant ears were also lower than the prospective cochlear implantees (children with sensorineural hearing loss who were candidates for CI but had not undergone surgery at the time of recording BC-VEMPs) and typically developing children with hearing and vestibular function within the normative limits. In a scoping review on air and bone conducted VEMPs, Ayas et al. (2024) noted that nearly 18% participants had a post-implantation change in asymmetry ratio by ≥30% on AC-cVEMPs as opposed to only about 8% demonstrating such a change on BC-cVEMP. While it is apparent that BC-VEMPs are less often affected than AC-VEMPs, there is considerable difference in the findings on BC-VEMPs among the studies, which makes it difficult to draw a conclusion about the extent of post-implantation otolith damage. Nonetheless, there is no doubting the potential of BC-VEMPs in deciphering a more realistic extent of cochlear implantation-inflicted otolith damage than AC-VEMPs.

In our clinical experience, BC-VEMPs are more reliable and effective for assessing post-implantation otolith function in children. We have observed an increased response rate, higher amplitude, and reduced asymmetry ratio in BC-cVEMPs and BC-oVEMPs compared to the corresponding AC-VEMPs. Moreover, we have also found a stronger correlation between PBS scores and abnormality on BC-VEMPs than on AC-VEMPs in children with cochlear implants. Therefore, BC-VEMPs have the potential to become a predictive measure for post-implantation behavioural balance function. Figure 21.2 illustrates the VEMP responses obtained using AC and BC stimulation in children with CIs, demonstrating the reduced asymmetry and increased amplitude. As we can appreciate from the waveforms, a clear asymmetry is seen for AC-VEMPs, while BC-VEMPs, both cVEMP and oVEMP, show normal responses. Absent BC responses offer confirmation of otolith dysfunction, whereas an absent AC-VEMP can leave us in jeopardy regarding whether the result is an indication of a vestibular dysfunction or emanates from changes in the middle ear impedance characteristics.

The electric stimulation via cochlear implants can also be used to evoke VEMPs. Parkes et al. (2017), although not exclusively on the paediatric population, investigated vestibular potentials in 53 CI recipients (8 unilateral, 38 bilateral sequential, and 7 bilateral simultaneous cochlear implantation) aged 7–27 years. An acoustic cVEMP was detected in 47% as opposed to electrical cVEMP in 35% implanted ears. Additionally, an acoustic oVEMP was elicited in 26% and electrical oVEMP in 35% implanted ears. In the ears non-responsive to acoustic stimuli, electrically evoked cVEMPs and oVEMPs were present in 27% and 25% ears, respectively. Further, electric VEMPs exhibited 2–3 ms shorter peak latencies than the corresponding acoustic VEMPs. While these findings suggest that electrical stimulation increases the response rate, further replication of this study is needed for conclusive inferences.

From the discussion above, it is apparent that there is considerable variability among the studies; nonetheless, loss of VEMP responses and reduction in their amplitude appears to show agreement among over 80% of studies. Emerging areas of work, such as BC-VEMPs and electrically evoked VEMPs, offer new avenues for the exploration of vestibular functioning in children post-implantation. However, current data sets are either too scanty for a worthy conclusion or do not align with each other to provide reliable conclusion in this regard. The vestibular health of the cochlear implantees must be monitored over a long period after the surgery to identify late onset changes.

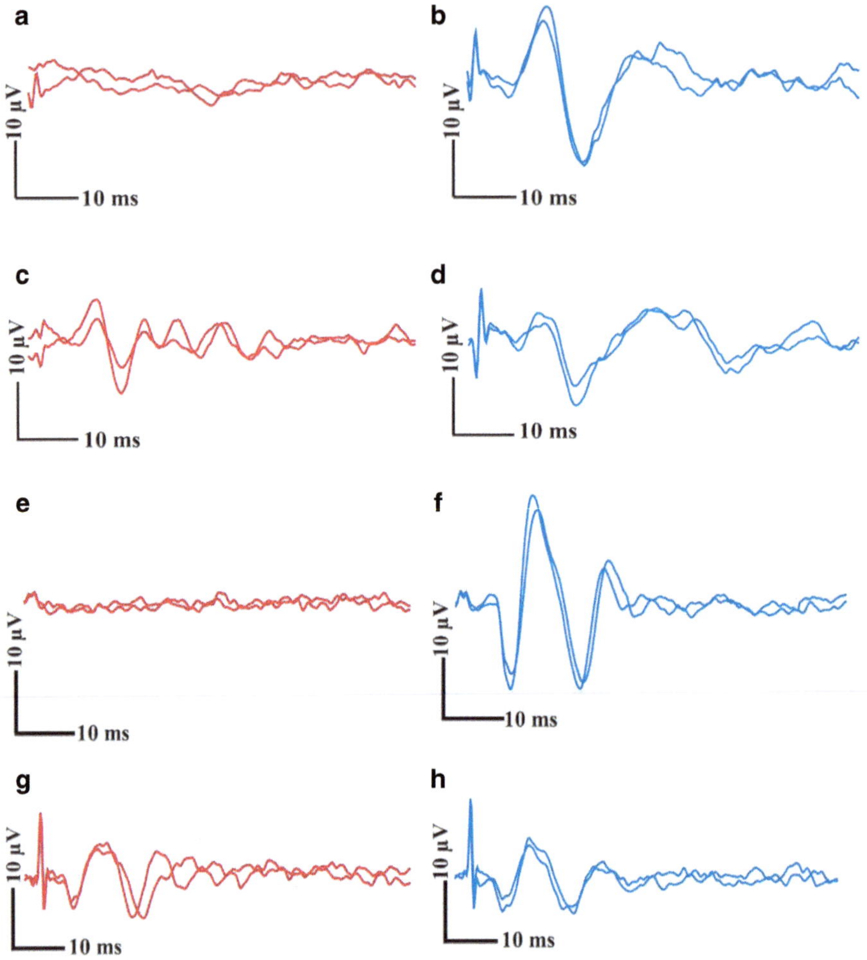

Fig. 21.2 The representative waveform of (**a**) AC-cVEMP in implant ear, (**b**) AC-cVEMP in non-implant ear, (**c**) BC-cVEMP in implant ear, (**d**) BC-cVEMP in non-implant ear, (**e**) AC-oVEMP in implant ear, (**f**) AC-oVEMP in non-implant ear, (**g**) BC-oVEMP in implant ear, (**h**) BC-oVEMP in non-implant ear

Assessment of Vestibulo-Ocular Reflex in Paediatric Cochlear Implantees

The section on adults with cochlear implantation has shown that vHIT, caloric test and Rotational chair test can give us a comprehensive assessment of VOR function before and after cochlear implantation. However, the complexity of use of these measures in children is further complicated by issues related to their development, both due to the physical ability to undergo a given test and the maturational aspects affecting the test outcomes. This section delves into the clinical findings of various tools to assess VOR in children before and after cochlear implantation.

Video Head Impulse Test (vHIT)

vHIT requires a child to sit with head erect, and therefore, it is not possible to administer this test until the child has achieved sitting, at least with support. Typically, this is achieved earliest by 6 months. Hence, vHIT should not be considered for children younger than 6 months of age. At present, children younger than 9 months are not being considered for cochlear implantation, and therefore, all children could be easily evaluated even preoperatively for their VOR assessment using vHIT, unless a child is developmentally delayed to an extent that sitting has not been acquired at the time of pre-implant evaluation. While histopathological evidence suggests that semicircular canals have little chance of being affected by the cochlear implantation surgery, some studies have observed post-implantation changes in vHIT (Dhondt et al., 2022; Janky & Patterson, 2020; Verrecchia et al., 2020). On the contrary, other studies found no significant post-implantation change in VOR gain or refixation saccades (Guan et al., 2021; Nassif et al., 2016; Dhondt et al., 2022; Janky & Patterson, 2020; Verrecchia et al., 2020).

Dhondt et al. (2022) reported ipsilateral loss of semicircular canal function in 5% ear after cochlear implantation. Long-term follow-up studies, such as that by Nassif et al. (2021), observed no significant long-term impact of unilateral and simultaneous/sequential bilateral cochlear implantation on the outcomes of vHIT, highlighting vHIT's reliability in children undergoing cochlear implantation. Janky and Patterson (2020) and Verrecchia et al. (2020) suggested that vHIT has a potential to be used as a primary screening test for VOR changes. Further, Strupp et al. (2017) noted that vHIT was beneficial in deciding the ear for implantation in children who demonstrated typical rotary chair responses on both sides and normal VOR gain on vHIT on one side but abnormally reduced gain on the other side.

We believe that vHIT could be an excellent tool for observing changes in VOR after cochlear implantation. The group data analysis in the way of some of the previous studies might be of little help as not all children show deficiencies in VOR after cochlear implantation. An example to prove our point is shown is Fig. 21.3. As can be seen in Fig. 21.3, the child had a bilateral normal VOR with no evidence of refixation saccades pre-operatively. The post-operative vHIT results show reduced VOR gain and presence of refixation saccades in the implant (left) ear, but no significant change in the non-implant (right) ear almost a month after the surgery (1 week after the device activation). After another 4 months, the VOR gain continues to be low with the presence of refixation saccades in the implant ear whereas the non-implant ear continues to maintain its pre-implant status. A close attention to the characteristics of the refixation saccades is an important take away from this case example. While the refixation saccades were largely scattered at the first post-implantation measurement and had a high latency, the ones at the 4-month follow-up show more clustered refixation saccades with shorter latencies than before. These changes are typically signs of central compensation against a unilateral vestibular damage, which in this case occurred during the cochlear implantation. Therefore, vHIT has not only the potential to show a post-implantation VOR dysfunction/hypofunction, it also has the potential to show long term compensatory changes, which might

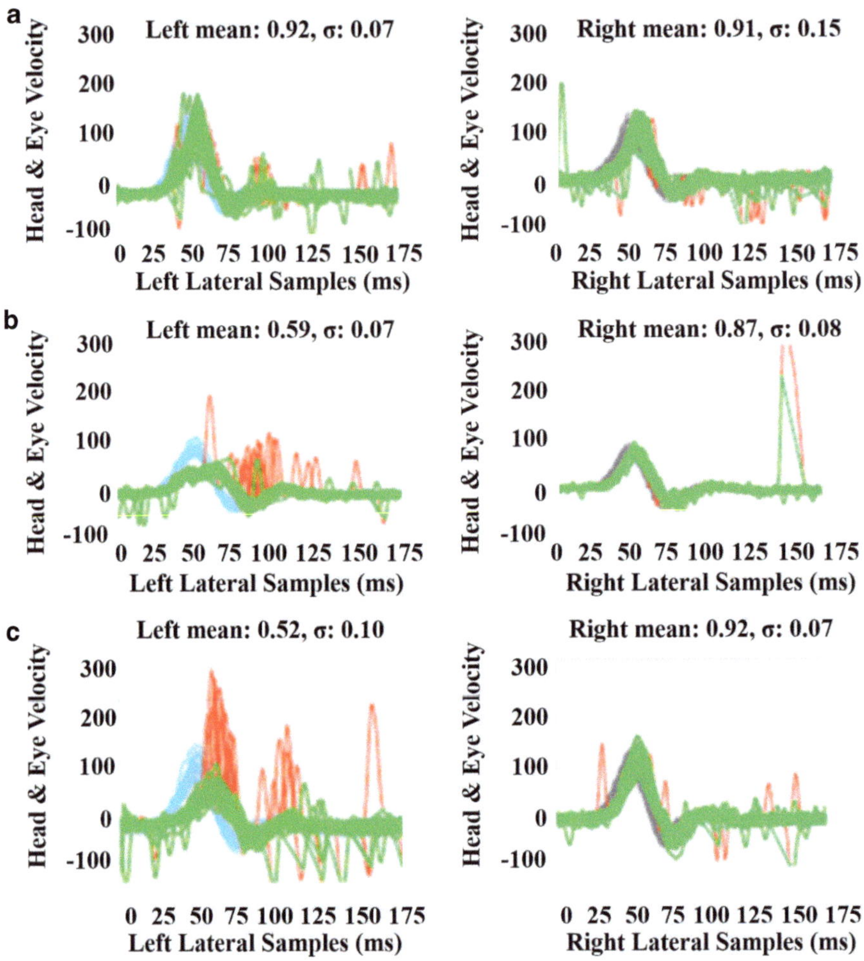

Fig. 21.3 Lateral canal vHIT results of a 4 years old child who underwent unilateral cochlear implantation in left ear; (**a**) pre-implantation vHIT; (**b**) post-implantation vHIT after a week of device activation; (**c**) post-implantation vHIT after 4 months of device activation

prove vital when documenting improvements when such children undergo active vestibular rehabilitation after cochlear implantation.

Similar to VEMPs, vHIT was assessed in cochlear implant users under different device conditions (switched-on or switched-off, with and without a sound input). Nassif et al. (2016) evaluated VOR using vHIT on 16 children (12 unilateral CI and 4 bilateral CI) aged 5–17 years. They observed significantly higher lateral canal VOR gain in both ears of unilaterally implanted children when the device was switched-on than when it was switched-off. However, this kind of a difference between the device switched-on and switched-off conditions was not observed in bilateral cochlear implantees. The authors suggested that the spread of excitation of electrodes in the basal turn of the cochlea, which are closest to the vestibule, may reach the vestibular labyrinth, potentially leading to an increase in VOR gain generated in the lateral semicircular canals. In a study from our lab, we observed an increase in refixation saccades when children using unilateral cochlear implant underwent lateral canal vHIT within a sound field of 80 dB SPL (Singh et al., 2016), likely due to current spread to Scarpa's ganglion. This suggests that vHIT could aid in determining C-levels, especially during initial mapping sessions when children cannot communicate vestibular symptoms voluntarily. Therefore, vHIT could play a crucial role in assessing semicircular canal function in children after cochlear implantation.

Caloric Testing

The caloric test, among all tests of VOR assessment, is probably the least tolerated test by children. Multiple water/air irrigations with varying temperature gradients make this test difficult to administer, especially below the age of 5–6 years. Adding to the difficulty is the time taken to complete this test, which is much longer than a vHIT or a rotational chair test. Achieving children's cooperation for about 30 minutes at a stretch is not easy, and this is the minimum duration a caloric test will require even in the most co-operative child. Therefore, most of the studies on caloric test findings before and/or after cochlear implantation are done on older, more co-operative children. Most of the studies on caloric test findings in children focus the analyses of unilateral weakness, although a few studies employed slow phase velocity due to its alignment with unilateral gain values of the vHIT and corrected amplitudes of the cervical vestibular-evoked myogenic potential (cVEMP). This approach is particularly relevant for simultaneous bilateral CI patients; as unilateral weakness assessment may be impractical. Another practical consideration could be to switch to monothermal caloric test to save time and achieve cooperation from more children. Among the studies using caloric test to investigate the lateral canal function, several studies have shown a negative impact of cochlear implantation on caloric responses (Devroede et al., 2016; Gupta & Raj, 2018; Jacot et al., 2009). On the contrary others reported no significant post-implantation change in caloric test results (Ajalloueyan et al., 2017; Dhondt et al., 2022).

Several studies have observed ipsilateral dwindling in response to caloric irrigation following unilateral cochlear implantation. Gupta and Raj (2018) conducted pre- and post-implantation assessments using monothermal caloric stimulation and noted post-implantation canal paresis in 15% (5/23) children, which included three post-implantation novel occurrences leading to an increased rate of post-implantation monothermal caloric asymmetry. Similar findings were reported by Devroede et al. (2016), where post-implantation changes in the caloric responses were observed in 32% children. The observed changes included decreased reactions, increased reactions possibly due to canal hyperexcitability, and absent reactions in some cases. Jacot et al. (2009) also observed varying vestibular responses in their study of 71 cases, with some patients showing no dysfunction while others exhibited complete ipsilateral areflexia or a statistically significant decrease or increase in the canal vestibulo-ocular reflex. Ice water caloric test was also used and found pathological in 14.3% and 11.4% in one of the studies (Verrecchia et al., 2020). In independent studies, Ajalloueyan et al. (2017) and Dhondt et al. (2022) reported no significant post-implantation change in caloric test findings in 13 and 10 children, respectively. These findings highlight the variability in semicircular canal damage post-implantation.

Among the studies administering caloric test as well as vHIT, abnormality on only one of these two tests have been found in a few children (Verrecchia et al., 2020). Therefore, a caloric test cannot be substituted by a lateral canal vHIT. The caloric testing may be more sensitive in detecting changes at an earlier stage, and in any case represents an entirely different frequency range to the vHIT. Hence, it is imperative to carefully choose, administer, and interpret caloric test pre- and post-implantation to accurately assess low frequency VOR dysfunction following the surgery.

Rotatory Chair Test

Rotatory chair testing (RCT) is probably the most easily administered test among the tests of VOR assessment in children, especially in children below 2 years of age. In fact, several children enjoy being swung in alternate directions. The challenge emanates from accurate positioning of the child in the chair, especially for very young children who cannot sit independently in the chair and therefore are seated in the parent or caregiver's lap, who in turn sits in the chair. In such cases, it is important to achieve a position of the child such that the earth-fixed vertical axis around which the rotation occurs passes right through the centre of the child's head. This is possible to achieve through careful seating of the parent or caregiver deep into the chair. However, if this aspect is not carefully dealt with, it could be a source for erroneous and variable outcomes. Similar to other assessments, there is variability in findings of RCT, with some researchers reporting no changes while others have observed alterations.

In a study involving 89 children with cochlear implantation, Jacot et al. (2009) reported no significant alteration for group as a whole despite the finding of vestibular dysfunction in other tests, including the caloric test. Similar results were noted by Dhondt et al. (2022). In contrast, Imai et al. (2019) observed changes in the RCT results in two out of 12 children. One child exhibited a decreased VOR gain, while another showed an increased gain after implantation. These tests were conducted at various intervals after surgery, spanning up to 7 years. Similarly, Shinjo et al. found that 70% of their 20 paediatric cochlear implant recipients exhibited normal responses during rotation in both directions. One patient had normal responses in one direction but poor responses in the opposite direction. Two patients had poor responses in both directions, and three showed no response in any direction.

In a recent study, Talaat et al. (2021) assessed the averaged gain and phase in children after cochlear implantation. They found significant differences in averaged gain at 0.02 Hz, while phase showed significant differences only at the low frequency of 0.01 Hz. Similarly, Dhondt et al. (2022) reported a significant postoperative deterioration of gain and phase measured at 0.04 Hz but not at 0.16 Hz rotations. These results suggest that lower-frequency (among the mid frequencies) semicircular canal function may be more susceptible to physiological changes in the inner ear following cochlear implantation. Although these findings align with those seen in adults, there is still a lack of comprehensive evaluation of these findings. Therefore, the extent of vestibular dysfunction after CI and the optimal test protocol for its assessment remains unclear. A test battery approach may provide clearer insights.

Quality of Life

The presence of vestibular dysfunction in children undergoing cochlear implantation can have far-reaching consequences beyond simple imbalance and reduced visual acuity. These issues can impede their ability to perform daily activities, ultimately diminishing their quality of life. While studies have documented reduced quality of life in adults with post-implantation vestibular dysfunction, similar investigations focusing on children are lacking.

Impact of Unrecognised Post-implantation Vestibular Dysfunction

From the discussion in all the above sections, it has become apparent that a post-implantation vestibular dysfunction is a reality; however, its extent within an individual and its incidence may vary due to several undiscovered factors, including the differences in testing and surgeons' expertise. Sometimes a patient does not have an overt manifestation of vestibular symptoms; however, the underlying vestibular hypofunction may still hamper him/her in more than one ways. The presence of post-implantation vestibular dysfunction in children can have far-reaching consequences beyond mere imbalance and reduced visual acuity. This short sub-section describes the repercussions of an unidentified post-implantation vestibular dysfunction in cochlear implantees, some specific to children or adults and some common to both age groups.

Motor Deficits

Keeping in mind the need for maximum availability of the sensitivity period that allows the best outcomes from auditory rehabilitation, the age of implantation in children is being increasingly brought down. The present FDA approval allows for implantation at 12 months or higher age. Nevertheless, several teams across the globe have successfully done cochlear implantation even at 9 months of age. During such young ages, the critical motor developments are still taking place. Literature is brimming with studies showing a significant association between vestibular dysfunction and delay in the achievement of motor milestones. Several studies have also shown vestibular dysfunction in cochlear implantees. Therefore, as mentioned in the section on symptoms of vestibular dysfunction post-CI in children, gross motor deficits resulting in delayed motor milestones in early implanted children with post-implantation vestibular dysfunction is a plausible finding (De Kegel et al., 2015). However, this hypothesis requires substantiation and findings will start emerging as more and more children undergo implantation within 12 months of age.

Increased Risk of Falls

A risk of fall is always lingering when a person develops a unilateral or bilateral vestibular dysfunction, with bilateral dysfunction increasing the risk of falls more than a unilateral one. Although the risk of falls is not specific to any age group, its impact could be variable across the age groups. Particularly, older adults could have an increased risk of falls, more so than young adults and children. A study reported a threefold higher risk of falls after cochlear implantation, especially in the first few days following surgery, despite a normal preoperative balance function (Stevens et al., 2014). However, these findings have not always been supported by other studies. While some studies have highlighted that the fall risk at the pre-implant stage is higher than the normal cohort, and though there is an increase in post-implantation risk of falls (1.25%), it was not statistically significant (Louza et al., 2018). Recently, Grimm et al. (2022) calculated the number of falls causing healthcare expenditure pre- and post-CI surgery in older adults, for a duration of 1 year on either side. They observed no significant increase in the number of falls requiring a medical expenditure. These observations do not confirm no increase in the falls, rather they suggest that the unrecognised vestibular loss might increase the fall risk, yet, the falls may not have been on the extreme end of the fall severity spectrum to necessitate hospital admission and medical expenditure. An increase in risk of falls even by a slight amount could be important to identify in older adults as even a single fall could land a severe blow to their quality of life, given the higher odds of hip fractures in this age group.

The risk of fall in children could have a different spectrum of impact. Our clinical experience suggests that children with vestibular dysfunction post-implantation have an increased risk of falls, especially while walking on uneven surfaces and in darkness, the situations in which a robust compensation does not typically occur due to lack of repeated exposure to such conditions. This is typically expressed during the post-implantation parental interviews.

Increased Likelihood of Hard Device Failure

The escalated imbalance and number of falls can have a major contribution to hard device failure (Cullen et al., 2008). According to Wolter et al. (2015), a higher proportion of CI children who experienced device failure also showed poor behavioral balance, horizontal canal dysfunction, and/or saccular dysfunction. There was a 7.6 times increase in the probability of device failure if the child was to have an absence of bilateral horizontal canal function. In the last 1 year, we have noted device failures following a fall in 1 out of 6 unilateral implantees with a bilateral vestibular loss found in the post-implant evaluation 2–3 weeks before the fall occurred. The pre-implant evaluation for vestibular function was not done in these 6 children. While it is speculative at best to assume that this child with a hard device failure had a preexisting congenital unilateral vestibular dysfunction and during the implantation process, the good ear (the ear with at least a residual vestibular function) lost its function. Alternatively, this child might have had a congenital bilateral vestibular dysfunction, leading to greater fall risk. Nonetheless, the parents reported increased instances of falls and stumbling behaviours after cochlear implantation, which suggests that the former scenario has a higher likelihood. The choice of ear could have been decided on the basis of pre-implant vestibular function assessment; unfortunately, it was not. This underscores the importance of thorough pre- and post-implantation evaluation and counselling regarding post-implantation care, especially considering the potential challenges in maintaining costly devices in children, compounded by a higher fall risk.

Cognitive Deficits

The research evidence gathered over the past two decades has highlighted the intricate connections between vestibular functioning and cognitive abilities, alongside the well-established link between hearing abilities and cognition. Several animal and human studies evaluating the effects of vestibular dysfunction on cognitive skills have found structural and functional deterioration, indicating cognitive decline secondary to vestibular dysfunction (Kremmyda et al., 2016; Bigelow & Agrawal, 2015; Gurvich et al., 2013; Smith & Zheng, 2013). Recent investigations have also found links between vestibular deficits and cognitive disorders like Alzheimer's disease (Bigelow & Agrawal, 2015; Yoon et al., 2020). Disruptions in vestibular inputs have emerged as potential contributors to cognitive deficits, particularly in visuospatial skills, executive functions, attention, and memory. While hypotheses linking the two have been proposed and supported by various studies, research on cochlear implantees with vestibular impairments remains limited. While there is scarcity of studies showing direct implications of the post-implantation vestibular deficits on the cognitive functioning in adults, the likelihood of the same cannot be eliminated, given the evidence supporting strong association between vestibular dysfunction and cognition in adult patients, albeit not in cochlear implantees. An inference in this regard can be drawn from a study by Tonini et al. (2019) who evaluated four patients with bilateral cochlear implants on balance conditions, including Romberg tests on medium-density compliant foam with eyes closed, with head stationary or moving in yaw or pitch plane. They carried out the investigation under different sound conditions ranging from no sound to delivery of foreign language stimuli. Head movements deteriorated when foreign-language or English words were presented. The sound condition did not influence standing balance skills, but when distractions were words, standing balance skills deteriorated only in adults with implants. Thus, distracted attention in adults post-CI can impair balance, not generally seen in adults without CI (Tonini et al., 2019). This indirectly implies compromised working memory and ability to perform dual tasking in individuals post-CI, likely due to vestibular deficits leading to secondary cognitive decline.

Cognition is important for all age groups; however, it is particularly important in children as it aids in the development of speech and language. Therefore, the possibility of post-implantation vestibular dysfunction could have a significant bearing on the outcomes with the cochlear implant. Although not on children with cochlear implants, a study on children with vestibular dysfunction revealed impairments in visuospatial skills, working memory, and space orientation, although attention remained unaffected (Lacroix et al., 2020). However, the evidence on children with cochlear implants seems to somewhat refute the above-mentioned hypothesis and contradict it by showing no significant effect of vestibular dysfunction on memory or executive functions in children with cochlear implants, although behavioural balance had a significant association with cognitive skills (Janky et al., 2022). These differences may stem from variations in sample characteristics and the predominant characterization of vestibular function using vHIT responses from semicircular canals rather than the otolith organs. Our clinical experience shows a strong correlation between post-implantation vestibular dysfunction (poor performance on PBS and abnormal BC-cVEMP) and cognitive abilities, particularly in visuospatial skills, memory, and executive functions. We have observed significantly poorer post-implantation non-verbal cognition in children who had a post-implantation vestibular dysfunction than in those without a post-implantation vestibular dysfunction. The cognitive deficits in children with a post-implantation vestibular dysfunction are particularly pronounced within the first 15 months of cochlear implantation. As the time since implantation increases, other factors, such as recovery and central compensation of the lost peripheral function, probably contribute to concealing of this difference. This underscores the importance of early identification and intervention in children with vestibular deficits to prevent potential impacts on cognitive skills and overall quality of life.

Speech and Language Deficits

Recent research indicates that speech perception skills and the vestibular system are directly related (Himi et al., 1997; Emami et al., 2012). Himi et al. (1997) found poorer speech recognition of consonants in adult CI users with caloric abnormality (areflexia). Further, consonant recognition correlated with distance of body sway on posturography. According to research on children with CI, behavioral balance is associated with cognitive ability (Janky et al., 2022). In their long-term study of language development and motor skills in children with language impairment, Sack et al. (2022) discovered that the cohort's long-term language skills were more accurately predicted by gross and fine motor skills. As cognition is essential to processing and comprehending auditory information, cognitive impairments can also impact how CI users perceive speech; and their speech and language development.

Self-concept

It is hypothesized that children with vestibular dysfunction might exhibit reduced self-concept beyond that associated with hearing loss, likely due to balance and visual acuity deficits (Janky et al., 2023). However, this study found that, on average, the self-concept scores of children post-implantation resembled those of children with normal hearing sensitivity. Interestingly, auditory-language factors such as speech perception and vocabulary predicted self-concept, while vestibular dysfunction did not significantly contribute to self-concept in children with cochlear implants. This suggests that children with vestibular dysfunction may not be fully aware that their symptoms are abnormal, influencing their self-perception. Nonetheless, it is plausible that the findings of the study were affected by high implant age (age since implantation), which may have led to central compensation, obscuring the vestibular effects on self-concept. We believe that children with cochlear implants have lower self-concept, as also shown by another study (Bantwal et al., 2021), and we have reasons to believe that vestibular dysfunction has a role to play in it, provided the effect is examined before a significant central compensation creeps in.

Now that we have discussed the findings of major vestibular tests, it is necessary to acknowledge the variable nature of test outcomes and the limitations of these tests. The variability among studies represents differences in methodology, criteria for defining normal/abnormal results, and variations in testing techniques, along with patient variables. In general, a statement can be made that CI surgery definitely has a greater impact on the VEMPs and caloric tests, mainly pointing towards damage to otoliths—majorly the Saccule and low-frequency response of the lateral semicircular canal (Guan et al., 2021). However, these tests have their own limitations. Air conduction VEMPs are abnormal not merely in presence of an otolith deficit but also in presence of a mere middle ear alteration. The calorics are affected by the temporal bone anatomy which is variable amongst patients and altered as a consequence of CI surgery (Ibrahim et al., 2017). The CI surgery has unique consequences on the vestibular apparatus in each individual. The horizontal canal function assessed using various methodologies, studied by Piker et al. (2020), led to the understanding that each individual might present with a unique finding. While statistical analysis failed to show any difference, the descriptive analysis yielded a post-CI vestibular abnormality in 30% individuals. Moreover, a case-by-case analysis revealed a deterioration in vestibular function in only one patient. Understanding each individual separately and using a battery of tests for understanding the vestibular function might help understand the individualistic changes post-CI.

References

Abdelghaffar, H., & Elshazly, M. (2011). Cochlear implants in children with vestibular hypofunction. *Egyptian Journal of Ear, Nose, Throat and Allied Sciences, 12*, 49–52.

Abramides, P. A., Bittar, R. S. M., Tsuji, R. K., & Bento, R. F. (2015). Caloric test as a predictor tool of postural control in CI users. *Acta Oto-Laryngologica, 135*(7), 685–691.

Ajalloueyan, M., Saeedi, M., Sadeghi, M., & Zamiri Abdollahi, F. (2017). The effects of cochlear implantation on vestibular function in 1-4 years old children. *International Journal of Pediatric Otorhinolaryngology, 94*, 100–103.

Ajallouyean, M., Amirsalari, S., Yousefi, J., Raeesi, M. A., Radfar, S., & Hassanalifard, M. (2011). A repot of surgical complications in a series of 262 consecutive pediatric cochlear implantations in Iran. *Iranian Journal of Pediatrics, 21*(4), 455–460.

Andries, E., Gilles, A., Topsakal, V., Vanderveken, O., Van de Heyning, P., Van Rompaey, V., & Mertens, G. (2022). The impact of cochlear implantation on health-related quality of life in older adults, measured with the Health Utilities Index Mark 2 and Mark 3. *European Archives of Oto-Rhino-Laryngology: official journal of the European Federation of Oto-Rhino-Laryngological Societies (EUFOS) : affiliated with the German Society for Oto-Rhino-Laryngology - Head and Neck Surgery, 279*(2), 739–750.

Arnvig, J. (1955). Vestibular function in deafness and severe hardness of hearing. *Acta Oto-Laryngologica, 45*(4), 283–288.

Ayas, M., Muzaffar, J., Phillips, V., Smith, M. E., Borsetto, D., & Bance, M. L. (2024). Effect of cochlear implantation on air conduction and bone conduction elicited vestibular evoked myogenic potentials—A scoping review. *Journal of Clinical Medicine, 13*(22), 6996.

Bantwal, A. R., Deshpande, R., Indurkar, R., Bhatnagar, S., Wadhera, M., Sridhara, A., Lalwani, N., Agarwal, A., Oza, R. K., Narayan, N., Sasidharan, P., Mallikarjun, B., Saha, C., Bhale, P., Deshpande, S., & Mandke, K. (2021). A study of self-perception and communication success as perceived by adolescents with cochlear implants and their significant others. *Cochlear Implants International, 22*, 203–215.

Basta, D., Todt, I., Goepel, F., & Ernst, A. (2008). Loss of saccular function after cochlear implantation: The diagnostic impact of Intracochlear electrically elicited vestibular evoked myogenic potentials. *Audiology and Neurotology, 13*(3), 187–192.

Batuecas-Caletrio, A., Klumpp, M., Santacruz-Ruiz, S., Gonzalez, F. B., Sánchez, E. G., & Arriaga, M. (2015). Vestibular function in cochlear implantation: Correlating objectiveness and subjectiveness. *The Laryngoscope, 125*(10), 2371–2375.

Baudhuin, J. L. (2008). *Balance function following cochlear implantation*. Independent Studies and Capstones. Paper 173. Program in Audiology and Communication Sciences, Washington University School of Medicine.

Bayat, A., Farhadi, M., Emamdjomeh, H., Nadimi, Z., Mirmomeni, G., & Saki, N. (2020). Influence of cochlear implantation on balance function in pediatrics. *The International Tinnitus Journal, 24*(1), xxx–xx.

Bigelow, R. T., & Agrawal, Y. (2015). Vestibular involvement in cognition: Visuospatial ability, attention, executive function, and memory. *Journal of Vestibular Research, 25*(2), 73–89.

Bigelow, R. T., Semenov, Y. R., Trevino, C., Ferrucci, L., Resnick, S. M., Simonsick, E. M., Xue, Q. L., & Agrawal, Y. (2015). Association between visuospatial ability and vestibular function in the Baltimore longitudinal study of aging. *Journal of the American Geriatrics Society, 63*(9), 1837–1844.

Birman, C. S., Gibson, W. P. R., & Elliott, E. J. (2015). Pediatric cochlear implantation. *Otology & Neurotology, 36*(2), 220–222.

Bittar, R. S. M., Sato, E., Ribeiro, D. J. S., Oiticica, J., Grasel, S. S., Mezzalira, R., Tsuji, R. K., & Bento, R. F. (2019). Video head impulse test relevance in the early postoperative period after cochlear implantation. *Acta Oto-Laryngologica, 139*(1), 6–10.

Black, F. O., Simmons, F. B., & Iii, C. W. (1980). Human Vestibulo-spinal responses to direct electrical eighth nerve stimulation. *Acta Oto-Laryngologica, 90*(1–6), 86–92.

Bodmer, D., Shipp, D. B., Ostroff, J. M., Ng, A. H. C., Stewart, S., Chen, J. M., & Nedzelski, J. M. (2007). A comparison of postcochlear implantation speech scores in an adult population. *The Laryngoscope, 117*(8), 1408–1411.

Bogle, J. M. M. (2010). *The effect of cochlear implantation on the vestibular evoked myogenic potential response in children and adult participants*. Doctoral dissertation. University of Colorado at Boulder.

Bozkurt, H. K., Yarali, M., & Aksoy, S. (2022). Static and dynamic equilibrium and postural control in adults with cochlear implants. *Kulak Burun Boğaz ve Baş Boyun Cerrahisi Dergisi, 30*(4), 207–215.

Brey, R. H., Facer, G. W., Trine, M. B., Lynn, S. G., Peterson, A. M., & Suman, V. J. (1995). Vestibular effects associated with implantation of a multiple channel cochlear prosthesis. *Otology & Neurotology, 16*(4), 424–430.

Buchman, C. A., Joy, J., Hodges, A., Telischi, F. F., & Balkany, T. J. (2004). Vestibular effects of cochlear implantation. *The Laryngoscope, 114*(S103), 1–22.

Čakrt, O., Slabý, K., Kučerová, K., Balatková, Z., Jeřábek, J., & Bouček, J. (2024). Subjective visual vertical and postural control in patients following cochlear implantation. *Journal of Vestibular Research, 33*(6), 403–409.

Carmona, S., Marquez, R., & Zalazar, G. (2018). Vestibular function in adults and children with cochlear implant surgery. *Journal of Otolaryngology-ENT Research, 10*(6), 368–371.

Chadha, N. K., James, A. L., Gordon, K. A., Blaser, S., & Papsin, B. C. (2009). Bilateral cochlear implantation in children with anomalous cochleovestibular anatomy. *Archives of Otolaryngology–Head & Neck Surgery, 135*(9), 903.

Chen, X., Chen, X., Zhang, F., & Qin, Z. (2016). Influence of cochlear implantation on vestibular function. *Acta Oto-Laryngologica, 136*(7), 655–659.

Clark, G. M., Shepherd, R. K., Franz, B. K. H., Dowell, R. C., Tong, Y. C., Blamey, P. J., Webb, R. L., Pyman, B. C., McNaughtan, J., Bloom, D. M., Kakulas, B. A., & Siejka, S. (1988). The histopathology of the human temporal bone and auditory central nervous system following cochlear implantation in a patient: Correlation with psychophysics and speech perception results. *Acta Oto-Laryngologica, 105*(sup448), 1–65.

Clarke, A. H., Schönfeld, U., & Helling, K. (2003). Unilateral examination of utricle and saccule function. *Journal of Vestibular Research, 13*(4–6), 215–225.

Colin, V., Bertholon, P., Roy, S., & Karkas, A. (2018). Impact of cochlear implantation on peripheral vestibular function in adults. *European Annals of Otorhinolaryngology, Head and Neck Diseases, 135*(6), 417–420.

Coordes, A., Basta, D., Götze, R., Scholz, S., Seidl, R. O., Ernst, A., & Todt, I. (2012). Sound-induced vertigo after cochlear implantation. *Otology & Neurotology, 33*(3), 335–342.

Cullen, R. D., Fayad, J. N., Luxford, W. M., & Buchman, C. A. (2008). Revision cochlear implant surgery in children. *Otology & Neurotology, 29*(2), 214–220.

Cushing, S. L., Chia, R., James, A. L., Papsin, B. C., & Gordon, K. A. (2008). A test of static and dynamic balance function in children with cochlear implants. *Archives of Otolaryngology–Head & Neck Surgery, 134*(1), 34.

Cushing, S. L., Gordon, K. A., Rutka, J. A., James, A. L., & Papsin, B. C. (2013). Vestibular end-organ dysfunction in children with sensorineural hearing loss and cochlear implants. *Otology & Neurotology, 34*(3), 422–428.

Dagkiran, M., Tuncer, U., Surmelioglu, O., Tarkan, O., Ozdemir, S., Cetik, F., & Kiroglu, M. (2019). How does cochlear implantation affect five vestibular end-organ functions and dizziness? *Auris Nasus Larynx, 46*(2), 178–185.

Danielian, A., Ishiyama, G., Lopez, I. A., & Ishiyama, A. (2021). Predictors of fibrotic and bone tissue formation with 3-D reconstructions of post-implantation human temporal bones. *Otology & Neurotology, 42*(7), e942–e948.

de Castro Vaz, F., Petrus, L., Martins, W. R., de Castro Silva, I. M., Lima, J. A. O., da Silva Santos, N. M., Turri-Silva, N., & Bahmad, F., Jr. (2022). The effect of cochlear implant surgery on vestibular function in adults: A meta-analysis study. *Frontiers in Neurology, 13.*

De Kegel, A., Maes, L., Van Waelvelde, H., & Dhooge, I. (2015). Examining the impact of cochlear implantation on the early gross motor development of children with a hearing loss. *Ear & Hearing, 36*(3), e113–e121.

Deng, J., Zhu, Q., Zhang, K., Xie, D., & Wu, W. (2022). Vestibular function in children with cochlear implant: Impact and evaluation. *Frontiers in Neurology, 13.*

Devroede, B., Pauwels, I., Le Bon, S.-D., Monstrey, J., & Mansbach, A.-L. (2016). Interest of vestibular evaluation in sequentially implanted children: Preliminary results. *European Annals of Otorhinolaryngology, Head and Neck Diseases, 133*, S7–S11.

Dhondt, C., Maes, L., Vanaudenaerde, S., Martens, S., Rombaut, L., Van Hecke, R., Valette, R., Swinnen, F., & Dhooge, I. (2022). Changes in vestibular function following pediatric cochlear implantation: A prospective study. *Ear & Hearing, 43*(2), 620–630.

Dumas, G., Perrin, P., & Schmerber, S. (2008). Nystagmus induced by high frequency vibrations of the skull in total unilateral peripheral vestibular lesions. *Acta Oto-Laryngologica, 128*(3), 255–262.

Ebrahimi, A.-A., Movallali, G., Jamshidi, A.-A., Haghgoo, H. A., & Rahgozar, M. (2016). Balance performance of deaf children with and without cochlear implants. *Acta Medica Iranica, 54*(11), 737–742.

Emami, S. F., Pourbakht, A., Sheykholeslami, K., Kamali, M., Behnoud, F., & Daneshi, A. (2012). Vestibular hearing and speech processing. *ISRN Otolaryngology, 2012*, 1–7.

Enticott, J. C., Tari, S., Koh, S. M., Dowell, R. C., & O'Leary, S. J. (2006). Cochlear implant and vestibular function. *Otology & Neurotology, 27*(6), 824–830.

Eustaquio, M. E., Berryhill, W., Wolfe, J. A., & Saunders, J. E. (2011). Balance in children with bilateral cochlear implants. *Otology & Neurotology, 32*(3), 424–427.

Filipo, R., Patrizi, M., La Gamma, R., D'Elia, C., La Rosa, G., & Barbara, >Maurizio. (2006). Vestibular impairment and cochlear implantation. *Acta Oto-Laryngologica, 126*(12), 1266–1274.

Genovese, E., Segato, E., Liberale, C., Zampieri, E., Monzani, D., Apa, E., Palma, S., & Nocini, R. (2024). Congenital deafness and vestibular disorders: A systematic literature review. *Frontiers in Neurology, 15.*

Gerdsen, M., Jorissen, C., Pustjens, D. C. F., Hof, J. R., Van Rompaey, V., Van De Berg, R., & Widdershoven, J. C. C. (2022). Effect of cochlear implantation on vestibular function in children: A scoping review. *Frontiers in Pediatrics, 10.*

Gnanasegaram, J. J., Parkes, W. J., Cushing, S. L., McKnight, C. L., Papsin, B. C., & Gordon, K. A. (2016). Stimulation from cochlear implant electrodes assists with recovery from asym-

metric perceptual tilt: Evidence from the subjective visual vertical test. *Frontiers in Integrative Neuroscience, 10.*
González-Navarro, M., Manrique-Huarte, R., Manrique-Rodríguez, M., Huarte-Irujo, A., & Pérez-Fernández, N. (2015). Long-term follow-up of late onset vestibular complaints in patients with cochlear implant. *Acta Oto-Laryngologica, 135*(12), 1245–1252.
Grimm, D. R., Fakurnejad, S., & Alyono, J. C. (2022). Cochlear implantation and risk of falls in older adults. *Otolaryngology–Head and Neck Surgery, 167*(3), 531–536.
Guan, R., Wang, Y., Wu, S., Zhang, B., Sun, J., Guo, X., & Sun, J. (2021). Vestibular function in children and adults before and after unilateral or sequential bilateral cochlear implantation. *Frontiers in Neurology, 12.*
Guigou, C., Toupet, M., Delemps, B., Heuschen, S., Aho, S., & Bozorg Grayeli, A. (2018). Effect of rotating auditory scene on postural control in normal subjects, patients with bilateral vestibulopathy, unilateral, or bilateral cochlear implants. *Frontiers in Neurology, 9.*
Gupta, A., & Raj, P. (2018). Compensated vestibular dysfunction post cochlear implantation in children with sensorineural hearing loss: A prospective study. *Indian Journal of Otolaryngology and Head & Neck Surgery, 70*(2), 200–204.
Gurvich, C., Maller, J. J., Lithgow, B., Haghgooie, S., & Kulkarni, J. (2013). Vestibular insights into cognition and psychiatry. *Brain Research, 1537*, 244–259.
Handzel, O., Burgess, B. J., & Nadol, J. B. (2006). Histopathology of the peripheral vestibular system after cochlear implantation in the human. *Otology & Neurotology, 27*(1), 57–64.
Hänsel, T., Gauger, U., Bernhard, N., Behzadi, N., Romo Ventura, M. E., Hofmann, V., Olze, H., Knopke, S., Todt, I., & Coordes, A. (2018). Meta-analysis of subjective complaints of vertigo and vestibular tests after cochlear implantation. *The Laryngoscope, 128*(9), 2110–2123.
Hansen, S., Anthonsen, K., Stangerup, S.-E., Jensen, J. H., Thomsen, J., & Cayé-Thomasen, P. (2010). Unexpected findings and surgical complications in 505 consecutive cochlear implantations: A proposal for reporting consensus. *Acta Oto-Laryngologica, 130*(5), 540–549.
Hartl, B. R. M., Mattingly, J. K., Greene, N. T., Jenkins, H. A., Cass, S. P., & Tollin, D. J. (2016). A preliminary investigation of the air-bone gap: Changes in intracochlear sound pressure with air- and bone-conducted stimuli after cochlear implantation. *Otology & Neurotology, 37*(9), 1291–1299.
Helmchen, C., Klinkenstein, J., Machner, B., Rambold, H., Mohr, C., & Sander, T. (2009). Structural changes in the human brain following vestibular neuritis indicate central vestibular compensation. *Annals of the New York Academy of Sciences, 1164*, 104–115.
Himi, T., Shintani, T., Yamaguchi, T., Harabushi, Y., Yoshioka, I., & Kataura, A. (1997). Relation between vestibular function and speech recognition in postlingually deafened adults with cochlear implantation. *Audiology and Neurotology, 2*(4), 223–230.
Ibrahim, I., da Silva, S. D., Segal, B., & Zeitouni, A. (2017). Effect of cochlear implant surgery on vestibular function: Meta-analysis study. *Journal of Otolaryngology – Head & Neck Surgery = Le Journal d'oto-rhino-laryngologie et de chirurgie cervico-faciale, 46*(1), 44.
Imai, T., Okumura, T., Ohta, Y., Oshima, K., Sato, T., Kamakura, T., & Inohara, H. (2019). Effects of cochlear implants on otolith function as evaluated by vestibulo-ocular reflex and vestibular evoked myogenic potentials. *Auris Nasus Larynx, 46*(6), 836–843.
Ishiyama, A., Doherty, J., Ishiyama, G., Quesnel, A. M., Lopez, I., & Linthicum, F. H. (2016). Post hybrid cochlear implant hearing loss and endolymphatic hydrops. *Otology & Neurotology, 37*(10), 1516–1521.
Ito, J. (1998). Influence of the multichannel cochlear implant on vestibular function. *Otolaryngology–Head and Neck Surgery, 118*(6), 900–902.
Jacobson, G. P., McCaslin, D. L., Piker, E. G., Gruenwald, J., Grantham, S., & Tegel, L. (2011). Insensitivity of the "Romberg test of standing balance on firm and compliant support surfaces" to the results of caloric and VEMP tests. *Ear & Hearing, 32*(6), e1–e5.
Jacot, E., Van Den Abbeele, T., Debre, H. R., & Wiener-Vacher, S. R. (2009). Vestibular impairments pre- and post-cochlear implant in children. *International Journal of Pediatric Otorhinolaryngology, 73*(2), 209–217.

Jafari, Z., & Asad Malayeri, S. (2011). The effect of saccular function on static balance ability of profound hearing-impaired children. *International Journal of Pediatric Otorhinolaryngology, 75*(7), 919–924.
Jang, D. H., Kang, S. S., Shim, H. J., & An, Y.-H. (2023). Re-fixation saccade at video-head impulse test in patients with sudden sensorineural hearing loss. *Research in Vestibular Science, 22*(2), 46–51.
Janky, K. L., & Givens, D. (2015). Vestibular, visual acuity, and balance outcomes in children with cochlear implants. *Ear & Hearing, 36*(6), e364–e372.
Janky, K. L., & Patterson, J. (2020). The relationship between rotary chair and video head impulse testing in children and young adults with cochlear implants. *American Journal of Audiology, 29*(4), 898–906.
Janky, K. L., Patterson, J., Thomas, M., Al-Salim, S., & Robinson, S. (2023). The effects of vestibular dysfunction on balance and self-concept in children with cochlear implants. *International Journal of Pediatric Otorhinolaryngology, 171*, 111642.
Janky, K. L., & Shepard, N. (2009). Vestibular evoked myogenic potential (VEMP) testing: Normative threshold response curves and effects of age. *Journal of the American Academy of Audiology, 20*(08), 514–522.
Janky, K. L., Thomas, M., Al-Salim, S., & Robinson, S. (2022). Does vestibular loss result in cognitive deficits in children with cochlear implants? *Journal of Vestibular Research, 32*(3), 245–260.
Jin, Y., Nakamura, M., Shinjo, Y., & Kaga, K. (2006). Vestibular-evoked myogenic potentials in cochlear implant children. *Acta Oto-Laryngologica, 126*(2), 164–169.
Jin, Y., Shinjo, Y., Akamatsu, Y., Ogata, E., Nakamura, M., Kianoush, S., Yamasoba, T., & Kaga, K. (2008). Vestibular evoked myogenic potentials evoked by multichannel cochlear implant—Influence of C levels. *Acta Oto-Laryngologica, 128*(3), 284–290.
Jin, Y., Shinjo, Y., Akamatsu, Y., Yamasoba, T., & Kaga, K. (2009). Vestibular evoked myogenic potentials of children with inner ear malformations before and after cochlear implantation. *Acta Oto-Laryngologica, 129*(11), 1198–1205.
Kaczmarczyk, K., Błażkiewicz, M., Wiszomirska, I., Pietrasik, K., Zdrodowska, A., Wit, A., Barton, G., & Skarżyński, H. (2019). Assessing gait stability before and after cochlear implantation. *BioMed Research International, 2019*, 1–8.
Kamath and Singh (2024). Otl*ithic Responses and Behavioural Balance in Children with and without Cochlear Implants* [Master's Dissertation, "All India Institute of Speech & Hearing].
Kardooni, M., Ahmadi, R., Saki Malehi, A., Kiani, A., & Saki, S. (2022). *Can video head impulse test determine the early effect of cochlear implantation on the semicircular canals function?* Auditory and Vestibular Research.
Katsiari, E., Balatsouras, D. G., Sengas, J., Riga, M., Korres, G. S., & Xenelis, J. (2013). Influence of cochlear implantation on the vestibular function. *European Archives of Oto-Rhino-Laryngology, 270*(2), 489–495.
Kaya, S., Schachern, P. A., Tsuprun, V., Paparella, M. M., & Cureoglu, S. (2017). Deterioration of vestibular cells in labyrinthitis. *Annals of Otology, Rhinology & Laryngology, 126*(2), 89–95.
Kelly, A., Liu, Z., Leonard, S., Toner, F., Adams, M., & Toner, J. (2018). Balance in children following cochlear implantation. *Cochlear Implants International, 19*(1), 22–25.
Khalil, L. H. (2017). Effects of cochlear implantation on vestibular pathway: Follow up study in cochlear implant children. *Global Journal of Otolaryngology, 8*(4).
Kluenter, H.-D., Lang-Roth, R., & Guntinas-Lichius, O. (2009). Static and dynamic postural control before and after cochlear implantation in adult patients. *European Archives of Oto-Rhino-Laryngology, 266*(10), 1521–1525.
Koka, K., Saoji, A. A., Attias, J., & Litvak, L. M. (2017). An objective estimation of air-bone-gap in cochlear implant recipients with residual hearing using electrocochleography. *Frontiers in Neuroscience, 11*.
Koyama, H., Kashio, A., Fujimoto, C., Uranaka, T., Matsumoto, Y., Kamogashira, T., Kinoshita, M., Iwasaki, S., & Yamasoba, T. (2021). Alteration of vestibular function in pediatric cochlear implant recipients. *Frontiers in Neurology, 12*.

Krause, E., Louza, J. P. R., Wechtenbruch, J., & Gürkov, R. (2010). Influence of cochlear implantation on peripheral vestibular receptor function. *Otolaryngology–Head and Neck Surgery, 142*(6), 809–813.

Krause, E., Wechtenbruch, J., Rader, T., & Gürkov, R. (2009). Influence of cochlear implantation on sacculus function. *Otolaryngology–Head and Neck Surgery, 140*(1), 108–113.

Krause E, Mayerhofer A, Gürkov R, Drexl M, Braun T, Olzowy B, Boetzel K. (2013). Effects of acoustic stimuli used for vestibular evoked myogenic potential studies on the cochlear function. *Otol Neurotol. 34*(7):1186–92. https://doi.org/10.1097/MAO.0b013e31829ce7b4. PMID: 23921920.

Kremmyda, O., Hüfner, K., Flanagin, V. L., Hamilton, D. A., Linn, J., Strupp, M., Jahn, K., & Brandt, T. (2016). Beyond dizziness: Virtual navigation, spatial anxiety and hippocampal volume in bilateral vestibulopathy. *Frontiers in Human Neuroscience, 10.*

Kuang, H., Haversat, H. H., & Michaelides, E. M. (2015). Impairment of caloric function after cochlear implantation. *Journal of Speech, Language, and Hearing Research, 58*(4), 1387–1395.

Kubo, T., Yamamoto, K., Iwaki, T., Doi, K., & Tamura, M. (2001). Different forms of dizziness occurring after cochlear implant. *European Archives of Oto-Rhino-Laryngology, 258*(1), 9–12.

Kusuma, S., Liou, S., & Haynes, D. S. (2005). Disequilibrium after cochlear implantation caused by a perilymph fistula. *The Laryngoscope, 115*(1), 25–26.

Lacroix, E., Edwards, M. G., De Volder, A., Noël, M.-P., Rombaux, P., & Deggouj, N. (2020). Neuropsychological profiles of children with vestibular loss. *Journal of Vestibular Research, 30*(1), 25–33.

le Nobel, G. J., Hwang, E., Wu, A., Cushing, S., & Lin, V. Y. (2016). Vestibular function following unilateral cochlear implantation for profound sensorineural hearing loss. *Journal of Otolaryngology - Head & Neck Surgery, 45*(1), 38.

Leng, Y., & Liu, B. (2020). Dissociation of caloric and video head impulse tests in patients with delayed endolymphatic hydrops. *Frontiers in Neurology, 11*, 362.

Li, H., Schart-Moren, N., Rajan, G., Shaw, J., Rohani, S. A., Atturo, F., Ladak, H. M., Rask-Andersen, H., & Agrawal, S. (2021). Vestibular organ and cochlear implantation–A synchrotron and micro-CT study. *Frontiers in Neurology, 12.*

Li, X., & Gong, S. (2020). The effect of cochlear implantation on vestibular evoked myogenic potential in children. *The Laryngoscope, 130*(12), E918–E925.

Licameli, G., Zhou, G., & Kenna, M. A. (2009). Disturbance of vestibular function attributable to cochlear implantation in children. *The Laryngoscope, 119*(4), 740–745.

Limb, C. J., Francis, H. F., Lustig, L. R., Niparko, J. K., & Jammal, H. (2005). Benign positional vertigo after cochlear implantation. *Otolaryngology–Head and Neck Surgery, 132*(5), 741–745.

Lin, Y.-S., Lee, F.-P., & Peng, S.-C. (2006). Complications in children with long-term cochlear implants. *ORL, 68*(4), 237–242.

Louza, J., Klappert, C. L., Ledderose, G., Gürkov, R., & Krause, E. (2018). Cochlear implant surgery and the risk of falls in an adult population. *Otology & Neurotology, 39*(2), e74–e79.

McSweeny, C., Cushing, S. L., Campos, J. L., Papsin, B. C., & Gordon, K. A. (2021). Functional consequences of poor binaural hearing in development: Evidence from children with unilateral hearing loss and children receiving bilateral cochlear implants. *Trends in Hearing, 25*, 233121652110512.

Meli, A., Aud, B. M., Aud, S. T., Aud, R. G., & Cristofari, E. (2016). Vestibular function after cochlear implant surgery. *Cochlear Implants International, 17*(3), 151–157.

Melvin, T.-A. N., Della Santina, C. C., Carey, J. P., & Migliaccio, A. A. (2009). The effects of cochlear implantation on vestibular function. *Otology & Neurotology, 30*(1), 87–94.

Merchant, G. R., Schulz, K. M., Patterson, J. N., Fitzpatrick, D., & Janky, K. L. (2020). Effect of cochlear implantation on vestibular evoked myogenic potentials and wideband acoustic Immittance. *Ear & Hearing, 41*(5), 1111–1124.

Migliaccio, A. A., Della Santina, C. C., Carey, J. P., Niparko, J. K., & Minor, L. B. (2005). The vestibulo-ocular reflex response to head impulses rarely decreases after cochlear implantation. *Otology & Neurotology, 26*(4), 655–660.

Mikkelsen, K. S., Ovesen, T., & Swan, C. Z. (2017). Pre- and post-operative dizziness, tinnitus, and taste disturbances among cochlear implant recipients. *The Journal of Laryngology & Otology, 131*(4), 309–315.

Miwa, T., Minoda, R., Matsuyoshi, H., & Takeda, H. (2019). The effect of cochlear implants on vestibular-evoked myogenic potential responses and postural stability. *Auris Nasus Larynx, 46*(1), 50–57.

Mohamed, S. T., Hazzaa, N., Abdel Rahman, T., Ezz Eldin, D. M., & Elhusseiny, A. M. (2024). Efficacy of vestibular rehabilitation program in children with balance disorders and sensorineural hearing loss. *International Journal of Pediatric Otorhinolaryngology, 179*, 111931.

Mujdeci, B., Önder, S., Alluşoğlu, S., Boynuegri, S., Kum, O., & Atan, D. (2021). The effects of age at cochlear implantation on balance in children: A pilot study. *The International Journal of Artificial Organs, 44*(6), 440–445.

Murray, D., Viani, L., Garvan, J., Murphy, A., Vance, R., Simoes-Franklin, C., Smith, J., & Meldrum, D. (2020). Balance, gait and dizziness in adult cochlear implant users: A cross sectional study. *Cochlear Implants International, 21*(1), 46–52.

Nair, S., Gupta, A., Nilakantan, A., Mittal, R., Dahiya, R., Saini, S., Prasad, R., & Vajpayee, D. (2017). Impaired vestibular function after cochlear implantation in children: Role of static posturography. *Indian Journal of Otolaryngology and Head & Neck Surgery, 69*(2), 252–258.

Nassif, N., Balzanelli, C., & Redaelli de Zinis, L. O. (2016). Preliminary results of video head impulse testing (vHIT) in children with cochlear implants. *International Journal of Pediatric Otorhinolaryngology, 88*, 30–33.

Nassif, N., Balzanelli, C., & Redaelli de Zinis, L. O. (2021). Long-Term lateral semicircular canal function in children with cochlear implants: results of video head impulse test. European *Journal of Investigation in Health, Psychology and Education, 11*(1):12–19.

Oikawa, K., Kobayashi, Y., Hiraumi, H., Yonemoto, K., & Sato, H. (2018). Body balance function of cochlear implant patients with and without sound conditions. *Clinical Neurophysiology, 129*(10), 2112–2117.

Oyewumi, M., Wolter, N. E., Heon, E., Gordon, K. A., Papsin, B. C., & Cushing, S. L. (2016). Using balance function to screen for vestibular impairment in children with sensorineural hearing loss and cochlear implants. *Otology & Neurotology, 37*(7), 926–932.

Parietti-Winkler, C., Lion, A., Montaut-Verient, B., Grosjean, R., & Gauchard, G. C. (2015). Effects of unilateral cochlear implantation on balance control and sensory organization in adult patients with profound hearing loss. *BioMed Research International, 2015*, 1–7.

Parkes, W. J., Gnanasegaram, J. J., Cushing, S. L., McKnight, C. L., Papsin, B. C., & Gordon, K. A. (2017). Vestibular evoked myogenic potential testing as an objective measure of vestibular stimulation with cochlear implants. *The Laryngoscope, 127*(2), E75–E81.

Piker, E. G., Riska, K., Garrison, D., & Kaylie, D. M. (2020). Vestibular function after cochlear implantation: A test battery and case-by-case approach. *Laryngoscope Investigative Otolaryngology, 5*(3), 560–571.

Psillas, G., Pavlidou, A., Lefkidis, N., Vital, I., Markou, K., Triaridis, S., & Tsalighopoulos, M. (2014). Vestibular evoked myogenic potentials in children after cochlear implantation. *Auris Nasus Larynx, 41*(5), 432–435.

Quimby, A. E., Wen, C. Z., Ruckenstein, M. J., Brant, J. A., & Bigelow, D. C. (2024). Caloric function as a predictor of cochlear implant performance. *Cochlear Implants International, 25*(1), 28–35.

Rah, Y. C., Park, J. H., Park, J. H., Choi, B. Y., & Koo, J.-W. (2016). Dizziness and vestibular function before and after cochlear implantation. *European Archives of Oto-Rhino-Laryngology, 273*(11), 3615–3621.

Rasmussen, K. M. B., West, N., Tian, L., & Cayé-Thomasen, P. (2021). Long-term vestibular outcomes in cochlear implant recipients. *Frontiers in Neurology, 12.*

Richard, C., Fayad, J. N., Doherty, J., & Linthicum, F. H. (2012). Round window versus cochleostomy technique in cochlear implantation. *Otology & Neurotology, 33*(7), 1181–1187.

Robard, L., Hitier, M., Lebas, C., & Moreau, S. (2015). Vestibular function and cochlear implant. *European Archives of Oto-Rhino-Laryngology, 272*(3), 523–530.

Rodriguez, A. I., Thomas, M. L. A., & Janky, K. L. (2019). Air-conducted vestibular evoked myogenic potential testing in children, adolescents, and young adults: Thresholds, frequency tuning, and effects of sound exposure. *Ear & Hearing, 40*(1), 192–203.
Sack, L., Dollaghan, C., & Goffman, L. (2022). Contributions of early motor deficits in predicting language outcomes among preschoolers with developmental language disorder. *International Journal of Speech-Language Pathology, 24*(4), 362–374.
Salem, M., Emara, A., Kolkaila, E., & Kotait, M. (2021). Vestibular evaluation using rotatory chair in children with cochlear implants. *Egyptian Journal of Ear, Nose, Throat and Allied Sciences, 22*(22), 1–7.
Sarac, E. T., Deniz, H., Okuyucu, S., Akoglu, E., & Berber, O. (2020). Vestibular function after cochlear implant surgery. *Turkish Journal of Audiology and Hearing Research.*
Schwab, B., Durisin, M., & Kontorinis, G. (2010). Investigation of balance function using dynamic posturography under electrical-acoustic stimulation in cochlear implant recipients. *International Journal of Otolaryngology, 2010*, 1–7.
Shah, J. (2013). Effect of motor control program in improving gross motor function and postural control in children with sensorineural hearing loss-A pilot study. *Pediatrics & Therapeutics, 03*(01).
Shetye, A. (2012). Benign paroxysmal positional vertigo in a child: An infrequent complication following a fairground ride and post-cochlear implant surgery. *Cochlear Implants International, 13*(3), 177–180.
Sheykholesami, K., Kaga, K., Megerian, C. A., & Arnold, J. E. (2005). Vestibular-evoked myogenic potentials in infancy and early childhood. *The Laryngoscope, 115*(8), 1440–1444.
Shupert, C. L. (2018). *Vestibular neuritis and labyrinthitis.*
Singh, N. K., Govindswamy, R., & Jagadish, N. (2016). *Undesirable vestibular stimulation in cochlear implant users.* Paper presented for oral presentation at Cochlear Implant group of India (CIGICON).
Singh, N. K., Keloth, N. K., & Sinha, S. (2019). Is there a safe level for recording vestibular evoked myogenic potential? Evidence from cochlear and hearing function tests. *Ear & Hearing, 40*(3), 493–500.
Singh, N. K., Sinha, S., Keshree, N. K., Kothari, S., Kumar, S., & Kumar, P. (2021). Relative efficacy of veria and mastoidectomy techniques of cochlear implantation in preservation of sound-induced saccular responses. *International Journal of Audiology, 60*(11), 858–866.
Situkho, M., Lutsenko, V., Antonov, Y., & Dolinay, V. (2023). Static posturography with nintendo balance board in children after cochlear implantation. In *Latest advances in cochlear implant technologies and related clinical applications.*
Smith, P. F., & Zheng, Y. (2013). From ear to uncertainty: Vestibular contributions to cognitive function. *Frontiers in Integrative Neuroscience, 7.*
Sosna-Duranowska, M., Tacikowska, G., Gos, E., Krupa, A., Skarzynski, P. H., & Skarzynski, H. (2021). Vestibular function after cochlear implantation in partial deafness treatment. *Frontiers in Neurology, 12.*
Stevens, M. N., Baudhuin, J. E., & Hullar, T. E. (2014). Short-term risk of falling after cochlear implantation. *Audiology and Neurotology, 19*(6), 370–377.
Stieger, C., Siemens, X., Honegger, F., Roushan, K., Bodmer, D., & Allum, J. (2018). Balance control during stance and gait after cochlear implant surgery. *Audiology & Neuro-Otology, 23*(3), 165–172.
Straumann, D. (2016). *Bedside examination* (pp. 91–101).
Strömberg, A.-K., Olofsson, Å., Westin, M., Duan, M., & Stenfelt, S. (2016). Changes in cochlear function related to acoustic stimulation of cervical vestibular evoked myogenic potential stimulation. *Hearing Research, 340*, 43–49.
Strupp, M., Kim, J.-S., Murofushi, T., Straumann, D., Jen, J. C., Rosengren, S. M., Della Santina, C. C., & Kingma, H. (2017). Bilateral vestibulopathy: Diagnostic criteria Consensus document of the Classification Committee of the Bárány Society1. *Journal of Vestibular Research, 27*(4), 177–189.

Suarez H, Angeli S, Suarez A, Rosales B, Carrera X, Alonso R. (2007). Balance sensory organization in children with profound hearing loss and cochlear implants. *Int J Pediatr Otorhinolaryngol. 71*(4):629--637. https://doi.org/10.1016/j.ijporl.2006.12.014. Epub 2007 Feb 2. PMID: 17275927

Suarez, A., Ferreira, E., Garcia Pintos, B., Arocena, S., & Suarez, H. (2021). Postural control characterization according to age and auditory input in cochlear implant users. *Cochlear Implants International, 22*(1), 29–34.

Su-Velez, B. M., Lopez, I. A., Ishiyama, A., & Ishiyama, G. (2020). Human temporal bone study of vestibular histopathology in cochlear implant patients with cochlear hydrops. *Otology & Neurotology, 41*(5), e607–e614.

Swain, S. K. (2022). Vertigo following cochlear implantation: A review. *International Journal of Research in Medical Sciences, 10*(2), 572.

Szirmai, Á., Ribári, O., & Répássy, G. (2001). Air caloric computer system application in monitoring vestibular function changes after cochlear implantation. *Otolaryngology–Head and Neck Surgery, 125*(6), 631–634.

Talaat, H. S., Chedid, A. I. F., Wageih, G. M., & Zein El-Abedein, A. M. (2021). Vestibular function assessment following cochlear implantation using rotatory chair testing. *European Archives of Oto-Rhino-Laryngology, 278*(7), 2253–2259.

Tan, E., Bester, C., Collins, A., Razmovski, T., & O'Leary, S. (2023). Four-point impedance and utricular dysfunction is associated with postoperative dizziness after cochlear implantation. *Otology & Neurotology, 44*(7), 688–695.

Tanyeri, O., Akdogan, M. V., Hizal, E., & Buyuklu, A. F. (2020). Assessment of vestibular function in adults with prelingual hearing loss using c/oVEMP tests. *The Journal of International Advanced Otology, 16*(1), 24–27.

Thierry, B., Blanchard, M., Leboulanger, N., Parodi, M., Wiener-Vacher, S. R., Garabedian, E.-N., & Loundon, N. (2015). Cochlear implantation and vestibular function in children. *International Journal of Pediatric Otorhinolaryngology, 79*(2), 101–104.

Tien, H., & Linthicum, F. H. (2002). Histopathologic changes in the vestibule after cochlear implantation. *Otolaryngology–Head and Neck Surgery, 127*(4), 260–264.

Todt, I., Basta, D., & Ernst, A. (2008). Does the surgical approach in cochlear implantation influence the occurrence of postoperative vertigo? *Otolaryngology–Head and Neck Surgery, 138*(1), 8–12.

Tonini, R., Cohen, H. S., Mulavara, A. P., & Sangi-Haghpeykar, H. (2019). Balance and sound conditions in adults with bilateral cochlear implants. *Biomedicine Hub, 4*(1), 1–9.

Truong, M., Bester, C., Orimoto, K., Vartanyan, M., Phyland, D., MacDougall, H., Tari, S., Rousset, A., Curthoys, I., & O'Leary, S. (2022). Cochlear implant surgery and perioperative dizziness is associated with utricular hyperfunction. *Journal of Vestibular Research, 32*(3), 295–304.

Valente, M., & McCaslin, D. L. (2011). Vestibular disorders and evaluation of the pediatric patient. *The ASHA Leader, 16*(3), 12–15.

Verrecchia, L., Galle Barrett, K., & Karltorp, E. (2020). The feasibility, validity and reliability of a child friendly vestibular assessment in infants and children candidates to cochlear implant. *International Journal of Pediatric Otorhinolaryngology, 135*, 110093.

Wagner, J. H., Basta, D., Wagner, F., Seidl, R. O., Ernst, A., & Todt, I. (2010). Vestibular and taste disorders after bilateral cochlear implantation. *European Archives of Oto-Rhino-Laryngology, 267*(12), 1849–1854.

Wang, R., Chao, X., Luo, J., Zhang, D., Xu, J., Liu, X., Fan, Z., Wang, H., & Xu, L. (2022). Objective vestibular function changes in children following cochlear implantation. *Journal of Vestibular Research, 32*(1), 29–37.

Wanna, G. B., Noble, J. H., Gifford, R. H., Dietrich, M. S., Sweeney, A. D., Zhang, D., Dawant, B. M., Rivas, A., & Labadie, R. F. (2015). Impact of intrascalar electrode location, electrode type, and angular insertion depth on residual hearing in cochlear implant patients. *Otology & Neurotology, 36*(8), 1343–1348.

Weinmann, C., Baumann, U., Leinung, M., Stöver, T., & Helbig, S. (2021). Vertigo associated with cochlear implant surgery: Correlation with vertigo diagnostic result, electrode carrier, and insertion angle. *Frontiers in Neurology, 12*.
West, N., Klokker, M., & Cayé-Thomasen, P. (2021). Video head impulse test saccades and loss of cervical vestibular evoked myogenic potentials are late vestibular footprints of cochlear implantation. *Journal of Vestibular Research, 31*(1), 61–67.
Wiszomirska, I., Zdrodowska, A., Tacikowska, G., Sosna, M., Kaczmarczyk, K., & Skarżyński, H. (2019). Does cochlear implantation influence postural stability in patients with hearing loss? *Gait & Posture, 74*, 40–44.
Wolter, N. E., Gordon, K. A., Papsin, B. C., & Cushing, S. L. (2015). Vestibular and balance impairment contributes to cochlear implant failure in children. *Otology & Neurotology, 36*(6), 1029–1034.
Wu, Q., Zhang, Q., Xiao, Q., Zhang, Y., Chen, Z., Liu, S., Wang, X., Xu, Y., Xu, X.-D., Lv, J., Jin, Y., Yang, J., & Zhang, Q. (2022). Vestibular dysfunction in pediatric patients with cochlear implantation: A systematic review and meta-analysis. *Frontiers in Neurology, 13*.
Xu, X.-D., Zhang, X.-T., Zhang, Q., Hu, J., Chen, Y.-F., & Xu, M. (2015). Ocular and cervical vestibular-evoked myogenic potentials in children with cochlear implant. *Clinical Neurophysiology, 126*(8), 1624–1631.
Yang, C. J., Lee, J. Y., Ahn, J. H., & Lee, K.-S. (2016). Value of pre-operative caloric test in predicting speech perception after cochlear implantation in adults with post-lingual hearing loss. *Acta Oto-Laryngologica, 136*(9), 912–918.
Yoon, B., Choi, S. H., Jeong, J. H., Park, K. W., Kim, E. J., Hwang, J., Jang, J. W., Kim, H. J., Hong, J. Y., Lee, J. M., Kang, J. H., & Yoon, S. J. (2020). Balance and mobility performance along the Alzheimer's disease spectrum. *Journal of Alzheimer's Disease, 73*(2), 633–644.
Young, Y.-H., Huang, T.-W., & Cheng, P.-W. (2003). Assessing the stage of Ménière's disease using vestibular evoked myogenic potentials. *Archives of Otolaryngology–Head & Neck Surgery, 129*(8), 815.
Zanetti, D., Barbara Campovecchi, C., Balzanelli, C., & Pasini, S. (2007). Paroxysmal positional vertigo after cochlear implantation. *Acta Oto-Laryngologica, 127*(5), 452–458.
Zawawi, F., Alobaid, F., Leroux, T., & Zeitouni, A. G. (2014). Patients reported outcome post-cochlear implantation: How severe is their dizziness? *Journal of Otolaryngology - Head & Neck Surgery, 43*(1), 49.
Zu Eulenburg, P., Stoeter, P., & Dieterich, M. (2010). Voxel-based morphometry depicts central compensation after vestibular neuritis. *Annals of Neurology, 68*(2), 241–249.

Chapter 22
Cortical Neuroplasticity in Deafness: Evidence from Children Fitted with Implantable Auditory Prostheses

Anu Sharma and Kayla Cormier

Abstract Neuroplastic brain changes occur across the lifespan, with a sensitive period of maximal central auditory system plasticity present in early childhood. Early intervention for hearing loss with amplification and/or electrical stimulation allows for cortical auditory maturation and language acquisition whereas delayed intervention may result in persistent atypical auditory processing, language and cognitive delays. Hearing loss also results in cross-modal plasticity, in which deprived auditory brain regions are recruited and repurposed by other intact sensory systems. Cross-modal reorganization in children and adults is partially reversible with timely intervention. Brain based biomarkers of neuroplastic changes have the potential to aid clinical decision-making.

Keywords Neuroplasticity · Auditory processing · Central auditory system · Cortical auditory evoked potential · Cochlear implants

Introduction

The human brain is dynamic in its capabilities and is able to change in response to experiences. *Neuroplasticity* is the ability of the brain to change at both a functional and structural level in response to intrinsic or extrinsic stimuli, which underlies behavioral changes. This incorporates alterations in the fundamental neural connections, pathways, and networks that arise from development, learning, sensory experiences, lack of sensory input, injury, and diseases. Neuroplasticity is a continual process affecting neural pathways at all levels and at all stages of life. When inputs

A. Sharma (✉) · K. Cormier
Speech Language and Hearing Science, University of Colorado Boulder, Boulder, CO, USA
e-mail: anu.sharma@colorado.edu

P. Kumar et al. (eds.), *Advances in Implantation Otology*,
https://doi.org/10.1007/978-981-96-8671-1_22

are inadequately received, such as when a person is deaf, compensatory neuroplastic changes occur. In this chapter, we will delve into both deprivations induced neuroplasticity in deafness and experience driven neuroplasticity after implantation with auditory prostheses like cochlear implants. Given that sufficient and high-quality auditory input is essential for typical development of the central auditory pathways, this chapter will focus on central auditory plasticity in deaf children. We will also discuss how neuroplasticity can be leveraged as a tool in the clinical treatment of deafness with implantable prostheses.

A variety of imaging techniques can be utilized to examine cortical development such as magnetic resonance imaging (MRI), positron emission tomography (PET) scans, and functional magnetic resonance imaging (fMRI) to name a few. However, auditory processing requires high temporal resolution, which makes the use of electroencephalography (EEG), a preferred choice when studying neuroplasticity-related changes before and after cochlear implantation. For this reason, in our laboratory, we use EEG to study neuroplasticity in children and adults with hearing loss. During high density EEG recordings, with the use of numerous electrodes, we can estimate and visualize the origins of brain responses using a sophisticated statistical modeling known as current density source reconstruction (CDR). These cortical sources can be projected on a 3-Dimensional image of the brain (structural MRI) with a graded color scale (F-Statistic) displaying the statistical likelihood of activation. While EEG lacks the fine spatial resolution of other neuroimaging methods such as fMRI, its superior temporal resolution, along with its inexpensive, silent and non-invasive nature, makes it an exceptional method when evaluating sensory changes in neuroplasticity in deaf populations fitted with cochlear implants.

Central Auditory System Maturation

Although the auditory system is structurally present at birth, development continues throughout childhood. Clinically, it is beneficial to understand the development patterns seen in typically developing children to inform our understanding of auditory system deficits in deafness and hearing loss. Typical auditory maturation is driven by both intrinsic plasticity and extrinsic plasticity (Sharma & Glick, 2016). This means that auditory experiences are needed for central auditory maturation to occur.

The obligatory Cortical Auditory Evoked Potential (CAEP) allows us an opportunity to monitor these developmental changes in a non-invasive and objective manner. The P1 component is the first positive peak in the CAEP, which is present at birth at a latency of around 200–300 ms (Fig. 22.1a1). Throughout development, P1 latency decreases, finally becoming adult-like in adolescence with a positive peak occurring around 60 ms (Fig. 22.1a2 and a3) (Sharma et al., 2002a). The P1 is followed by a negative trough called the N1 and a positivity called the P2, often referred to as the N1P2 complex (Fig. 22.1a3). The N1 and P2 are indicative of higher-level auditory cortex maturation including secondary auditory cortex, while the P1 component is representative of thalamic and primary auditory cortex

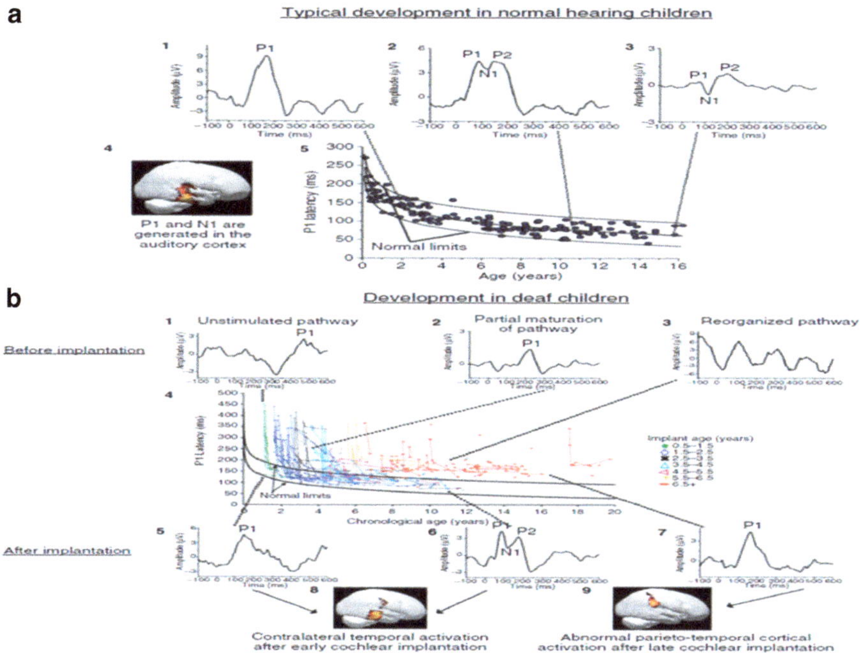

Fig. 22.1 Central auditory maturation in normal hearing children and in children receiving cochlear implants. The P1 cortical auditory evoked potential (P1 CAEP) is a biomarker of auditory cortex maturation. In normal hearing children (**a**), the CAEP morphology changes with typical development. The P1 component is the primary response during infancy and early childhood (**a1**). As children mature, the N1 and P2 components emerge (**a2** and **a3**). Source localization via high-density EEG shows that the P1 component originates from the primary auditory cortex, while the N1P2 components involve higher-level auditory cortical regions (**a4** and **a5**). Over the first 2 years of life, typical development is marked by a rapid decrease in P1 latency, which continues to decline more slowly into adolescence. In contrast, (**b**) depicts the development of central auditory pathways in deaf children prior to and after receiving a CI. Before implantation, 231 deaf children show distinct CAEP patterns not seen in normal hearing children. Younger children typically show abnormal CAEP patterns like "deprivation negativity" (**b1**), indicating an unstimulated auditory system, or a delayed P1 response due to partial auditory stimulation (**b2**). In older children, a polyphasic CAEP morphology emerges, suggesting central auditory reorganization (**b3**). When children receive a CI before 3.5 years of age, they develop age-appropriate P1 latencies within 6–8 months (**b5**) and show N1P2 components in later childhood, paralleling normal hearing development (**b6**). However, children implanted after 7 years have significantly delayed P1 latencies and may not develop the N1P2 components, even after years of CI use (**b7**). High-density EEG in early-implanted children shows activation in the auditory cortex similar to that of normal hearing children (**b8**), whereas late-implanted children exhibit atypical activation in parietotemporal regions, indicative of cortical reorganization (**b9**). This data collectively highlights the importance of early CI implantation during a sensitive developmental window to support typical central auditory pathway maturation. (Reproduced from Kral and Sharma (2012))

development (Fig. 22.1a4) (Eggermont & Ponton, 2003; Sharma et al., 1997, 2005, 2015; Kral & Sharma, 2012).

From an examination of 136 normal hearing subjects ranging in age from infancy to adulthood, our group created normative P1 latency data (Sharma et al., 2002a). Ninety-five percent confidence intervals were created around this data to allow for comparison of individual P1 latencies to age-appropriate normative data (Fig. 22.1a5). Therefore, P1 latencies falling outside of this 95% confidence interval indicate delayed auditory system maturation. Normative data allows not only analysis of normal versus abnormal auditory maturation but can play a key role in examining the effectiveness of treatment on cortical maturation (Sharma et al., 2002a, b).

The emergence of the N1 component has been examined across development. It has been reported that in normal hearing children between the ages of three and six years, this negativity is present in about 57% of children, while in children between the ages of six and nine years, the N1 is observed in 71%. By age nine, this response was noted in 100% of normal hearing children (Sharma et al., 2015). This pattern can be examined in deaf children to determine if higher-order cortical maturation can be inferred based on the presence or absence of the N1 response (Sharma et al., 2015).

Previous research has displayed differing morphology patterns in CAEPs when comparing children and adults. In infants and toddlers only a large P1 response is observed (Fig. 22.1a1). In early childhood, children display a bifid morphology pattern including an invagination of the emerging N1 response (Fig. 22.1a2). This pattern develops into the adult canonical morphology pattern with a small P1, and a more defined N1 and P2 component (Fig. 22.1a3). N1 development is driven by auditory experiences, while the P1 component does not require extrinsic plasticity to be initially observed (Sharma et al., 2005). Distinct morphologic patterns have also been observed in under-stimulated auditory systems in deaf children. A large negativity prior to the observed P1 peak suggests an unstimulated central auditory system (Fig. 22.1b1), a delayed latency P1 response suggests a partially stimulated auditory pathway (Fig. 22.1b2) and a polyphasic morphology suggests a central pathway which is unlikely to be responsive to auditory stimulation (Fig. 22.1b3) (Sharma et al., 2005; Sharma et al., 2002a). In this manner, both latency and morphology markers for central auditory development and plasticity have been documented.

A Brief Sensitive Period for Central Auditory Maturation

During a short window of development, external auditory input rapidly changes the structural neural circuits underlying our hearing abilities, often referred to as a sensitive period in the auditory system (Knudsen, 2004; Kral & Sharma, 2012). CAEP measures have allowed researchers to demonstrate and characterize this sensitive period in the human central auditory system (Sharma et al., 2002a; Sharma et al., 2005, 2015; Kral & Sharma, 2012; Cardon & Sharma, 2013). Through a series of studies, our group has established that the central auditory system is sufficiently sensitive up to around 3.5 years of age, during which the plasticity of the auditory cortex is maximal for good outcomes with cochlear implantation. We recorded P1 responses from 245 congenitally deaf children fitted with cochlear implants (CI) and compared them with the 95% confidence intervals created based on P1 latencies of normal hearing children. The congenitally deaf children fell into three groups of P1 responses, which were characterized by the age of cochlear implantation. Overall, almost all children who obtained a CI before the age of 3.5 years exhibited latencies within normal limits comparable to their normal hearing peers. Among the children implanted between the ages of 3.5 and 6.5 years, approximately two-third (66%) demonstrated delayed P1 latencies. The vast majority (95%) of children who received a CI after the age of 7 years showed abnormal or delayed latencies compared to the age-matched normative data. These results suggest that after 3.5 years of auditory deprivation, the plasticity of the auditory system decreases, and stimulation of the auditory pathway may no longer be able to overcome the effects of sensory deprivation (Sharma et al., 2002a, 2005, 2009; Dorman et al., 2007). In 231 congenitally deaf CI children, we have also assessed the P1 CAEP biomarker longitudinally to examine individual developmental trajectories. Results from this study are indicated in Fig. 22.1b4. Children who are congenitally deaf and receive CIs before the age of 3.5 years (early implanted) often display delayed P1 latencies before implantation (see Fig. 22.1b1). However, after receiving the implants, these children typically experience a swift reduction in P1 latency within the initial months of use (see Fig. 22.1b4), ultimately achieving P1 latencies within the 95% confidence interval after 6–8 months of use (refer to Fig. 22.1b5) and developing an N1P2 response as they continue to develop. In contrast, although children who are implanted later (receiving CI > age 7 years) showed reductions in P1 latencies with CI use (Fig. 22.1b4), these children also continued to exhibit delayed P1 CAEP latencies and absent N1P2 responses even 7–10 years after CI use (see Fig. 22.1b7) (Sharma et al., 2002a, b, 2007, Eggermont & Ponton, 2003; Dorman et al., 2007).

The aforementioned pattern of central auditory development has been noted in studies of speech and language outcomes in children such that children implanted within the sensitive period tend to show better speech and language abilities in comparison to children implanted later (Dunn et al., 2014; Geers, 2006; Harrison et al., 2005; Holt & Svirsky, 2008; Niparko et al., 2010; Robbins et al., 2004; Svirsky et al., 2004; Wang et al., 2008). In a large study examining 117 children who received a CI within the sensitive period, speech outcomes were not significantly different between those implanted at 1, 2, or 3 years of age when accounting for their years of experience with the implant (Tajudeen et al., 2010). The results for a sensitive period in cochlear implanted children are consistent with animal studies demonstrating abnormal cortical activation patterns in response to cochlear implantation outside of a brief developmental sensitive period for congenitally deaf cats (Kral & Sharma, 2012; Kral et al., 2016, 2019). Animal studies have shown that auditory deprivation beyond this sensitive period results in altered connectivity and a decoupling between the primary auditory cortex and higher order auditory cortex, as well as, between the auditory system and other sensory systems, and higher order cognitive regions of the brain that may result in a lack of top-down cognitive modulation of incoming bottom-up auditory input (Kral et al., 2016, 2019). Due to a partial or complete decoupling between primary and higher-order auditory cortex, when implanted after 7 years of age, congenitally deaf children are no longer able to utilize the auditory input they are being provided from their CI meaningfully to acquire oral speech and language (Sharma et al., 2015).

While the P1 reflects deficits in primary auditory cortical maturation, abnormalities in higher-order cortical maturation in late implanted CI children are evidenced by the N1 component. The emergence pattern of the N1 appears at later ages with longer periods of auditory deprivation. While early implanted children show similar N1 responses to age-matched typical hearing peers by age 6 years (Fig. 22.1b6), N1 responses are not typically noted in late implanted children (Fig. 22.1b7). Children who receive a CI after the age of 7 years are unlikely to develop the N1 component, suggesting deficits in development of higher order auditory cortex and reduced connectivity between primary auditory and higher order cortical areas (Sharma et al., 2015; Eggermont & Ponton, 2003) consistent with the decoupling hypothesis of Kral et al. (2016, 2019). Thus, results from both animal studies and children with CIs highlight the importance of early access to sounds to allow for proper cortical auditory development.

Finally, it is interesting to note that the aforementioned sensitive period for good outcomes with cochlear implantation may not be the same in all clinical populations. In a study from our group, we examined P1 latencies of children with Auditory Neuropathy Spectrum Disorder (ANSD), a kind of hearing loss which affects synchrony of neural firing in the central auditory pathways (Cardon & Sharma, 2013). In children with ANSD who received CIs, it was found that 72% of those implanted before 2 years of age showed normal P1 latencies following treatment, while only 23% of those implanted after 2 years of age demonstrated normal P1 latencies. This suggests that the sensitive period may be shorter for children with ANSD (Cardon & Sharma, 2013).

Sequential Versus Simultaneous Cochlear Implantation

Central auditory maturation has also been examined as a function of sequential versus simultaneous implantation, in which sequential implantation involves implanting the CIs in each ear at different times, and simultaneous implantation refers to implanting both ears during the same surgical procedure. Children who obtain simultaneous CIs rather than sequential CIs, show more typical central auditory maturation patterns (Bauer et al., 2006; Gordon et al., 2010, 2007, 2008, 2011, 2013; Jiwani et al., 2016). Sequentially implanted children are more likely to show a significant difference between evoked potential responses from each ear, while most of those children who received simultaneous implantation have a higher likelihood of showing similar responses between the ears (Gordon et al., 2007, 2008, 2011; Bauer et al., 2006; Sparreboom et al., 2014). Furthermore, even after a year of bilateral CI usage, the differences between ears were still prevalent, and only those with minimal inter-implant delays (<1.5 years) demonstrated significantly greater benefit from bilateral CI use in quiet and in noise compared with unilateral CI use (Gordon et al., 2007, 2008, 2011). In comparison to normal hearing peers, unilateral CI users, for more than 1.5 years, exhibited greater activation of the contralateral auditory cortices relative to the first CI side. However, when stimulating the second implant, these children showed less contralateral activation, which was also associated with worse speech outcomes with the second implant. These unusual lateralization patterns continued in these children following 3–4 years of bilateral CI usage. In children with minimal or no delay between receiving implants, cortical activation levels were not significantly different from that of their normal-hearing peers (Gordon et al., 2013). This suggests that, in addition to the sensitive period for central auditory maturation, there is a window of 1.5-years from the first implant a child receives to their second for typical binaural maturation to occur, beyond which the risk of abnormal cortical activation patterns increases (Gordon et al., 2013). Overall, this section underscores a needed emphasis on early implantation within the 3.5-year sensitive period, but best by age 1 year, when the underlying neuroplasticity is likely at its peak for acquisition of oral speech and language. Furthermore, bilateral implantation within the sensitive period, with as minimal an inter-implantation delay as possible, results in the best cortical maturational outcomes.

Cross-Modal Reorganization

Another form of compensatory plasticity which occurs with sensory deprivation is called cross-modal plasticity. This refers to the reallocation of neural networks in the brain when there is a prolonged lack of sensory input, such as audition (Bavelier & Neville, 2002). Specifically, cross-modal plasticity is thought to arise from an unmasking or strengthening of neural inputs from other intact senses (Kral & Sharma, 2023). In individuals with prolonged or congenital deafness who have not used amplification, auditory cortical areas can be recruited and begin processing information from other intact modalities such as vision and/or somatosensation (Glick & Sharma, 2017, 2020; Campbell & Sharma, 2016; Cardon & Sharma, 2019, Levänen & Hamdorf, 2001; Rosemann & Thiel, 2020; Schürmann et al., 2006). Cross-modal plasticity, in the face of deafness, is thought to occur as a possible compensatory action, which increases the capabilities of the intact sensory systems to help construe degraded auditory input by utilizing the resources of the sensory system that is deprived of input (Sharma et al., 2015).

Animal studies have confirmed recruitment of deprived auditory areas by both the visual and somatosensory systems (Lomber et al., 2010; Meredith & Lomber, 2011; Kral et al., 2003; Land et al., 2016). Cross-modal recruitment is typically not demonstrated in the primary auditory area, rather higher-order sensory cortices are considered more susceptible to recruitment by the visual modality (Kral & Sharma, 2012, 2023; Kral et al., 2003). Land et al. (2016) demonstrated that congenitally deaf cats' auditory responsiveness is maintained in response to auditory stimuli when cross-modal recruitment of higher order areas is present (Land et al., 2016). Animal studies highlight that the brain does not entirely lose the ability to respond to auditory stimuli in the face of cross-modal reorganization; however, this higher order reorganization seen both in deaf animals and in humans may explain some of the individual differences in outcomes after cochlear implantation.

In a study in our laboratory examining cross-modal recruitment by vision in deaf children, children with CIs demonstrated greater visual evoked potential (VEP) amplitudes for the N1a and P2b components, as well as earlier latencies and amplitudes for the N1 component compared to age-matched normal hearing children (Campbell & Sharma, 2016). Additionally, auditory processing areas (superior temporal gyrus, medial temporal gyrus, inferior temporal gyrus, and Brodmann Area 22) in right temporal cortex were activated in response to a visual stimulus only in children with CIs, which was not observed in normal hearing children (Fig. 22.2a1 and a2). This pattern of results was considered evidence for cross-modal reorganization of auditory cortex by the visual modality. In the same study, a greater degree of visual cross-modal reorganization (as evidenced by earlier latencies) was associated with worse speech perception in noise in children with CIs (Fig. 22.2b) (Campbell & Sharma, 2016). We have also recorded somatosensory evoked potentials (SSEP) using a vibrotactile stimulus in children with CIs and age-matched normal hearing children (Cardon & Sharma, 2019). CI children had significantly earlier latencies for the P50 SSEP component in the right temporal lobe and overall exhibited more robust peak components than normal hearing children. While children with CI showed the typical cortical activation (i.e., post-central gyrus) associated with the somatosensory stimulation, they also demonstrated additional activation of auditory areas in the temporal cortex (superior temporal gyrus, transverse temporal gyrus, supramarginal gyrus, angular gyrus, superior frontal gyrus, paracentral lobule, and insula) (Fig. 22.2d1 and d2). These results indicate that a cross-modal reorganization by the somatosensory system occurs with auditory deprivation (Cardon & Sharma, 2019). Furthermore, like the VEPs in the aforementioned study, earlier SSEP latencies were correlated with worse speech-in-noise outcomes (Fig. 22.2e). Both studies indicate a negative association between speech perception and cross-modal plasticity, such that children who had greater difficulty perceiving speech-in-noise via their CI, also showed greater cross-modal reorganization, presumably due to their greater reliance on multimodal cues to comprehend the degraded speech input.

Additionally, our laboratory recently demonstrated that cross-modal reorganization by vision and somatosensation were positively correlated with each other. Specifically, in children with CIs, greater cross-modal reorganization of one sensory modality (for example, vision) was associated with greater cross-modal reorganization of another sensory modality (for example, touch). Both types of cross-modal reorganization were related to worse speech-in-noise abilities. This may suggest that cross-modal reorganization, independent of sensory modality, could underlie CI children's variable benefit when comprehending speech-in-noise (Hennesy et al., 2022).

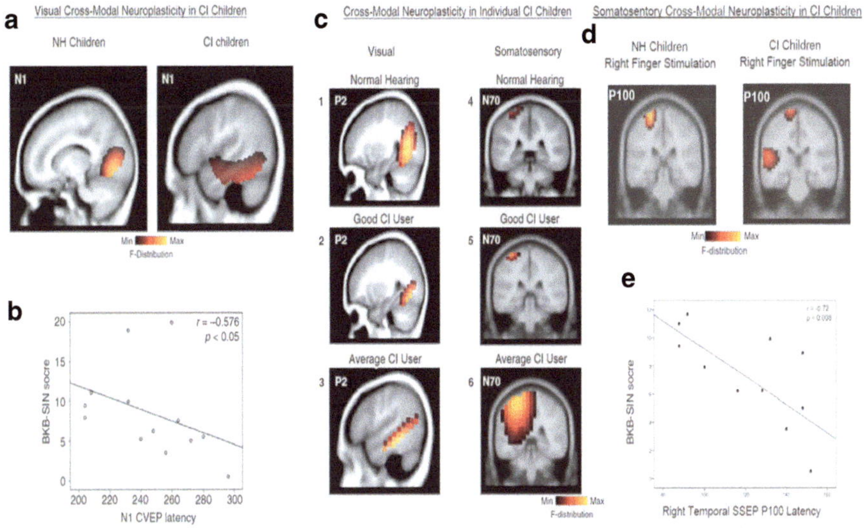

Fig. 22.2 Cross-modal reorganization in cochlear implanted children. Current density source reconstructions (CDRs) of visual and somatosensory evoked potentials in children with normal hearing and children with CI. The F-Distribution color scale indicates the likelihood of cortical activation, with the associated color scale of maximum (yellow) through the minimum (black), in a particular cortical region. (**a**) Comparison of the VEP N1 component CDRs in a group of normal hearing children ($n = 41$) and children with CI ($n = 14$). In response to visual motion processing, normal children demonstrate occipital cortex activation (**a1**). Children with CI demonstrate additional temporal cortex activation (**a2**), suggestive of cross-modal reorganization of auditory regions by the visual system. (**b**). BKB-SIN speech perception scores plotted against VEP N1 latencies. Using a speech-in-noise test (BKB-SIN), earlier N1 latencies in the temporal cortex, suggestive of greater cross-modal reorganization, was correlated with poorer speech-in-noise perception. (**c**) CDRs in individual children ($n = 6$) of the VEP P2 component and SSEP N70 component. Speech perception in quiet were measured using the Consonant Nucleus Consonant (CNC), Multi-syllabic Lexical Neighborhood Test (MLNT), or Lexical Neighborhood Test (LNT) to determine a percent correct score. The normal hearing children obtained a score of 100%, the good CI users obtained scores of 96% and 94%, while the average CI user obtained scores of 67% and 76%. The two good CI users exhibited activation in the occipital cortex when processing a visual motion stimulus (**c2**) and activation in the parietal cortex when processing a vibrotactile stimulus (**c5**). These same activation patterns were noted in the children with normal hearing (**c1** and **c4**). (**d**) Comparison of the SSEP P100 component CDRs in a group of normal hearing children ($n = 17$) and children with CI ($n = 12$). In response to right index finger vibrotactile stimulation, normal hearing children displayed parietal cortex activation (**d1**), while children with CI display cross-modal reorganization through additional temporal cortex activation (**d2**). (**b**) BKB-SIN speech perception scores plotted against SSEP P100 latencies. Earlier P100 latencies in the temporal cortex were correlated with poorer speech-in-noise perception. This suggests that greater cross-modal reorganization is associated with worse speech outcomes. (Reproduced from Campbell and Sharma (2016); Sharma et al. (2015); and Cardon and Sharma (2019))

Studies examining positron emission tomography (PET) testing have also demonstrated cross-modal reorganization and functional outcomes. Examining the blood flow and metabolic rate in early implanted children (3–4 years of age) and late implanted children (6–7 years of age) demonstrated differences in cross-modal plasticity and behavioral outcomes. Cross-modal recruitment of the auditory cortex was observed in children with longer durations of auditory deprivation, while early implantation did not allow for this recruitment to take place. Additionally, in line with aforementioned results, cross-modal reorganization was associated with poorer outcomes post cochlear implantation (Lee et al.,2005, 2007). The greater potential for cross-modal reorganization with longer periods of auditory deprivation further highlights the importance of early intervention. Additionally, cross-modal recruitment could provide valuable insight into individual differences in outcomes with CIs.

Sharma et al. (2015) described cross-modal reorganization in children with CIs as a function of their varying speech perception abilities. A typical hearing child and a CI child with excellent speech perception abilities (score of 96% on the Lexical Neighborhood Test) showed only expected visual (occipital) cortex activation to visual stimuli (Fig. 22.2c1 and c2); however, an average performing child with a CI (score of 67% on the Multisyllabic Lexical Neighborhood Test), demonstrated activation of auditory cortical areas in response to a visual stimulus (Fig. 22.2c3) suggestive of cross-modal recruitment. Similarly, a normal hearing child and a child with good speech perception with the CI (score of 94% on the Consonant Nucleus Consonant test) showed only the expected somatosensory cortex (post central gyrus) activation to vibrotactile stimulation (Fig. 22.2c4 and c5). However, a CI child with average speech perception scores (score of 76% on the Consonant Nucleus Consonant test) demonstrated cross-modal recruitment via activation of auditory processing areas in temporal cortex by vibrotactile stimuli (Fig. 22.2c6). These results were further explored in a group of children with CIs. In five CI children with better speech-in-noise abilities compared to eight CI children with worse speech-in-noise abilities visual motion stimuli were found to elicit more cortical activity in auditory and frontal brain regions in those with worse speech-in-noise abilities. However, no differences were noted in cortical activation patterns by the vibrotactile stimulus. Thus, it may be that children with CIs demonstrate a greater reliance on compensatory input from vision than that of somatosensation (Hennesy et al., 2022). Taken together with the aforementioned group data, cross-modal reorganization can afford insight into realistic expectations for individual CI users. In the future, examining cross-modal reorganization may aid in decisions regarding whether specific aural rehabilitation and practices should be emphasized for children with different cross-modal reorganization patterns.

Cross-modal plasticity may have some functional benefits. CI users have been shown to have better visual only and auditory-visual perception abilities than normal hearing peers (Bergeson et al., 2005; Tyler et al., 1997; Schorr et al., 2005). In a study examining facial processing in 21 post-lingually deafened adults with unilateral CI both brain changes within the visual system and the presence of cross-modal reorganization were found when compared to an age-matched normal hearing control group. Greater activation of auditory brain areas resulted in better face recognition and lip-reading abilities in CI users (Stropahl et al., 2015). In pre-lingual hearing loss, results in humans and animals have also demonstrated enhanced visual motion abilities (Hauthal et al., 2013; Shiell et al., 2014; Shiell et al., 2016; Lomber et al., 2010). Therefore, this cross-modal reorganization in both pre-and post-lingually deafened adults may demonstrate an adaptive mechanism that could be beneficial in functional, multimodal speech processing. However, this adaptive mechanism may come at the cost of auditory only speech processing abilities.

CI users who demonstrate more visual recruitment of auditory cortices tend to demonstrate poorer auditory only speech outcomes with their CIs (Strelnikov et al., 2013; Kim et al., 2016; Doucet et al., 2006). In a recent study, Sun et al. (2021) examined the predictive nature of cross-modal reorganization and speech perception outcomes in 94 cochlear implantees with long-term profound hearing loss and compared their findings to 37 age-matched sudden sensorineural hearing loss cases. The study used MRI to evaluate the cross-modal reorganizations. CI participants underwent imaging a minimum of 3 years post implantation, while those with sudden sensorineural hearing loss underwent imaging within 2 weeks of the onset of hearing loss. Lower gray matter volume was noted in auditory and language regions of the brain in the CI group compared with the sudden sensorineural hearing loss group. Furthermore, in the CI group recovery of this gray matter, suggestive of non-auditory activation, was noted in all auditory and language regions, except for the middle temporal cortical area. Gray matter volume recovery is, therefore, suggestive of cross-modal reorganization resulting from non-auditory stimuli activating these secondary auditory brain regions. However, this reorganization does not take place within the primary auditory brain regions, indicating that these regions can still be stimulated by auditory input following a period of auditory deprivation. This non-auditory activation of auditory and language regions was positively correlated with duration of deafness. Greater gray matter recovery in the thalamus and superior temporal region was negatively related to post-CI speech comprehension abilities. Meanwhile, less loss of gray matter volume in the middle temporal area, which houses the primary auditory cortex, predicted good speech outcomes (Sun et al., 2021). This study further demonstrates the link between poorer speech outcomes and greater cross-modal reorganization in post lingually deafened adults. These findings point to the possible usage of measuring cross-modal reorganization to obtain better post-implant expectations. It is possible that utilizing these techniques clinically could also lead to better tailoring of auditory rehabilitation following CIs; however, additional research is needed in this area to determine how best to support these individuals.

Neurocognition

In the last decade, hearing loss has been identified as a risk factor for cognitive decline (Lin, 2011). Both auditory deprivation and treatment of this deprivation can alter neural networks within the brain, influencing cognitive processing (Kral et al., 2016; Kral & Sharma, 2023). Research on congenitally deaf children with CIs revealed that their rate of executive functioning difficulties was three to four times higher than that of their peers with normal hearing, without this being related to the age of implantation (Kronenberger et al., 2014). Even for children who were implanted within the sensitive period, verbal working memory abilities remained weaker compared to their normal-hearing peers. However, when recalling words in a verbal learning task, children with CIs performed similar to their normal-hearing counterparts in terms of the number of words recalled. Interestingly, while the performance was similar, the strategies differed between these children. In early trials, children with normal hearing were more likely to recall words in the exact order presented, a tendency that declined after the second trial. Conversely, children with CIs showed an increasing tendency to recall words in the presented order as the task continued (Kronenberger et al., 2018).

While cognitive outcomes in children with CIs have been previously examined, fewer studies have examined young adult CI users who were implanted as children. Given that CIs were first approved for use in children within the sensitive period in 1990, it is important to consider long-term outcomes in these now young adults. When examining young adults who were implanted within the sensitive period, there were no significant differences on tests of executive function shifting, inhibitory control, episodic memory, working memory, or processing speed in comparison to young adults who were implanted outside of the sensitive period. Significant differences were found in terms of American Sign Language (ASL) competency, with the later implanted young adults demonstrating greater ASL competency. These findings may suggest that early access to language regardless of modality supports cognitive development (Kartheiser et al., 2024).

Additionally, in a subset of these young adult CI users cross-modal plasticity was examined as a function of those who received their CIs within versus outside of the sensitive period. Consistent with previous studies, there was greater cross-modal reorganization in those who received their CI after 3.5 years of age. It is interesting to note that these differences in neuroplasticity did not appear to have an effect on cognitive development. This indicates that cross-modal reorganization, which may have emerged in development, continues to be present into young adulthood (Kartheiser et al., 2024).

The aforementioned results suggest that even brief periods of auditory deprivation can lead to differences in cognitive strategies and higher-order cognitive abilities in children with CIs, even when implantation occurs early. However, given the significant individual variability in cognitive processes, a personalized approach to evaluating cognition in this population may be necessary (Kral et al., 2016). The area of neurocognition with implanted prostheses is still emerging, and further research is needed to examine neurocognitive plasticity in implanted children to determine what rehabilitative support facilitates better cognitive outcomes.

Clinical Assessment of Neuroplastic Changes in Patients with Hearing Loss

Cortical evoked potential testing provides not only a glimpse into the cortical maturation of those with hearing loss but allows an objective measurement of how deaf children with CI are processing auditory input in comparison to their peers. This allows a way to examine hearing treatments and make appropriate recommendations on an individual basis. Sufficiently intense and high-quality auditory input can be determined by comparing a CI patient's P1 latencies and morphology to the normative data, as described previously in this chapter. Using CAEP results with hearing aids, CI candidacy can be aided based on the determination of sufficient or insufficient auditory input being provided to the system to allow for central auditory maturation. CAEP results can also be employed as a counseling tool for parents of children who inconsistently utilize amplification.

In clinical testing in our lab, CAEPs are recorded using the speech syllable /ba/. Tone burst stimuli may also be used in CAEP testing; however, it is essential to consider the configuration and degree of hearing loss in the context of which frequency tone burst is selected. Stimuli are presented at a conversational level via sound field at a 45-degree angle to the ear(s) of interest. This allows for testing with the amplification device in use. An active electrode is placed at Cz with a reference electrode located on one mastoid. Eyeblinks are monitored using a bipolar electrode montage with the lateral outer canthus referenced to the superior orbit. Eyeblinks occur in the same frequency range as the P1 response and must be monitored to ensure the response is not obscured. CI artifacts can also obscure or mimic the P1 response. To reduce CI artifact, multiple active electrodes can be positioned across the forehead in addition to the Cz electrode (Gilley et al., 2006). At least 200–300 sweeps of at least two replicable runs are obtained and grand-averaged to examine the P1 response. This latency can then be compared to the 95% confidence interval to establish age-appropriate cortical maturation outcomes, to demonstrate how CAEP responses can be utilized to determine CI candidacy and monitor the effects of treatment (Sharma et al., 2005; Campbell et al., 2011).

We find testing of the P1 CAEP biomarker for establishing CI candidacy particularly useful in children with co-morbidities such as Auditory Neuropathy Spectrum Disorder, in addition to hearing loss (Cardon & Sharma, 2013; Roland et al., 2012; Sharma & Cardon, 2015; Campbell et al., 2011; Sharma et al., 2013; Cardon et al., 2012). ANSD is characterized by the inability of the auditory system to send synchronous neural signals. It is marked by the presence of otoacoustic emissions (OAE) or a cochlear microphonic indicative of normal auditory hair cell function, with an abnormal auditory brainstem response (ABR) reflecting the lack of synchrony (Rance, 2005). However, CAEP measures can be obtained in this population. Hearing aids are a relatively controversial treatment for children with ANSD (Rance et al., 2002; Sharma et al., 2011; Cardon et al., 2012; Sharma & Cardon, 2015; Berlin et al., 1998; Hood, 1998). Sharma et al. (2011) showed that approximately only a third of ANSD children had a normally developing P1 response with the use of hearing aids (Sharma et al., 2011) and several children showed decreased coherence of cortical responses after treatment with hearing aids (Cardon & Sharma, 2021). However, in a study examining CAEP results pre- and post-CI in 11 children with ANSD, Cardon and Sharma (2013) were able to document the effectiveness of treatment with CIs. Almost all of these children (91%) showed latency improvements or normal P1 latencies after implantation. In this sample, 27% of the children had a normal P1 latency response with the use of a hearing aid and continued to have normal latencies with the use of a CI. Those children who had delayed or abnormal P1 responses with hearing aids demonstrated improvements in P1 latencies 6 months post activation of the CI. This suggests that CIs may help overcome some of the dys-synchrony by providing adequate auditory input into the central auditory system (Buss et al., 2002; Cardon & Sharma, 2013; Martinho de Carvalho et al., 2011; Harrison et al., 2015). Additionally, P1 latencies were found to be correlated with speech development scores such that earlier latencies corresponded with higher language development scores in children with ANSD (Cardon & Sharma, 2013).

The following two cases describe how we use the P1 biomarker in clinical decision-making in pediatric cases of ANSD that are referred to our laboratory: Case 1 was a child who failed his newborn hearing screening bilaterally and was diagnosed with ANSD before the age of 3 months. His birth history revealed the use of supplemental oxygen. At 8 months of age, the child received bilateral hearing aids. He was referred to our laboratory for P1 testing before and after intervention with bilateral hearing aids. Figure 22.3 depicts P1 CAEP waveforms prior to hearing-aid fitting. A robust and replicable P1 response was present; however, when plotted against 95% confidence intervals for normal P1 latency development, the child's response was delayed for his age, indicating delayed cortical auditory maturation (Fig. 22.3). Figure 22.3b depicts the child's P1 CAEP waveforms after several months of hearing aid use. After intervention, a robust and replicable P1 response could be observed, and the latency of this response fell within normal limits for the child's age (Fig. 22.3), consistent with the child's progress in listening and spoken language after hearing aid fitting.

Case 2 was born prematurely, presented with several high-risk factors for hearing loss, including hyperbilirubinemia requiring blood transfusion, and prolonged mechanical ventilation while in the neonatal intensive care unit for a 7-week period. Absent ABR and present distortion product otoacoustic emissions (DPOAE) led to a diagnosis of ANSD before the age of 3 months. The child was fitted with bilateral hearing aids at 4 months of age and was referred for P1 testing in our laboratory due to concerns about significant delays in speech and language development. Figure 22.4 depicts P1 CAEP waveforms obtained with hearing aids. As can be seen, no replicable P1 response could be observed, indicating that the hearing aids were providing inadequate auditory input to allow for normal auditory cortical maturation. The P1 results were taken into consideration while deciding on candidacy for cochlear implantation for this child. The child received a CI in the left ear at 21 months of age. Figure 22.4 shows the child's P1 CAEP waveforms after several months of implant use. The P1 latencies recorded following CI use were within the 95% confidence interval for the child's age, indicating age-appropriate development of the central auditory pathways. In this case, electrical stimulation from the CI

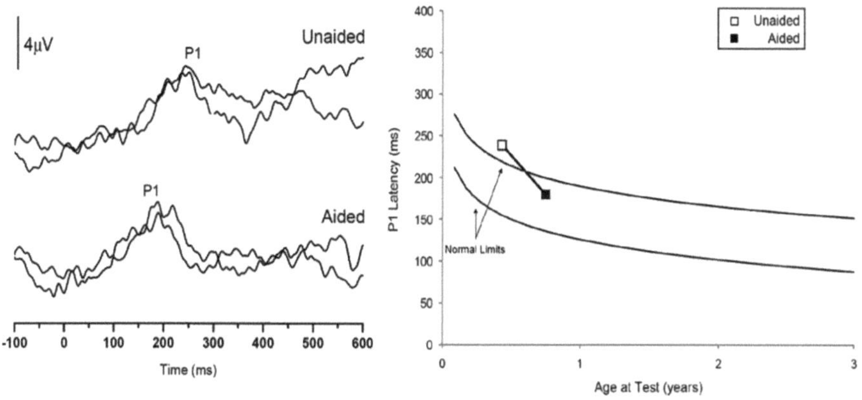

Fig. 22.3 P1 CAEP waveforms (with replications) for an ANSD child prior to hearing aid use (left panel top) and several months after bilateral hearing aid use (left panel). Averaged P1 CAEP latencies in the unaided and aided conditions are plotted against 95% confidence intervals for normal P1 latencies. Results indicate delayed P1 latency prior to hearing aid use. Within several months of hearing aid use, the P1 latency was age appropriate. (Reproduced from Cardon et al. (2012))

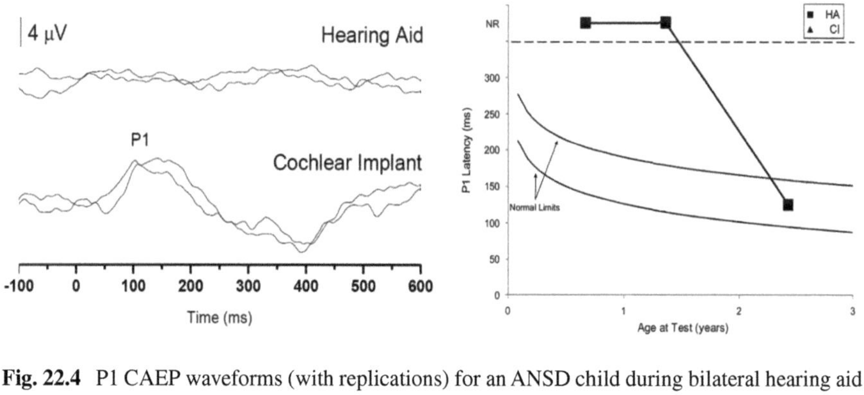

Fig. 22.4 P1 CAEP waveforms (with replications) for an ANSD child during bilateral hearing aid use (Left panel top) and several months after cochlear implantation of the left ear (Left panel bottom). Averaged P1 CAEP latencies hearing aid and cochlear implant (CI) conditions are plotted against 95% confidence intervals for normal P1 latency (Right panel). Results indicate absent P1 responses during hearing aid use. Within several months after left-ear cochlear implantation, P1 latency was age-appropriate. (Reproduced from Cardon et al. (2012))

appeared to facilitate rapid progress toward age-appropriate auditory cortical development.

Furthermore, we have demonstrated the feasibility of monitoring of the P1 biomarker in children with hearing loss and a wide array of additional disabilities (Lamminmäki et al., 2023). It is not uncommon for children with hearing loss to present with an additional disability (Cupples et al., 2018; Picard, 2004; Birman et al., 2012; Johnson & Wiley, 2009). In children with additional disabilities, audiologic behavioral testing may be unreliable, necessitating an objective measure to aid in hearing loss treatment decision making, such as CI candidacy. Recently our laboratory has examined CAEP responses in children with treated hearing loss and additional disabilities (e.g., Charge syndrome, cleft palate, gross motor difficulties, Cytomegalovirus, etc.) pre- and post- approximately 6 months of additional speech therapy in comparison to a cohort of children with only hearing loss. The children with additional disabilities were found to have comparable P1 responses pre- and post- the additional therapy to their peers with only hearing loss. Additionally, language scores at either time point did not significantly differ between these groups of children. Overall, in these children with hearing loss and a wide range of additional disabilities the presence of an additional disability did not lead to further delays in language skills and auditory cortical maturation, when hearing rehabilitation and language therapy were provided. Additionally, P1 latencies were significantly correlated to language abilities in this study further demonstrating the clinical utility of the P1 biomarker in this population. Results such as these suggest that the P1 biomarker could aid in clinical decision making and counseling on patient expectations in potentially difficult to test populations (Lamminmäki et al., 2023).

The above studies highlight how the P1 biomarker may be used to determine what kind of intervention method may be best suited in difficult pediatric cases. These case examples also highlight the importance of the P1 biomarker in assessing whether and to what extent the benefits derived from the intervention is providing the necessary stimulation for the auditory cortex to develop.

Monitoring of treatment outcomes with P1 testing can also be utilized with other implantable devices. Pantelemon et al. (2019) reported a case study of a 38-month-old female who presented with bilateral ear canal stenosis and left ossicular chain deformity resulting in a moderate to severe mixed hearing loss. Optimal treatment was determined to be a bone conduction hearing aid (BAHA) being utilized via a soft band. After 27 months of bone conduction hearing aid use this child's P1 latency was found to be within an age-appropriate range with expected morphology. These results coincided with overall improvements in the Denver Developmental Screening Test II, which examines gross motor, fine motor, language, and personal-social abilities in young children (Pantelemon et al., 2019). In this case, P1 testing with the BAHA allowed both the hearing professionals and parents to make informed decisions regarding the option for implantation of a bone conduction hearing aid once the child is at appropriate age for this procedure.

When children present with auditory nerves that are not viable for cochlear implantation, an auditory brainstem implant (ABI) can be considered. ABIs bypass the auditory nerve and deliver direct electrical stimulation to the cochlear nucleus. Very little research to date has examined neuroplastic changes in ABI recipients. In a series of studies by He et al. (2015, 2018), electrically evoked cortical auditory potentials were examined in 5 pre-lingually deafened children fitted with an ABI. Two distinct morphological responses were noted with the first morphological response showing a single positive peak occurring between 40 and 100 ms. This response type was similar to that seen in children with CIs, demonstrating appropriate maturation of the cortical auditory pathway. The second response type demonstrated multiple positive peaks between 25 and 700 ms. These responses varied greatly between the children and between different electrodes. Electrically evoked cortical auditory potentials were noted to change over the course of 41 months of ABI usage, but central auditory maturation could not account for all the changes seen in this study. However, one participant, who exhibited no initial response, showed the emergence of a response similar to that seen in children with CIs followed by the first indications of auditory perception, which may suggest that auditory development could be objectively tracked using the P1 biomarker in children with ABIs (He et al., 2015, 2018).

Auditory deprivation leads to neuroplastic brain changes throughout the lifespan. These neuroplastic changes may contribute to individual differences seen with audiologic treatment outcomes. Timely intervention with amplification and/or electrical stimulation within a sensitive period of 3.5 years is essential for the acquisition of age-appropriate auditory development. Following this age, implantation may not result in typical central auditory maturation even after long periods of CI use. Providing CIs within the sensitive period limits deprivation induced neuroplastic changes that arrest functional developmental processes. Sensitive periods also exist for typical binaural development of the auditory system. If the inter-implant delay is longer than 1.5 years, an atypical strengthening of the contralateral auditory pathway occurs. Auditory deprivation can also drive compensatory cross-modal reorganization allowing auditory brain regions to be recruited by the other intact sensory systems impacting functional outcomes with implantable devices.

When implantable prostheses are fitted in deaf patients, and rehabilitation programs allow these patients to reach optimal performance after treatment—these processes are subserved by underlying neuroplastic changes. As discussed in this chapter, harnessing cortical neuroplasticity has enabled us to develop tools (i.e., brain-based biomarkers like the P1 CAEP) for investigating appropriate treatments for hearing loss. The same biomarkers enable us to optimize intervention and rehabilitation in individual patients and allow us to assess how well the chosen intervention or rehabilitation is working or whether a different intervention is needed. Future research, that underscores a better understanding of cortical neuroplasticity that accompanies deafness, will also allow us to incorporate improvements in the design and fitting of hearing prostheses to allow them to better accommodate altered cortical processing.

References

Bauer, P. W., Sharma, A., Martin, K., & Dorman, M. (2006). Central auditory development in children with bilateral cochlear implants. *Archives of Otolaryngology–Head & Neck Surgery, 132*(10), 1133–1136.

Bavelier, D., & Neville, H. J. (2002). Cross-modal plasticity: Where and how? *Nature Reviews Neuroscience, 3*(6), 443–452.

Bergeson, T. R., Pisoni, D. B., & Davis, R. A. (2005). Development of audiovisual comprehension skills in prelingually deaf children with cochlear implants. *Ear and Hearing, 26*(2), 149–164.

Berlin, C. I., Bordelon, J., St John, P., Wilensky, D., Hurley, A., Kluka, E., & Hood, L. J. (1998). Reversing click polarity may uncover auditory neuropathy in infants. *Ear and Hearing, 19*(1), 37–47.

Birman, C. S., Elliott, E. J., & Gibson, W. P. (2012). Pediatric cochlear implants: Additional disabilities prevalence, risk factors, and effect on language outcomes. *Otology & Neurotology, 33*(8), 1347–1352.

Buss, E., Labadie, R. F., Brown, C. J., Gross, A. J., Grose, J. H., & Pillsbury, H. C. (2002). Outcome of cochlear implantation in pediatric auditory neuropathy. *Otology & Neurotology: Official Publication of the American Otological Society, American Neurotology Society [and] European Academy of Otology and Neurotology, 23*(3), 328–332.

Campbell, J. D., Cardon, G., & Sharma, A. (2011). Clinical application of the P1 cortical auditory evoked potential biomarker in children with sensorineural hearing loss and auditory neuropathy spectrum disorder. *Seminars in Hearing, 32*(2), 147–155.

Campbell, J., & Sharma, A. (2016). Visual cross-modal re-organization in children with cochlear implants. *PLoS One, 11*(1), e0147793.

Cardon, G., Campbell, J., & Sharma, A. (2012). Plasticity in the developing auditory cortex: Evidence from children with sensorineural hearing loss and auditory neuropathy spectrum disorder. *Journal of the American Academy of Audiology, 23*(6), 396–495.

Cardon, G., & Sharma, A. (2013). Central auditory maturation and behavioral outcome in children with auditory neuropathy spectrum disorder who use cochlear implants. *International Journal of Audiology, 52*(9), 577–586.

Cardon, G., & Sharma, A. (2021). Cortical neurophysiologic correlates of auditory threshold in adults and children with normal hearing and auditory neuropathy spectrum disorder. *American Journal of Audiology, 30*(1), 28–42.

Cardon, G., & Sharma, A. (2019). Somatosensory cross-modal reorganization in children with cochlear implants. *Frontiers in Neuroscience, 13*, 469.

Cupples, L., Ching, T. Y. C., Button, L., Leigh, G., Marnane, V., Whitfield, J., Gunnourie, M., & Martin, L. (2018). Language and speech outcomes of children with hearing loss and additional disabilities: Identifying the variables that influence performance at five years of age. *International Journal of Audiology, 57*(sup2), S93–S104.

Dorman, M. F., Sharma, A., Gilley, P., Martin, K., & Roland, P. (2007). Central auditory development: Evidence from CAEP measurements in children fit with cochlear implants. *Journal of Communication Disorders, 40*(4), 284–294.

Doucet, M. E., Bergeron, F., Lassonde, M., Ferron, P., & Lepore, F. (2006). Cross-modal reorganization and speech perception in cochlear implant users. *Brain: A Journal of Neurology, 129*(Pt 12), 3376–3383.

Dunn, C. C., Walker, E. A., Oleson, J., Kenworthy, M., Van Voorst, T., Tomblin, J. B., Ji, H., Kirk, K. I., McMurray, B., Hanson, M., & Gantz, B. J. (2014). Longitudinal speech perception and language performance in pediatric cochlear implant users: The effect of age at implantation. *Ear and Hearing, 35*(2), 148–160.

Eggermont, J. J., & Ponton, C. W. (2003). Auditory-evoked potential studies of cortical maturation in normal hearing and implanted children: Correlations with changes in structure and speech perception. *Acta Oto-Laryngologica, 123*(2), 249–252.

Geers, A. E. (2006). Factors influencing spoken language outcomes in children following early cochlear implantation. *Advances in Oto-Rhino-Laryngology, 64*, 50–65.

Gilley, P. M., Sharma, A., Dorman, M., Finley, C. C., Panch, A. S., & Martin, K. (2006). Minimization of cochlear implant stimulus artifact in cortical auditory evoked potentials. *Clinical Neurophysiology: Official Journal of the International Federation of Clinical Neurophysiology, 117*(8), 1772–1782.

Glick, H. A., & Sharma, A. (2020). Cortical neuroplasticity and cognitive function in early stage, mild-moderate hearing loss: Evidence of neurocognitive benefit from hearing aid use. *Frontiers in Neuroscience, 14*, 93.

Glick, H., & Sharma, A. (2017). Cross-modal plasticity in developmental and age-related hearing loss: Clinical implications. *Hearing Research, 343*, 191–201.

Gordon, K. A., Jiwani, S., & Papsin, B. C. (2011). What is the optimal timing for bilateral cochlear implantation in children? *Cochlear Implants International, 12*(Suppl 2), S8–S14.

Gordon, K. A., Valero, J., & Papsin, B. C. (2007). Binaural processing in children using bilateral cochlear implants. *Neuroreport, 18*(6), 613–617.

Gordon, K. A., Valero, J., Van Hoesel, R., & Papsin, B. C. (2008). Abnormal timing delays in auditory brainstem responses evoked by bilateral cochlear implant use in children. *Otology & Neurotology: Official Publication of the American Otological Society, American Neurotology Society [and] European Academy of Otology and Neurotology, 29*(2), 193–198.

Gordon, K. A., Wong, D. D., & Papsin, B. C. (2010). Cortical function in children receiving bilateral cochlear implants simultaneously or after a period of interimplant delay. *Otology & neurotology: Official Publication of the American Otological Society, American Neurotology Society [and] European Academy of Otology and Neurotology, 31*(8), 1293–1299.

Gordon, K. A., Wong, D. D., & Papsin, B. C. (2013). Bilateral input protects the cortex from unilaterally-driven reorganization in children who are deaf. *Brain: A Journal of Neurology, 136*(Pt 5), 1609–1625.

Harrison, R. V., Gordon, K. A., & Mount, R. J. (2005). Is there a critical period for cochlear implantation in congenitally deaf children? Analyses of hearing and speech perception performance after implantation. *Developmental Psychobiology, 46*(3), 252–261.

Harrison, R. V., Gordon, K. A., Papsin, B. C., Negandhi, J., & James, A. L. (2015). Auditory neuropathy spectrum disorder (ANSD) and cochlear implantation. *International Journal of Pediatric Otorhinolaryngology, 79*(12), 1980–1987.

Hauthal, N., Sandmann, P., Debener, S., & Thorne, J. D. (2013). Visual movement perception in deaf and hearing individuals. *Advances in Cognitive Psychology, 9*(2), 53–61.

He, S., Teagle, H. F., Ewend, M., Henderson, L., & Buchman, C. A. (2015). The electrically evoked cortical auditory event-related potential in children with auditory brainstem implants. *Ear and Hearing, 36*(3), 377–379.

He, S., Teagle, H., McFayden, T. C., Ewend, M., Henderson, L., He, N., & Buchman, C. A. (2018). Longitudinal changes in electrically evoked auditory event-related potentials in children with auditory brainstem implants: Preliminary results recorded over 3 years. *Ear and Hearing, 39*(2), 318–325.

Hennesy, T., Cardon, G., Campbell, J., Glick, H., Bell-Souder, D., & Sharma, A. (2022). Cross modal reorganization from both visual and somatosensory modalities in cochlear implanted children and its relationship to speech perception. *Otology & Neurotology, 43*(8), e872–e879.

Holt, R. F., & Svirsky, M. A. (2008). An exploratory look at pediatric cochlear implantation: Is earliest always best? *Ear and Hearing, 29*(4), 492–511.

Hood, L. J. (1998). An overview of neural function and feedback control in human communication. *Journal of Communication Disorders, 31*(6), 461–553.

Jiwani, S., Papsin, B. C., & Gordon, K. A. (2016). Early unilateral cochlear implantation promotes mature cortical asymmetries in adolescents who are deaf. *Human Brain Mapping, 37*(1), 135–152.

Johnson, K. C., & Wiley, S. (2009). Cochlear implantation in children with multiple disabilties. In *Clinical management of children with cochlear implants* (1st ed., pp. 573–632). Plural Pub.

Kartheiser, G., Cormier, K., Bell-Souder, D., Dye, M., & Sharma, A. (2024). Neurocognitive outcomes in young adults with cochlear implants: The role of early language access and crossmodal plasticity. *Hearing Research, 451*, 109074.

Kim, M. B., Shim, H. Y., Jin, S. H., Kang, S., Woo, J., Han, J. C., Lee, J. Y., Kim, M., Cho, Y. S., Moon, I. J., & Hong, S. H. (2016). Cross-modal and intra-modal characteristics of visual function and speech perception performance in postlingually deafened, cochlear implant users. *PLoS One, 11*(2), e0148466.

Knudsen, E. I. (2004). Sensitive periods in the development of the brain and behavior. *Journal of Cognitive Neuroscience, 16*(8), 1412–1425.

Kral, A., Dorman, M. F., & Wilson, B. S. (2019). Neuronal development of hearing and language: Cochlear implants and critical periods. *Annual Review of Neuroscience, 42*, 47–65.

Kral, A., Kronenberger, W. G., Pisoni, D. B., & O'Donoghue, G. M. (2016). Neurocognitive factors in sensory restoration of early deafness: A connectome model. *The Lancet Neurology, 15*(6), 610–621.

Kral, A., Schröder, J. H., Klinke, R., & Engel, A. K. (2003). Absence of cross-modal reorganization in the primary auditory cortex of congenitally deaf cats. *Experimental Brain Research, 153*(4), 605–613.

Kral, A., & Sharma, A. (2012). Developmental neuroplasticity after cochlear implantation. *Trends in Neurosciences, 35*(2), 111–122.

Kral, A., & Sharma, A. (2023). Crossmodal plasticity in hearing loss. *Trends in Neurosciences, 46*(5), 377–393.

Kronenberger, W. G., Beer, J., Castellanos, I., Pisoni, D. B., & Miyamoto, R. T. (2014). Neurocognitive risk in children with cochlear implants. *JAMA Otolaryngology–Head & Neck Surgery, 140*(7), 608–615.

Kronenberger, W. G., Henning, S. C., Ditmars, A. M., Roman, A. S., & Pisoni, D. B. (2018). Verbal learning and memory in prelingually deaf children with cochlear implants. *International Journal of Audiology, 57*(10), 746–754.

Lamminmäki, S., Cormier, K., Davidson, H., Grigsby, J., & Sharma, A. (2023). Auditory cortex maturation and language development in children with hearing loss and additional disabilities. *Children, 10*(11), 1813.

Land, R., Baumhoff, P., Tillein, J., Lomber, S. G., Hubka, P., & Kral, A. (2016). Cross-modal plasticity in higher-order auditory cortex of congenitally deaf cats does not limit auditory responsiveness to cochlear implants. *The Journal of Neuroscience: The Official Journal of the Society for Neuroscience, 36*(23), 6175–6185.

Lee, H. J., Giraud, A. L., Kang, E., Oh, S. H., Kang, H., Kim, C. S., & Lee, D. S. (2007). Cortical activity at rest predicts cochlear implantation outcome. *Cerebral Cortex, 17*(4), 909–917.

Lee, H. J., Kang, E., Oh, S. H., Kang, H., Lee, D. S., Lee, M. C., & Kim, C. S. (2005). Preoperative differences of cerebral metabolism relate to the outcome of cochlear implants in congenitally deaf children. *Hearing Research, 203*(1–2), 2–9.

Levänen, S., Hamdorf, D. (2001) Feeling vibrations: enhanced tactile sensitivity in congenitally deaf humans. *Neuroscience Letters, 301*(1), 75–77. https://doi.org/10.1016/S0304-3940(01)01597-X

Lin, F. R. (2011). Hearing loss and cognition among older adults in the United States. *The Journals of Gerontology. Series A, Biological Sciences and Medical Sciences, 66*(10), 1131–1136.

Lomber, S. G., Meredith, M. A., & Kral, A. (2010). Cross-modal plasticity in specific auditory cortices underlies visual compensations in the deaf. *Nature Neuroscience, 13*(11), 1421–1427.

Martinho de Carvalho, A. C., Bevilacqua, M. C., Sameshima, K., & Filho, O. (2011). Auditory neuropathy/auditory dyssynchrony in children with cochlear implants. *Brazilian Journal of Otorhinolaryngology, 77*(4), 481–487.

Meredith, M. A., & Lomber, S. G. (2011). Somatosensory and visual crossmodal plasticity in the anterior auditory field of early-deaf cats. *Hearing Research, 280*(1–2), 38–47.

Niparko, J. K., Tobey, E. A., Thal, D. J., Eisenberg, L. S., Wang, N. Y., Quittner, A. L., Fink, N. E., & CDaCI Investigative Team. (2010). Spoken language development in children following cochlear implantation. *JAMA, 303*(15), 1498–1506.

Pantelemon, C., Necula, V., Livint Popa, L., Palade, S., Strilciuc, S., & Muresanu, D. F. (2019). The potential use of P1 CAEP as a biomarker for assessing central auditory pathway maturation in hearing loss and associated disabilities: A case report. *Journal of Medicine and Life, 12*(4), 457–460.

Picard, M. (2004). Children with permanent hearing loss and associated disabilities: Revisiting current epidemiological data and causes of deafness. *Volta Review, 104*(4), 221–236.

Rance, G., Cone-Wesson, B., Wunderlich, J., & Dowell, R. (2002). Speech perception and cortical event related potentials in children with auditory neuropathy. *Ear and Hearing, 23*(3), 239–253.

Rance, G. (2005). Auditory neuropathy/dys-synchrony and its perceptual consequences. *Trends in Amplification, 9*(1), 1–43.

Robbins, A. M., Green, J. E., & Waltzman, S. B. (2004). Bilingual oral language proficiency in children with cochlear implants. *Archives of Otolaryngology–Head & Neck Surgery, 130*(5), 644–647.

Roland, P., Henion, K., Booth, T., Campbell, J. D., & Sharma, A. (2012). Assessment of cochlear implant candidacy in patients with cochlear nerve deficiency using the P1 CAEP biomarker. *Cochlear Implants International, 13*(1), 16–25.

Rosemann, S., & Thiel, C. M. (2020). Neural signatures of working memory in age-related hearing loss. *Neuroscience, 429*, 134–142.

Schorr, E. A., Fox, N. A., Van Wassenhove, V., & Knudsen, E. I. (2005). Auditory-visual fusion in speech perception in children with cochlear implants. *Proceedings of the National Academy of Sciences of the United States of America, 102*(51), 18748–18750.

Schürmann, M., Caetano, G., Hlushchuk, Y., Jousmäki, V., & Hari, R. (2006). Touch activates human auditory cortex. *NeuroImage, 30*(4), 1325–1331.

Sharma, A., Kraus, N., McGee, T.J., Nicol, T.G. (1997) Developmental changes in P1 and N1 central auditory responses elicited by consonant-vowel syllables. *Electroencephalography and Clinical Neurophysiology/Evoked Potentials Section, 104*(6), 540–545. https://doi.org/10.1016/S0168-5597(97)00050-6

Sharma, A., Nash, A.A., Dorman, M. (2009) Cortical development plasticity and re-organization in children with cochlear implants. *Journal of Communication Disorders, 42*(4), 272–279. https://doi.org/10.1016/j.jcomdis.2009.03.003

Sharma, A., Campbell, J., & Cardon, G. (2015). Developmental and cross-modal plasticity in deafness: Evidence from the P1 and N1 event related potentials in cochlear implanted children. *International Journal of Psychophysiology, 95*(2), 135–144.

Sharma, A., & Cardon, G. (2015). Cortical development and neuroplasticity in Auditory Neuropathy Spectrum Disorder. *Hearing Research, 330*(Pt B), 221–232.

Sharma, A., Cardon, G., Henion, K., & Roland, P. (2011). Cortical maturation and behavioral outcomes in children with auditory neuropathy spectrum disorder. *International Journal of Audiology, 50*(2), 98–106.

Sharma, A., Dorman, M. F., & Kral, A. (2005). The influence of a sensitive period on central auditory development in children with unilateral and bilateral cochlear implants. *Hearing Research, 203*(1–2), 134–143.

Sharma, A., Dorman, M. F., & Spahr, A. J. (2002a). A sensitive period for the development of the central auditory system in children with cochlear implants: Implications for age of implantation. *Ear and Hearing, 23*(6), 532–539.

Sharma, A., Dorman, M. F., & Spahr, A. J. (2002b). Rapid development of cortical auditory evoked potentials after early cochlear implantation. *Neuroreport, 13*(10), 1365–1368.

Sharma, A., & Glick, H. (2016). Cross-modal re-organization in clinical populations with hearing loss. *Brain Sciences, 6*(1), 4.

Sharma, A., Glick, H., Campbell, J., & Biever, A. (2013). Central auditory development in children with hearing loss: Clinical relevance of the P1 CAEP biomarker in hearing -impaired children with multiple disabilities. *Hearing, Balance and Communication, 11*(3), 110–120.

Shiell, M. M., Champoux, F., & Zatorre, R. J. (2014). Enhancement of visual motion detection thresholds in early deaf people. *PLoS One, 9*(2), e90498.

Shiell, M. M., Champoux, F., & Zatorre, R. J. (2016). The right hemisphere planum temporale supports enhanced visual motion detection ability in deaf people: Evidence from cortical thickness. *Neural Plasticity, 2016*, 7217630.

Sparreboom, M., Beynon, A. J., Snik, A. F., & Mylanus, E. A. (2014). Auditory cortical maturation in children with sequential bilateral cochlear implants. *Otology & Neurotology, 35*(1), 35–42.

Strelnikov, K., Rouger, J., Demonet, J. F., et al. (2013). Visual activity predicts auditory recovery from deafness after adult cochlear implantation. *Brain, 136*(Pt 12), 3682–3695.

Stropahl, M., Plotz, K., Schönfeld, R., Lenarz, T., Sandmann, P., Yovel, G., De Vos, M., & Debener, S. (2015). Cross-modal reorganization in cochlear implant users: Auditory cortex contributes to visual face processing. *NeuroImage, 121*, 159–170.

Sun, Z., Seo, J. W., Park, H. J., Lee, J. Y., Kwak, M. Y., Kim, Y., Lee, J. Y., Park, J. W., Kang, W. S., Ahn, J. H., Chung, J. W., & Kim, H. (2021). Cortical reorganization following auditory deprivation predicts cochlear implant performance in postlingually deaf adults. *Human Brain Mapping, 42*(1), 233–244.

Svirsky, M. A., Teoh, S. W., & Neuburger, H. (2004). Development of language and speech perception in congenitally, profoundly deaf children as a function of age at cochlear implantation. *Audiology & Neuro-Otology, 9*(4), 224–233.

Tajudeen, B. A., Waltzman, S. B., Jethanamest, D., & Svirsky, M. A. (2010). Speech perception in congenitally deaf children receiving cochlear implants in the first year of life. *Otology & Neurotology, 31*(8), 1254–1260.

Tyler, R. S., Fryauf-Bertschy, H., Kelsay, D. M., Gantz, B. J., Woodworth, G. P., & Parkinson. (1997). Speech perception by prelingually deaf children using cochlear implants. *Otolaryngology–Head and Neck Surgery, 117*(3 Pt 1), 180–187.

Wang, N. Y., Eisenberg, L. S., Johnson, K. C., Fink, N. E., Tobey, E. A., Quittner, A. L., Niparko, J. K., & CDaCI Investigative Team. (2008). Tracking development of speech recognition: Longitudinal data from hierarchical assessments in the childhood development after cochlear implantation study. *Otology & Neurotology, 29*(2), 240–245.

Chapter 23
Auditory Brainstem Implants: Audiological Perspectives

Niraj Kumar Singh, Prawin Kumar, and Neevita Narayan

Abstract Auditory brainstem implant (ABI) is a bio-electronic neuroprosthetic device that directly stimulates the second order neurons of the Cochlear Nucleus Complex (CNC) at the brainstem, bypassing the cochlea and auditory nerve. The ABIs were first implemented in patients with Neurofibromatosis Type 2 (NF2) to reinstate hearing. Later, they were also used in children and adults with hearing loss due to pathologies other than NF2, such as cochlear or auditory nerve aplasia and cochlear ossification, in whoma cochlear implantation was not feasible. This chapter highlights evolution of the ABI, candidacy, fitting of the device and its benefits.

Keywords Auditory brainstem implants · ABI · Cochlear nucleus · Neurofibromatosis · Electrode array · Electrode peddle · Penetrating ABI

Introduction

Cochlear implants, possibly the biggest invention of the century gone by, reinstates hearing in individuals with severe to profound degree of hearing impairment. As discussed in the chapters on cochlear implants in this book, cochlear implantation has been a main reason behind successful rehabilitation in a large majority of children and adults suffering from congenital or acquired severe to profound sensorineural hearing loss. However, several conditions of the cochlea or those that affect the Vestibulocochlear nerve contraindicate cochlear implantation due to anatomic constraints that allow minimal or no benefit possibility from this prosthetic device. Cochlear ossification, aplasic cochlea or cochlear nerve, hypoplastic cochlear nerve, severing of the cochlear nerve due to a temporal bone injury or during temporal

N. K. Singh (✉) · P. Kumar
Department of Audiology, All India Institute of Speech and Hearing, University of Mysore, Mysore, India

N. Narayan
SpHear Speech & Hearing Clinics, G-32, New Delhi, India

P. Kumar et al. (eds.), *Advances in Implantation Otology*,
https://doi.org/10.1007/978-981-96-8671-1_23

bone surgeries, bilateral vestibular schwannomas (as might be evidenced in people with Neurofibromatosis Type 2) etc. are such anatomic constraints that contraindicate cochlear implantation. A ray of hope for regaining auditory sensation in such people could be an Auditory Brainstem Implant (ABI), although work on other possible options such as auditory midbrain implants (AMI) has begun promisingly just over a decade ago. However, the AMI outcomes are in nascence (more details in Chapter 25), and until at such times when it shows better outcomes than the time tested ABI, ABI remains the best option for these patients.

ABI, like the cochlear implant, is a bio-electronic neuroprosthetic device. It directly stimulates the second order neurons of the Cochlear Nucleus Complex (CNC) at the brainstem, bypassing the cochlea and auditory nerve. An ABI was first implanted in patients with Neurofibromatosis Type 2 (NF2) to reinstate hearing. Later, they were also used in pathological conditions other than NF2, wherein the cochlear implantation was not feasible.

In a Cochlear Implant, the electrical device is surgically implanted in the cochlea, whereas in ABI, the device is implanted in the CNC at the brainstem. The cochlear nucleus is the site of choice for electrode placement due to its anatomy and function. The ABIs are designed to circumvent the cochlea and the auditory nerve to directly stimulate the cochlear nucleus. This makes ABI an option to regain hearing in individuals in whom a cochlear implantation was contraindicated due to severely aberrant anatomies. Owing to the findings of growing incidence of congenital cochlear and cochlear nerve anomalies, which deprives several of such patients from cochlear implantation, ABI has brought hope for providing them auditory sensation.

The fundamental mechanism of an ABI is similar to that of a Cochlear Implant. The difference is that the ABI uses a flat paddle-shaped electrode array to stimulate the surface of the cochlear nucleus, whereas the spiral ganglion neurons (SGNs) in the cochlear region are stimulated using the CI electrode array that spirals along the Scala tympani. While the coding strategies are similar, the mode of stimulation can vary between CI and ABI. Auditory brainstem implant is mostly stimulated using bipolar stimulation whereas in CI the monopolar mode of stimulation is preferred.

The question here is what was the reason to create an ABI electrode differently to the cochlear implant? The answer lies in the hugely varied anatomy between the structures where the electrode arrays of the two devices are to be instated. The cochlear nucleus complex, as the name suggests, is a congregation of three different parts joined together into one structure. These parts are: the Dorsal Cochlear Nucleus (DCN), the Anteroventral Cochlear Nucleus (AVCN) and the Posteroventral Cochlear Nucleus (PCVN), with the latter two combining to form the Ventral Cochlear Nucleus (VCN). These different nuclei of CNC are innervated by the auditory nerve fibers constituted by the axons of SGNs. Each of these CNC nuclei has its own unique tonotopic organization (Kandler et al., 2009). In stark contrast to the cochlea, which has a more straight-forward two dimensional tonotopic arrangement with frequencies reducing systematically from the base to apex, the tonotopic map within the CNC is a 3-dimensional arrangement with frequencies arranged like pages in book (layered manner) such that each page has a separate characteristic frequency (Luo et al., 2009). Further, unlike a well-defined structure in to which a CI electrode array is inserted, CNC has a very small and less defined surface area, making it difficult to precisely identify and locate its boundaries (more on the anatomy of the CNC is described in Chapter 2). While these anatomical differences are the reason for a major difference in the electrode design between the ABI and the CI, mere differences in the electrode design cannot completely offshoot the differences. As the cochlea is a highly tonotopically organised structure with tonotopic gradient spread across the length of the basilar membrane in the cochlear lumen, an electrode array traversing below the basilar membrane within the scala tympani can stimulate the SGNs along the basilar membrane in a tonotopic manner. However, in ABI, the three-dimensional CNC is to be stimulated by a two dimensional surface electrode paddle, and therefore, while an auditory stimulation is achieved with electrically stimulating the CNC surface, it is hard to achieve tonotopic stimulation using an electrode design paradoxical to the tonotopicity within the CNC.

Components of Auditory Brainstem Implant

At present, there are two major manufactures of the ABI system in the world. The Nucleus Auditory Brainstem Implant System, is manufactured by Cochlear Corporation, Australia, whereas the Med EL ABI system is manufactured by Med EL Elektromedizinische Geräte Gesellschaft m.b.H., Austria. Irrespective of the manufacturer and the model, an ABI system has external components that are worn outside, appearing similar to a behind-the-ear (BTE) hearing aid to naive observer, although off-the-ear (OTE) external component is now also available. The ABI also has surgically implantable internal components.

External components of ABI consist of a sound processor, transmitting coil and battery. Two major designs of sound processors exist on the basis of the style (place) of wearing: BTE sound processor and OTE sound processor (Fig. 23.1). Historically,

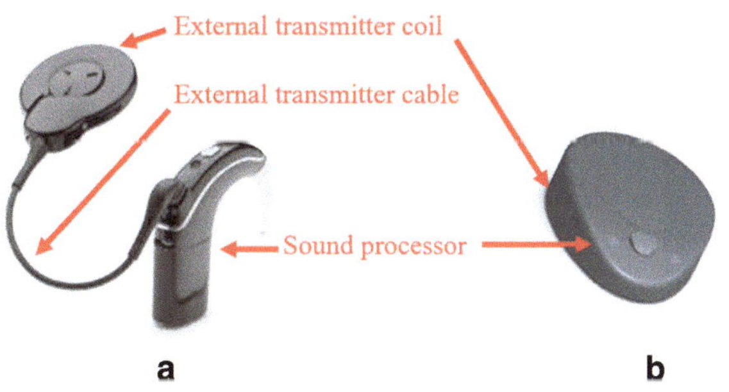

Fig. 23.1 Types of modern-day external sound processors: (**a**) Behind the Ear (BTE) sound processor; (**b**) Off the Ear (OTE) sound processor (Pictures published with permission from the manufacturer)

body worn sound processors were also available; however, this style has become extinct with no manufacturer offering it currently. The BTE sound processor, which also houses the battery compartment in it, is worn behind the ear and the transmitting coil is connected to the processor by a cable. In the OTE sound processor, the three major components are all housed in a single unit, which is placed on the temporal part of the skull over the receiver-stimulator of the internal implant. Irrespective of the style, the overall functioning of the external components of ABI remains the same. The sound processor has an in-built directional microphone on it, which converts the picked up acoustic signals to electrical signals. The sound processor then converts these analog signals into digital signals which are used to modulate radio frequency waves and sent to the external transmitting coil via the transmitter cable. The external transmitter coil emits these radiofrequency waves to the internal receiver stimulator. The external transmitting coil and the internal receiver stimulator have a magnet each to secure the external transmitting coil over the skin overlying the internal receiver-stimulator. However, it is possible to remove the magnet of an ABI system, in which case the external coil is kept in place with the help of an adhesive disk or a headband. This is particularly important in patients with NF2 who have undergone ABI but may need periodic monitoring using the Magnetic resonance imaging (MRI).

An electrode paddle and the receiver stimulator constitute the internal components of an ABI system. The receiver and the electrode paddle are connected to each other by insulated micro wires. These internal components are surgically placed in their desired locations -- the receiver stimulator on the temporal bone under the skin surface and the electrode paddle over the surface of CNC. The details about the ABI surgery are discussed in Chaper 24.

The electrode paddle design has been created keeping in mind not only the neuroanatomy of CNC and its surrounding structures but also charge density requirements to safely stimulate the neurons in the region. Depending on the manufacturer and model, 12–24 active platinum contacts embedded in a flat oval-shaped silicone paddle constitute the electrode paddle. The soft electrode paddle has a pre-shaped curvature which allows it to seamlessly hug the curved surface of the brainstem. The presence of a polyester mesh embedded in silicone allows tissue growth which helps with further stabilization of the electrode array on the surface of the brainstem in order to minimize the possibility of electrode migration. The internal components of ABI, with their specific dimensions, are depicted in Figs. 23.2, and 23.3. A schematic representation of various external and internal components and their interrelationship to accomplish the electrical stimulation of the CNC surface is shown in Fig. 23.3.

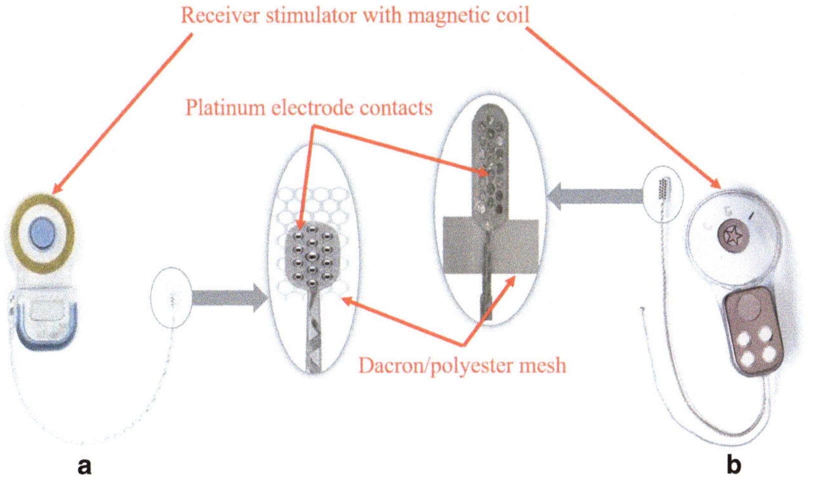

Fig. 23.2 Internal components of an ABI system manufactured by (**a**) Med EL, Austria (**b**) Cochlear Ltd., Australia. (Picture reproduced with permission from Med EL, Austria and Cochlear Ltd., Australia)

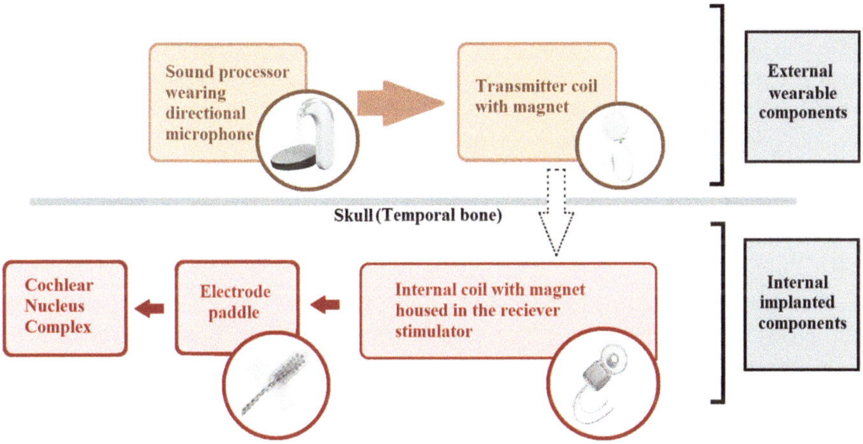

Fig. 23.3 Schematic representation of an ABI's components and their inter-relationships

Evolution of Auditory Brainstem Implant

During the development in the initial years, significant contributions came from several corners. The device itself evolved from being a single channel prototype to the present day masterpiece. This section describes the history of ABI, tracing its evolution along the way.

Single-Channel ABI System

Dr. William House, a neuro-otologist of the House Ear Institute at Los Angeles, is credited with the invention of the ABI concept in the year 1979. Dr. House and his neurosurgeon colleague William Hitselberger at the House Ear Institute could demonstrate auditory percept after placing dual platinum ball-electrodes on the cochlear nucleus of a patient with severely damaged cochlear nerve due to NF2 (Brackmann et al., 1993; Hitselberger et al., 1984). Subsequently, 24 NF2 patients at the House Ear Institute were implanted with a single-channel ABI system until 1991. Among them, 19 were implanted with a two-plate electrode design whereas the last five received a three-plate electrode design (Brackmann et al., 1993). Among 25 patients (including the first one) with the above-mentioned single channel ABI systems, several patients faced medical and technical issues. While a revision surgery due to device failure was needed in only three patients, others experienced broken wires (n = 2), percutaneous electrical plug connector infections (n = 4), postoperative meningitis which was treated with antibiotics (n = 2), and cerebrospinal fluid leaks requiring treatment with mastoid pressure dressings, surgical exploration and repacking, or lumbar drainage (n = 9) (Brackmann et al., 1993). Nonetheless, as far as the audiometric outcomes are concerned, a majority of these patients received environmental sound awareness and perceived subjective auditory benefit from their ABIs. Because of the success with the single channel ABI system, Dr. House and his team, in collaboration with Cochlear Ltd., developed a multi-channel ABI system. Many years later in the 1990s and early 2000s, the other major manufacturer of the cochlear implants, Med-EL also developed ABI systems.

Penetrating Electrode Auditory Brainstem Implant

The development of the penetrating electrode ABI (PABI) was another strategy to improve the auditory performance with an ABI. The PABI was designed bearing in mind the 3-dimensional (sheet-like) tonotopic organization of the CNC. It consisted of multiple needle-shaped microelectrodes of varying lengths that allowed the electrodes to penetrate the CNC up to a depth of 1–2 mm which enabled stimulation of deeply sheeted neural pathways that had remained inaccessible to the standard surface electrodes. After experimenting for a while, the final experimental device, which had a combination of 8–10 penetrating microneedle electrodes and 10–12 surface electrodes, saw the daylight in the early part of the 1990s. This experimental device was a collaborative work of Huntington Medical Research Institutes (Pasadena, CA, United States) and Cochlear Ltd. (Sydney, Australia), and was developed at the House Ear Institute.

A prospective clinical trial of PABI on 10 patients with NF2 reported that the penetrating electrodes required substantially lower charge levels to achieve auditory thresholds, produced a markedly broader electrode-specific pitch sensation range and greatly reduced inter-electrode interference in compparison to the surface electrodes (Schwartz et al., 2008; Otto et al., 2008). The clinical outcomes were variable across the patients; however, the overall speech comprehension in the PABI patients remained comparable to the ABI patients with the traditional surface electrodes. On the flip side, less than 25% of the penetrating electrodes yielded auditory sensation as opposed to the auditory percept with nearly 60% of the surface electrodes (Schwartz et al., 2008). However, observation of several serious side effects ensured against further continuation with PABI.

Multi-Channel ABI System with Surface Electrodes

The year 1991 was witness to the development of a multichannel ABI system by Laszig et al. in collaboration with Cochlear Ltd. (Sydney, Australia). While the basic design of the electrode array included a polyethylene terephthalate mesh that had three platinum plates mounted on it, it was later developed in two versions: a 21-electrode version for Europe (Laszig & Aschendorff, 1999) and an 8-electrode version for the North America (Otto et al., 2002). It allowed for coding of different frequencies on the basis of differences in the pattern of electrode activations.

The evolution of ABI into a multi-channel device evidenced its wide use in the Northern Americas and Europe with the University of Verona (Italy) alone accounting for 27 recipients of the European version of the Nucleus multichannel ABI device (Nevison et al., 2002). No participant of this first ever cohort of multi-channel ABI device recipients had any major surgical complication, and a majority of them demonstrated environmental sound awareness and better pattern recognition to aid lip reading than those using the predecessor single-channel ABI. In fact, at least two recipients could even follow regular conversations even without being aided by lip reading, clearly demonstrating supremacy of performance with the multi-channel ABI over the single-channel ABI. The outcomes from the North American version (8-electrode) Nucleus multi-channel ABI were very similar to the Italian study (Schwartz et al., 2008), with most of the 71 patients with NF2 showing closed-set word recognition scores above the chance level.

The outcomes from the twin studies in Europe and the North Americas paved the way for first ever FDA approval for an ABI device (Nucleus 24 ABI) in the year 2000 (Otto et al., 2002) and its successor (Nucleus ABI 541), which had an all-improved receiver-stimulator and accommodated a removable magnet to support serial MRIs, in the year 2016. This proved to be a shot in the arm for the manufacturers, surgeons and the prospective recipients who could now begin to believe in the safety and efficacy of an ABI device. When stimulated with an ABI today, a majority of the NF2 patients demonstrate clear environmental sound awareness and some ability for phoneme discrimination, although only a few become capable of open set speech discrimination (Ramsden et al., 2016). Despite a major improvement from the single-channel ABI, the overall performance even with the multichannel ABI remains inferior to that from even a unilateral cochlear implantation. It is believed that trauma to the brainstem structures could be responsible for the large spectrum of outcomes from ABI in patients of NF2. The major reason for this hypothesis percolates from the outcomes of studies on ABI in non-NF2 patients such as those with congenital cochlear nerve aplasia, temporal bone fractures involving the cochlea or internal auditory canal, labyrinthine ossification due to bacterial meningitis, and otosclerosis involving a major section of the cochlea (Colletti et al., 2007; Colletti & Shannon, 2005). For example, the non-NF2 cohort showed higher proportion of patients with open-set speech discrimination than did the NF2 cohort. Additional reasons for the variability could emanate from a number of factors such as, but not limited to, the accuracy of surgical positioning of the electrodes on the surface of the cochlear nucleus, duration of hearing loss, the number of electrodes producing a pitch percept, perceptual levels, and the stimulation rate used in the ABI system.

The potentials to use electrically-evoked auditory brainstem responses (eABRs) to verify near precise placement of the ABI electrode paddle was explored in the mid 1990s, and the study reported that the intraoperative monitoring using eABRs ensured accurate placement of the electrode paddle at the CNC surface (Waring, 1995). This was particularly beneficial because the surgeon places the array in a "blind" fashion as the CNC is obscured from the direct visual field during the process. Soon, intraoperative eABRs became essential to the success in accurately positioning the electrode array and ensuring against its shifting during closure of the dura and soft tissue (Kaplan et al., 2015). However, even with the extensive use of eABR for intraoperative monitoring, the three-dimensional multiplanar reconstruction have shown high degree of variability in electrode array positioning among patients (Barber et al., 2017).

Candidacy for ABI

Candidacy evaluation of ABI is usually performed by a multidisciplinary team involving neuro-otologist, audiologist, neuro-surgeon, speech language pathologist, radiologist, and neuropsychologist. Originally, the ABI was indicated as an appropriate treatment option for patients with post-lingual hearing impairment as a consequence of NF2. Although the Food and Drug Administration (FDA) in the United

States continues to approve adults with NF2 as the sole population to undergo ABI, several European countries and a few Asian countries, including India, have been practicing auditory brainstem implantation for children who do not fulfil the cochlear implantation candidacy. In fact, a few years ago, Med-EL received CE-mark approval for much broader ABI candidacy due to which patients 12 months or older, who do not fulfil the cochlear implantation candidacy due to non-functional auditory nerves, can now be considered for ABI.

Indications for an auditory brainstem implant (ABI) can be broadly classified based on the timing of deafness onset, either pre-lingual or post-lingual. In post-lingually hearing-impaired patients, the indications may include tumor-related conditions such as bilateral vestibular schwannomas in the context of NF2, as well as non-tumor-related conditions, such as severe cochlear ossification, fractures of the cochlea or internal auditory meatus, or purposeful/iatrogenic resection of the auditory nerve, all of which contraindicate cochlear implantation. In the case of pre-lingual hearing-impairment, congenital inner ear malformations are the primary cause of sensorineural deafness in children, with these malformations potentially being unilateral or bilateral in nature. People with bilateral cochlear aplasia or cochlear nerve aplasia can be considered for ABI; however, a complete absence of cochlear nerve on both sides cannot be ascertained using the modern-day radiological techniques. Additionally, studies have shown that despite non-visualization of cochlear nerves on both sides during the radiological evaluation, acceptable outcomes, often better than those with ABI, could be obtained after cochlear implantation (Choe et al., 2022, 2023; Han et al., 2019). This obviously means that the modern-day radiological techniques are still failing to identify some very thin or obscured fibers. Therefore, the radiological evidence for a well-developed cochlea in cases with suspected auditory nerve aplasia warrants a failed cochlear implantation before considering ABI. Sennaroglu and colleagues divided the indicators for ABI into 'Definite' and 'Probable' indicators (Sennaroglu et al., 2013). The 'Definite' indicators of ABI are constituted by the presence of one or more among complete labyrinthine aplasia (Michel Aplasia), cochlear aplasia, cochlear nerve aplasia and cochlear aperture aplasia (Sennaroglu et al., 2013). On the other hand, hypoplastic cochlea with hypoplastic cochlear aperture, common cavity with incomplete partition (IP) I with a present nerve, and hypoplastic cochlear nerve constitute the 'Probable' indicators for ABI. These conditions are kept under the 'probable' indicators category because they create a dilemma for the implant team, as it is difficult to determine whether or not a sufficient amount of neural tissue is travelling to CNC. Although not included in the criteria proposed by Sennaroglu et al. (2013), the ABI criteria have been expanded to also include children or adults with a bilateral complete cochlear ossification, the kinds often encountered after a bacterial meningitis. ABI is considered an option for individuals with no psychological contraindications. Those in whom hearing loss is the main reason for speech-language delay and those who belong to families having realistic expectation of the outcomes in speech and language functions post-ABI should be considered for ABI, pending fulfilment of the other ABI candidacy criteria.

Preoperative and Intraoperative Audiological Investigations

The above section makes it clear that those in whom a cochlear implantation is contraindicated become probable candidates for ABI and should be evaluated further for its suitability. Although there is no specific guideline on audiological findings that indicate the need for an ABI, the corollaries drawn from cochlear implantation candidacy could prove useful, as ABI is typically done on those who do not fulfil the cochlear implantation candidacy despite having a severe-to-profound hearing impairment. The audiological investigation involved in candidacy selection for ABI includes the routine audiological test battery, inclusive of behavioral and electrophysiological tests to determine a severe to profound degree of hearing loss. Further, Oto-acoustic emissions (OAE), Electrocochleography (ECochG) and Auditory Brainstem Responses (ABR) are useful tests in non-tumor patients as they can be helpful in ruling out the presence of auditory neuropathy spectrum disorders (ANSD) and other conditions associated with a neuronal degenerative disease. This could be vital, as these kinds of pathologies are not detectable through radiological investigations due to essentially normal structure, but could prove potentially detrimental to the outcomes from an ABI due to poor neural function at the brainstem level and beyond.

Electrically-evoked Auditory Brainstem Response (eABR) can be an additional audiological tool while assessing the audiological candidacy for an ABI. It can be performed pre-operatively by placing the electrode on the round window or promontory to determine the extent of excitability of the auditory nerve and brainstem. While the presence of eABR could push the case in favor of a CI rather than an ABI, a no response on eABR defies neither the cochlear implant candidacy nor the candidacy for an ABI.

An eABR can also be performed intraoperatively to measure the responses of cochlear nucleus and brainstem when the stimulus is delivered through the ABI system. As mentioned before, this has utility in intra-operative monitoring of the auditory function. It is also used to guide the surgeon on optimum positioning of the electrode array on the CNC surface. Positioning of the ABI on the cochlear nucleus is paramount for good outcome (Colletti et al., 2013). When the electrode contacts of the electrode paddle are placed on the cochlear nucleus, they elicit auditory responses. These are popularly called auditory electrodes. When the electrode array is placed outside the cochlear nucleus and no electrode makes contact with CNC, they only produce non-auditory percepts. These are often called non-auditory electrodes. When a few electrodes are in contact with CNC but others are placed outside the cochlear nucleus, they may elicit auditory as well as non-auditory percepts. The presence of non-auditory sensation in response to an auditory stimulus is among the biggest concerns when dealing with patients undergoing ABI. It is possible to reduce or arrest the non-auditory sensation by identifying the electrodes producing non-auditory sensation. While most adult ABI recipients can reliably indicate the body part receiving a sensation when an auditory stimulus is delivered through an ABI system, it can be a difficult task for most children and even some adults. In such scenarios, the post-operative eABR could prove valuable when programming the sound processor.

Studies have analyzed the characteristics of intra-operative and post-operative eABR in children with ABI and investigated the correlation of eABR thresholds with the behavioral T and C levels (Herrmann et al., 2015; O'Driscoll et al., 2011; Waring, 1995; Wong et al., 2020). Across these studies, the morphology of the eABR waveform varied from having a single vertex positive peak in certain patients to as many as four vertex positive peaks in others. The differences in the number of eABR peaks can also be observed between the electrodes used to deliver the current pulses at CNC. The electrodes yielding discernible eABR, irrespective of the number of peaks, are considered auditory electrodes because the mere presence of eABR illustrates that a portion of the auditory tissue on the cochlear nucleus surface is stimulated to evoke a brainstem response. Therefore, the presence of an eABR during the intra-operative session should be considered a marker to localize electrodes that provide auditory sensations. This has been confirmed by the finding of a greater number of auditory electrodes during device activation in patients who had evidence of eABR from larger number of electrodes intra-operatively. The effects of maturation can also be evidenced in the eABR responses. Generally, as the implant age increases, the latencies of various eABR peaks decrease.

A key to using the eABR information is understanding its relationship with the behavioural perception. The electrodes in certain areas produce eABRs; however, the behavioral responses for stimulation of these electrodes can be non-auditory, possibly indicating a higher eABR threshold than the level needed for non-auditory sensation. Also, sometimes higher current levels result in stimulation of adjacent sites due to the spread of electrical current to these areas. This may also be a cause of coexisting auditory and non-auditory sensations for the same stimulus. Therefore, one needs to be careful when using intense current levels. Further, the post-operative eABR thresholds correlate positively with the behavioral T and C levels, and often fall between the T and the C levels. Therefore, the post-operative eABR threshold level can be used in the initial fitting in the difficult to test population.

Post-operative Switch-on and Programming of ABI

The device activation or switch-on of the ABI, where the external sound processor is fitted and internal implant is stimulated for the first time with the patient in a non-anaesthetized state, must be done in an Intensive Care Unit. The switch-on in a typical patient is done 6–8 weeks after the surgery. During switch-on, monitoring of vital parameters is important as the ABI is placed at the surface of CNC, and several lower cranial nerves pass through this region. Stimulation of lower cranial nerve nuclei can cause non-auditory signs and symptoms which need close monitoring. In particular, vagal nerve stimulation can lead to significant cardio-respiratory events and may even prove fatal, if unattended. Therefore, complete caution must be ensured during the switch-on of an ABI device. A few common side effects after

ABI activation are watering of eyes, tingling sensation, facial muscle movement, eye twitch, and leg movement.

In an adults ABI recipient, the programming procedure for ABI is similar to those used for cochlear implants. However, unlike cochlear implants, the pitch percepts generated by the different electrodes in the ABI are highly variable. This variability significantly complicates the programming process. The initial programming process involves setting threshold and comfort levels. At the same time, it is also important that the clinician evaluates for the presence of non-auditory stimulation and manages it by turning off the non-auditory electrodes. For the auditory electrodes, performing pitch scaling is important. A monopolar stimulation is preferred to begin with. It is applied to one electrode at a time, and while doing so the clinician must check on the level and pitch of the auditory percept. If the non-auditory percepts also accompany the auditory percepts, stimulation parameters can be adjusted to reduce non-auditory responses while preserving sound quality. In case all adjustments fail to reduce the non-auditory percepts, a bipolar stimulation may be tried. And if nothing works, such electrodes can be deactivated. The electrodes that generate only auditory responses are used for pitch scaling. This can be a herculean task to assign specific pitch values to the electrodes in the initial session. If a patient finds the task of pitch scaling hard, he/she may be encouraged to describe its quality by associating with certain environmental sounds like bell or drum. Later, pairwise pitch comparisons between the electrodes can be performed to facilitate pitch assignments and the electrodes can be ranked in the order of their pitch. During the initial stimulation, some patients may find the quality of their auditory sensation unsatisfactory; however, they can be reassured that with continued use and experience with the ABI, sound quality is likely to improve, and any residual non-auditory sensations typically diminish over time.

Among children and some adults too, an eABR based fitting is primarily conducted in cases they cannot provide reliable behavioural responses. In any grown-up child or an adult, eABR responses are correlated with behavioral responses and a MAP is created. It is important to activate only those number of electrodes which show presence of reliable auditory response either behaviourly or electrophysiologically on eABR.

Electrically-evoked compound action potential (eCAP) is widely used in the mapping of cochlear implants; however, reliable eCAPs cannot be measured from the cochlear nucleus. Therefore, eABR remains the only reliable objective measure to assist in ABI mapping. A few children, due to changes in electrophysiological properties because of tissue growth and healing process, may show changes in their eABR responses over time. Therefore, it is pertinent that the eABR thresholds be measured in serial sessions over time and reprogramming of the processor be done on its basis. This may be particularly useful in cases of delay or deterioration of unknown origin.

The use of eABR in the fitting protocol of ABI was initially proposed by Colletti and colleagues, who selected the electrodes to be retained in active mode and programmed the ABI device using the information from the intra-operative eABR (Colletti et al., 2001). The patients (n = 2) in their study were non-tumor patients with radiographic evidence for cochlear deformity concomitant with the auditory nerve aplasia. When compared to the NF2 patients, a substantially larger number of auditory electrodes could be traced using eABR. One month after the first programming using eABR information, over 80% of the Ling's 6-sounds and over 70% of the onomatopoeic sounds were detectable in patient 1 and 65% of the Ling's 6-sounds and 40% of onomatopoeic sounds were detectable by patient 2. To put this in perspective, the authors informed that the performance of these children was better than those who had similar anomalies of the cochlea and auditory nerve but had undergone cochlear implantation. Even though the study reported outcomes on only 2 patients, the evidence showed that the information derived from eABR was effective in appropriate mapping of the ABI device. These findings paved the way for these measures to be considered effective objective tools for ABI mapping, especially in children or other patients in whom behavioural responses are unreliable or difficult to obtain.

Later, Polak et al. (2018) demonstrated eABR's effectiveness as an objective tool for mapping the ABIs of children with congenital inner ear malformations. They used a criteria of the presence of eABR on 75% or more electrodes for an appropriate positioning of the electrode paddle; in case of no eABRs from any of the electrodes, the electrode paddle was repositioned until a response was obtained. They recommended to use the presence of eABR to determine the auditory electrodes during the device activation and to use the presence of non-auditory side effects, irrespective of the eABR finding of that electrode, to disable electrodes. The maximum and the minimum levels of stimulation were determined based on the responses obtained from eABR, and an eABR based map was created. For each electrode, Polak observed that the eABR threshold was at a point about 60% of the dynamic range. In their study, they found that best outcomes were achieved when setting a dynamic range of 12 dB on all electrodes that elicited a clear waveform on the eABR. The literature reporting the use of eABR in post-operative device programming is scanty. The matter is further compounded by limited number of subjects and lack of clear information on the objective determination of the electrode nature in the studies that have used eABR for post-operative mapping of ABI. Therefore, there is a lack of definite protocol on eABR's use for mapping thus far.

Assessment of Benefits with ABI

During the ABI surgery, a surgeon places the electrode on the CNC surface; however, the extent of information that the ABI electrodes can transduce to the CNC and the extent to which the neurons of the CNC can process and propel the information further along the central auditory nervous system decides how a recipient progresses after an ABI. While a multitude of factors can influence the outcomes, it is important to understand the auditory outcomes of the average ABI user to estimate the effectiveness of this neuroprosthetic device in auditory rehabilitation. Over the years, both subjective assessments and objective measures have been used to document the outcomes from an ABI.

In a performance report of the Med-EL ABI system recipient, obtaining 80% score on multisyllabic words five choice test has been documented (Dhanasingh & Hochmair, 2021). Following 6-weeks of device usage, the recognition of words with lip reading improved from a pre-implantation baseline of 5% to 80% after it.

Rajeswaran and Kameswaran (2020) reported the performance on several tests after ABI in a group of children who were followed-up up to 24 months from the first fit. The tests used included Listening Progress Profile (LIP), Meaningful Auditory Integration Scale (MAIS), Meaningful Use of Speech Scale (MUSS), Monosyllabic Trochee Polysyllabic (MTP) words test, Categories of Auditory Performance (CAP), Speech Intelligibility Rating (SIR), the Little Ears Auditory Questionnaire (LEAQ) and Checklist of auditory communication skills. In the first 12 months of the first fit, significant improvement was observed on all tests, except MTP 6 and MTP 12 (the numbers indicate the number of picture cards from which the target word was to be identified; for example, MTP 6 means that the target word was to be identified from among six picture cards). While the next 12 months (12–24 months) witnessed stable performance on LIP, MTP 3, MTP 6, MTP 12 and CAP, with significant improvements observed on MAIS, MUSS, SIR, LEAQ and checklist for auditory skills communication during the same period. LEAQ was reported in comparison to normal curve of German speaking normal hearing children and regression curve of children with CI. They noted that within the first 24 months after the first fitting with ABI, the performance of a few non-tumor children with ABI was comparable to children with normal hearing (Rajeswaran & Kameswaran, 2020).

In a study reporting outcome of 16 adults (6 NF2, 1 acoustic neuroma, and 9 non-tumor patients) and 8 (all non-tumor patients) children who continued follow-up with the center over a period of 10 years, Veronese et al. (2023) reported variable outcomes from ABI among children as well as adults. In their study, 9 (56.25%) adults and 6 (75%) children received appreciable benefit from ABI. They categorized their performance in three different levels where at least 60% correct detection of sounds and words presented at 65 dBA constituted Level 1, a minimum of 60% closed-set disyllabic word identification amounted to a performance at Level 2, and participants obtaining at least 60% open-set word and sentence recognition were categorized as Level 3. Among the adult ABI recipients, 4 (25%) reached Level 1, 2 (12.5%) performed at Level 2 and further 2 (12.5%) nudged Level 3. In the children's group, 2 (25%) achieved Level 2, and 4 (50%) functioned at Level 3. Further, the study also compared the perceptual outcomes after ABI of the tumor and non-tumor adults. Among the adult ABI recipients with a substantial benefit from ABI, 4 had tumors whereas 5 did not. Among the tumor patients with a significant benefit from ABI, 2 performed at Level 1, and one each reached Level 2 and Level 3. Among the non-tumor patients showing significant benefits from ABI, 2 performed at Level 1, 2 achieved Level 2, and one functioned at Level 3. Therefore, 57% of tumor patients and 55% of non-tumor patients showed substantial benefits from ABI. Overall, despite having lesser number of active electrodes than adults, children had better perceptual outcomes. The authors believed that two factors may have played a part in this difference in the perceptual outcomes between children and adults- (1) uncompromised neural substrate in children (Colletti et al., 2014), as the children in their study were devoid of tumors or neurodegenerative diseases; (2) greater neural plasticity allowing more malleability in children than adults (Fallon et al., 2008). Although the first assumption has been used in several previous studies to justify lesser benefits from ABI in tumor patients than non-tumor patients (Colletti et al., 2009; Noij et al., 2015; Shannon, 2019), the data from Veronese et al. (2023) shows comparable performance between adults with and without tumor, thereby refuting the first hypothesis. Hence, it appears that greater neural plasticity than adults probably lead to better perceptual outcomes in children.

Generally, patients with ABI show poorer results on the perceptual outcome measures than those with cochlear implants. In a recent study, Dornhoffer et al. (2024) compared CI users and ABI users, all with vestibular schwannomas associated with NF2, on open-set speech perception, consonant-nucleus-consonant word scores, and AzBio sentence in quiet scores. They reported significantly superior performance in CI users than ABI users. Open-set speech perception was achieved by 77% CI users as against only 12% among the ABI users. On the consonant-nucleus-consonant test and AzBio sentences in quiet, the median performance was documented at 31% and 57%, respectively, among the CI users as against 0% on both these measures among the ABI users. Based on these findings, it can be concluded that several patients with NF2-associated vestibular schwannoma receive auditory perceptual benefit with either CI or ABI; nonetheless, the outcomes among CI recipients, despite the vestibular schwannomas, is far better in CI than ABI users. However, these performances were compared after 2 years of implantation. Given that vestibular schwannomas are slow growing, it is hard to predict on how much longer the performance with CI would continue to be better than ABI. When the surgical excision of the tumor becomes unavoidable, one does not know whether the performance with CI will continue to stay better.

A final consideration on the outcome measure could be the use of eABR. As elaborated in earlier sections of this chapter, patients with larger number of electrodes demonstrating the presence of eABR response show a tendency of better performance than do those with a smaller number of electrodes eliciting eABR responses. Hence, eABR can also be used as a tool to predict outcome. This could bring down the time required to assess the outcome, especially among children, until the child can start producing reliable conditioned responses.

From the discussion in this chapter, it is apparent that ABI is a promising solution for people, both children and adults, in whom a cochlear implantation is contraindicated. The outcomes in both groups are variable; however, children tend to perform better than adults. However, this performance in most cases is limited to environmental sound awareness and aid to lip-reading, but in some cases closed-set speech recognition can be achieved.

References

Barber, S. R., Kozin, E. D., Remenschneider, A. K., Puram, S. V., Smith, M., Herrmann, B. S., et al. (2017). Auditory brainstem implant array position varies widely among adult and pediatric patients and is associated with perception. *Ear and Hearing, 38*(6), e343.

Brackmann, D. E., Hitselberger, W. E., Nelson, R. A., Moore, J., Waring, M. D., Portillo, F., et al. (1993). Auditory brainstem implant: I. Issues in surgical implantation. *Otolaryngology-Head and Neck Surgery, 108*(6), 624–633.

Chao, X., Luo, J., Wang, R., Hu, F., Wang, H., Fan, Z., & Xu, L. (2023). Long-term auditory and speech outcomes of cochlear implantation in children with cochlear nerve aplasia. *Ear and Hearing, 44*(3), 558–565.

Choe, G., Kim, Y. S., Oh, S. H., Lee, S. Y., & Lee, J. H. (2022). Functional outcomes of cochlear implantation in children with bilateral cochlear nerve aplasia. *Medicina (Kaunas, Lithuania), 58*(10), 1474.

Colletti, V., & Shannon, R. V. (2005). Open set speech perception with auditory brainstem implant? *The Laryngoscope, 115*(11), 1974–1978.

Colletti, V., Fiorino, F., Sacchetto, L., Miorelli, V., & Carner, M. (2001). Hearing habilitation with auditory brainstem implantation in two children with cochlear nerve aplasia. *International Journal of Pediatric Otorhinolaryngology, 60*(2), 99–111.

Colletti, V., Shannon, R., Carner, M., Sacchetto, L., Turazzi, S., Masotto, B., & Colletti, L. (2007). The first successful case of hearing produced by electrical stimulation of the human midbrain. *Otology and Neurotology, 28*(1), 39–43.

Colletti, V., Shannon, R., Carner, M., Veronese, S., & Colletti, L. (2009). Outcomes in nontumor adults fitted with the auditory brainstem implant: 10 years' experience. *Otology and Neurotology, 30*(5), 614–618.

Colletti, L., Wilkinson, E. P., & Colletti, V. (2013). Auditory brainstem implantation after unsuccessful cochlear implantation of children with clinical diagnosis of cochlear nerve deficiency. *The Annals of Otology, Rhinology, and Laryngology, 122*(10), 605–612.

Colletti, L., Shannon, R. V., & Colletti, C. (2014). The development of auditory perception in children after auditory brainstem implantation. *Audiology and Neurotology, 19*(6), 386–394.

Dhanasingh, A., & Hochmair, I. (2021). ABI-auditory brainstem implant. *Acta Otolaryngologica, 141*(supl), 63–81.

Dornhoffer, J. R., Plitt, A. R., Lohse, C. M., Driscoll, C. L. W., Neff, B. A., Saoji, A. A., Van Gompel, J. J., Link, M. J., & Carlson, M. L. (2024). Comparing speech recognition outcomes between cochlear implants and auditory brainstem implants in patients with NF2-related schwannomatosis. *Otology & Neurotology, 45*(1), 29–35.

Fallon, J. B., Irvine, D. R., & Shepherd, R. K. (2008). Cochlear implants and brain plasticity. *Hearing Research, 238*(1–2), 110–117.

Han, J. J., Suh, M. W., Park, M. K., Koo, J. W., Lee, J. H., & Oh, S. H. (2019). A predictive model for cochlear implant outcome in children with cochlear nerve deficiency. *Scientific Reports, 9*(1), 1154.

Herrmann, B. S., Brown, M. C., Eddington, D. K., Hancock, K. E., & Lee, D. J. (2015). Auditory brainstem implant: electrophysiologic responses and subject perception. *Ear and Hearing, 36*(3), 368–376.

Hitselberger, W. E., House, W. F., Edgerton, B. J., & Whitaker, S. (1984). Cochlear nucleus implant. *Otolaryngology–Head and Neck Surgery, 92*(1), 52–54.

Kandler, K., Clause, A., & Noh, J. (2009). Tonotopic reorganization of developing auditory brainstem circuits. *Nature Neuroscience, 12*(6), 711–717.

Kaplan, A. B., Kozin, E. D., Puram, S. V., Owoc, M. S., Shah, P. V., Hight, A. E., Sethi, R. K. V., Remenschneider, A. K., & Lee, D. J. (2015). Auditory brainstem implant candidacy in the United States in children 0-17 years old. *International Journal of Pediatric Otorhinolaryngology, 79*(3), 310–315.

Laszig, R., & Aschendorff, A. (1999). Cochlear implants and electrical brainstem stimulation in sensorineural hearing loss. *Current Opinion in Neurology, 12*(1), 41–44.

Luo, F., Wang, Q., Farid, N., Liu, X., & Yan, J. (2009). Three-dimensional tonotopic organization of the C57 mouse cochlear nucleus. *Hearing research., 257*(1–2), 75–82.

Nevison, B., Laszig, R., Sollmann, W. P., Lenarz, T., Sterkers, O., Ramsden, R., et al. (2002). Results from a European clinical investigation of the Nucleus® multichannel auditory brainstem implant. *Ear and Hearing, 23*(3), 170–183.

Noij, K. S., Kozin, E. D., Sethi, R., Shah, P. V., Kaplan, A. B., Herrmann, B., Remenschneider, A., & Lee, D. J. (2015). Systematic review of nontumor pediatric auditory brainstem implant outcomes. *Otolaryngology--Head and Neck Surgery: Official Journal of American Academy of Otolaryngology-Head and Neck Surgery, 153*(5), 739–750.

O'Driscoll, M., El-Deredy, W., & Ramsden, R. T. (2011). Brain stem responses evoked by stimulation of the mature cochlear nucleus with an auditory brain stem implant. *Ear and Hearing, 32*(3), 286–299.

Otto, S. R., Brackmann, D. E., Hitselberger, W. E., Shannon, R. V., & Kuchta, J. (2002). Multichannel auditory brainstem implant: update on performance in 61 patients. *Journal of Neurosurgery, 96*(6), 1063–1071.

Otto, S. R., Shannon, R. V., Wilkinson, E. P., Hitselberger, W. E., McCreery, D. B., Moore, J. K., & Brackmann, D. E. (2008). Audiologic outcomes with the penetrating electrode auditory brainstem implant. *Otology & Neurotology: Official Publication of the American Otological Society, American Neurotology Society [and] European Academy of Otology and Neurotology, 29*(8), 1147–1154.

Polak, M., Colletti, L., & Colletti, V. (2018). Novel method of fitting of children with auditory brainstem implants. *European Annals of Otorhinolaryngology, Head and Neck Diseases, 135*(6), 403–409.

Rajeswaran, R., & Kameswaran, M. (2020). Auditory brainstem implantation (ABI) in children without neurofibromatosis type II (NF2): communication performance and safety after 24 months of use. *Cochlear Implants International, 21*(3), 127–135.

Ramsden, R. T., Freeman, S. R. M., Lloyd, S. K. W., King, A. T., Shi, X., Ward, C. L., et al. (2016). Auditory brainstem implantation in neurofibromatosis type 2: experience from the Manchester programme. *Otology & Neurotology, 37*(9), 1267–1274.

Schwartz, M. S., Otto, S. R., Shannon, R. V., Hitselberger, W. E., & Brackmann, D. E. (2008). Auditory brainstem implants. *Neurotherapeutics: The journal of the American Society for Experimental NeuroTherapeutics, 5*(1), 128–136.

Sennaroglu, L., Sennaroglu, G., & Atay, G. (2013). Auditory brainstem implantation in children. *Current Otorhinolaryngology Reports, 1*(2), 80–91.

Shannon, R. V. (2019). The auditory brainstem implant. In Oxford University Press eBooks (pp. 759–770).

Veronese, S., Cambiaghi, M., Tommasi, N., Sbarbati, A., & Galvin, J. J. I. I. I. (2023). Ten-year follow-up of auditory brainstem implants: From intraoperative electrical auditory brainstem responses to perceptual results. *PLoS ONE, 18*(3), e0282261.

Waring, M. D. (1995). Auditory brain-stem responses evoked by electrical stimulation of the cochlear nucleus in human subjects. *Electroencephalography and Clinical Neurophysiology, 96*(4), 338–347.

Wong, K., Kiringoda, R., Kanumuri, V. V., Barber, S. R., Franck, K., Sahani, N., Brown, M. C., Herrmann, B. S., & Lee, D. J. (2020). Effect of anesthesia on evoked auditory responses in pediatric auditory brainstem implant surgery. *The Laryngoscope, 130*(2), 507–513.

Chapter 24
Auditory Brainstem Implants: Surgical Perspectives

Ameet Kishore, Neevita Narayan, and Pranav Kumar

Abstract Auditory brainstem implant surgery has gained worldwide popularity because it offers a chance for hearing to many patients who might otherwise remain deaf. For over two decades, ABIs have been used primarily in patients with neurofibromatosis type 2 (NF2) who have bilateral vestibular schwannomas. The main goal in these cases is to provide hearing sensation after reducing or removing the tumours. Recent evidence also shows that ABIs are highly effective for non-tumour patients, especially pre-lingually deaf children with severe cochlear abnormalities that make them unsuitable for cochlear implantation.

Keywords Auditory brainstem implant · Cochlear nucleus · Cochlear aplasia · eABR · Intraoperative monitoring · Meningitis

Introduction

You have already learnt in Chap. 23 that Auditory Brainstem Implant (ABI) is an electronic device designed to bypass the cochlea and VIIIth cranial nerve to transmit sound directly to the cochlear nucleus (Liu et al., 2019). You have also learnt that the ABI system was designed to restore a degree of hearing sensation to patients who have bilateral dysfunction of the auditory nerve. This is achieved by direct electrical stimulation of the cochlear nucleus complex in the brainstem (Deep et al., 2019). Unlike the cochlea, which is a well-defined bony structure, the cochlear nucleus is more difficult to locate. Precise placement of the ABI electrodes is thus essential to

A. Kishore (✉)
Department of ENT, Indraprastha Apollo Hospital, Sarita Vihar, New Delhi, Delhi, India

N. Narayan
SpHear Speech & Hearing Clinics, G-32, New Delhi, India

P. Kumar
Department of Neurosurgery, Indraprastha Apollo Hospital, Sarita Vihar, New Delhi, India

P. Kumar et al. (eds.), *Advances in Implantation Otology*,
https://doi.org/10.1007/978-981-96-8671-1_24

yield auditory perception. The aim of ABI surgery is to insert the electrode paddle into the lateral recess of Fourth Ventricle of the brainstem, so that it lies on its floor, over the Cochlear Nucleus. This is achieved by entering the lateral recess through its foramen, the Foramen of Lushka (Puram & Lee, 2015; Kuroki & Moller, 1995). This chapter will describe the medical and radiological candidacy and surgical techniques involved in ABI.

Candidacy Selection

During its initial years, ABI was done only on the tumour patients. However, as the years passed by, several non-tumour conditions emerged in which cochlear implantation was either not an option or produced limited benefits. Chapter 23 has already described the audiological candidacy details for ABI. This section of this chapter will focus mainly on the medical and radiological indications for ABI.

ABI in Tumour Patients

The ABIs have been traditionally used in patients with a diagnosis of Neurofibromatosis Type 2 (NF 2), with bilateral vestibular schwannomas (Laszig 1997). The recipients must be 12 years of age or older and medically and psychologically suitable (Peng 2018). ABI in patients of neurofibromatosis type 2 poses additional sets of challenges. Needless to say, the tumour needs to be excised before the implant placement. The pre-operative audiologic work-up has an important role to play in deciding the side of the implant placement (Wilkinson et al., 2014). The details on the pre-operative audiologic work-up have been covered in Chap. 23.

The ABI can be done during first-or second-side tumour removal, or it may even be performed as a separate procedure. Due to possible injury to the cochlear nucleus or necrosis resulting from radiotherapy treatment, and anatomic distortion and fibrosis, prospective ABI recipients who have undergone gamma knife radiation should be considered with extreme caution (Marangos et al., 1999; Deep & Roland, 2020). The presence of very large vestibular schwannomas should also be considered a contraindication for ABI because large tumours might be associated with brainstem distortion or could have damaged the midbrain / pons, which could negate effective forward transmission of signals beyond the level of the brainstem (Colletti, 2006).

ABI in Non-tumor Patients

Although the ABIs have been traditionally used to provide auditory sensation to NF-2 patients having very high degree of sensorineural hearing loss following tumour excision, over the years the indication has been expanded to include even the non-tumour patients (Rutherford 2019). The non-tumour patients with bilateral profound sensorineural hearing loss, who cannot receive a CI, are being considered for ABI (Sennaroglu et al., 2016; Noij et al., 2015). The unaidable SNHL in these patients could be due to absence / hypoplasia of cochlea, cochlear nerve aplasia / hypoplasia or meningitis resulting in a severely ossified cochlea and with no benefit from CI. Often the decision has to be made between CI and ABI in children with complex inner malformations (Sennaroglu et al., 2016).

In a consensus statement regarding the use of ABI in non-tumour patients, Sennaroglu et al. (2011) categorized the non-NF2 patients into two major categories. The first category of patients included those with pre-lingual hearing loss associated with inner ear malformations and cochlear nerve hypoplasia/aplasia. The second category included patients with post-lingual hearing loss because of meningitis, temporal bone fractures with cochlear nerve avulsion, otosclerosis with gross cochlear destruction, or unmanageable facial nerve stimulation with CI. He then recommended further dividing them into 3 main-subcategories on the basis of radiological indications shown in Table 24.1.

In addition to the criteria proposed by Sennaroglu et al. (2011), to undergo ABI surgery, the recipients must be in the age 18-months to 5-years (for the pre-lingual group), or 5-years to 21-years (for the post-lingual group) (Aslan et al., 2020). There must be no medical contraindications, and diagnosed cognitive or developmental

Table 24.1 Radiologic indications for ABI on the basis of a consensus statement (Sennaroglu et al., 2011)

Well-defined congenital indications	Possible congenital indications	Acquired indications
Complete labyrinthine aplasia (Michel aplasia) Cochlear aplasia Cochlear nerve aplasia Cochlear aperture aplasia	Hypoplastic cochleas with cochlear aperture hypoplasia Common cavity and incomplete partition type 1 cases with an absent cochlear nerve or those with the presence of nerve but CI fails to elicit auditory percept. The presence of an unbranched cochleo-vestibular nerve. The hypoplastic cochlear nerve (nerve size <50% of the usual size or less than the diameter of the facial nerve) such that a sufficient amount of neural tissue cannot be followed into the cochlear space.	Post-lingual deafness due to meningitis is associated with severe cochlear ossification; nonetheless, the visualization of a patent cochlea on T2 MRI should be considered to prioritise CI over ABI. Bilateral temporal bone transverse fractures with cochlear nerve avulsion Cochlear otosclerosis with gross destruction of the cochlea, or cochlear otosclerosis with post-implantation facial nerve stimulation despite attempts to eliminate it during mapping sessions, or complete cochlear ossification (labyrinthitis ossificans).

delays. The recipient needs to have strong family support and the expectations of family must be reasonable (Asfour et al., 2018; Monsanto et al., 2014).

Candidacy Considerations and Work-Up

The Audiological and Radiological criteria as related to the cochlear and cochlear nerve anatomy have been covered in the previous chapter (Chap. 23). For the purpose of this section, let us assume that the patient will not obtain benefits from a cochlear implant.

Medical, Neurosurgical and Neuro-radiological Aspects

The recipient must be medically fit to undergo a neurosurgical procedure. As is routine with all surgical procedures, appropriate preoperative tests and anaesthetic clearances are obtained. The pre-operative CT scan should be examined for the bony anatomy and integrity of the temporal bone, especially the squamous and the petrous parts and the occipital bone. One should also look at the cranio-vertebral junction for any anomaly / instability. In the MRI, one should look for locations or any aberrations in the course of the transverse sinus, the sigmoid sinus, the jugular bulb and major arteries of the posterior fossa on the proposed side of the surgery. The gross anatomy of the cerebellum and the brainstem should also be studied. MRI would also reveal if the patient has any hydrocephalus or Arnold-Chiari malformation (Puram & Lee, 2015; Shah et al., 2016; Haber et al., 2020).

The Recommended Experience for an ABI Team

The team must have experienced multi-disciplinary professionals including otology, neurosurgery, electrophysiology, audiology, and speech pathology. The surgeons must have extensive surgical experience with cochlear implants also in addition to the translabyrinthine and retrosigmoid routes of surgery. A team with expertise in monitoring of cranial nerves Vth, VIIth, VIIIth, IXth, Xth, and XIth must be present to ensure appropriate cranial nerve monitoring. The audiologists and rehabilitation professionals must have prior experience of being in an established cochlear implant program with significant experience in advanced device programming and habilitation techniques.

Surgical Approaches

ABI is more challenging than CI because of the involvement of surgery at the level of brainstem and cerebrospinal fluid (CSF) in the posterior fossa in the background of a pulsatile field for implantation. Knowledge of the anatomical landmarks and variants in anatomy of the brainstem is vital for ABI surgery. For anatomical landmarks and variants in anatomy of the brainstem, please refer to Chap. 2 of this book. Another crucial aspect is the side selection for ABI. The side selection for ABI is vital in both tumour and non-tumour cases. One can consider implanting based on the development and ease of accessibility. One should choose the side (1) with a better development of the lateral recess; (2) which allows a more favourable entry to the lateral recess; (3) which necessitates lesser cerebellar retractions while accessing the lateral recess; (4) with a better development of neural structures. While it is not a given, the side with the presence of facial nerve (if facial nerve is present on only one side), or the side that has a more prominent vestibular nerve or the cochleo-vestibular nerve, could have higher likelihood of a better developed cochlear nucleus and the area adjoining it than the other side).

The surgery for ABI should be performed in a neurosurgical operation theatre under general anaesthesia. One among translabyrinthine, retrolabyrinthine and retrosigmoid approaches are used for reaching the cochlear nucleus, the site for the placement of ABI electrode. In the situation of NF2 tumours, the choice between the two surgical approaches depends on the tumour characteristics; however, the preference of the surgical team also plays a part in this selection. In non-tumour cases, the retrosigmoid approach is often preferred. During the entire surgical process, keeping in mind the proximity of several other cranial nerves, the penetrating needle electrodes are placed for intraoperative monitoring of the VIIth (facial), VIIIth (vestibulocochlear nerve), IXth (glossopharyngeal), Xth (vagus), and XIth (spinal accessory) cranial nerves.

Retrosigmoid (Sub-occipital) Craniotomy Approach

The patient is placed in a lateral position and the head is fixed in a rigid, Mayfield-Kees head fixator with clamps in park-bench position or in a supine position with head-rest to expose the retro-auricular surgical field adequately. The head and neck should be flexed which will allow the surgeon good exposure of the occipital and retro-mastoid regions (Fig. 24.1).

A large retro-auricular reverse hockey stick type incision or extended curvilinear incision is made such that it not only exposes the temporo-parietal bone where the receiver of the implant device will be placed but also the occipital squama (Fig. 24.2).

A sub-occipital craniotomy, extending up to the margins of the transverse and the sigmoid sinus, is carried out. Mastoid air cells, if opened inadvertently, should be sealed at this point. Dura is incised along the sigmoid sinus and its edges are

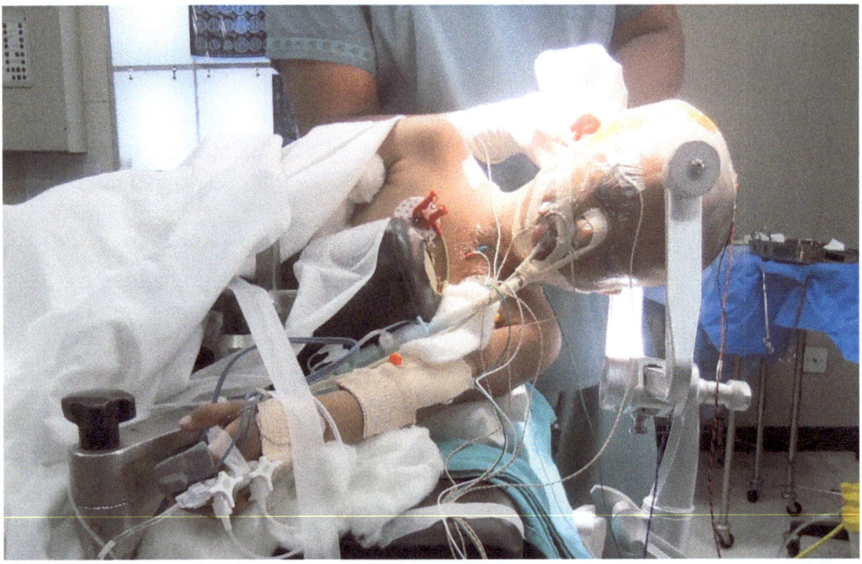

Fig. 24.1 Patient position for a Retrosigmoid (suboccipital) craniotomy approach

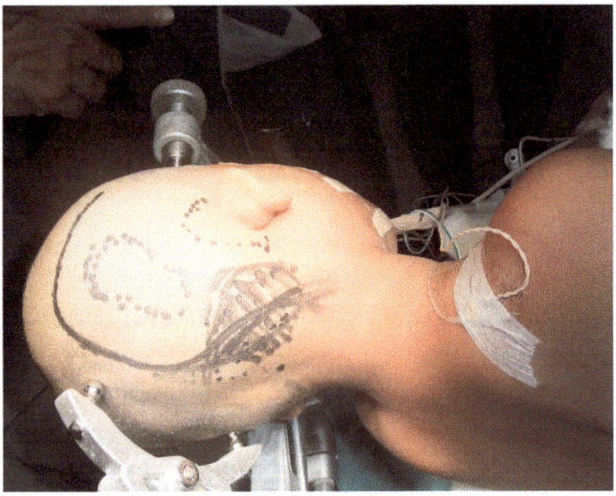

Fig. 24.2 Markings for incision and position of Receiver stimulator and craniotomy site

retracted. Drainage of CSF through an opening made in the cisterna magna makes the cerebellum extremely lax, which not only obviates the need of a cerebellar retractor, but also avoids risk of cerebellar contusion. The cerebellum falls away from the petrous bone once adequate amount of CSF is drained. In cases of NF2, the tumor excision should take place at this point of time. Once the tumor is excised, the VIIth, IXth, Xth, and XIth cranial nerves are identified. The next step is to locate the Foramen of Luschka. The IXth cranial nerve is traced medially to the point of its origin from the brainstem, which is a good landmark to the foramen of Luschka. Small fronds of choroid plexus can be seen protruding out of the foramen. These may have to be fulgurated. Some surgeons also preserve a stump of the cochlear nerve to aid in identification of the cochlear nucleus. They follow the cochlear nerve medially as it enters the lateral recess of the fourth ventricle. To reach the floor of the fourth ventricle, further dissection is done. Here lies a constant vein, also called the straight vein, which leads to the site of the cochlear nucleus (Raghunandhan & Kameswaran, 2010).

The receiver-stimulator of the ABI device is fixed in a bed over of the temporo-parietal bone at least 10 mm behind the edge of the auricle and above the cantho-meatal line and is angled 30 to 45 degrees postero-superiorly, in a way similar to the cochlear implantation (Fig. 24.3). Tie-down holes are made on either side of the receiver-stimulator to fasten it to prevent its migration. The precision of electrode site identification and insertion of the electrode at the optimum place is paramount. One can use the egress of CSF during the Valsalva maneuver to locate the lateral recess. While not essential, it can be a good practice to pass a dummy test electrode pad through the foramen of Luschka to the floor of the fourth ventricle as a trial to check optimal positioning of electrodes. Once convinced, the surgeon can then insert the permanent electrode paddle gently via the same route, such that it lies over the dorsal cochlear nucleus. While placing the electrodes, it is important to ensure that the active electrode side remains in contact with the brainstem (Fig. 24.4). The optimal placement of the electrode paddle is subsequently verified by the audiologist by administering Electrically-evoked Auditory Brainstem Response (eABR), Early Electrically-evoked Middle Latency Response (eMLR) and Device Telemetry (DT). Depending upon the responses obtained on these evoked potentials, the

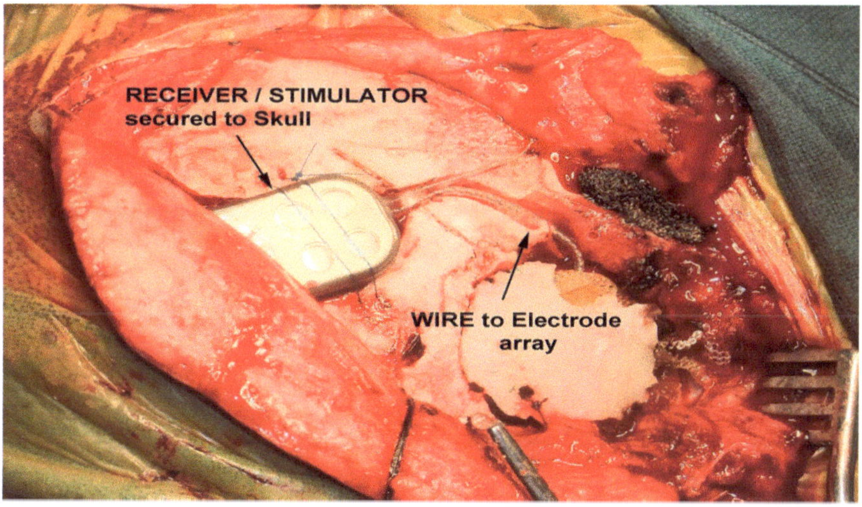

Fig. 24.3 The receiver-stimulator secured in a bed created for it with the lead wire to the electrode paddle going through the craniotomy

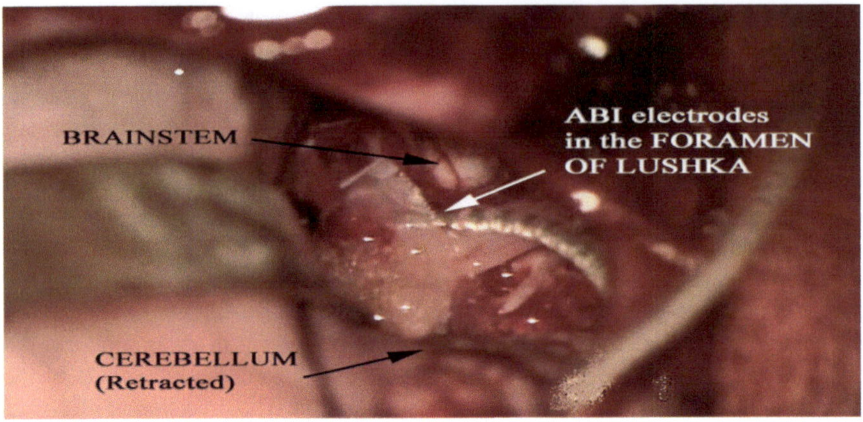

Fig. 24.4 A view of the Electrode paddle placed into the fourth ventricle through the Foramen of Lushka

placement of the electrode-array may need to be adjusted slightly. Once satisfied with the responses, fibrin sealant (biological glue) and hemostatic bio-absorbable gauze consisting of oxidized regenerated cellulose may have to be used to anchor the electrode-array in place and the ground electrode is placed under the temporalis muscle, A water-tight dural closure is carried out, and the wound is closed in layers (Shah et al., 2016; Hochmair & Dhanasingh, 2021).

The ABI surgery is a blind sac procedure because the cochlear nucleus is invisible from the opening created during this procedure. Nonetheless, if one pays attention to and uses four major anatomical landmarks, guiding the electrode towards the cochlear nucleus will be nearly accurate in a majority of patients (Goyal et al., 2017). These anatomical landmarks are as follows:

A. The Choroid plexus is present at the entrance of the lateral recess whereas the taenia travels along the roof of the lateral recess.
B. The Flocculus of the cerebellum forms an operculum (a flap) that covers the entrance of lateral recess of the fourth ventricle.
C. The cranial nerves VIIth, VIIIth and IXth exiting the cerebellopontine angle and the lateral parts of the medulla form a triangle of about 5–6 mm, which could be helpful in identifying the entrance of the lateral recess of the fourth ventricle.
D. The Straight vein, which runs from cranial nerve complex IXth, Xth, or XIth to the cranial nerve complex VIIth or VIIIth, forms floor of lateral recess and heads towards the entrance of the foramen of Luschka.

Translabyrinthine Craniotomy Approach

Hitselberger and House (1966) introduced a surgical technique that took transtemporal route to the cerebellopontine angle, referred to as the translabyrinthine pathway. This technique involves the complete removal of the labyrinthine block, offering a wide access route that facilitates identification of the facial nerve while minimizing trauma to the brainstem, cerebellum, and surrounding blood vessels. The translabyrinthine craniotomy allows easy access to and provides better visibility of the lateral recess of the fourth ventricle and its adjoining structures (Monsell et al., 1987). Despite minimal cerebellar retraction, it allows a clear visualization of structures posterior to the cochlear nucleus and the lateral recess. An early identification of the facial nerve during this approach augments complete tumor removal from the fundus of the internal auditory meatus by avoiding facial nerve traction. It also allows a surgeon a relatively easy grafting option in case the facial nerve has been injured (Brackmann et al., 1993).

One can reach the cochlear nucleus through the foramen of Luschka, which marks the end of the lateral recess of the fourth ventricle. The lateral recess, which is bordered superiorly by the roots of the seventh and eighth cranial nerves, and inferiorly by the root of the glossopharyngeal nerve, can be seen when one extends the choroid plexus from the fourth ventricle through the foramen of Luschka. To confirm whether the structures being visualized are indeed the foramen of Luschka and the lateral recess, a Valsalva maneuver can be used which will cause the egress of the cerebrospinal fluid. Going ahead, the electrode is blindly inserted into the lateral recess near the presumed location of the cochlear nucleus. Subsequently, intraoperative electrophysiological monitoring is conducted to verify the presence of eABRs. At this point, the surgery team should also inspect for the presence of any unintended stimulation of other nearby cranial nerves or potential hemodynamic instability. Depending on the findings on these investigations, the electrode array should be adjusted to allow for a more optimal stimulation (no non-auditory stimulation with best recordable eABRs), which is achieved by a trial-and-error method. Once the electrode placement is satisfactory, a small piece of fat or Teflon felt is used to secure the electrode array in place. After detaching the magnet, the receiver-stimulator is placed firmly fixed in to the bony well, which was drilled into the lateral skull. The excess free coils of the electrode array should be tucked into the mastoid cavity gently while ensuring no displacement of the electrode. The ground electrode is positioned beneath the temporalis muscle. Fat tissue is harvested from the abdominal wall, and this is used to pack the mastoid cavity. The surgical site is sutured ensuring a watertight closure, and this is followed by a pressure dressing. It is crucial to note that monopolar cautery should be avoided after auditory brainstem implant placement.

Retrolabyrinthine Surgical Approach

The two most popular surgical techniques for ABI, the retrosigmoid and translabyrinthine approaches, come with their own set of disadvantages. While the translabyrithine approach sacrifices the labyrinth, which compromises the patient's vestibular function, the retrosigmoid approach has higher potential for cerebellar injury as it requires cerebellum retraction. A third surgical technique, the retrolabyrinthine approach, which is a derivative of the translabyrinthine approach, can help preserve vestibular function of the patients, as it does not involve labyrinthectomy. Elsewhere, this technique is called presigmoid retrolabyrinthine approach (Bento & Lopes, 2021), infralabyrinthine approach (Hitselberger & Pulec, 1972) or transmastoidretrolayrinthine approach (Bento et al., 2002).

During the surgery, the patient is placed under general anesthesia; however, the use of muscle relaxants must be avoided so that accurate monitoring of the facial, glossopharyngeal, vagus and spinal accessory cranial nerves during the surgery. The patient is positioned supine, with the side to be operated facing upward. An incision running from a point just above helix to approximately 3 cm above the auricle, moving tangentially to the plane of the posterior wall of the external auditory canal and extending about 5 cm from the postauricular groove to the tip of the mastoid. Once the incision is done, the soft tissue is elevated above the periosteum, and an osteoperiosteal flap is created using the cortical bone near the mastoid, which is preserved for the final stages of the surgery. A horseshoe-shaped incision is made starting just above the pinna, extending posteriorly from the zygomatic root to the inion, and terminating about 1 cm below and slightly anterior to the tip of the mastoid bone. Further, the attachments of the sternocleidomastoid and splenius capitus muscles to the tip of the mastoid bone are exposed and preserved. A mastoidectomy is performed using the canal wall-up procedure and the posterior bony part of the external auditory canal is drilled to thin it out while still keeping it intact. During mastoidectomy, the groove of the digastric muscle is exposed, which provides not only an important anatomical landmark near the stylomastoid foramen, but is also a precise location for the exit of the vertical segment of the facial nerve. At this point, careful inspection is done to clearly identify the location of the incus, as well as the lateral and posterior semicircular canals. Identifying the sigmoid sinus, and the descending and mastoid segments of the facial nerve is equally important. The bone in the sigmoid venous sinus region is excavated from the sinodural angle to the jugular bulb while retaining a bony section in the central portion of the sinus, which will aid in retractor placement. The posterior fossa dura is exposed and incisions are made between the posterior canal, sigmoid sinus, and jugular bulb, and another incision is made in the region just anterior to the sigmoid sinus. In order to achieve clear visualization of the glossopharyngeal, vagus and spinal accessory cranial nerves, the bone between the posterior semicircular canal and the jugular bulb is drilled inferiorly. In a minority of cases, despite drilling the space between posterior semicircular canal and the jugular bulb, the clear visibility of these cranial nerves is not achieved. Such cases necessitate drilling of the posterior semicircular canal and obliteration of the crura. After the posterior fossa dural incision, the cisternal CSF is released by opening the subarachnoid space. This is followed by slight retraction of the cerebellum to enable visibility of the nerve roots at the cerebellopontine angle.

The surgeon needs to identify the anatomical structures in the vicinity of the cochlear nucleus and use them as reference to place the electrode paddle in an assumed position of the cochlear nucleus complex, as the complex itself is concealed from clear field of visibility. The dorsal cochlear nucleus lies superior to the lateral recess of the fourth ventricle, while the ventral cochlear nucleus is covered by the cerebellar peduncle. The foramen of Luschka is the ideal site for placement of the electrode paddle. This area is located medial to the entry of the glossopharyngeal nerve in an area between the glossopharyngeal and facial nerves. Further confirmation can be achieved by identifying the vestibulocochlear nerve when it reaches close to the glossopharyngeal nerve. The entry into the fourth ventricle through the foramen of Luschka can be identified by the choroid plexus, which envelops the cerebellar flocculus. After removing the venous and arterial networks and the arachnoid over the foramen of Luschka, the cerebellar floculus and the choroid plexus are retracted to reach the lateral recess; the testimony to its correct identification is the egress of CSF. The electrode array is inserted into the lateral recess using small forceps. The electrode's correct position is verified with intraoperative electrically evoked auditory brainstem responses and neural response telemetry, delineated later in this chapter. Once the surgery team is satisfied regarding the optimal electrode paddle positioning, a temporalis fascia graft is used with fibrin glue to close the dural opening. As the final steps, the fat graft harvested from the iliac fossa of the abdominal wall on the left side is used to obliterate the mastoid cavity. The periosteum, muscule, and skin, in that order, are sutured, and a pressure dressing is done. An ICU stay is typically needed until the patient's condition become stable after the surgery.

Intraoperative Auditory Nerve Electrophysiology for ABI Device Placement

During an ABI surgery, a surgeon can only see bulges, veins, colourations, stumps, adjacent nerve groups and surrounding structures which lead to the opening of the lateral recess of the fourth ventricle. There is no solid structure upon which one can accurately mark the periphery of the CN complex. The lack of visibility of the entire surface of the cochlear nucleus can induce errors in optimum placement of the electrode paddle even from the skilled and experienced surgeons. The so-called 'normal anatomical variations' make the task more difficult, and the matter gets further complicated by the presence of a distorted anatomy caused by a large tumour removal. Therefore, the surgeon must rely on the findings of eABR, eMLR and/or Device Telemetry to fathom the accuracy of his/her electrode positioning.

The value of intraoperative eABR lies in its ability to predict the post-operative auditory percepts (not speech perception). It validates the optimum placement of the electrode paddle on the cochlear nucleus by providing the highest number of peaks in the recording (Herrmann et al., 2015; Teagle et al., 2018). One might argue that knowing the anatomy ensures correct placement of the electrode array and that multiple repositioning only risks traumatizing the cochlear nucleus complex thereby reducing eventual benefit. However, proper placement of the electrode array also reduces the risk of non-auditory sensations when the ABI is in use (Anwar et al., 2017).

The EABR can be obtained intra operatively which makes it suitable for intraoperative real-time analysis of the forward moving signals to cochlear nucleus and beyond. Although it is also possible to use ECAPs as a measure, the responses could be from any neural population, not necessarily from the auditory pathway; hence, eABR is preferred over ECAPs for intraoperative evaluation of the accuracy of electrode placement. This is the primary reason an audiologist being a necessity in the operation theatre. The audiologist must be available from the beginning of the surgery as the recording electrodes must be placed before the patient is draped. Once the surgery begins, adjust or repositioning of the recording electrodes is not possible. The surgery for ABI requires a number of other monitors; hence, to avoid interference in recording, it is advisable to set up the evoked-potential system opposite to the surgery side. The details on the equipment used, electrode placement, stimulations, and recording are discussed in the Chap. 18 of this book, and therefore, will not be discussed here again.

The waveform of eABR should be viewed keeping in mind the site of stimulus delivery. Since the electrode paddle is placed on the cochlear nucleus, waves I and II of the auditory brainstem response cannot be recorded. In several instances, even the wave III cannot be visualized. Wave V remains the most robust and therefore, the audiologist looks for wave V (sometimes wave III, if it is present) as shown in Fig. 24.5. The audiologist will need to measure eABRs from different combinations of electrodes to provide crucial information on the position of the electrode array.

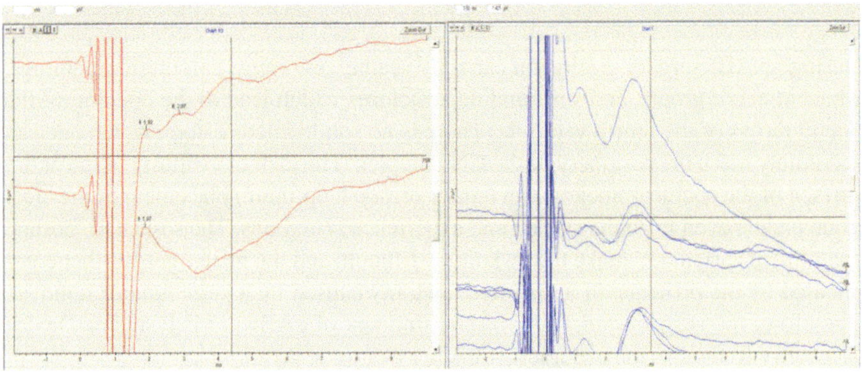

Fig. 24.5 Typical intraoperative eABR responses obtained from ABI

The decision on retention of or change in position of the electrode paddle depends completely based on the presence of wave V (in some cases waves III & V). The readjustment to the electrode paddle position is needed when eABR shows no replicable waves in the waveform. Once the gross position of the electrode array is fixed, the response from other electrode combinations are checked for co-stimulation of other organs, in which case the event and the electrode number is noted (Narayan, N. 2013). This electrode/combination may require turning-off at the time of switch-on. Monitoring of neighbouring cranial nerves serves to detect activity that indicates misplacement of the electrode array (Kuroki & Moller, 1995).

Positioning of the ABI Device

Performing eABR and obtaining identifiable waves V (possibly also wave III) in the waveform helps confirm that the implanted electrode array delivered electrical signals are travelling along the ascending auditory pathway, which is a desired outcome (Nevison et al., 2002). From an ABI device, the number of electrodes elicit usable auditory sensation varies greatly from one patient to the other. One can find a huge improvement in the outcome by altering the electrode paddle position by merely few millimetres. The assurance that the electrodes can effectively stimulate the auditory system is enhanced through the use of electrophysiological guidance during the placement of the implanted electrode paddle. This technique involves stimulating individual electrode and recording eABR as an aid in positioning the electrode array. By using this approach, it is possible to place most electrodes over the cochlear nucleus, minimizing the stimulation of other cranial nerves and thereby reducing the risk of undesirable side effects. (Fig. 24.5). When the electrode paddle is correctly positioned, it elicits an eABR response with between 1 and 4 waves in the waveform whose average latencies are approximately 0.7 ms (0.4–0.9 ms), 1.5 ms (1.2–1.9 ms), 2.7 ms (2.1–3.4 ms) and 3.7 ms (3.4–4.0 ms). These waves are likely associated with waves III-VI of the traditional acoustically-evoked ABRs. While inspecting the waveform, one should decipher a present eABR condition to there being no additional peaks within a 10-ms window and no clear signs of other cranial nerves being stimulated. Stimulation of bipolar combinations of electrodes at lateral, medial, and distal positions offers insights into the insertion depth.

Obtaining the EABR Recordings

Paired sub-dermal needle electrodes are generally used to obtain stable position with low impedances. Electrode montage that uses vertex (Cz) as positive, neck hairline (on the midline) as ground, C7 (on the spine, midline) as negative. Short, platted or twisted recording electrode wires are used to reduce electrical interference. The electrode wires are connected directly into an electrode head-box that is connected to the main amplifier. The electrode montage for EABR during ABI operations is different from that used for recording regular ABR or cochlear implant EABR, which typically uses vertex (Cz) or upper forehead as positive, ipsilateral mastoid as ground, contralateral mastoid as negative. The use of the traditional ABR montage for recording an EABR, both with ABI and CI, will result in a larger stimulus artifact than the montage described above. The electrical stimulus generates a large potential immediately preceding the neural response. This has two specific complicating effects: (1) The stimulus artifact may extend in time and overlap with the response, (2) The amplitude of the stimulus (which is orders of magnitude greater than the response) may cause the amplifiers to become overloaded or 'saturated', obscuring any response which should occur within the first milliseconds after the stimulus. Both of the above phenomena can be managed by a combination of: (a) electrode montage, (b) filtering, (c) gain settings, and (d) stimulus control.

It is preferable not to filter the input signal as much as when recording ABR. Filter cut-offs should be in the 1–10 Hz range (high-pass filter) to 5–10 kHz (low pass filter) range. Too high a setting of the high-pass filter, for example to 100 Hz or above, can adversely affect the recording. (Nevison et al., 2002; Polak et al., 2018).

The stimuli are generated by the ABI programming system, which also provides a trigger signal for the evoked potential machine that is used for EABR recordings. Typically, approximately 1000 responses must be averaged to achieve an acceptable signal to noise ratio. Post-stimulus delays should be set to 0 ms as it can be helpful to see the stimulus on the screen in order to better interpret the response. Other features such as artifact rejection can be enabled provided they are set not to reject anything within the first 2 ms after the stimulus. The manufacturer's programming software will allow for the set-up of the stimulus to be used during surgery. It is important to use bipolar electrode combinations. Monopolar stimulation creates much larger stimulus artifacts and may stimulate tissue other than the CN. The stimulus must be increased from a low starting intensity and increased until a clear multi-peaked EABR waveform is observed. The threshold provides a measure of the excitability of the CN complex. Lower thresholds indicate that the tested electrode is in a good position on the surface of the CN and that any adjacent structures are less likely to be stimulated. Confirming the approximate placement of an electrode array is best achieved with a relatively wide bipolar stimulation path across most of the array (Nevison et al., 2002).

The wider modes are more likely to stimulate nearby cranial nerves, which then can be detected provided that the cranial nerves in question are monitored. If this occurs with low stimulus current levels, it is a strong indication to change the position of the electrode array. For more accurate placement of the electrode array, a combination of electrodes across the array should be stimulated. Each position should be tested and the responses compared before making any decision about advancing or retracting the electrode array. Rotational and/or sideways positioning is far more difficult in practice because of the limited space available. In cases where the lateral recess is wide, combinations of electrodes along the sides of the array should be stimulated, since 1 mm of sub-optimal placement in this direction could

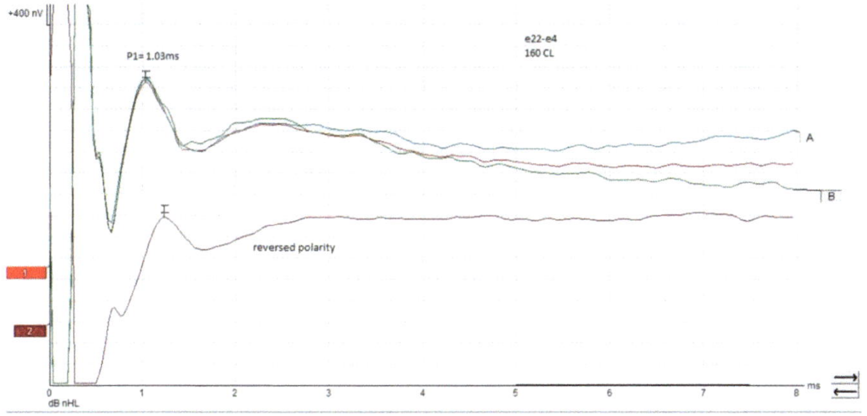

Fig. 24.6 Reversal of Stimulus Polarity and no reversal of response confirms that the response is not an artefact. (Figure courtesy Dr. William Shapiro, NYU)

make 7 electrodes non-functional compared to only 3 electrodes for incorrect placement in the lateral-medial direction.

After examining a response, the stimulus polarity should be inverted and a second response obtained, making sure that only the stimulus artifact inverts and not the response (Fig. 24.6). When responses are small and noisy, this is the best indicator that the observed potential is biological and neither noise stimulus artifacts nor an artifact of the filtering. Stimulation at high current levels has the possibility to stimulate the vagus nerve and may cause heart arrest.

Characterising the Response

The waveform of the recorded EABRs differ considerably among patients. This individual variation might indicate that either different auditory pathways are activated in different patients or that the state of the auditory pathway differs among patients, and especially those who have a tumour or have had surgery to remove them. Normally between 1 and 4 positive waves can be identified within a window of approximately 4 ms from the start of the stimulus. No dominant component normally occurs in the remainder of the observation window (typically 10 ms). Any response beyond 5 ms is likely to be a myogenic response (Fig. 24.7a). It is more common to see 2- or 3-peak responses than 1 or 4 peaks (Fig. 24.7c, d). The most dominant and reliable positive peak occurs at a latency of approximately 1.5 ms (1.2–1.9 ms).

There are many different sources of electrical interference in an operating room and electrical interference can obscure the recorded responses. For example, cautery/diathermy machines tend to produce interference even in standby. It is important that such interference is brought to a minimum before a recording is begun. If

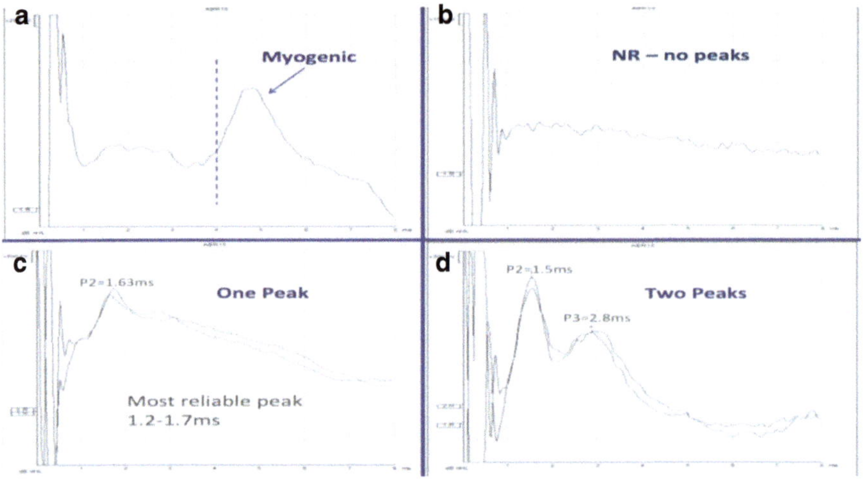

Fig. 24.7 Different types of EABR responses (**a**) Myogenic (**b**) No response (**c**) single peak audiotory response (**d**) Double peak auditory response. (Figure courtesy Dr. William Shapiro, NYU)

the waveforms are saturated by a large, decaying stimulus artifact, consider widening the stimulus pulse width to lower the stimulus current requirements, lower the high-pass filter cut-off and reduce the amplification. Alternatively, try electrode combinations that have a different orientation to that initially chosen. If no clear response is obtained (Fig. 24.7b), this may be due to lack of excitability of the CN, inaccurate positioning of the electrode array or poor contact with the CN surface are likely causes of the failure to obtain a response. Repositioning or repacking behind the ABI array may be options to consider (Anwar et al., 2017;Nevison et al., 2002).

Post-operative Care

Careful wound management is essential for preventing infections, reducing the risk of cerebrospinal fluid (CSF) leaks that can lead to meningitis, and avoiding post-surgical complications such as device exposure or biofilm formation. Postoperative imaging, including plain X-rays or CT scans, is required to verify the device's position in the brainstem (see Fig. 24.8a, b). Device activation typically occurs 6–8 weeks later. Unlike CI, which can be switched-on in an OPD set-up, it is imperative to monitor vital signs and potential non-auditory effects. Typically, the initial device activation, or "switch-on," is performed in an ICU setting where the neurological monitoring of the VIIth, VIIIth, and lower cranial nerves is feasible. Proper preparation for active CPR is crucial due to the risk of unintended stimulation of other brainstem nuclei and vital centers. If side effects occur, the stimulation intensity is adjusted until hearing is achieved without adverse effects. If this adjustment is not feasible, the problematic channel is deactivated. Common side effects include facial

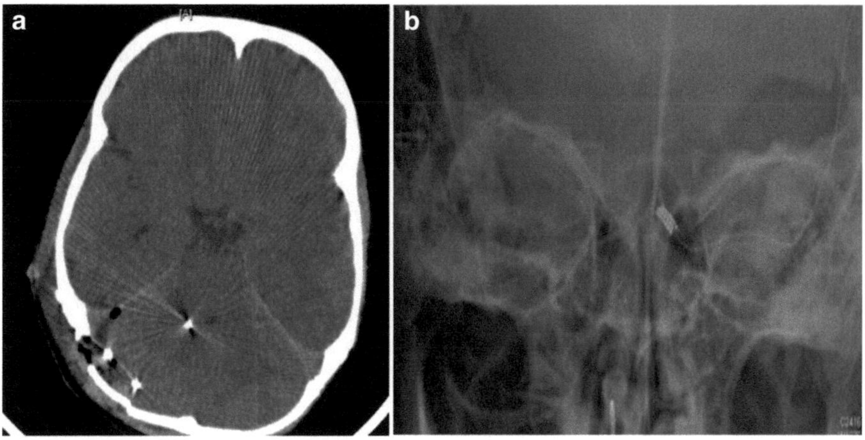

Fig. 24.8 (**a**, **b**) Post operative CT scan (5**a**) and Xray (5**b**) of an ABI in situ

nerve stimulation, nystagmus, vagal stimulation, dizziness, and gait changes, most of which should improve over time (Brackmann et al. 2010; Raghunandhan & Kameswaran, 2010).

Risks, Side Effects and Complications of ABI

The complexity of the surgery, the delicate nature of the brainstem, and the proximity of critical neural structures mean that the procedure carries potential complications. Therefore, surgery for ABI requires high precision and careful planning. Despite that, some forms of major complications have been observed in <15% of the ABI recipients. The complications have been more often found in adults, and more so in in adults with NF2 In fact, studies have shown that the complications observed in patients undergoing ABI were not significantly more than those undergoing surgery only for the tumor removal. This is despite the fact that ABI increases the surgery time by a fair amount, requires more manipulations of the brainstem and cerebellum, and requires insertion of an additional hardware within the nervous system (Colletti et al., 2010). In a recent systematic review, Garcia et al. (2024) classified the side effects according to their type and location. The type was classified as sensory, motor, and unspecified, whereas the locations were mapped to eyes, face, head, vestibular, throat, body, arms, and legs. The congregated data in their study revealed side effects in nearly one-third (24 out of 67) patients in the non-tumor cohort. In stark contrast, almost 81% (165 out of 204) tumor patients had side effects. Irrespective of the group and location, 18.0% side effects were sensory whereas motor side effects constituted just over 4% of patients. Almost 78% patients had unspecified side effects. Vertigo observed in 22.5% patients was the most common side effect within the non-tumor cohort. Nearly 19% non-tumor patients reported facial twitching, numbness, and unspecified facial sensations and just over 16% patients reported pain, tingling, unspecified sensations in the throat (Goffi-Gomez et al., 2012; Choi et al., 2011; Jung et al., 2017; Raghunandhan et al., 2019; Rajeswaran & Kameswaran, 2020; Sennaroglu et al., 2016; Malerbi et al., 2018). In the tumor cohort, the problems in the head region such as headache, pressure, head pain, ear pain, tingling, pounding was found in 31.5% patients. Tingling, vibration, motor response, and unspecified responses in the rest of the body was found in 18.2% tumor patients whereas vertigo was evidenced in 10.9% tumor patients (Sanna et al., 2012; Nevison et al., 2002; Matthies et al., 2013; Goffi-Gomez et al., 2012; Otto et al., 2002; Ramsden et al., 2016; Briggs et al., 2000; Jackson et al., 2002; Lenarz et al., 2001; Lesinski-Schiedat et al., 2000; Maini et al., 2009; Marangos et al., 2000). The details of specific risks and complications are given below:

Mortality

Most of the studies on ABI have reported no fatal consequences directly linked to the procedure itself. In a study by Colletti et al. (2010), the authors reported no intraoperative mortality among their patient group consisting of 83 adults and 31 children. However, postoperative mortality, which was unrelated to ABI, occurred in three adults all of whom had NF2. Myocardial infarction after one moth of the implant activation was the cause of death in one patient. Another one succumbed to cardiopulmonary complications one year after ABI activation, while the third patient passed away seven months post-activation due to pontine myelinolysis, which resulted from an overly rapid administration of hyperosmolar sodium chloride at a different clinic while being treated for dehydration associated with flu-induced fever and vomiting.

Facial Nerve Injury

The facial nerve is one of the most commonly injured structures during ABI surgery. The facial nerve lies in close proximity to the cochlear nucleus, and the risk of damage increases during the dissection and electrode placement phases of the surgery. The facial nerve can have direct trauma during dissection or electrode insertion, especially if the nerve is unusually positioned or adherent to surrounding structures. Further, incorrect placement of the electrode array can result in direct contact with the facial nerve or irritation of the nerve. Additionally, excessive retraction of the cerebellum or brainstem during surgery may increase the risk of facial nerve injury. Facial nerve injury can lead to facial weakness, paralysis, or dyskinesia, which may be temporary or permanent. Colletti et al. (2010) reported of relatively temporary facial palsy in 8 NF2 adults, which resolved within 1–8 weeks with use of tear substitutes, lubricants, and eye protection. Others have also reported transient, yet clinical facial palsy on the ipsilateral side of the surgery in a few patients after the ABI (Madhav et al., 2018). A permanent facial palsy was evidenced in one patient after tumor excision. Early recognition and careful intraoperative monitoring, such as electromyographic (EMG) monitoring of the facial nerve, can help minimize this risk. In some cases, facial nerve decompression or surgical intervention may be required (Fisch & Moffat, 2015).

Cerebellar Injury

The cerebellum, which controls coordination and balance, lies adjacent to the surgical site and can be at risk if the brainstem or posterior fossa needs to be retracted during the surgery. Cerebellar injury can occur due to excessive or forceful retraction, or prolonged pressure leading to contusion, ischemia and tissue damage. Additionally, cerebellar edema can result from prolonged surgical manipulation or ischemia. Irrespective of how the cerebellar damage has occurred, it can result in neurological deficits, such as ataxia, balance problems, or even more severe motor dysfunction. Colletti et al. (2010) reported 2 patients with cerebellar injury in their series of 114 patients undergoing ABI. Among them, one was an adult with NF2 whereas the other one was a non-tumor child. The NF2 adult had a cerebellar contusion with infarction and hydrocephalus, requiring partial surgical removal of the cerebellum, and placement of a ventriculoperitoneal shunt. In the non-tumor child, an intracerebellar clot was found on the CT scan. Surgical removal of the clot resulted in complete recovery, even the restoration of eABR that had deteriorated following the clot formation. While secondary surgical interventions have been found to yield encouraging results, it is essential to minimize cerebellar retraction by using delicate techniques and instruments so as to prevent cerebellar complications in the first place. Intraoperative monitoring of cerebellar function could play a pivotal part in preventing damage (Mastoid et al., 2016). Sometimes, the patient may need ventilator support for a few days. In fact, Madhav et al. (2018) reported that a few of their study population were placed on ventilator support for 2 days after the surgery due to transient cerebellar oedema.

Infection and Meningitis

As with any surgery involving the brain and spinal cord, there is a risk of infection, including the potential for meningitis. Infection can arise from bacterial contamination during surgery, post-surgical wound infection, or cerebrospinal fluid (CSF) leaks. In some cases, an unintended leak of cerebrospinal fluid during the dural opening or following craniotomy can increase the risk of infection. Among the 114 patients, Colletti et al. (2010) reported development of meningitis in 4 patients.

Among these 4, one NF2 adult developed meningitis in the postoperative period whereas mastoiditis nearly 2 years after ABI activation led to meningitis in 2 non-tumor adults and 1 non-tumor child, all of whom had severe cochlear malformations. Teagle et al. (2018) also reported that one out of their series of five non-tumor children developed aseptic bacterial meningitis on postoperative day 10 with complete resolution after 6 weeks intravenous administration of Vancomycin and Ceftriaxone. Prophylactic antibiotics should be administered before and after surgery to minimize the risk of infection. The other kinds of infections could the infection to the surgical incisions, surgical flap, and infections around the implant itself. Colletti et al. (2010) reported infections of the surgical incision in 5 patients (2 adults with NF2, 2 non-tumor adults, and 1 non-tumor child), infection of the surgical flap in 2 NF2 adults and 1 non-tumor adults, and infections with intact skin around their implants in 2 adults with NF2 and one non-tumor adult. Howver, all of them were easily treated with suitable antibiotics and minor procedures. Infection and meningitis can have severe consequences, including sepsis or permanent neurological deficits. If meningitis or infection occurs, it may require antibiotic treatment, drainage of any abscesses, and sometimes additional surgical interventions to repair CSF leaks (Berenholz & Gacek, 2017).

Lesions of Other Lower Cranial Nerves

Lower cranial nerve (LCN) lesions can occur after auditory brainstem implantation (ABI) and can cause symptoms like dysphagia, dysarthria, and hoarseness, and may also increase the risk of aspiration. Colletti et al. (2010) reported postoperative dysphonia and swallowing difficulties in two adults with NF2, who had large schwannomas of the Glossopharyngeal nerve (CN IX) and Vagus nerve (CN X). Among others, Schwartz et al. (2008) noted pathological function of the contralateral lower cranial nerves leading to a far higher incidence of aspiration and dysphagia in patients undergoing ABI than in the acoustic neuroma population as a whole.

Hydrocephalus

Hydrocephalus of temporary or permanent nature can be a less frequently observed complication after ABI than some of the others. In a study reporting various complications of ABI, Colletti et al. (2010) reported postoperative hydrocephalus in two adults, one with NF2 and the other one a non-tumor patient, both requiring shunt placement. They also observed temporary hydrocephalus in one non-tumor adult and seven adults with NF2; however, no one needed a shunt placement.

Cerebrospinal Fluid Leak

Cerebrospinal fluid (CSF) leaks can occur during the surgical procedure, particularly when the dura is opened or when there is a tear during the craniotomy. In patients with elevated CSF pressure or underlying conditions that affect CSF dynamics, the risk of leaks increases. CSF leaks can increase the risk of infection, especially meningitis. In a study on 19 patients who underwent ABI, two were reported to have CSF-related complications that required further surgical measure for resolution (Dastagirzada et al., 2024). Before this, Colletti et al. (2010) had reported CSF leaks after ABI in nearly 18% of the NF2 adults (6 out of 34) and about 0.5% (1 out of 49) non-tumor adults. None of the two NF2 children and 29 non-tumor children had a CSF leak. In a leak is found, the surgeon must seal the leak with sutures or a synthetic dural patch. In more severe cases, additional procedures may be required to repair the leak (Sanna & Mancini, 2010).

Pseudo Meningocele

Two NF2 patients developed a pseudo meningocele that was treated with drainage and application of a mastoid pressure dressing medication Colletti et al. (2010). More recently, Teagle et al. (2018) reported that 1 out of their series of 5 non-tumor children developed stridor and cough induced a pseudomeningocele at the surgery site which was transpired in CSF wound leakage that necessitated a second surgery to reinforce the closure and placement of a lumbar drainage. This was a child with CHARGE Syndrome who had subglottic stenosis with mild stridor even preoperatively. Colletti et al. (2021) reported that among 103 patients who underwent ABI between the years 2000 and 2014, one patient undergoing bilateral simultaneous ABI using the retrosigmoid approach developed pseudomeningocele, which was successfully managed through the use of fat grafting and resorbable cranioplasty plates during the revision surgery. A much higher incidence of postoperative pseudomeningocele has been reported by Madhav et al. (2018). The reported pseudomeningocele in 4 (≈17%) children after ABI using a retrosigmoid approach of surgery, all of whom were successfully treated with pressure dressing, aspiration and intra venous antibiotics.

Electrode Malposition and Failure

Accurate placement of the electrode array within the cochlear nucleus is pivotal to the success with ABI. Misplacement of the electrode or improper stimulation may result in inadequate hearing restoration or device failure. Postoperative CT scans can help identify electrode placement issues. One needs to use of eABR for intraoperative monitoring and using the information from it to position the electrodes to minimize this risk. This has been covered in detail in Chap. 23. In some cases, a revision surgery may be required to reposition the electrode or replace the device (Buchman & Roush, 2012).

Cerebrovascular Complications

The brainstem and posterior fossa are rich in vascular structures, and there is a risk of vascular injury during ABI surgery, particularly to the posterior inferior cerebellar artery or other smaller vessels. Additionally, there could be a chance that excessive retraction or pressure on the brainstem can compromise the blood supply, resulting in ischemia and potential neurological deficits. Intraoperative vigilance and careful dissection near vascular structures are essential to minimize the risk of bleeding or vascular injury. Surgical hemostasis and possible embolization techniques can be employed to control bleeding (Moffat & McHugh, 2014).

Wound Seroma

Seroma refers to the atypical buildup of serous fluid within a dead space, which consists of plasma and lymphatic fluid (Agrawal et al., 2006; Van Bemmel et al., 2011; Kuroi et al., 2006). The exact cause of seroma formation after any surgery is not fully understood, but it is believed to result from the disruption of lymphatic and vascular drainage due to extensive soft tissue dissection, leading to the accumulation of serum and potentially inflammatory exudate within a dead space (Kuroi et al., 2005; Andrades et al., 2007). In a study in 2010, Colletti et al. reported wound seroma in 4 adults with NF2 and 6 non-tumor patients (2 adults and 4 children). In all of them, aspiration and pressure dressing helped in successful management, and in none of them it necessitated device extrusion.

Balance Problems

The relatively temporary balance problems have been reported to occur after ABI. Colletti et al. (2010) reported temporary balance problems in 14 patients, which included 11 adults with NF2, 2 non-tumor adults and 1 non-tumor child. In the NF2 adults, the balance problems lasted for a slightly longer duration (5–23 days) than the non-tumor patients in whom the issue lasted 2–4 days. In the non-tumor child, the postoperative dizziness spontaneously resolved within 5 days. Raghunandhan et al. (2019) also reported postoperative balance issues in 2 non-tumor children which resolved within a few months. Natarajan et al. (2021) reported post-ABI vestibular disturbances in 16.7% of 48 patients with bilateral cochlear and cochlear nerve aplasia. These vestibular disturbances were evidenced in patients who had either a Grade 3 or a Grade cerebellar flocculus, where retraction of cerebellum was required for visualization of root entry zone of lower cranial nerves. Therefore, the balance issues in them was possibly related to the manipulations of the parts of the cerebellum.

Headache

Headaches after a brain surgery not uncommon. It can also a side effect of ABI. Headaches lasting a few days has been reported in ABI recipients after the surgery in 9 adults of whom 7 had NF2 whereas 2 patients were non-tumor adults (Colletti et al., 2010). Relatively lesser proportion of patients (1 non-tumor adult and 1 adult with NF2) experienced persistent headache long after the surgery.

Bradycardia

A drop in heart rate below the acceptable norms, called Bradycardia, is a side effect typically associated with the ABI device activation. A vagal nerve monitoring is therefore an essential component of the device activation. Nonetheless, bradycardia has also been observed as a post-surgical complication. In a study by Raghunandhan et al. (2019), the authors reported evidence of post-surgery bradycardia with drop in the heart rate to 50/minute in 2 patients. While one of them was treated using atropine (0.5 mg), the resolution in the other required a reduction in the stimulation current level for the electrodes.

Infections Around the Implant

The infections around the implant are different from wound seroma. Colletti et al. (2010) reported infections around the implants, despite the intact skin, in 2 adults with NF2 and one non-tumor adult. In their study, one non-tumor adult, who developed an abscess requiring subsequent incision and drainage, had an unknown catgut allergy that was not informed to the surgical team before the surgery. In another study, one implantee underwent a revision surgery due to bio-film formation with subsequent implantation on the contralateral side after a gap of one and a half year (Madhav et al., 2018).

Non-auditory Side Effects

The critical location of the ABI electrodes in the vicinity of several key structures and cranial nerves causes some of the electrodes to elicit non-auditory percepts (Behr et al., 2007). Typically, the non-auditory side effects are caused by an unintentional stimulation of the cerebellar flocculus, cerebellar peduncles, long sensory tracts, and/or facial nerve. Studies have reported non-auditory stimulations in 35–60% of the ABI patients (Matthies et al., 2013; Polak et al., 2018). The non-auditory sensations are almost always benign but could cause considerable amount of discomfort to certain patients. These sensations have been documented to affect various body parts such as head (headache/knocking, pressure sensation, dizziness, or tickling sensation), temple (tactile or pain), ear (twitching, tickling, or pressure), eyes (eyebrow twitching/tickling, eye movement, blurred vision, or diplopia), chin (irritation), arms (unpleasant sensation or twitching), chest (tickling or unpleasant sensation), legs (twitching), and abdomen (twitching) (Matthies et al., 2013; Polak et al., 2018). The non-auditory side effects are not limited to NF2 patients alone (Fig. 24.9). Colletti et al. (2010) reported the presence of one or more non-auditory percepts in 73% NF2 adults, 32% non-tumor adults, and nearly 23% non-tumor children (Fig. 24.9). The non-auditory side effects are generally minimised by deactivating or reconfiguring the electrode channels. Use of eABR to identify the electrodes generating auditory responses and deactivating the remaining electrodes can be also helpful.

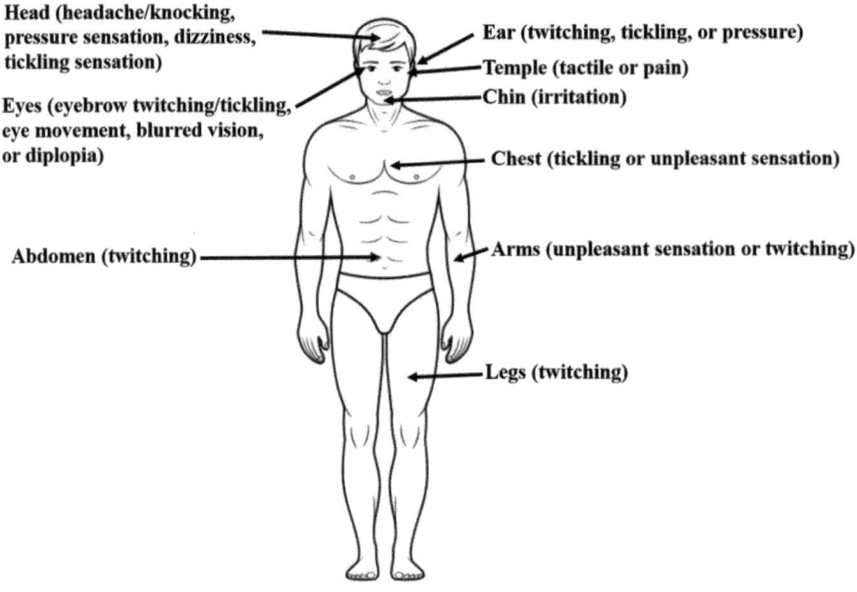

Fig. 24.9 Site and type of non-auditory percepts created on the basis of the information from earlier publications (Colletti et al., 2010; Matthies et al., 2013; Polak et al., 2018)

Contraindications for ABI include a history of stereotactic radiotherapy, which carries the risk of radiation-induced necrosis in the cochlear nucleus area, as well as anatomical distortion and fibrosis that may lead to pontine hypoplasia (Kameswaran et al., 2005).

Auditory brainstem implant surgery has gained worldwide popularity because it offers a chance for hearing to many patients who might otherwise remain deaf. For over two decades, ABIs have been used primarily in patients with neurofibromatosis type 2 (NF2) who have bilateral vestibular schwannomas. The main goal in these cases is to restore hearing after reducing or removing the tumours. Recent evidence also shows that ABIs are highly effective for non-tumour patients, especially prelingually deaf children with severe cochlear abnormalities that make them unsuitable for cochlear implantation. Regardless of whether the patient has a tumour or not, intraoperative recording of eABR during ABI electrode paddle positioning provides crucial information about the electrodes' ability to activate neurons in the cochlear nucleus. This information can help adjust the electrode paddle's position during the surgery and enhance the possibility of effective stimulation of the cochlear nucleus complex by as many electrodes as possible. However, even with good intraoperative eABR results, only a few auditory electrodes might function after surgery, potentially due to shifting of the electrode paddle during the wound closure. Monitoring other cranial nerves during the ABI procedure is also valuable and is particularly important in surgeries for removing vestibular schwannomas, which often precede the implantation of the ABI electrode paddle.

References

Agrawal, A., Ayantunde, A. A., & Cheung, K. L. (2006). Concepts of seroma formation and prevention in breast cancer surgery. *ANZ Journal of Surgery, 76*(12), 1088–1095.

Andrades, P., Prado, A., Danilla, S., Guerra, C., Benitez, S., Sepulveda, S., Sciarraffia, C., & De Carolis, V. (2007). Progressive tension sutures in the prevention of postabdominoplasty seroma: A prospective, randomized, double-blind clinical trial. *Plastic and Reconstructive Surgery, 120*(4), 935–946.

Anwar, A., Singleton, A., Fang, Y., Wang, B., Shapiro, W., Roland, J. T., & Waltzman, S. B. (2017). The value of intraoperative EABRs in auditory brainstem implantation. *International Journal of Pediatric Otorhinolaryngology, 101*((Anwar, Singleton, Fang, Wang, Shapiro, Roland, Waltzman) New York University School of Medicine, NYU Langone Medical Center, United States), 158–163.

Asfour, L., Friedmann, D. R., Shapiro, W. H., Roland, J. T., & Waltzman, S. B. (2018). Early experience and health related quality of life outcomes following auditory brainstem implantation in children. *International Journal of Pediatric Otorhinolaryngology, 113*((Asfour, Friedmann, Shapiro, Roland, Waltzman) New York University School of Medicine, 550 1st Ave, NY NY 10016, United States), 140–149.

Aslan, F., Ozkan, H. B., Yucel, E., Sennaroglu, G., Bilginer, B., & Sennaroglu, L. (2020). Effects of age at auditory brainstem implantation: Impact on auditory perception, language development, speech intelligibility. *Otology & Neurotology: Official Publication of the American Otological Society, American Neurotology Society [and] European Academy of Otology and Neurotology, 41*(1), 11–20.

Behr, R., Müller, J., Shehata-Dieler, W., et al. (2007). The high rate CIS auditory brainstem implant for restoration of hearing in NF-2 patients. *Skull Base, 17*(2), 91–107.

Bento, R. F., & Lopes, P. T. (2021). Surgery for ABI: Retrolabyrinthine approach. In E. P. Wilkinson & M. S. Schwartz (Eds.), *Auditory brainstem implants*. Thieme Publishers.

Bento, R. F., De Brito, R. V., Sanchez, T. G., & Miniti, A. (2002). The transmastoid retrolayrinthine approach in vestibular schwannoma surgery. *Otolaryngology—Head & Neck Surgery, 127*(5), 437–441.

Berenholz, L. P., & Gacek, R. R. (2017). Infection and cerebrospinal fluid leaks in auditory brainstem implantation. *Journal of Neurosurgery, 126*(3), 756–762.

Brackmann, D. E., Hitselberger, W. E., & Nelson, R. A. (1993). Auditory brainstem implant: I. Issues in surgical implantation. *Otolayngology—Head and Neck Surgey, 108*(6), 624–633.

Brackmann, D. E., Shelton, C., & Arriaga, M. A. (2010). Auditory brainstem implants. In *Otologic surgery* (3rd ed., pp 591–602). W.B. Saunders Company.

Briggs, R. J. S., Fagan, P., Atlas, M., et al. (2000). Multichannel auditory brainstem implantation: The Australian experience. *The Journal of Laryngology and Otology. Supplement, 114*(S27), 46–49.

Buchman, C. A., & Roush, P. A. (2012). Electrode placement and efficacy in auditory brainstem implantation. *Otology & Neurotology, 33*(5), 902–908.

Choi, J. Y., Song, M. H., Jeon, J. H., Lee, W. S., & Chang, J. W. (2011). Early surgical results of auditory brainstem implantation in nontumor patients. *The Laryngoscope, 121*(12), 2610–2618.

Colletti, V. (2006) Auditory outcomes in tumor vs. non-tumor patients fitted with auditory brainstem implants. *Advances in Otorhinolaryngol, 64*, 167–85.

Colletti V, Shannon RV, Carner M, Veronese S, Colletti L. (2010). Complications in auditory brainstem implant surgery in adults and children. *Otol Neurotol, 31*(4):558–64.

Colletti, V., Mandala, M., Colletti, G., & Colletti, L. (2021). Pediatric auditory brainstem implantation: Colletti team experience and special considerations. Ento Key. Retrieved online on 28.11.2024 from https://entokey.com/9-pediatric-auditory-brainstem-implantation-colletti-team-experience-andspecial-considerations/#b923a976_32

Dastagirzada, Y. M., Eremiev, A., Wisoff, J. H., Kay-Rivest, E., Shapiro, W. H., Unterberger, A., Waltzman, S. B., Roland, J. T., Golfinos, J. G., & Harter, D. H. (2024). Auditory brainstem implantation: surgical experience and audiometric outcomes in the pediatric population. *Journal of Neurosurgery: Pediatrics, 33*(5), 496–504.

Deep, N. L., & Roland, J. T. (2020). Auditory brainstem implantation: Candidacy evaluation, operative technique, and outcomes. *Otolaryngologic Clinics of North America, 53*(1), 103–113.

Deep, N. L., Roland, J. T., & Choudhury, B. (2019). Auditory brainstem implantation: An overview. *Journal of Neurological Surgery, Part B: Skull Base, 80*(2), 203–208.

Fisch, U., & Moffat, D. A. (2015). Facial nerve preservation in auditory brainstem implantation using the retrosigmoid approach. *The Laryngoscope, 125*(2), 343–349.

Garcia A, Haleem A, Poe S, Gosh D, Christian Brown M, Herrmann BS, Lee DJ. (2024). Auditory Brainstem Implant Outcomes in Tumor and Nontumor Patients: A Systematic Review. *Otolaryngol Head Neck Surg, 170*(6):1648–1658.

Goffi-Gomez, M. V. S., Magalhães, A. T., Brito Neto, R., Tsuji, R. K., Gomes, M. Q. T., & Ferreira Bento, R. (2012). Auditory brainstem implant outcomes and MAP parameters: Report of experiences in adults and children. *International Journal of Pediatric Otorhinolaryngology, 76*(2), 257–264.

Goyal, S., Krishnan, S. K., Kameswaran, M., Vasudevan, M. C., Rajeswaran, R., & Natarajan, K. (2017). Does cerebellar flocculus size affect subjective outcomes in pediatric auditory brainstem implantation. *International Journal of Pediatric Otorhinolaryngol, 97*, 30–34.

Haber, K., Burzynska-Makuch, M., & Mierzwinski, J. (2020). The role of preoperative imaging for auditory implants in children. *Otolaryngologia Polska, 74*(6), 1–5.

Herrmann, B. S., Brown, M. C., Eddington, D. K., Hancock, K. E., & Lee, D. J. (2015). Auditory brainstem implant: Electrophysiologic responses and subject perception. *Ear and Hearing, 36*(3), 368–376.

Hitselberger, W. E., & House, W. F. (1966). A combined approach to the cerebellopontine angle: A suboccipital-petrosal approach. *Archives of Otolaryngology, 84*(3), 267–285.

Hitselberger, W. E., & Pulec, J. L. (1972). Trigemial nerve (posterior root) retrolabyrinthine selective section: Operative procedure for intractable pain. *Archives of Otolryngology, 96*(5), 412–415.

Hochmair, I., & Dhanasingh, A. (2021). ABI-auditory brainstem implant. *Acta Oto-Laryngologica, 141*(S1), 63–81.

Jackson, K. B., Mark, G., Helms, J., Mueller, J., & Behr, R. (2002). An auditory brainstem implant system. *American Journal of Audiology, 11*(2), 128–133.

Jung, N. Y., Kim, M., Chang, W. S., Jung, H. H., Choi, J. Y., & Chang, J. W. (2017). Favorable long-term functional outcomes and safety of auditory brainstem implants in nontumor patients. *Operative Neurosurgery, 13*(6), 653–660.

Kameswaran, M. C., Vasudevan, R. S., Anandkumar, N., Jawahar, N., Kiran, S., & Raghunandhan, S. (2005). Auditory brainstem implantation: The first Indian experience. *Indian Journal of Otolaryngology and Head and Neck Surgery, 57*(1), 58–63.

Kuroi, K., Shimozuma, K., Taguchi, T., Imai, H., Yamashiro, H., Ohsumi, S., & Saito, S. (2005). Pathophysiology of seroma in breast cancer. *Breast Cancer, 12*(4), 288–293.

Kuroi, K., Shimozuma, K., Taguchi, T., Imai, H., Yamashiro, H., Ohsumi, S., & Saito, S. (2006). Effect of mechanical closure of dead space on seroma formation after breast surgery. *Breast Cancer, 13*(3), 260–265.

Kuroki, A., & Moller, A. R. (1995). Microsurgical anatomy around the foramen of Luschka in relation to intraoperative recording of auditory evoked potentials from the cochlear nuclei. *Journal of Neurosurgery, 82*(6), 933–939.

Laszig, R., Marangos, N., Soilmann, P., Ramsden, R., Fraysse, B., Lenarz, T., Rask- Andersen, H., Bredberg, G., Sterkers, O., Manrique, M., & Nevison, B. (1997). Initial results from the clinical trial of the nucleus 21-channel auditory brain stem implant. *American Journal of Otology, 18*(6 SUPPL), S160.

Lenarz, T., Moshrefi, M., Matthies, C., et al. (2001). Auditory brainstem implant: part I. Auditory performance and its evolution over time. *Otology & Neurotology, 22*(6), 823–833.

Lesinski-Schiedat, A., Frohne, C., Illg, A., et al. (2000). Auditory brainstem implant in auditory rehabilitation of patients with neurofibromatosis type 2: Hannover. *The Journal of Laryngology and Otology, 114*(S27), 15–17.

Liu, C. C., Horn, D. L., & Anne, S. (2019). Advances in management of pediatric sensorineural hearing loss. *Otolaryngologic Clinics of North America, 52*(5), 847–861.

Madhav, K., Kumar, R. S., Vadivu, S., Natarajan, K., & Kameswaran, M. (2018). Paediatric auditory brainstem implantation (ABI): A journey through surgery and outcomes. *Otolaryngology: Open Access, 8*(3), 350.

Maini, S., Cohen, M. A., Hollow, R., & Briggs, R. (2009). Update on longterm results with auditory brainstem implants in NF2 patients. *Cochlear Implants International, 10*(sup 1), 33–37. https://doi.org/10.1179/cim.2009.10.supplement-1.33

Malerbi, A. F. S., Goffi-Gomez, M. V. S., Tsuji, R. K., Gomes, M. Q. T., Brito Neto, R., & Bento, R. F. (2018). Auditory brainstem implant in postmeningitis totally ossified cochleae. *Acta Oto-Laryngologica, 138*(8), 722–726.

Marangos, N., Sollmann, W.-P., Ramsden, R. T., & Laszig, R. (1999). Central electrical stimulation of the auditory pathway in neurofibromatosis type 2. *Ear, Nose and Throat Journal, 78*(2), 110–117.

Marangos, N., Stecker, M., Sollmann, W.-P., & Laszig, R. (2000). Stimulation of the cochlear nucleus with multichannel auditory brainstem implants and long-term results: Freiburg patients. *The Journal of Laryngology and Otology, 114*(S27), 27–31.

Mastoid, S., Goudy, S. L., & Brown, S. (2016). Impact of cerebellar retraction on neurological outcomes in auditory brainstem implantation using the retrosigmoid approach. *Otology & Neurotology, 37*(5), 578–585.

Matthies, C., Brill, S., Kaga, K., et al. (2013). Auditory brainstem implantation improves speech recognition in neurofibromatosis type II patients. *ORL: Journal for Otorhinolaryngology and Its Related Specialties, 75*(5), 282–295.

Moffat, D. A., & McHugh, J. (2014). Management of cerebrovascular complications in auditory brainstem implantation. *Journal of Neurosurgery, 120*(2), 250–258.

Monsanto, R. C., Bittencourt, A. G., Neto, N. J. B., Beilke, S. C. A. S. B., Salomone, R., & Lorenzetti, F. T. M. (2014). Indications, results, and new frontiers of auditory brainstem implants in children. *Otolaryngology - Head and Neck Surgery (United States), 151*(1 SUPPL. 1), P210.

Monsell, E. M., McElveen, J. T., Jr., Hitselberger, W. E., & House, W. F. (1987). Surgical approaches to the human cochlear nucleus complex. *American Journal of Otology, 8*(5), 450–455.

Narayan, N. (2013). Management of Auditory Brainstem Implant Recipients. In *The cochlear implant—An overview* (Vol. 13, pp. 113–119). ISHA Monograph.

Natarajan, K., et al. (2021). Vestibular dysfunction after cochlear and auditory brainstem implantation: Madras ENT Research Foundation experience. *International Journal of Otorhinolaryngology and Head and Neck Surgery, 7*(3), 513–519. http://www.ijorl.com

Nevison, B., Laszig, R., Sollmann, W.-P., Lenarz, T., Sterkers, O., Ramsden, R., Fraysse, B., Manrique, M., Rask-Andersen, H., Garcia-Ibanez, E., Colletti, V., & von Wallenberg, E. (2002). Results from a European clinical investigation of the nucleus(R) multichannel auditory brainstem implant. *Ear and Hearing, 23*(3), 170–183.

Noij, K. S., Kozin, E. D., Sethi, R., Shah, P. V., Kaplan, A. B., Remenschneider, A., Lee, D. J., & Herrmann, B. (2015). Systematic review of nontumor pediatric auditory brainstem implant outcomes. *Otolaryngology-Head and Neck Surgery, 153*(5), 739–750.

Otto, S. R., Brackmann, D. E., Hitselberger, W. E., Shannon, R. V., & Kuchta, J. (2002). Multichannel auditory brainstem implant: Update on performance in 61 patients. *Journal of Neurosurgery, 96*(6), 1063–1071.

Peng, K. A., Otto, S. R., Brackmann, D. E., Wilkinson, E. P., & Lorenz, M. B. (2018). Cochlear implantation and auditory brainstem implantation in neurofibromatosis type 2. *Laryngoscope, 128*(9), 2163–2169.

Polak, M., Colletti, L., & Colletti, V. (2018). Novel method of fitting of children with auditory brainstem implants. *European Annals of Otorhinolaryngology, Head and Neck Diseases, 135*(6), 403–409.

Puram, S. V., & Lee, D. J. (2015). Pediatric auditory brainstem implant surgery. *Otolaryngologic Clinics of North America, 48*(6), 1117–1148.

Raghunandhan, S., & Kameswaran, M. (2010). Auditory brainstem implants. *Otorhinolaryngology Clinics: An International Journal, 2*(2), 151–155.

Raghunandhan, S., Madhav, K., Senthilvadivu, A., Natarajan, K., & Kameswaran, M. (2019). Paediatric auditory brainstem implantation: The South Asian experience. *European Annals of Otorhinolaryngology, Head and Neck Diseases, 136*(3), S9–S14.

Rajeswaran, R., & Kameswaran, M. (2020). Auditory brainstem implantation (ABI) in children without neurofibromatosis type II (NF2): Communication performance and safety after 24 months of use. *Cochlear Implants International, 21*(3), 127–135.

Ramsden, R. T., Freeman, S. R. M., Lloyd, S. K. W., et al. (2016). Auditory brainstem implantation in neurofibromatosis type 2: Experience from the Manchester programme. *Otology & Neurotology, 37*(9), 1267–1274.

Rutherford, S. A., Hammerbeck-Ward, C. L., Freeman, S. R., Lloyd, S. K., Henderson, L., & O'Driscoll, M. P. (2019). Hearing outcomes with auditory brainstem implantation in children with aplastic and hypoplastic cochlear nerves. *British Journal of Neurosurgery, 33*(4), 472.

Sanna, M., & Mancini, F. (2010). Cerebrospinal fluid leaks following auditory brainstem implantation surgery. *Laryngoscope Investigative Otolaryngology, 120*(5), 1145–1150.

Sanna, M., Di Lella, F., Guida, M., & Merkus, P. (2012). (2012). Auditory brainstem implants in NF2 patients: Results and review of the literature. *Otology & Neurotology, 33*(2), 154–164. https://doi.org/10.1097/MAO.0b013e318241bc71
Schwartz, M. S., Otto, S. R., Shannon, R. V., Hitselberger, W. E., & Brackmann, D. E. (2008). Auditory brainstem implants. *Neurotherapeutics, 5*(1), 128–136.
Sennaroglu, L., Colletti, V., Manrique, M., Laszig, R., Offeciers, E., Saeed, S., Ramsden, R., Sarac, S., Freeman, S., Andersen, H. R., Zarowski, A., Ziyal, I., Sollmann, W. P., Kaminsky, J., Bejarano, B., Atas, A., Sennaroglu, G., Yucel, E., Sevinc, S., Colletti, L., et al. (2011). Auditory brainstem implantation in children and non-neurofibromatosis type 2 patients: A consensus statement. *Otology and Neurotology, 32*(2), 187–191.
Sennaroglu, L., Sennaroglu, G., Yucel, E., Bilginer, B., Atay, G., Bajin, M. D., Mocan, B. O., Yaral, M., Aslan, F., Cnar, B. C., Ozkan, B., Batuk, M. O., Kirazl, C. E., Karakaya, J., Atas, A., Sarac, S., & Ziyal, I. (2016). Long-term results of ABI in children with severe inner ear malformations. *Otology and Neurotology, 37*(7), 865–872.
Shah, P. V., Kozin, E. D., Kaplan, A. B., & Lee, D. J. (2016). Pediatric auditory brainstem implant surgery: A new option for auditory habilitation in congenital deafness? *Journal of the American Board of Family Medicine, 29*(2), 286–288.
Teagle, H. F. B., Henderson, L., He, S., Ewend, M. G., & Buchman, C. A. (2018). Pediatric auditory brainstem implantation: Surgical, electrophysiologic, and behavioral outcomes. *Ear and Hearing, 39*(2), 326–336.
Van Bemmel, A. J., van de Velde, C. J., Schmitz, R. F., & Liefers, G. J. (2011). Prevention of seroma formation after axillary dissection in breast cancer: A systematic review. *European Journal of Surgical Oncology, 37*(10), 829–835.
Wilkinson, E. P., Schwartz, M. S., Otto, S. R., & Brackmann, D. E. (2014). Surgery for auditory brainstem implantation. *Operative Techniques in Otolaryngology - Head and Neck Surgery, 25*(4), 327–332.

Chapter 25
Auditory Midbrain Implants

Anindya Nayak, Preetam Chappity, Anurita Swarup, and Sanjay Kumar Behera

Abstract An Auditory midbrain implant (AMI) is an attempt to improve speech outcomes in individuals unsuitable for a CI by implanting a neural prosthetic device in the midbrain. Cochlear implants have revolutionized the management of deafness. In the subset of patients who do not benefit from Cochlear implants due to a lack of robust neural connection between the cochlea and the brain, Auditory brainstem implants have been used with variable outcomes. This chapter focuses on various aspects of AMI, a possible alternative to auditory brainstem implants.

Keywords Auditory midbrain implant · Inferior colliculus · Neurofibromatosis type 2 · NF2 · Midbrain

Introduction

The ability of any living being to hear is vital for survival. Language and speech development is what makes the human superior to other life creatures. Therefore, any impairment in hearing is potentially debilitating and needs rehabilitation. Hearing loss can be divided in various ways. One of them is based on which part of the auditory pathway is involved, i.e., the conductive pathway, the sensoryneural pathway or a combination of both. These can be managed in multiple ways. Auditory implants constitute one such intervention.

An implant is a medical device that replaces, supports or enhances the functioning of a damaged biological structure, or assumes the role of a missing biological structure. The invention with cochlear implant as a neuroprosthetic device

A. Nayak
Department of ENT, Medanta Medicity Hospital, Gurugram, Haryana, India

P. Chappity (✉)
Department of ENT, Launceston General Hospital, Launceston, Australia

A. Swarup · S. K. Behera
Department of ENT, All India Institute of Medical Sciences (AIIMS), Bhubaneswar, India

P. Kumar et al. (eds.), *Advances in Implantation Otology*,
https://doi.org/10.1007/978-981-96-8671-1_25

revolutionized the management of people with severe to profound hearing loss. Over the years, the implant and the surgeries have developed to such an extent that recipients are able to lead near-normal lives with good speech comprehension, auditory awareness, and discrimination.

Despite the huge progress made in the cochlear implant technology, the fact remains that the implant benefits only those who have an intact auditory nerve. A significant challenge in improving cochlear implant performance seems to be restricted by the number of independent information channels the implant can provide. Central auditory implants have been developed as an alternative to overcome these limitations.

Rationale

The first device to be implanted at a structure in the central auditory nervous system was the Auditory Brainstem Implant (ABI), which was implanted in 1979 at the House Ear Institute in Los Angeles, California, by William Hitselberger and William House. This device, which featured two ball electrodes supported by a fabric backing, was developed in collaboration with Douglass McCreery from the Huntington Medical Research Institutes in Pasadena, California. The ABI was placed on the surface of the cochlear nucleus (Schwartz et al., 2008). The device was developed for patients with neurofibromatosis type 2 (NF2), associated with bilateral acoustic neuromas. Severe damage to the auditory nerves during the tumor resection surgery left these patients deaf and unable to benefit from cochlear implants (CIs). However, since the cochlear nucleus was already accessed during tumor removal, placing electrodes on its surface involved minimal additional surgical risk. Inspite of the early promise, the response obtained from ABIs was found to be highly variable with unpredictable audiometric outcomes (Colletti et al., 2014; Behr et al., 2014). While some patients reported good closed-set speech perception, majority had problems in sound awareness. The precise reason for such variable outcomes is not well understood. Surgical trauma to the nerve or the centres involved in speech processing during the tumor resection was thought to be a major contributing factor (Colletti et al., 2014; Behr et al., 2014).

The Auditory midbrain implant (AMI) was thus developed as a possible solution to overcome this problem. Stimulation of the central auditory nucleus, which is quite distant from the surgical site is the key concept of AMI. The midbrain presents with an easier and better surgical accessibility than does the cochlear nucleus located in the lateral recess (Lim et al., 2009). The AMI targets the inferior colliculus, particularly its central nucleus. The central nucleus of inferior colliculus (ICC) exhibits a well-defined tonotopic organization, making it a highly suitable structure for stimulation using an auditory neuroprosthesis. As the primary convergence center of the central auditory system, the ICC receives both monaural and binaural inputs from various brainstem nuclei, with these projections thought to remain partially segregated up to and within the ICC. Stimulating different regions of the midbrain is expected to produce distinct directional percepts. Notably, the stimulation of ICC offers lower thresholds, wider dynamic range, and highly localized, more frequency-specific cortical activation than even the stimulation through a cochlear implant (CI).

Surgical Technique

The primary motivation for the first AMI clinical trial was to offer an alternative hearing solution to the ABI for NF2 patients. Research and development of AMI began around the year 2000. A fruitful association between Thomas Lenarz from the Hannover Medical School, Minoo Lenarz (currently at the University of Berlin-Charité) and James Patrick's team from Cochlear Limited, who worked on the creation of an electrode array for human use, eventually culminated in to the development of AMI (Lim et al., 2009). The AMI electrode array features a single shank linearly spaced electrodes, designed to align with the tonotopic arrangement within the central nucleus of Inferior Coliculus. The AMI array is 6.4 mm in length and has a diameter of 0.4 mm. The array includes 20 equispaced platinum ring electrodes to stimulate different frequency layers of the ICC (Fig. 25.1). A Dacron mesh is used to anchor the electrode array onto the neural structures. A receiver-stimulator bed, which is made in the temporoparietal skull region near the craniotomy site, houses the receiver-stimulator (Lim et al., 2009). The external components of the device have resemblance to cochlear implants and intraoperative/postoperative verification of accurate placement of the electrode array on ICC using latency responses remains important. The monitoring of other cranial nerves is also paramount. The first clinical trial, conducted between 2006 and 2008, was done on five adult NF2 patients who were implanted with the AMI device. The animal studies conducted before the human trial had demonstrated that the stimulation of ICC using the AMI

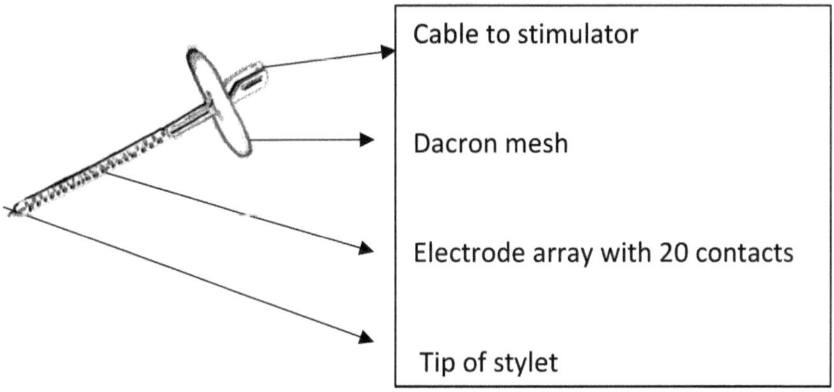

Fig. 25.1 Human prototype AMI electrode array (COCHLEAR LTD.): a diagrammatic representation

electrode array yielded frequency-specific auditory activation with low-thresholds, that, on occasions superseded the ones produced by the cochlear implant stimulation (Lenarz et al., 2006). Since the trials were initially done on the NF2 patients, the surgical approach for electrode implantation had accommodated additional ways to ensure the safe removal of vestibular schwannomas within the same surgical session. Additionally, the approach needed to facilitate the correct angle for implanting the AMI array along the tonotopic gradient of the ICC. The lateral suboccipital approach, a well-established technique for the safe removal of large vestibular schwannomas, that also facilitates hearing preservation, could allow for both these procedures to be performed with relative ease, and was therefore deemed the most suitable (Samii et al., 2007). It can be easily extended to a lateral supra-cerebellar infratentorial approach, which provides surgical access to the inferior colliculus and allows for the insertion of the AMI electrode array along the tonotopic gradient of the ICC. Reconstructed images of the prototype AMI used in human trials, the landmarks created for the suboccipital approach on the skull, and the route taken to expose the ICC are shown in Figs. 25.1, 25.2, and 25.3, respectively.

In brief, the array implantation procedure is performed with the patient in a semi-sitting position. The tumor removal at the brainstem level is accomplished using a modified lateral suboccipital approach, which requires the cerebellum to be retracted medially to reveal the tumor. Once the tumor is excised, the cerebellum naturally descends due to gravity, the same craniotomy window allows direct visualization of the surface inferior colliculus (Samii et al., 2007). During the first clinical trial, the authors reported that the primary difficulty emanated out of the small size of the craniotomy, which obscured the key anatomical landmarks defining the outer

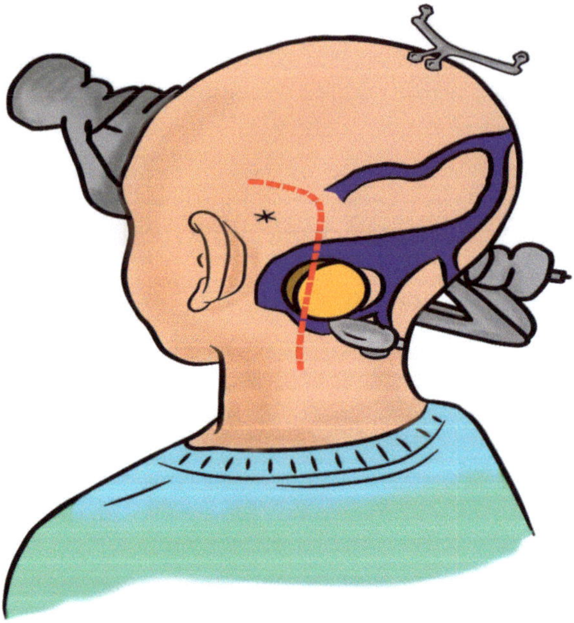

Fig. 25.2 The skin incision (red dotted line), approximate location for receiver-stimulator (star) and the location of the lateral craniotomy exposing the transverse and sigmoid sinus

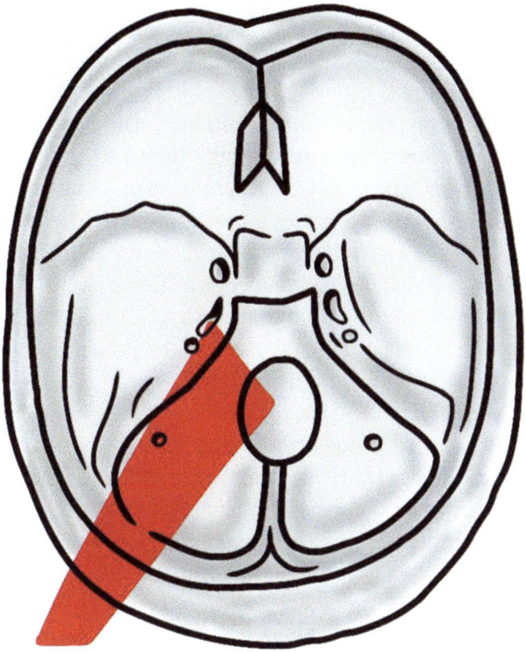

Fig. 25.3 Diagram depicting the exposure route via the ipsilateral cerebellopontine angle and dorsolateral aspect of the mesencephalon

boundaries of the IC. This made the task of accurate positioning of the array in relation to the surface of IC more challenging during its insertion (Lim & Lenarz, 2015). These landmarks obscured from the direct vision were the rostral edge of the IC, which comes in contact with the superior colliculus, the midline between the ICs from the two sides, and caudal border of IC near the exit point of the trochlear nerve.

Outcomes

In the above discussed first clinical trial, five patients of Neurofibromatosis 2 were implanted with an AMI during the same surgical session in which the tumour was removed. The most encouraging aspect of this trial was the safety outcome, with no post-surgical complications reported in any of the five patients (Lim & Lenarz, 2015). Although the results were encouraging, the responses were highly variable with even the best performer failing to achieve open set speech perception in the absence of lip-reading cues (Lenarz et al., 2006). However, the use of AMI resulted in perceivable betterment of their lip-reading abilities and auditory awareness of environmental sounds, with small improvements speech perception. The performance of these patients were within the same bracket as achieved by a majority of NF2 patients after undergoing auditory brainstem implantation (Lim et al., 2009; Schwartz et al., 2008; Sennaroglu & Ziyal, 2012), despite achieving accurate surgical placement of the electrode array along the tonotopic gradient of ICC in only one of five patients in this trial. This patient had the best outcomes of the five who were implanted. He also had a clear distinction in pitch perception across the electrode sites (Lim et al., 2009; Lim et al., 2013). In the remaining four patients, the AMI array, the obscuring of clear vision of the structures led to an inadvertent location in the adjoining regions, such as the lateral lemniscus, brachium of IC, dorsal IC and rostral IC. The researchers concluded that while stimulation of the auditory midbrain provides a broad range of level, spectral, and temporal cues, each important for understanding of speech, these cues probably do not fuse sufficiently to assist open-set speech perception (Lenarz et al., 2006). Additionally, suppression effects in the neurons due to the use of a single shank could have contributed to the limited outcomes, probably even in the patient in whom the AMI array was placed along the tonotopic gradient (Dyballa et al., 2022). Nonetheless, it cannot be refuted that wrongly located electrodes may have contributed to less than expected outcomes from previous animal and human experiments (De Martino et al., 2013; Geniec & *Morest*, 1971; Malmierca et al., 2008; Ress & Chandrasekaran, 2013; Schreiner & *Langner*, 1997). The researchers believed that with more opportunities to conduct these surgeries exposure, they would become better at a more precise identification of the caudal edge of the IC and the structures around the midline. Surface stimulation of the IC could then help pinpoint the start of the brachium of the IC and surface locations that correspond to the correct trajectories into specific regions of the ICC. This approach is expected to enhance the overall accuracy of the AMI (Lenarz et al., 2006).

Second Clinical Trial

The primary surgical limitation in the first clinical trial arose due to a small craniotomy, which obscured several key anatomical landmarks surrounding the ICC, making it difficult to accurately identify them. In order to overcome this challenge in the second clinical trial, the surgical approach was revised on the basis of the studies conducted on cadavers (Lim & Lenarz, 2015). The revised approach still employed a modified version of the lateral suboccipital exposure; however, the skull opening had added extension towards the midline. The expanded exposure not only provided an easier access to the lateral recess for the tumour removal but also enabled a rather panoramic view to the midline structures, thereby allowing easier identification of the key landmarks not identifiable clearly during the first clinical trial. For patients not requiring tumour excision, a more traditional paramedian approach is recommended, which will minimize the extent of the skull opening. After opening the dura along the sinuses and retracting the cerebellum downward, the IC can be visualized after gently displacing the arachnoid covering and blood vessels. The structures in sight are then confirmed using CT-MRI guided brain navigation. The direct view of the midline of the brain helps determine the sagittal plane angle for precise positioning of the AMI electrode array into the IC. These new steps are expected to enhance the accuracy of electrode placement along the tonotopic gradient of the ICC compared to the first clinical trial (Lim & Lenarz, 2015).

A new AMI device, consisting of two penetrating arrays (called shanks) with 11 electrode contacts on each, has been developed to overcome the limitation imposed by the use of single shank that probably led to suppression effects in the neurons. The change from a single shank design of the previous version AMI array to the two-shank design in the new AMI array was based on the studies in animal models which demonstrated reduction of the suppression effects when the stimulation within the same frequency layer in the ICC was alternated in two electrode arrays parallelly (Dyballa et al., 2022). A second clinical trial using this new AMI device, which was funded by the National Institutes of Health, ran from 2017 to 2019. This trial was conducted at Hannover Medical School in collaboration with Cochlear Limited and the University of Minnesota, and involved implanting the new two-shank AMI device in five adult NF2 patients who could not sufficiently benefit from a CI or ABI. The initial results on pitch perception and speech perception were encouraging, and so were the measurements of the suppression effects. A clearly evidenced difference in the new device compared to its predecessor is the perception of stable loudness even when using as short a pulse interval as 17.5 μs. This suggests that the two-shank device is assured of providing stable auditory perceptions.

AMI is a new kid on the block. It has come into vogue as a viable alternative to stimulate the central auditory system in cases where CI and ABI are unusable. Although the device is still in its nascence, the preliminary outcomes, including the safety concerns, seem to be encouraging. The results of the second trial, if found positive in the long run, could go a long way in explaining the pathways involved in central auditory processing and the functional auditory cortex.

References

Behr, R., Colletti, V., Matthies, C., Morita, A., Nakatomi, H., Dominique, L., Darrouzet, V., Brill, S., Shehata-Dieler, W., Lorens, A., & Skarzynski, H. (2014). New outcomes with auditory brainstem implants in NF2 patients. *Otology and Neurotology, 35*(10), 1844–1851.

Colletti, L., Shannon, R. V., & Colletti, V. (2014). The development of auditory perception in children after auditory brainstem implantation. *Audiology & Neuro-Otology, 19*(6), 386–394.

De Martino, F., Moerel, M., van de Moortele, P. F., Ugurbil, K., Goebel, R., Yacoub, E., & Formisano, E. (2013). Spatial organization of frequency preference and selectivity in the human inferior colliculus. *Nature Communications, 4*, 1386.

Dyballa, K. H., Nogueira, W., Samii, A., Salcher, R., Timm, M., McKay, C., Lim, H., & Lenarz, T. (2022). Clinical test results on patients with a novel electrical hearing prosthesis: The two-shank Auditory Midbrain Implant (AMI). *Laryngo-Rhino-Otologie, 101*(S 02), S243–S244.

Geniec, P., & Morest, D. K. (1971). The neuronal architecture of the human posterior colliculus. A study with the Golgi method. *Acta Oto-Laryngologica. Supplementum, 295*, 1–33.

Lenarz, T., Lim, H. H., Reuter, G., Patrick, J. F., & Lenarz, M. (2006). The auditory midbrain implant: A new auditory prosthesis for neural deafness-concept and device description. *Otology and Neurotology, 27*(6), 838–843.

Lim, H. H., Lenarz, M., Joseph, G., & Lenarz, T. (2013). Frequency representation within the human brain: Stability versus plasticity. *Scientific Reports, 1474*.

Lim, H. H., & Lenarz, T. (2015). Auditory midbrain implant: Research and development towards a second clinical trial. *Hearing Research, 322*, 212–223.

Lim, H. H., Lenarz, M., & Lenarz, T. (2009). Auditory midbrain implant: A review. *Trends in Amplification, 13*(3), 149–180.

Malmierca, M. S., Izquierdo, M. A., Cristaudo, S., Hernandez, O., Perez-Gonzalez, D., Covey, E., & Oliver, D. L. (2008). A discontinuous tonotopic organization in the inferior colliculus of the rat. *The Journal of Neuroscience, 28*, 4767–4776.

Ress, D., & Chandrasekaran, B. (2013). Tonotopic organization in the depth of human inferior colliculus. *Frontiers in Human Neuroscience, 7*, 586.

Samii, A., Lenarz, M., Majdani, O., Lim, H. H., Samii, M., & Lenarz, T. (2007). Auditory midbrain implant: A combined approach for vestibular schwannoma surgery and device implantation. *Otology and Neurotology, 28*(1), 31–38.

Schreiner, C. E., & Langner, G. (1997). Laminar fine structure of frequency organization in auditory midbrain. *Nature, 388*, 383–386.

Schwartz, M. S., Otto, S. R., Shannon, R. V., Hitselberger, W. E., & Brackmann, D. E. (2008). Auditory brainstem implants. *Neurotherapeutics: the journal of the American Society for Experimental Neuro Therapeutics, 5*(1), 128–136.

Sennaroglu, L., & Ziyal, I. (2012). Auditory brainstem implantation. *Auris, Nasus, Larynx, 39*, 439–450.

Chapter 26
Vestibular Implants: The Present Status and Future Prospects

Mustafa Karabulut, Alexander van Soest, Joost J. A. Stultiens, Nils Guinand, Angélica Perez Fornos, Raymond van de Berg, and Elke M. J. Devocht

Abstract Vestibular implant (VI) is a device designed to restore peripheral vestibular function in patients with bilateral vestibulopathy. It comprises three key components: gyroscopes and/or accelerometers, an external processor, and an implanted stimulator. The VI compensates for bilateral vestibular loss, by electrically stimulating the vestibular system. Candidates for implantation typically experience disabling chronic symptoms such as unsteadiness and oscillopsia. Multiple research groups demonstrated the feasibility of the vestibular implant in humans. It was shown that a VI is able to partially restore the vestibulo-ocular reflex, otolith responses, and improve quality of life.

Keywords Vestibular implant · Bilateral vestibulopathy · Vestibular system · Utricle · Saccule

Introduction

Bilateral vestibulopathy (BVP) is a heterogeneous condition that frequently results from bilaterally decreased peripheral vestibular function (Hain et al., 2013; Lucieer et al., 2016). BVP may be diagnosed using criteria determined by the Bárány Society (Strupp et al., 2017), which include a combination of vestibular symptoms and vestibular test results. The most reported symptoms in BVP patients are chronic unsteadiness and oscillopsia (Guinand et al., 2012a; Lucieer et al., 2018). However,

M. Karabulut (✉) · A. van Soest · J. J. A. Stultiens · R. van de Berg · E. M. J. Devocht
Division of Balance Disorders, Department of Otorhinolaryngology and Head and Neck Surgery, School for Mental Health and Neuroscience, Maastricht University Medical Center, Maastricht, The Netherlands
e-mail: mustafa.karabulut@mumc.nl

N. Guinand · A. Perez Fornos
Service of Otorhinolaryngology and Head and Neck Surgery, Department of Clinical Neurosciences, Geneva University Hospitals, Geneva, Switzerland

P. Kumar et al. (eds.), *Advances in Implantation Otology*,
https://doi.org/10.1007/978-981-96-8671-1_26

the vestibular system also contributes to various other activities such as spatial orientation and motion perception (Smith & Darlington, 2013; Smith & Zheng, 2013). Besides these physical symptoms, BVP patients also report that their vestibular loss has a negative impact on their cognitive and social functioning (Lucieer et al., 2020). Consequently, BVP can decrease quality of life and have adverse socioeconomic effects (Guinand et al., 2012a; Sun et al., 2014). The current documented prevalence of BVP ranges between 28 and 81 in 100,000 adults, but this might be an underestimation (Van De Berg et al., 2015b; Ward et al., 2013). It can present with various clinical pictures, and is therefore often misdiagnosed (Miffon & Guyot, 2015; Van De Berg et al., 2015b).

BVP can have many different etiologies such as meningitis, hereditary conditions, autoimmune disorders, neurodegenerative diseases, or ototoxicity (e.g., aminoglycosides) (Lee et al., 2020; Miffon & Guyot, 2015; Requena et al., 2014). Finding the true cause for BVP can be challenging. A definite or probable etiology may only be established in 49–80% of the cases. In other cases, the etiology remains idiopathic (Rinne et al., 1998; Zingler et al., 2009). Unfortunately, currently there is no adequate treatment for restoring vestibular function. Treatment of BVP is mainly focused on rehabilitation strategies, generally using physiotherapy (Porciuncula et al., 2012). However, despite intensive balance training and vestibular exercises, they often have a low yield, and BVP cannot be treated adequately in most cases (Porciuncula et al., 2012). In the 1960s, it was demonstrated by Cohen and Suzuki that compensatory eye movements and postural responses could be elicited by selective electrical stimulation of the ampullary branches of the vestibular nerve in monkeys and cats (Cohen & Suzuki, 1963; Cohen et al., 1965). Ever since the first signs of success by Gong and Merfeld (2000), research has shown that rotational cues can be transmitted to the central nervous system by electrical stimulation of the vestibular nerves (Dai et al., 2011a; Lewis et al., 2013; Migliaccio et al., 2011; Phillips et al., 2016; Thompson et al., 2012).

Based on the results obtained in animal studies and the growing success of cochlear implants (CIs), the concept of a vestibular implant (VI) arose. The aim of the VI, similar to a CI, is to bypass the dysfunctional sensory end-organ by directly stimulating its sensory nerves. This neuroprosthesis was developed and implanted during several clinical trials since 2007 (Guyot et al., 2011b). In this chapter, the general aspects of the VI will be discussed.

The Vestibular System

The inner ear, located in the temporal bone, consists of the vestibular organ and the cochlea. The vestibular organ contains five sensory structures, which are able to sense head accelerations and gravity. Three semicircular canals (SCCs, i.e., the lateral, superior and posterior) capture rotational accelerations around three orthogonal axes. Two otolith organs (i.e., the utricle and saccule) mainly sense linear accelerations and gravity. By regulating the firing rate of the vestibular nerves, these five sensory structures supply head motion information to the central nervous system, leading to several reflexes and self-motion perception (Bogle & Burkard, 2020).

The vestibular nerves can be divided into regular-firing nerve fibres and irregular-firing nerve fibres which have different characteristics. Irregular-firing nerve fibres, when compared to regular-firing nerve fibres, are more sensitive to natural stimulation of the end organs and to electrical stimulation of the efferent system (Goldberg et al., 1984). The regular-firing nerve fibres have a resting discharge firing rate (baseline firing rate) of about 90 action potentials per second (pps). Head movements can change this firing rate. For example, a yaw rotation to the left leads to an increase in the firing rate of the nerve fibres in the lateral SCC (excitatory response). Depending on the velocity, the firing rate can go up to around 400 pps (Faan et al., 2010). In contrast, a yaw rotation to the right leads to a decrease in the firing rate of these nerve fibres (inhibitory response). Depending on the velocity, the firing rate can become as low as 0 pps (Brontë-Stewart & Lisberger, 1994). The lateral SCC on the contralateral side shows an inverse response to the same movements. The two vestibular organs work in unison to provide information about head movements to the brain (push-pull system).

The motion-controlled modulation of the firing rate provides necessary information for several processes. The vestibulo-ocular reflex (VOR) generates compensatory eye movements upon head movements, providing gaze stabilization in dynamic situations, such as during walking and running. The vestibulospinal reflex (VSR) and vestibulocollic reflex (VCR) generate rapid compensatory body and neck movements to enable postural control and balance (Kingma & Van de Berg, 2016). Additionally, the vestibular system contributes to self-motion perception and spatial navigation. These processes require a complex integration of inputs not only from the vestibular system but also from the visual and somatosensory system (Dupuits et al., 2019; Merfeld et al., 1999). Finally, the multiple vestibular projections are known to influence emotions, memory and cognition (Fuller et al., 2004; Smith & Zheng, 2013). Refer to Chap. 3 for more details about the anatomy and physiology of the vestibular system.

General Aspects of the Vestibular Implant

The aim of the VI is to restore vestibular function by detecting head motion information and processing this into electrical signals that stimulate the vestibular nerves. By directly stimulating these nerves, it bypasses the vestibular end-organs and is able to restore vestibular function in BVP patients (Parkes et al., 2017). Although different designs exist, the VI generally consists of four key components:

1. Gyroscopes and/or accelerometers, which sense head motion.
2. An external motion processor that converts head motion signals into electrical signals for stimulation.

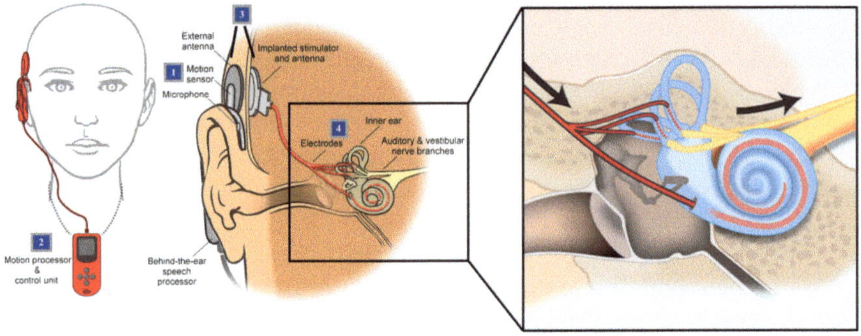

Fig. 26.1 Vestibulocochlear implant (VCI). A VCI comprises vestibular and cochlear implant parts. The VI part includes three main components: (1) Motion sensor (gyroscopes) senses head motion; (2) External motion processor converts head motion signals into electrical signals for stimulation; (3) External antenna sends electrical signals to implanted stimulator by radio frequency; (4) Electrodes implanted in the vestibular organ directly stimulate the vestibular nerves. In order to restore vestibular function and hearing function at the same time, a VI can also be combined with a cochlear implant, which is referred to as VCI. (This figure was created in collaboration with the *"Swiss Foundation For Innovation And Training In Surgery"*)

3. An external antenna, which transmits electrical signals to implanted stimulator by radio frequency.
4. Electrodes implanted in the vestibular organ, which directly stimulate the vestibular nerves (see Fig. 26.1).

The implanted stimulator generally consists of electrodes inserted into the SSC or otolith organs, or a combination of both. The electrical signals modulate the firing rate and/or amplitude of the vestibular nerve fibres. This information is perceived as a head movement by the central nervous system. Through this process, the vestibular function can be artificially restored (Guinand et al., 2015). In order to restore vestibular function and hearing function at the same time, a VI can also be combined with a cochlear implant, which is then referred to as a vestibulocochlear implant (VCI) (see Fig. 26.1). Most VI prototypes have been based on modified commercially available cochlear implant types.

Fundamentals of the Vestibular Implant

In order to restore vestibular function with the VI, a baseline firing rate is created using electrical stimulation (Guyot et al., 2011b; Perez Fornos et al., 2014). This baseline firing rate can then be modulated to generate vestibular responses (Davidovics et al., 2012; Guyot et al., 2016). In the case of SCC stimulation, these responses include, among others, eye movements in both directions along each SCC plane.

Modification of the Baseline Firing Rate

Human VI research is currently limited to unilateral vestibular implantation. Unilateral stimulation leads to an asymmetry in response since the natural baseline firing rate (90 pps) is below the middle of the stimulation range (0–400 pps). This causes a stronger excitatory response compared to the inhibitory response. For this reason, baseline stimulation of a vestibular implant can artificially be set higher (supraphysiological baseline) (Gong et al., 2008; Lewis et al., 2013; Merfeld et al., 2006). Using a supraphysiological baseline, corresponding to 50% of the total dynamic range, increases the inhibitory responses but reduces the excitatory responses, leading to a more symmetrical response.

This (supraphysiological) baseline firing rate will initially be interpreted by the brain as an excitatory stimulus, resulting in nystagmus. Furthermore, symptoms of vertigo and/or nausea can occur (Guyot et al., 2011b). These undesired symptoms mainly disappear within 30 minutes of continuous baseline stimulation due to adaptation (Guyot et al., 2011b). Turning off the device after baseline adaptation can again initiate vertigo, nausea, and nystagmus, but in the opposite direction (Guinand et al., 2011; Guyot et al., 2011b). The central nervous system (CNS) is, however, able to adapt and habituate to switching between both conditions (electrical stimulation on and off) which is often referred to as *dual state adaptation* (Gong & Merfeld, 2002; Guinand et al., 2011; Guyot et al., 2011b). This implies that after several off-to-on and on-to-off transitions of electrical stimulation, the intensity of the nystagmus becomes less, and adaptation to the new baseline happens more quickly. Eventually, (almost) no significant undesired nystagmus is triggered anymore by transitions between VI conditions "on" and "off" (Guyot et al., 2011b; Lewis et al., 2010; Merfeld et al., 2006). The adaptation time gradually becomes longer if the device remains deactivated for longer periods (Guinand et al., 2011). The *dual state adaptation* would allow VI recipients to switch their device on or off without any significant side effects (for example, when changing batteries, taking a shower, or sleeping).

Motion Modulation

After adaptation to the supraphysiological baseline firing rate has been established, motion-based modulation is applied. The baseline firing rate is modulated up and down depending on the direction and velocity of the head movements. For example, when a patient (with a VI on the right side, adapted to the supraphysiological baseline) makes a yaw rotation to the right, stimulation of the right lateral ampullary nerve increases. The amount of increase depends on the velocity of the movement—a slow head movement leads to a smaller increase in stimulation than a fast head movement. A head movement in the opposite direction (to the left in this case) leads to an inverse response. The amount of increase (or decrease) of stimulation for a

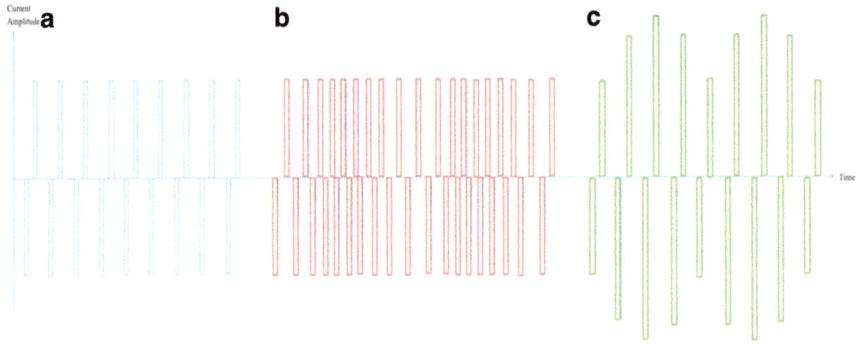

Fig. 26.2 Baseline stimulation with motion modulation. Motion modulation can consist of pulse rate modulation and/or pulse amplitude modulation: (**a**) *Unmodulated baseline*—electrical stimulation by cathodic-first, charge-balanced, biphasic, rectangular pulses; (**b**) *Pulse rate modulation*—the amplitude of the electrical stimulation remains the same, but the frequency of pulses is altered over time; (**c**) *Pulse amplitude modulation*—the frequency of the electrical stimulation remains the same, but the amplitude of pulses is altered over time

given angular velocity is called the *modulation sensitivity*, and it can artificially be set for each electrode.

Motion modulation around a supraphysiological baseline firing rate can be executed with pulse rate modulation, pulse amplitude modulation, or a combination of both (Davidovics et al., 2012; Guyot et al., 2011b; Nguyen et al., 2016) (see Fig. 26.2). Pulse rate modulation is similar to the natural neural coding of the vestibular system (Fernandez & Goldberg, 1971). However, recent studies have demonstrated that pulse amplitude modulation is more effective than pulse rate modulation in evoking eye movements (Nguyen et al., 2016; Perez Fornos et al., 2014). Animal studies have shown that co-modulation evokes significantly larger eye movement responses than amplitude or rate modulation alone (Davidovics et al., 2012; DiGiovanna et al., 2016; Nguyen et al., 2016).

Electrical Stimulation

The optimal electrical stimulation paradigm is not yet determined. The most commonly used pulse shape is the charge-balanced, biphasic, rectangular, cathodic-first current pulse (Dai et al., 2011b; Della Santina et al., 2007; Guyot et al., 2011b; Wall III et al., 2007). Stimulation parameters (current intensity, pulse rate, phase width, current range, etc.) can vary depending on the research setting (Boutabla et al., 2020).

The fitting process of VI shows similarities with the fitting of a CI. First, the dynamic range is determined by finding the lower and the upper stimulation threshold. This is done by increasing the stimulation step by step. The lowest current level where a vestibular response can be observed is considered the lower threshold. The vestibular response can be the onset of nystagmus or the perception of a vestibular sensation. As a next step, the current level is further increased until stimulation causes discomfort to the patient (upper comfortable level) or leads to stimulation of off-target nerves (upper threshold; for example, facial nerve stimulation). Lower and upper thresholds are determined for each of the electrodes separately and are patient specific. The available dynamic range, which is the range between the lower and the upper stimulation level, can vary between electrodes. It can, for example, be as wide as 550 μA or as narrow as 25 μA (Guinand et al., 2015). Electrode position, the integrity of the targeted neurons and interpatient variability of anatomy and physiology are parameters known to influence the dynamic range of stimulation (Guinand et al., 2015).

Candidacy Evaluation

In the past, research teams used different implantation criteria for their subjects (Boutros et al., 2019; Golub et al., 2014; Guinand et al., 2015). Recently, in order to facilitate better comparison between studies, research teams jointly published an opinion statement about vestibular implantation criteria. These VI implantation criteria are shown in Table 26.1, adapted from Van De Berg et al. (2020).

The VI-implantation criteria include severe loss of vestibular function based on disabling chronic symptoms (chronic imbalance and oscillopsia) together with objective signs of decreased or absent vestibular function in both ears. In contrast to the diagnostic criteria of BVP (Strupp et al., 2017), the caloric test, the rotatory chair test and the video head impulse test, all need to show abnormalities. Furthermore, not only the lateral SCC but also vertical SCCs should also show deficits. Vestibular-evoked myogenic potentials are included on indication. The main reasons for these changes to the diagnostic criteria of BVP are:

1. Vestibular implantation can cause damage to vestibular structures in the inner ear, which might be irreversible. The diagnosis should therefore be verified by more than one vestibular test.
2. Implantation is not restricted to the lateral semicircular canals but can also include the other SSCs and otolith organs. Therefore, impairment of the structures to be implanted should be demonstrated.
3. VI surgery can impair residual vestibular function (for example, by surgical plugging of the SCCs and/or inducing local trauma). VI-implantation should not damage the vestibular system more than it can restore (Feigl et al., 2009; Van De Berg et al., 2012).

In the future, based on study-related outcomes, these criteria might be revised for clinical use, and other indications for implantation might be evaluated as well (for example, unilateral vestibulopathy).

Table 26.1 Vestibular implantation criteria for research

A. Chronic Vestibular Syndrome with the following disabling symptoms	Unsteadiness when walking or standing	Movement-induced blurred vision or oscillopsia during walking or quick head/ body movements[a]	[a]Worsening of unsteadiness in darkness and/or on uneven ground			
B. Symptoms greatest during head movement						
C. Major criteria for bilaterally reduced or absent angular VOR function[b]	Bilaterally pathological lateral angular VOR gain =0.6 and at least bilaterally one vertical angular VOR gain <0.7, measured by the video-HIT or scleral-coil technique	Reduced caloric response (sum of bithermal max. peak SPV on each side =6°/sec for 30 sec water stimuli or <10°/sec for 60 sec water or air stimuli)	Reduced lateral angular VOR gain =0.1 upon sinusoidal stimulation on a rotatory chair (0.1 Hz, Vmax = 50°/ sec) and a phase lead >68° (time constant <5 sec)			
C. Obligatory for otolith implantation	Bilaterally absent cVEMP and oVEMP responses					
D. Minor criteria for bilaterally reduced or absent angular VOR function[c]	Bilaterally pathological VOR gains of at least two semicircular canals <0.7, measured by the video-HIT or scleral-coil technique	Reduced caloric response (sum of bithermal max. peak SPV on each side <10°/sec for water and air stimuli of =30 sec)	Reduced lateral angular VOR gain <0.2 upon sinusoidal stimulation on a rotatory chair (0.1 Hz, Vmax = 50°/ sec)			

(continued)

Table 26.1 (continued)

E. Symptoms are not better accounted for by another disease						
F. Additional requirements	Age 18 years and above	BVP results most likely from a peripheral origin	Vestibular function and symptoms are unlikely to significantly improve, according to the duration of symptoms and clinicians' estimations	Patent vestibular end-organ and intact vestibular nerve	Ability to use the device and follow a personalized rehabilitation program	Ability to undergo the surgery
G. No current psychological or psychiatric disorder that could significantly interfere with use or evaluation of the VI						

[a]At least one of these two symptoms should be applicable
[b]At least one item has to be met
[c]In case only one or two major criteria (C) are met, (and also criterion C' is matched in case of otolith stimulation), the remaining test(s) should comply with the following items

Surgical Approaches

Basically two surgical approaches have been used for vestibular implantation: the intralabyrinthine approach and the extralabyrinthine approach (Van De Berg et al., 2012). Both surgical approaches have been successfully carried out and have been shown to selectively stimulate the ampullary nerves.

The most commonly used approach is the intralabyrinthine approach (Fridman et al., 2010; Gong et al., 2008; Gong & Merfeld, 2002; Lewis et al., 2002; Merfeld et al., 2006; J. Rubinstein et al., 2012). In this approach, a cortical mastoidectomy is performed, the labyrinth is opened, and electrodes are inserted in the semicircular canals and/or the otoliths, as close to the sensory epithelium as possible (see Fig. 26.3). Advantages of this approach are that the surgery is less challenging for most surgeons, and middle ear structures are preserved (Feigl et al., 2009; Guyot et al., 2011a; Wall III et al., 2007). Risks and challenges include possible

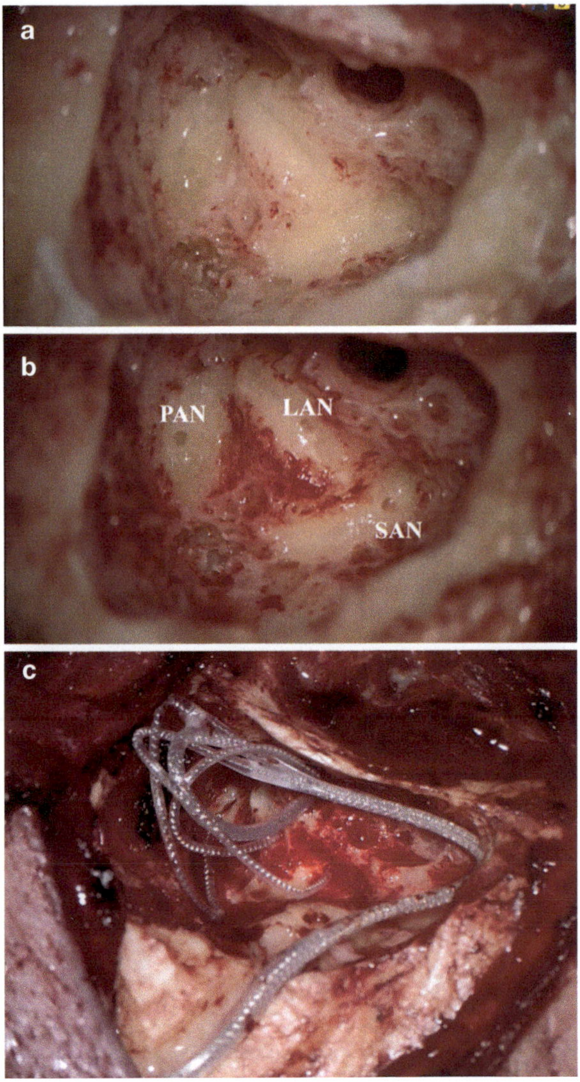

Fig. 26.3 Stepwise images during vestibular implant surgery using the intralabyrinthine approach: (**a**) Semicircular canals are blue-lined adjacent to their ampullary nerves; (**b**) Fenestrations are performed for each semicircular canal (SAN, LAN, PAN) to allow selective intralabyrinthine access; (**c**) Electrodes are inserted in the semicircular canals nearby the sensory epithelium

sensorineural hearing loss due to opening the labyrinth and inserting electrodes, and difficulty in getting the electrodes as close as possible to the sensory epithelium (Dai et al., 2011b; Fridman et al., 2010; Tang et al., 2009).

In the extralabyrinthine approach, the electrodes are directly placed on the posterior, lateral and superior ampullary nerves close to the labyrinth without opening the semicircular canals and the vestibule. This approach consists of two pathways: (1) the posterior ampullary nerve (PAN) access, and (2) the superior ampullary nerve (SAN) and lateral ampullary nerve (LAN) access. The PAN access is reached by drilling the round window niche. The PAN is identified, and an electrode is placed in contact with the nerve. The LAN and SAN pathway is created by removing the head of the malleus and the incus. By drilling superiorly from the facial nerve, the SAN and LAN can be identified, and an electrode is placed in contact with the nerves. It should be noted that the LAN and SAN cannot yet be stimulated separately since they are located very close to each other. The main advantage of this approach is the fact that the labyrinth does not need to be opened, minimizing the risk of sensorineural hearing loss. Risks and challenges of the extralabyrinthine approach include accidentally opening the labyrinth (causing a sensorineural hearing loss), facial nerve damage, inability to correctly fixate the electrodes or failure to reach the nerve canals (mainly applicable to the PAN approach) (Feigl et al., 2009).

Intraoperative Measurements

During VI surgery, intraoperative monitoring is performed to evaluate the integrity of the implant and to provide appropriate placement of the electrodes (Nguyen et al., 2017). It seems that electrode placement should be as close as possible to the sensory epithelium of the ampulla (Hedjoudje et al., 2019). Several strategies are being investigated to achieve optimal electrode position:

1. Fluoroscopy, a real-time radiation-based imaging technique, can be utilized to improve the placement of the electrodes into the SSCs. It has been previously applied in CI surgery to provide direct feedback on the location of the CI electrodes (Stultiens et al., 2020). In this way, electrodes are visualized within the SCCs in real-time, enabling more precise placement of the electrodes in the SCCs (Fishman et al., 2003) (see Fig. 26.4).
2. Eye movement responses as a result of direct electrical stimulation can be observed during surgery. By manipulating the electrode position until the favorable eye movements (correct magnitude and angle) are obtained, the best electrode position can be determined. However, general anaesthesia is known to alter and suppress the nystagmic response. Surgery under local anaesthesia may improve this procedure so that it can be used to indicate optimal placement.

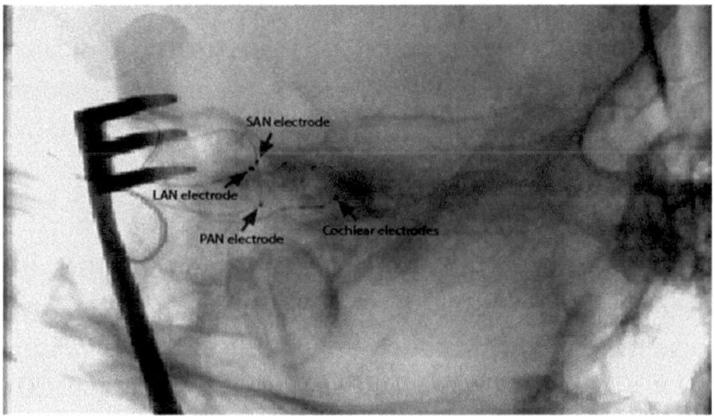

Fig. 26.4 Fluoroscopy. A real-time radiation-based imaging technique. Black dots represent electrode contacts in each semicircular canal as well as the cochlear array. **Abbreviations:** SAN, Superior Ampullary Nerve; LAN, Lateral Ampullary Nerve; PAN, Posterior Ampullary Nerve

3. The synchronous response of the vestibular nerve fibres (Phillips et al., 2015a, b) can be used to characterize the direct effect of vestibular electrical stimulation at a certain electrode position. This neural potential is referred to as the vestibular electrically evoked compound action potential (veCAP), in analogy with the auditory eCAP in CIs. These measures can be performed intraoperatively as well as postoperatively (fitting information and follow-up tool). Anaesthetics may have less impact compared to eye movement responses, but current spread between electrodes can hamper interpretation of the results.

Until now, no strategy has been proven to be infallible. Further research is currently being conducted to optimize these strategies as well as to possibly find alternatives.

Outcomes with Vestibular Implant

In the 1960s, it was demonstrated that a nystagmic response could be generated in monkeys by electrical stimulation of the vestibular nerves. Since the beginning of this century, many feasibility studies on animals have demonstrated the effectiveness of chronic electrical stimulation (Dai et al., 2013; Davidovics et al., 2012, 2013) and how different stimulation parameters can be optimized (Lewis et al., 2010; Mitchell et al., 2016). After obtaining promising results from animal studies, studies on humans were initiated. Results obtained in individuals fitted with a vestibular implant prototype are discussed below.

(a) **Vestibular Reflexes**

The VOR, VCR and VSR have all been used to evaluate the effect of VI stimulation. Regarding the VOR, it was found that it is possible to partially restore the low and high-frequency VOR with a VI in patients with BVP (Guinand et al., 2017; Perez Fornos et al., 2014) (see Fig. 26.5). The electrically-evoked VOR increases with increasing stimulation, it shows a natural frequency-dependency (Van De Berg et al., 2015a), and the eye movements can be aligned with the plane of the stimulated canal, although misalignment can occur (Boutros et al., 2019).

As for VSR and VCR, it was demonstrated that it is possible to generate controlled postural responses with a VI in patients with BVP (Fornos et al., 2019; Phillips et al., 2013). In general, these results indicate that electrical stimulation of the vestibular end-organ in humans enables both compensatory eye movements and compensatory body and neck movements, potentially restoring gaze stabilization and postural control, respectively.

(b) **Functional Improvements**

One of the main symptoms of BVP is oscillopsia, the loss of visual acuity during head movements (Lucieer et al., 2020). Visual acuity in dynamic conditions (like head movements), referred to as *dynamic visual acuity* (DVA), can be compared to the visual acuity in static conditions (Guinand et al., 2012b). Measuring DVA allows

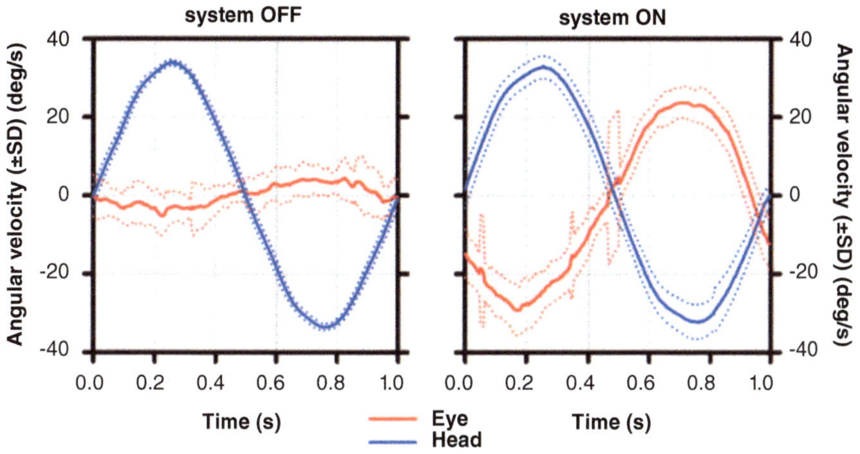

Fig. 26.5 Vestibulo-ocular reflex restoration with vestibular implant. Vestibular ocular reflex gain is almost absent (eye velocity (in grey) around zero) with the vestibular implant turned OFF (left panel) while it normalizes (eye velocity (grey) mirroring head velocity (black)) when the vestibular implant is turned ON (right panel). (Obtained from (Perez Fornos et al., 2014))

the above-mentioned improvement in VOR gain to be evaluated on a more functional level. It was found that VI stimulation significantly improved dynamic visual acuity when walking and during fast-passive head movements (Guinand et al., 2016; Starkov et al., 2020; Versino et al., 2014).

Alongside oscillopsia, imbalance is also an often-reported symptom of BVP (Lucieer et al., 2020). Therefore, posture and gait have been examined to investigate whether the electrically-evoked VSR and VCR can result in functional benefits for the patient. Outcome measures for posture (Bruininks-Oseretsky Test of Motor proficiency) and gait (Dynamic Gait Index) in long-term users of a VI prototype indicated improvement compared to a control situation without electrical stimulation (Chow et al., 2021). These results demonstrate the potential of the VI to improve balance.

(c) **Subjective outcomes**

Various subjective outcome measures have been used in order to demonstrate the effects of a VI in daily life. Regarding qualitative measurements, more stable vision and increased postural responses were reported by VI recipients. Besides, some patients reported that the VI increased their ability to perform daily life activities safely (for example, abandoning the use of walking sticks, increased ability to walk in darkness, increased ability to walk on uneven ground, and being able to carry weight) (Boutros et al., 2019). As for the quantitative measurements, improvements were demonstrated by the quality of life questionnaires (Short Form 36, Health Utility Index 3) (Chow et al., 2021). In general, patients report an increased quality of life.

(d) **Undesirable Consequences of VI**

Apart from the positive results obtained in VI trials, hearing loss is an often-reported side-effect of VI implantation surgery. Most likely due to a combination of the surgical drilling and the insertion of electrodes into the inner ear, hearing loss was reported for most patients with functional hearing in the implanted ear prior to surgery (Chow et al., 2021; Phillips et al., 2015b). Efforts are being made to reduce this risk by investigating different surgical strategies (for example, the extralabyrinthine approach) and soft-surgery techniques. Due to this risk, several research groups are currently only implanting patients with complete hearing loss in the ear to be implanted. In this light, the Geneva-Maastricht and Washington (Rubinstein et al., 2020) groups are using a combined vestibular and cochlear implant (VCI) to restore both modalities simultaneously (Guyot et al., 2016).

Future Prospective

The VI concept presented in this chapter has the potential to be the first clinically available treatment aimed at restoring vestibular function loss. Although promising, several aspects can still be improved.

Regarding the surgery, the overall goal is to get the VI electrodes as safely as possible at the desired location, using a technique which does not require extensive training. Therefore, the implant design and surgical techniques should allow easy placement of the electrodes, with one of the main goals being the preservation of inner ear structures and therefore hearing function. Intra-operative monitoring (either imaging-based, via neural monitoring or VOR-based) might facilitate this goal.

Accurate neural stimulation is vital for the functioning of a VI. A more extensive understanding of the physiology of the vestibular neurons and their response to electrical stimulation, together with central vestibular processing within the reflex and perception pathways, is probably important to optimize the stimulation algorithms. Although previous research in animals indicated the capacity of the brain to adapt to suboptimal (i.e., misaligned) stimulation (Della Santina et al., 2007), mapping the electro-dynamics inside the inner ear might create a better understanding on how to improve stimulation algorithms, including current steering and the influence of spatial and temporal coding of the stimulus signal.

Another aspect is to improve or create outcome measures to evaluate the vestibular system. This will aid in substantiating any claims on VI efficacy while also giving insights into the complex integration of sensory modalities for balance and motion perception. This also includes subjective outcome measures explicitly aimed at the BVP population to quantify symptoms, disease burden and overall quality of life.

Besides the above-mentioned goals, future efforts will be aimed at the usability of the device and its effective integration into standard clinical practice. This includes increasing the wearability and concealability of the device, improving battery life and making it easy to use, both for patients and clinicians. Furthermore, VI-specific rehabilitation programs need to be developed.

Currently, the VI is mainly aimed at patients with severe BVP, but other indications for VI implantation (e.g., uncompensated unilateral vestibulopathy) and the possible added value of bilateral vestibular implantation will be evaluated in the future.

References

Bogle, J. M., & Burkard, R. F. (2020). Practical anatomy and physiology of the vestibular system. *Balance Function Assessment and Management, 69.*

Boutabla, A., Cavuscens, S., Ranieri, M., Crétallaz, C., Kingma, H., van de Berg, R., et al. (2020). Simultaneous activation of multiple vestibular pathways upon electrical stimulation of semicircular canal afferents. *Journal of Neurology, 267*(1), 273–284.

Boutros, P. J., Schoo, D. P., Rahman, M., Valentin, N. S., Chow, M. R., Ayiotis, A. I., et al. (2019). Continuous vestibular implant stimulation partially restores eye-stabilizing reflexes. *JCI Insight, 4*(22).

Brontë-Stewart, H., & Lisberger, S. G. (1994). Physiological properties of vestibular primary afferents that mediate motor learning and normal performance of the vestibulo-ocular reflex in monkeys. *Journal of Neuroscience, 14*(3), 1290–1308.

Chow, M. R., Ayiotis, A. I., Schoo, D. P., Gimmon, Y., Lane, K. E., Morris, B. J., et al. (2021). Posture, gait, quality of life, and hearing with a vestibular implant. *New England Journal of Medicine, 384*(6), 521–532.

Cohen, B., & Suzuki, J.-I. (1963). Eye movements induced by ampullary nerve stimulation. *American Journal of Physiology-Legacy Content, 204*(2), 347–351.

Cohen, B., Suzuki, J.-I., & Bender, M. B. (1965). Nystagmus induced by electric stimulation of ampullary nerves. *Acta Oto-Laryngologica, 60*(1–6), 422–436.

Dai, C., Fridman, G. Y., Chiang, B., Davidovics, N. S., Melvin, T.-A., Cullen, K. E., & Della Santina, C. C. (2011a). Cross-axis adaptation improves 3D vestibulo-ocular reflex alignment during chronic stimulation via a head-mounted multichannel vestibular prosthesis. *Experimental Brain Research, 210*(3–4), 595–606.

Dai, C., Fridman, G. Y., Chiang, B., Rahman, M. A., Ahn, J. H., Davidovics, N. S., & Della Santina, C. C. (2013). Directional plasticity rapidly improves 3D vestibulo-ocular reflex alignment in monkeys using a multichannel vestibular prosthesis. *Journal of the Association for Research in Otolaryngology, 14*(6), 863–877.

Dai, C., Fridman, G. Y., & Della Santina, C. C. (2011b). Effects of vestibular prosthesis electrode implantation and stimulation on hearing in rhesus monkeys. *Hearing Research, 277*(1–2), 204–210.

Davidovics, N. S., Fridman, G. Y., & Della Santina, C. C. (2012). Co-modulation of stimulus rate and current from elevated baselines expands head motion encoding range of the vestibular prosthesis. *Experimental Brain Research, 218*(3), 389–400.

Davidovics, N. S., Rahman, M. A., Dai, C., Ahn, J., Fridman, G. Y., & Della Santina, C. C. (2013). Multichannel vestibular prosthesis employing modulation of pulse rate and current with alignment precompensation elicits improved VOR performance in monkeys. *Journal of the Association for Research in Otolaryngology, 14*(2), 233–248.

Della Santina, C. C., Migliaccio, A. A., & Patel, A. H. (2007). A multichannel semicircular canal neural prosthesis using electrical stimulation to restore 3-D vestibular sensation. *IEEE Transactions on Biomedical Engineering, 54*(6), 1016–1030.

DiGiovanna, J., Nguyen, T., Guinand, N., Pérez-Fornos, A., & Micera, S. (2016). Neural network model of vestibular nuclei reaction to onset of vestibular prosthetic stimulation. *Frontiers in Bioengineering and Biotechnology, 4*, 34.

Dupuits, B., Pleshkov, M., Lucieer, F., Guinand, N., Pérez Fornos, A., Guyot, J. P., et al. (2019). A new and faster test to assess vestibular perception. *Frontiers in Neurology, 10*, 707.

Faan, R. W. B. M., Dmsc, V. H. M., Kerber, K., & Kerber, K. A. (2010). *Baloh and Honrubia's clinical neurophysiology of the vestibular system.*

Feigl, G. C., Fasel, J. H., Anderhuber, F., Ulz, H., Rienmüller, R., Guyot, J.-P., & Kos, I. M. (2009). Superior vestibular neurectomy: A novel transmeatal approach for a denervation of the superior and lateral semicircular canals. *Otology & Neurotology, 30*(5), 586–591.

Fernandez, C., & Goldberg, J. M. (1971). Physiology of peripheral neurons innervating semicircular canals of the squirrel monkey. II. Response to sinusoidal stimulation and dynamics of peripheral vestibular system. *Journal of Neurophysiology, 34*(4), 661–675.

Fishman, A. J., Roland, J. T., Alexiades, G., Mierzwinski, J., & Cohen, N. L. (2003). Fluoroscopically assisted cochlear implantation. *Otology & Neurotology, 24*(6), 882–886.

Fornos, A. P., van de Berg, R., Armand, S., Cavuscens, S., Ranieri, M., Crétallaz, C., et al. (2019). Cervical myogenic potentials and controlled postural responses elicited by a prototype vestibular implant. *Journal of Neurology, 266*(1), 33–41.

Fridman, G. Y., Davidovics, N. S., Dai, C., Migliaccio, A. A., & Della Santina, C. C. (2010). Vestibulo-ocular reflex responses to a multichannel vestibular prosthesis incorporating a 3D coordinate transformation for correction of misalignment. *Journal of the Association for Research in Otolaryngology, 11*(3), 367–381.

Fuller, P., Jones, T., Jones, S., & Fuller, C. (2004). Evidence for macular gravity receptor modulation of hypothalamic, limbic and autonomic nuclei. *Neuroscience, 129*(2), 461–471.

Goldberg, J., Smith, C. E., & Fernandez, C. (1984). Relation between discharge regularity and responses to externally applied galvanic currents in vestibular nerve afferents of the squirrel monkey. *Journal of Neurophysiology, 51*(6), 1236–1256.

Golub, J. S., Ling, L., Nie, K., Nowack, A., Shepherd, S. J., Bierer, S. M., et al. (2014). Prosthetic implantation of the human vestibular system. *Otology & Neurotology: official publication of the American Otological Society, American Neurotology Society [and] European Academy of Otology and Neurotology, 35*(1), 136–147.

Gong, W., Haburcakova, C., & Merfeld, D. M. (2008). Vestibulo-ocular responses evoked via bilateral electrical stimulation of the lateral semicircular canals. *IEEE Transactions on Biomedical Engineering, 55*(11), 2608–2619.

Gong, W., & Merfeld, D. M. (2000). Prototype neural semicircular canal prosthesis using patterned electrical stimulation. *Annals of Biomedical Engineering, 28*(5), 572–581.

Gong, W., & Merfeld, D. M. (2002). System design and performance of a unilateral horizontal semicircular canal prosthesis. *IEEE Transactions on Biomedical Engineering, 49*(2), 175–181.

Guinand, N., Boselie, F., Guyot, J.-P., & Kingma, H. (2012a). Quality of life of patients with bilateral vestibulopathy. *Annals of Otology, Rhinology & Laryngology, 121*(7), 471–477.

Guinand, N., Guyot, J.-P., Kingma, H., Kos, I., & Pelizzone, M. (2011). *Vestibular implants: The first steps in humans.* Paper presented at the 2011 Annual International Conference of the IEEE Engineering in Medicine and Biology Society.

Guinand, N., Pijnenburg, M., Janssen, M., & Kingma, H. (2012b). Visual acuity while walking and oscillopsia severity in healthy subjects and patients with unilateral and bilateral vestibular function loss. *Archives of Otolaryngology–Head & Neck Surgery, 138*(3), 301–306.

Guinand, N., Van de Berg, R., Cavuscens, S., Ranieri, M., Schneider, E., Lucieer, F., et al. (2017). The video head impulse test to assess the efficacy of vestibular implants in humans. *Frontiers in Neurology, 8*, 600.

Guinand, N., Van de Berg, R., Cavuscens, S., Stokroos, R., Ranieri, M., Pelizzone, M., et al. (2016). Restoring visual acuity in dynamic conditions with a vestibular implant. *Frontiers in Neuroscience, 10*, 577.

Guinand, N., van de Berg, R., Cavuscens, S., Stokroos, R. J., Ranieri, M., Pelizzone, M., et al. (2015). Vestibular implants: 8 years of experience with electrical stimulation of the vestibular nerve in 11 patients with bilateral vestibular loss. *ORL, 77*(4), 227–240.

Guyot, J.-P., Fornos, A. P., Guinand, N., van de Berg, R., Stokroos, R., & Kingma, H. (2016). Vestibular assistance systems: Promises and challenges. *Journal of Neurology, 263*(1), 30–35.

Guyot, J.-P., Sigrist, A., Pelizzone, M., Feigl, G. C., & Kos, M. I. (2011a). Eye movements in response to electrical stimulation of the lateral and superior ampullary nerves. *Annals of Otology, Rhinology & Laryngology, 120*(2), 81–87.

Guyot, J.-P., Sigrist, A., Pelizzone, M., & Kos, M. I. (2011b). Adaptation to steady-state electrical stimulation of the vestibular system in humans. *Annals of Otology, Rhinology & Laryngology, 120*(3), 143–149.

Hain, T. C., Cherchi, M., & Yacovino, D. A. (2013). *Bilateral vestibular loss.* Paper presented at the Seminars in neurology.

Hedjoudje, A., Hayden, R., Dai, C., Ahn, J., Rahman, M., Risi, F., et al. (2019). Virtual Rhesus Labyrinth Model predicts responses to electrical stimulation delivered by a vestibular prosthesis. *Journal of the Association for Research in Otolaryngology, 20*(4), 313–339.

Kingma, H., & Van de Berg, R. (2016). Anatomy, physiology, and physics of the peripheral vestibular system. In *Handbook of clinical neurology* (Vol. 137, pp. 1–16). Elsevier.

Lee, S. U., Kim, H. J., & Kim, J. S. (2020). Bilateral vestibular dysfunction. *Seminars in Neurology, 40*(1), 40–48.

Lewis, R. F., Gong, W., Ramsey, M., Minor, L., Boyle, R., & Merfeld, D. M. (2002). Vestibular adaptation studied with a prosthetic semicircular canal. *Journal of Vestibular Research, 12*(2, 3), 87–94.

Lewis, R. F., Haburcakova, C., Gong, W., Lee, D., & Merfeld, D. (2013). Electrical stimulation of semicircular canal afferents affects the perception of head orientation. *Journal of Neuroscience, 33*(22), 9530–9535.

Lewis, R. F., Haburcakova, C., Gong, W., Makary, C., & Merfeld, D. M. (2010). Vestibuloocular reflex adaptation investigated with chronic motion-modulated electrical stimulation of semicircular canal afferents. *Journal of Neurophysiology, 103*(2), 1066–1079.

Lucieer, F., Duijn, S., Van Rompaey, V., Pérez Fornos, A., Guinand, N., Guyot, J. P., et al. (2018). Full spectrum of reported symptoms of bilateral vestibulopathy needs further investigation—A systematic review. *Frontiers in Neurology, 9*, 352.

Lucieer, F., Vonk, P., Guinand, N., Stokroos, R., Kingma, H., & van de Berg, R. (2016). Bilateral vestibular hypofunction: Insights in etiologies, clinical subtypes, and diagnostics. *Frontiers in Neurology, 7*, 26.

Lucieer, F. M., Van Hecke, R., van Stiphout, L., Duijn, S., Perez-Fornos, A., Guinand, N., et al. (2020). Bilateral vestibulopathy: Beyond imbalance and oscillopsia. *Journal of Neurology, 267*(1), 241–255.

Merfeld, D. M., Gong, W., Morrissey, J., Saginaw, M., Haburcakova, C., & Lewis, R. F. (2006). Acclimation to chronic constant-rate peripheral stimulation provided by a vestibular prosthesis. *IEEE Transactions on Biomedical Engineering, 53*(11), 2362–2372.

Merfeld, D. M., Zupan, L., & Peterka, R. J. (1999). Humans use internal models to estimate gravity and linear acceleration. *Nature, 398*(6728), 615–618.

Miffon, M., & Guyot, J.-P. (2015). Difficulties faced by patients suffering from total bilateral vestibular loss. *ORL, 77*(4), 241–247.

Migliaccio, A. A., Meierhofer, R., & Della Santina, C. C. (2011). Characterization of the 3D angular vestibulo-ocular reflex in C57BL6 mice. *Experimental Brain Research, 210*(3–4), 489–501.

Mitchell, D. E., Della Santina, C. C., & Cullen, K. E. (2016). Plasticity within non-cerebellar pathways rapidly shapes motor performance in vivo. *Nature Communications, 7*(1), 1–13.

Nguyen, T., Cavuscens, S., Ranieri, M., Schwarz, K., Guinand, N., Van De Berg, R., et al. (2017). Characterization of cochlear, vestibular and cochlear-vestibular electrically evoked compound action potentials in patients with a vestibulo-cochlear implant. *Frontiers in Neuroscience, 11*, 645.

Nguyen, T., DiGiovanna, J., Cavuscens, S., Ranieri, M., Guinand, N., Van De Berg, R., et al. (2016). Characterization of pulse amplitude and pulse rate modulation for a human vestibular implant during acute electrical stimulation. *Journal of Neural Engineering, 13*(4), 046023.

Parkes, W. J., Gnanasegaram, J. J., Cushing, S. L., McKnight, C. L., Papsin, B. C., & Gordon, K. A. (2017). Vestibular evoked myogenic potential testing as an objective measure of vestibular stimulation with cochlear implants. *The Laryngoscope, 127*(2), E75–E81.

Perez Fornos, A., Guinand, N., van de Berg, R., Stokroos, R., Micera, S., Kingma, H., et al. (2014). Artificial balance: Restoration of the vestibulo-ocular reflex in humans with a prototype vestibular neuroprosthesis. *Frontiers in Neurology, 5*, 66.

Phillips, C., DeFrancisci, C., Ling, L., Nie, K., Nowack, A., Phillips, J. O., & Rubinstein, J. T. (2013). Postural responses to electrical stimulation of the vestibular end organs in human subjects. *Experimental Brain Research, 229*(2), 181–195.

Phillips, C., Ling, L., Oxford, T., Nowack, A., Nie, K., Rubinstein, J. T., & Phillips, J. O. (2015a). Longitudinal performance of an implantable vestibular prosthesis. *Hearing Research, 322*, 200–211.

Phillips, C., Shepherd, S. J., Nowack, A., Nie, K., Kaneko, C. R., Rubinstein, J. T., et al. (2016). Loss of afferent vestibular input produces central adaptation and increased gain of vestibular prosthetic stimulation. *Journal of the Association for Research in Otolaryngology, 17*(1), 19–35.

Phillips, J. O., Ling, L., Nie, K., Jameyson, E., Phillips, C. M., Nowack, A. L., et al. (2015b). Vestibular implantation and longitudinal electrical stimulation of the semicircular canal afferents in human subjects. *Journal of Neurophysiology, 113*(10), 3866–3892.

Porciuncula, F., Johnson, C. C., & Glickman, L. B. (2012). The effect of vestibular rehabilitation on adults with bilateral vestibular hypofunction: A systematic review. *Journal of Vestibular Research, 22*(5, 6), 283–298.

Requena, T., Espinosa-Sanchez, J. M., & Lopez-Escamez, J. A. (2014). Genetics of dizziness: Cerebellar and vestibular disorders. *Current Opinion in Neurology, 27*(1), 98–104.

Rinne, T., Bronstein, A., Rudge, P., Gresty, M., & Luxon, L. (1998). Bilateral loss of vestibular function: Clinical findings in 53 patients. *Journal of Neurology, 245*(6–7), 314–321.

Rubinstein, J., Bierer, S., Fuchs, A., Kaneko, C., Ling, L., & Nie, K. (2012). Prosthetic implantation of the semicircular canals with preservation of rotational sensitivity: A "hybrid" vestibular implant. *Otology & Neurotology, 33*(5), 789–796.

Rubinstein, J. T., Ling, L., Nowack, A., Nie, K., & Phillips, J. O. (2020). Results from a second-generation vestibular implant in human subjects: Diagnosis may impact electrical sensitivity of vestibular afferents. *Otology & Neurotology, 41*(1), 68–77.

Smith, P., & Darlington, C. (2013). Personality changes in patients with vestibular dysfunction. *Frontiers in Human Neuroscience, 7*, 678.

Smith, P., & Zheng, Y. (2013). From ear to uncertainty: Vestibular contributions to cognitive function. *Frontiers in Integrative Neuroscience, 7*, 84.

Starkov, D., Guinand, N., Lucieer, F., Ranieri, M., Cavuscens, S., Pleshkov, M., et al. (2020). Restoring the high-frequency dynamic visual acuity with a vestibular implant prototype in humans. *Audiology and Neurotology, 25*(1–2), 91–95.

Strupp, M., Kim, J.-S., Murofushi, T., Straumann, D., Jen, J. C., Rosengren, S. M., et al. (2017). Bilateral vestibulopathy: Diagnostic criteria Consensus document of the Classification Committee of the Bárány Society. *Journal of Vestibular Research, 27*(4), 177–189.

Stultiens, J. J. A., Postma, A. A., Guinand, N., Fornos, A. P., Kingma, H., & van de Berg, R. (2020). Vestibular implantation and the feasibility of fluoroscopy-guided electrode insertion. *Otolaryngologic Clinics of North America, 53*(1), 115–126.

Sun, D. Q., Ward, B. K., Semenov, Y. R., Carey, J. P., & Della Santina, C. C. (2014). Bilateral vestibular deficiency: Quality of life and economic implications. *JAMA Otolaryngology–Head & Neck Surgery, 140*(6), 527–534.

Tang, S., Melvin, T.-A. N., & Della Santina, C. C. (2009). Effects of semicircular canal electrode implantation on hearing in chinchillas. *Acta Oto-Laryngologica, 129*(5), 481–486.

Thompson, L. A., Haburcakova, C., Gong, W., Lee, D. J., Wall, C., III, Merfeld, D. M., & Lewis, R. F. (2012). Responses evoked by a vestibular implant providing chronic stimulation. *Journal of Vestibular Research, 22*(1), 11–15.

Van De Berg, R., Guinand, N., Guyot, J.-P., Kingma, H., & Stokroos, R. (2012). The modified ampullar approach for vestibular implant surgery: Feasibility and its first application in a human with a long-term vestibular loss. *Frontiers in Neurology, 3*, 18.

Van De Berg, R., Guinand, N., Nguyen, T., Ranieri, M., Cavuscens, S., Guyot, J.-P., et al. (2015a). The vestibular implant: Frequency-dependency of the electrically evoked vestibulo-ocular reflex in humans. *Frontiers in Systems Neuroscience, 8*, 255.

Van De Berg, R., Ramos, A., Van Rompaey, V., Bisdorff, A., Perez-Fornos, A., Rubinstein, J. T., et al. (2020). The vestibular implant: Opinion statement on implantation criteria for research. *Journal of Vestibular Research, 30*, 213–223.

Van De Berg, R., van Tilburg, M., & Kingma, H. (2015b). Bilateral vestibular hypofunction: Challenges in establishing the diagnosis in adults. *ORL, 77*(4), 197–218.

Versino, M., Colagiorgio, P., Sacco, S., Colnaghi, S., Quaglieri, S., Manfrin, M., et al. (2014). Reading while moving: The functional assessment of VOR. *Journal of Vestibular Research, 24*(5, 6), 459–464.

Wall, C., III, Kos, M. I., & Guyot, J.-P. (2007). Eye movements in response to electric stimulation of the human posterior ampullary nerve. *Annals of Otology, Rhinology & Laryngology, 116*(5), 369–374.

Ward, B. K., Agrawal, Y., Hoffman, H. J., Carey, J. P., & Della Santina, C. C. (2013). Prevalence and impact of bilateral vestibular hypofunction: Results from the 2008 US National Health Interview Survey. *JAMA Otolaryngology–Head & Neck Surgery, 139*(8), 803–810.

Zingler, V. C., Weintz, E., Jahn, K., Huppert, D., Cnyrim, C., Brandt, T., & Strupp, M. (2009). Causative factors, epidemiology, and follow-up of bilateral vestibulopathy. *Annals of the New York Academy of Sciences, 1164*(1), 505–508.

MIX
Papier aus verantwortungsvollen Quellen
Paper from responsible sources
FSC® C105338

If you have any concerns about our products,
you can contact us on
ProductSafety@springernature.com

In case Publisher is established outside the EU,
the EU authorized representative is:
Springer Nature Customer Service Center GmbH
Europaplatz 3, 69115 Heidelberg, Germany

Printed by Libri Plureos GmbH
in Hamburg, Germany